Clinical Decisions in
**Neuro-Ophthalmology**

# Clinical Decisions in
# Neuro-Ophthalmology

## Ronald M. Burde, M.D.

Professor and Chairman, Department of Ophthalmology and Visual Sciences,
Professor of Neurology and Neurological Surgery,
Albert Einstein College of Medicine and Montefiore Medical Center,
University Hospitals, Bronx, New York

## Peter J. Savino, M.D.

Director, Neuro-Ophthalmology Service, Wills Eye Hospital;
Chairman, Department of Ophthalmology, The Graduate Hospital;
Professor of Ophthalmology, Thomas Jefferson University;
Clinical Professor of Ophthalmology, University of Pennsylvania,
Philadelphia, Pennsylvania

## Jonathan D. Trobe, M.D.

Professor of Ophthalmology, Associate Professor of Neurology,
University of Michigan School of Medicine, Ann Arbor, Michigan

SECOND EDITION

*with 252 illustrations, including 10 four-color plates*

*Illustrations:*
**Christopher J. Burke, A.M.I.**

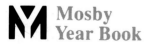
Mosby
Year Book

St. Louis   Baltimore   Boston   Chicago   London   Philadelphia   Sydney   Toronto

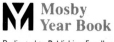
**Mosby**
**Year Book**
Dedicated to Publishing Excellence

Editor: Kimberly M. Kist
Developmental Editor: Emma Dankoski
Project Manager: Gayle May Morris
Production Editor: Judith Bange

**SECOND EDITION**

Printed in the United States of America

Mosby–Year Book, Inc.
11830 Westline Industrial Drive
St. Louis, Missouri 63146

**Library of Congress Cataloging-in-Publication Data**

Burde, Ronald M.
    Clinical decisions in neuro-ophthalmology/Ronald M. Burde, Peter
J. Savino, Jonathan D. Trobe; illustrations [by] Christopher J.
Burke.
        p.    cm.
    Includes bibliographical references and index.
    ISBN 0-8016-0694-2
    1. Neuroophthalmology—Decision making—Outlines, syllabi, etc.
I. Savino, Peter J.   II. Trobe, Jonathan D.   III. Title.
    [DNLM: 1. Decision Theory. 2. Eye Diseases—diagnosis. 3. Eye
Diseases—therapy. 4. Nervous System Diseases—diagnosis.
5. Nervous System Diseases—therapy.   WW 140 B949c]
RE725.B87   1992
617.7'3—dc20
DNLM/DLC
for Library of Congress                                          91-32514
                                                                      CIP

        96  CL/UN/MY  9 8 7 6 5 4

The inspiration for this book came to one of us
at the 60th birthday celebration of a revered teacher:
*Jerome Y. Lettvin, M.D., Ph.D.*

*Collectively, we would like to dedicate this book
to our loving families, without whose support
we could not have completed this task,
and to our teachers in ophthalmology and neuro-ophthalmology who,
we trust, will approve our efforts.*

**R.M. Burde/P.J. Savino/J.D. Trobe**

# *Preface*

. . . . . . . . . . . . . . . . . .

When the first edition of this book appeared 7 years ago, decision trees were a novel device in medical teaching texts, and there were none in ophthalmology. We are proud to find that we are no longer alone.

But, as we suspected at the time of initial publication, some of our original decision trees were too awkward to survive into the second edition. Readers who remember the first edition will recognize that a great deal of pruning and grafting has occurred in response to their helpful comments and as a result of new clinical information.

The basic format of the book remains the same. Unlike most medical textbooks, which present disease entities followed by their attributes, we lead with symptoms and signs. That is, after all, how physicians face clinical problems. The trail leads to a series of diagnoses according to various test results.

The decision-making process is encoded into decision trees in which symptoms or signs are contained in boxes ( ▢ ), and inputs or maneuvers are contained in ovals ( ⬭ ). The outcome of each maneuver determines the next step until a diagnosis ( ▤ ) is reached.

The first—and most common—clinical problem is visual loss. We present a decision tree for investigating *unexplained visual loss,* or visual loss that cannot be accounted for by abnormalities within the globe. In the succeeding chapters on prechiasmal, chiasmal, and postchiasmal visual loss, we provide the core clinical information needed to manage those entities. Transient visual loss has its own decision tree because its evaluation is based on very different principles. In response to numerous requests, we have added an entirely new chapter on visual illusions and hallucinations.

The decision tree on the abnormal optic disc has remained largely unchanged. Readers have accepted the logic of dividing this problem into the abnormal swollen disc and the abnormal flat disc.

Ocular motility problems are divided into three parts based on their presentations: gaze, alignment, and oscillatory disturbances. The chapter on gaze disturbances does not lend itself to a decision tree; instead, we dwell on how the brain controls eye movements.

The diagnosis of pupillary disturbances ought to be easy but is not. The decision tree reflects the complexities, although it is markedly simplified as compared with our first try.

The workup of ptosis, lid retraction, and blepharospasm makes up the next section. The biggest change here is the dramatic success of botulinum toxin in the treatment of blepharospasm. Neurectomy and myectomy—so important in the last edition—are virtually gone.

The decision tree on proptosis aims at the distinction between Graves' disease and orbital and periorbital masses. An understanding of imaging is ever more critical here.

The last chapter deals with one of the most frustrating clinical problems—headache. We have held to our formulation that divides headache into distinctive and nondistinctive syndromes. Most of the changes in this chapter have to do with new concepts and management in migraine.

If this edition weighs more than the last, it is because the decision trees are more densely foliated. As time goes on, the management of nearly every entity appears to have more options. To accommodate these developments, we have expanded the text and illustrations, and introduced more MRI scans and computer-assisted perimetry results. Where a critical management issue confronts the clinician, we have capsulized our approach in a highlighted "management box."

We thank our mentors and colleagues for their suggestions and support.

Ronald M. Burde, M.D.
Peter J. Savino, M.D.
Jonathan D. Trobe, M.D.

# Contents

1  *Unexplained Visual Loss*, 1

2  *Prechiasmal Visual Loss*, 41

3  *Chiasmal Visual Loss*, 74

4  *Postchiasmal Visual Loss*, 104

5  *Transient Visual Loss*, 117

6  *Visual Illusions and Hallucinations*, 145

7  *Abnormal Optic Discs*, 173

8  *Gaze Disturbances*, 200

9  *Diplopia and Similar Sensory Experiences*, 224

10  *Incomitant Ocular Misalignment*, 239

11  *Comitant Ocular Misalignment*, 282

12  *Nystagmus and Other Ocular Oscillations*, 289

13  *Anisocoria and Abnormal Pupillary Light Reactions*, 321

14  *Eyelid Disturbances*, 347
    PART I: PTOSIS, 347
    PART II: LID RETRACTION, 362
    PART III: BLEPHAROSPASM, 365

15  *Proptosis and Adnexal Masses*, 379

16  *Headache*, 417

# Color Plates

· · · · · · · · · · · · · · · ·

1  **A,** Map-dot-fingerprint corneal dystrophy. **B,** Keratoconus. **C,** After cataract. **D,** Central serous chorioretinopathy. **E** and **F,** Cystoid macular edema, 20

2  **A,** Surface-wrinkling maculopathy. **B,** Multiple evanescent white dot syndrome (MEWDS). **C,** Acute multifocal placoid pigment epitheliopathy (AMPPE). **D,** Macular star figure (Leber's stellate neuroretinopathy). **E** and **F,** Nonarteritic ischemic optic neuropathy, 20

3  **A,** Lymphomatous infiltration of optic nerve. **B,** Radiation-induced retinopathy and optic neuropathy. **C** and **D,** Leber's optic neuropathy, acute. **E,** Central retinal artery occlusion, acute. **F,** Branch retinal artery occlusion, acute, 52

4  **A,** Retinal intravascular (Hollenhorst) plaque. **B,** Venous stasis retinopathy. **C,** Cotton-wool spot. **D,** Roth spot. **E,** Sea fan in sickle cell retinopathy. **F,** Ischemic ocular syndrome, 132

5  **A** to **D,** Congenitally anomalous optic discs without elevation, 180

6  **A** to **F,** Congenitally anomalous optic discs with elevation, 180

7  **A** to **F,** Stages of papilledema, 180

8  Disc elevation not secondary to increased intracranial pressure. **A,** Optociliary shunt. **B,** Papillitis. **C,** Diabetic papillopathy. **D,** Ischemic optic neuropathy. **E,** Central retinal vein occlusion. **F,** Papillophlebitis, 180

9  **A** and **B,** Graves' ophthalmopathy. **C,** Carotid-cavernous fistula. **D,** Dural fistula. **E,** Diffuse scleral injection. **F,** Marked conjunctival chemosis, 388

10  Color Doppler orbital image. **A,** Normal superior ophthalmic vein. **B,** Carotid-cavernous fistula, 388

Clinical Decisions in
**Neuro-Ophthalmology**

# CHAPTER 1

# Unexplained Visual Loss

· · · · · · · · · · · · · · · · · · · · · · · · ·

One of the most challenging problems a physician faces is the diagnosis of visual loss when no structural abnormalities in the eye are apparent. If this *unexplained visual loss* has an organic cause, the lesion is presumed to lie somewhere behind the eye. However, careful inspection of the globe often reveals previously overlooked abnormalities, which we consider legitimate causes of unexplained visual loss.

This problem may confront the physician in one of three forms: (1) abnormal visual acuity, (2) abnormal visual field, or (3) "normal" visual acuity and visual fields in a patient who insists that vision is disturbed. In this chapter we will explore primarily the diagnosis of unexplained visual acuity loss. The other presentations are discussed briefly here and in Chapters 2 through 5.

## A Decision Tree Approach to the Evaluation of Unexplained Visual Acuity Loss

To investigate the problem of *unexplained visual acuity loss*, the decision tree (Chart 1-1) is divided conceptually into two branches: (1) *optical disturbances* and (2) *neuroretinal disturbances*. Optical disturbances arise from refractive errors and abnormalities of the ocular media—the tear film, cornea, lens, and vitreous. Neuroretinal disturbances involve the retina, optic nerve, chiasm, optic tract, optic radiations, and visual cortex.

If the patient still has subnormal visual acuity after refraction *(subnormal best-corrected acuity)*, the *potential acuity* tests are used to separate optical from neuroretinal disease. Should the potential acuity tests improve visual acuity, then the examiner must presume that an optical problem is responsible. Otherwise, the examiner investigates neuroretinal disease and performs the *swinging light pupil test* in search of a *relative afferent pupillary defect* (RAPD). The swinging light pupil test is positioned early in the sequence of tests because it provides an objective means of separating asymmetric optic nerve disease (or, less commonly, retinal disease) from other forms of visual pathway disease and psychogenic visual loss.

1

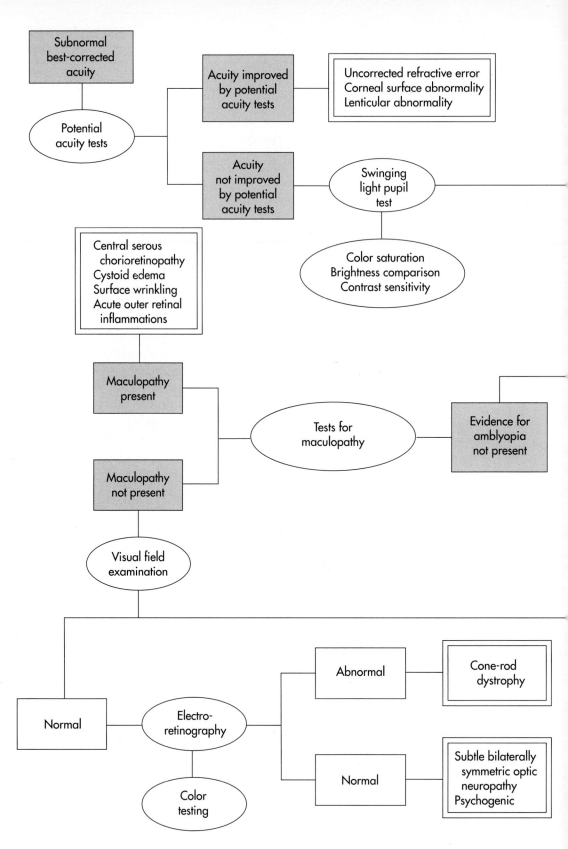

*Chart 1-1*

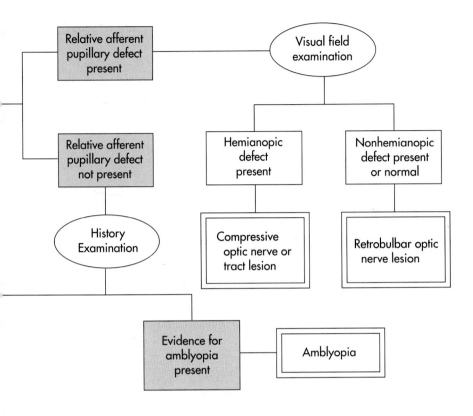

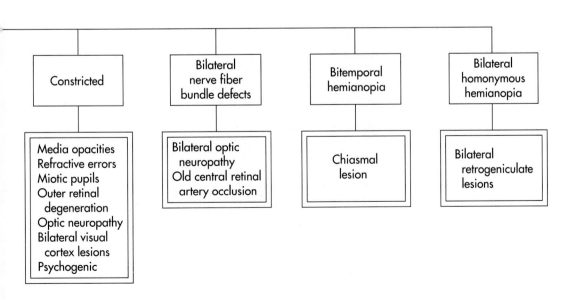

■ Subnormal best-corrected acuity

Understood in the concept of unexplained visual loss is that a skilled refraction has failed to eliminate subnormal acuity. *Best-corrected acuity* means that no further improvement in acuity can be obtained by altering the spectacle prescription. However, even the most skilled refractionist may make an error. If potential acuity tests demonstrate an acuity substantially better than that obtained with refraction, the examiner must conclude that either (1) the refraction was in error or (2) a media aberration is responsible for the subnormal best-corrected acuity.

○ *Potential acuity tests.* Potential acuity tests consist of the pinhole, the potential acuity meter, and laser interferometer tests.

The *pinhole test* (Fig. 1-1) is an effective (but not perfect) means of separating out visual dysfunction caused by aberrations of the optical media. It will improve acuity in uncorrected refractive errors and in tear film, corneal, and lenticular abnormalities by selecting a narrow central light ray that produces a small blur circle on the retina. It does not always work, however. Children under age 6 and elderly patients, particularly those who are infirm or demented, may not be

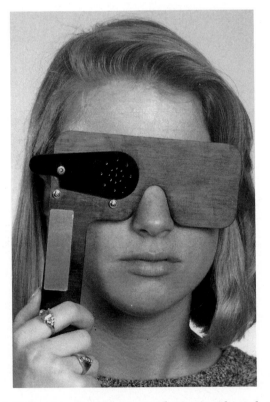

*Fig. 1-1.* Pinhole test. If visual acuity improves with viewing through a multiple pinhole, either uncorrected refractive error or ocular media abnormalities contribute to subnormal acuity.

able to "find the hole" and therefore may not show improvement in acuity. Furthermore, if the media are sufficiently disrupted, the pinhole may not find a clear optical path. On the other hand, false-positive results are rare, especially if a positive result is considered to be an improvement in visual acuity of at least two Snellen lines. We recommend the multiple pinhole test with hole diameters between 2 and 2.5 mm, which minimizes the degradation from diffraction (smaller than 2 mm) and surface aberrations (larger than 2.5 mm).[1]

Because the pinhole test has some limitations, two other tests have been used as alternatives: the *potential acuity meter* (PAM)[2] and the *laser interferometer.*[3] The laser interferometer has not received wide clinical use because of its high cost. When tested with the PAM, the patient views a miniaturized Snellen chart projected onto the retina from a box mounted on the slit lamp biomicroscope (Fig. 1-2). By projecting such a small image, the PAM is often able to bypass the eye's refractive and media aberrations. Its advantage over the pinhole test is that

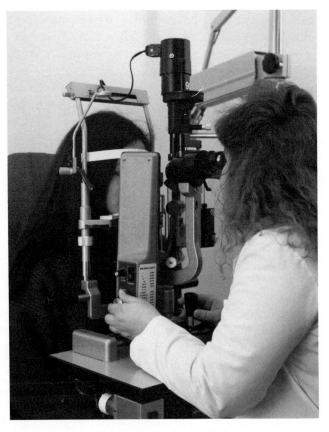

*Fig. 1-2.* Potential acuity meter (PAM) test. Box mounted on slit lamp biomicroscope projects miniaturized Snellen chart onto retina, bypassing any refractive and media aberrations.

it does not require a steady hand from the patient. Its disadvantage is that the instrument is expensive and requires some examiner expertise. Results have been generally accurate, with the notable exception of cystoid macular edema,[4] wherein the PAM may overestimate the patient's maximum visual acuity. Although we acknowledge this limitation, we consider the PAM a valuable adjunct in deciding whether subtle media abnormalities account for subnormal best-corrected acuity.

## Acuity improved by potential acuity tests

### Uncorrected refractive error

If the potential acuity tests show improvement in acuity, the examiner must first recheck the refraction to be sure that no error has been made. If that is not the explanation, a defect of the ocular media may be present.

### Corneal surface abnormality

A minor disturbance in the integrity of the corneal epithelium can have a marked effect on visual acuity. Fortunately, topical fluorescein will readily stain areas of denuded epithelium, but not areas of redundant or irregular thickening such as often occur in the **epithelial dystrophies,** particularly the common "map-dot-fingerprint" dystrophy[5,6] (Plate 1, *A*). To detect these changes, the examiner must pay attention to the pattern of tearfilm breakup.

An irregular retinoscopic reflex may be a clue to diagnosis of an early **keratoconus,**[7] a dystrophic thinning of the cornea that results in steepening of its curvature (Plate 1, *B*). Although keratoconus usually becomes symptomatic in youth, indolent cases come to attention only in adulthood. The diagnosis is made definitively by examination with the keratometer, Placido disc, and slit lamp biomicroscope. Alterations in the corneal curvature may also arise from pressure from eyelid masses, and from conjunctival and corneal scarring. A helpful way to rule out irregular astigmatism as the cause of unexplained visual acuity loss is to see if a trial hard contact lens placed on the cornea markedly improves acuity.

### Lenticular abnormality

Cataract is rarely overlooked as a cause of unexplained visual acuity loss. Nevertheless, **nuclear sclerosis, lenticular water clefts,** or mildly **opacified posterior lens capsules** (Plate 1, *C*) can degrade acuity to a surprising degree. When lenticular abnormalities are at fault, the patient will often report not only blurred vision, but a second, "ghost" image. This "ghosting" may mistakenly be interpreted as a symptom of ocular misalignment (see Chapter 9). Although perhaps not easily seen with the slit lamp, the lenticular abnormalities may be suspected when retinoscopy produces irregular reflexes.

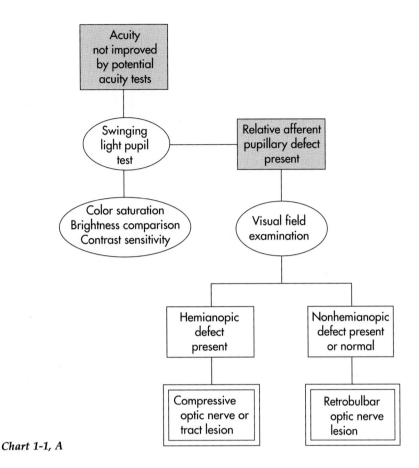

*Chart 1-1, A*

 Acuity not improved by potential acuity tests (Chart 1-1, A)

○ *Swinging light pupil test.*[8,9]. Seat the patient in a room with the least amount of background illumination that permits observation of the unstimulated pupils. Have the patient fixate at a distance to provide maximal relaxation of the iris sphincter muscle. (A near target would evoke miosis associated with the *synkinetic near reflex*.) Use a bright light stimulus, but not so bright as to produce photophobia or extreme miosis.[10] Be guided by the response of the pupil; that is, if neither pupil constricts very much, try a more potent light source (the indirect ophthalmoscope). Direct the light from below the level of the eyes so as not to provoke miosis from the patient's fixing on the light. Move the light briskly and rhythmically from eye to eye several times. (Hold the light over each eye for a fast count of three.) This pace is necessary to distinguish the consistent (although often minimal) differences in pupillary dynamics that characterize a true RAPD from the irregular "bouncing" sphincter movements unrelated to the light stimulus that characterize physiologic pupillary unrest. The affected pupil need not dilate

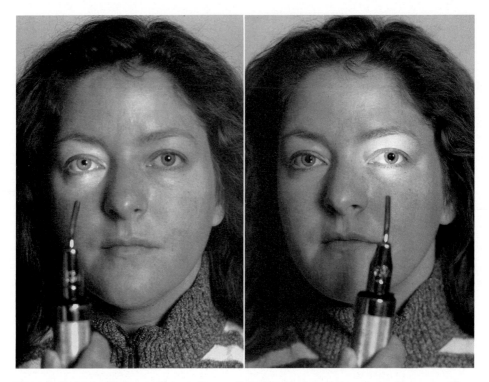

*Fig. 1-3.* Swinging light pupil test. Strong light directed at right eye produces pupillary constriction in both eyes *(left)*. When light is directed at left eye *(right)*, both pupils dilate, indicating a left RAPD.

to reflect an RAPD. The pupil may merely show reduced amplitude of constriction and an accelerated recovery from contraction (escape) as compared with the "control" eye.

Patients with no anterior visual pathway disease should have little or no pupillary constriction on the first or second pass. That is because the direct and consensual pupillary reactions are normally equal. (The only reason for slight constriction is that the light input is briefly interrupted as the flashlight passes over the nasal bridge. If the light is moved quickly enough, that constriction should be negligible.)

If the pupil dilates on either the first or second pass (but not both), then the patient has an RAPD on the side of the dilating pupil (Fig. 1-3). For the most part, an RAPD indicates the presence of unilateral or asymmetric optic nerve disease. Less commonly, macular lesions, widespread retinal lesions, or optic tract lesions may be responsible.

One may quantitate the RAPD by placing progressively higher neutral density filters over the normal eye until the RAPD is eliminated.[11] We find the filters particularly useful when the RAPD is equivocal. In such cases place the lowest filter (0.3 log units) over each eye consecutively and perform the swinging light test. If no RAPD is present, the pupil of the eye covered by the filter will dilate slightly to direct light; if the RAPD is minimal, the filter placed over the ipsilateral eye will enhance it, whereas the filter placed over the contralateral eye will neutralize it.

The swinging light pupil test is useful even if only one iris sphincter muscle is operational. Constriction of the pupil in the control eye as the light is swung toward it is equivalent to pupillary dilatation in the contralateral eye and represents an RAPD in the contralateral eye.

The finding of an RAPD generally indicates a lesion of the ipsilateral optic nerve. Lesions may be present in both optic nerves, but the intensity of the RAPD correlates linearly with the difference in the density of the visual field defects corresponding to those lesions.[12,13] The RAPD is less tightly correlated with differences in visual acuity.

An RAPD does not always indicate optic nerve disease. Lesions that damage the retinal nerve fiber layer (retinal artery occlusion) may be responsible, as may be widespread chorioretinal lesions or retinal detachment. Lesions limited to the macula tend to cause an RAPD only when acuity is depressed to 20/200 or worse.[14] Amblyopia is reported to cause a minimal RAPD.[15] Even so, we believe that *an RAPD should not be attributed to amblyopia unless optic nerve disease has been excluded.* Finally, an RAPD may be found either ipsilateral or contralateral to an optic tract lesion[16] (see Compressive Optic Nerve or Tract Lesion).

Because an RAPD so often occurs when asymmetric optic nerve disease is present, its absence virtually rules out such a condition, provided that proper technique has been followed.

○ *Color saturation, brightness comparison, and contrast sensitivity.* The color saturation, brightness comparison, and contrast sensitivity tests provide support for the results of the swinging light pupil test. Although limited by their subjectivity, these tests are nevertheless helpful in confirming unilateral or asymmetric optic neuropathy uncovered by the RAPD.

For the color saturation test, present a red stimulus to each eye sequentially and ask the patient if he or she notes any difference in the saturation or brightness of the red color (Fig. 1-4). If the patient says no and has clearly understood the question, then the result is interpreted as negative. If the patient does notice a difference, ask the patient to describe the appearance of the red stimulus in each eye. On the side of the more defective optic nerve, the patient will report that the red appears either faded, orange, pink, gray, or brown and will be describing a relative reduction in the saturation or brightness of the color. A response of orange, pink, or faded implies reduced saturation; the color appears to contain less of its spectral hue and more white. A response of gray or brown indicates loss of brightness. If reproducible, this discrepancy in color perception signifies asymmetric optic nerve disease. It is not noted in macular disease unless involvement is severe and therefore funduscopically evident.

For the brightness test, shine a flashlight into each of the patient's eyes sequentially and ask the patient to note any difference in the brightness of the light (Fig. 1-5). Be certain that the patient is responding to the intensity rather than the clarity of the stimulus. If the patient notes a difference, this can be

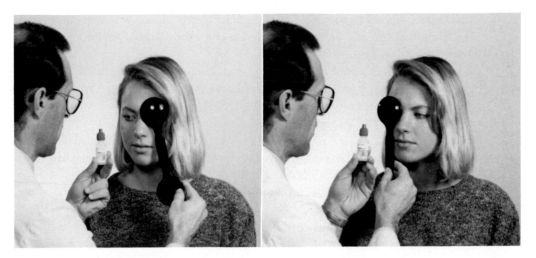

*Fig. 1-4.* Color saturation test. As red bottle cap is viewed first by right eye *(left)* and then by left eye *(right),* patient is asked to report any difference in color.

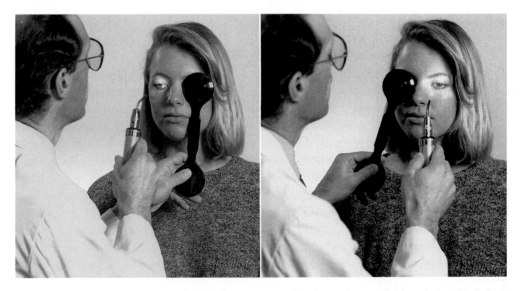

*Fig. 1-5.* Brightness test. As bright light is viewed first by right eye *(left)* and then by left eye *(right),* patient is asked if there is any difference in light brightness (or intensity).

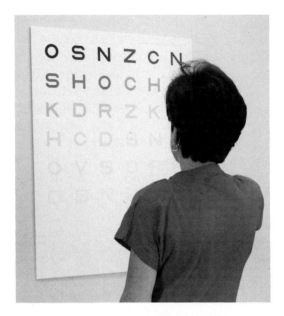

*Fig. 1-6.* Contrast sensitivity test. Patient is asked to identify letters from an array of equal-sized letters of diminishing contrast relative to white background. One of many contrast sensitivity tests, this one, designed by Pelli and Robson, was selected for use in Optic Neuritis Treatment Trial.

quantitated by assigning the normal side a value of 100 and asking the patient to give a value to the abnormal side. In our experience, the patient rarely notes clear-cut desaturation in the absence of an RAPD. Where the responses are discrepant, we are guided by the objective RAPD.

Because Snellen acuity measures discriminative vision at only one spatial frequency and at 100% contrast, it may not be sensitive to subtle deficits in visual function. Contrast sensitivity tests (Fig. 1-6), which can be manipulated to test various spatial frequencies and contrast levels, have uncovered deficits in patients who have visual pathway lesions and normal Snellen acuity.[17] Their reliability and sensitivity are yet to be verified in large patient groups.[18] At this time, we are uncertain of their utility.

### Relative afferent pupillary defect present

When an RAPD accompanies visual loss, the evaluation proceeds according to the results of visual field examination.

*Visual field examination.* The major purpose of visual field examination (see Appendix at the end of this chapter) is to localize the neuroretinal lesion, which in turn often suggests its nature. If the field defect has a nerve fiber bundle configuration, the lesion may be in either the retinal nerve fiber layer or in that portion of the optic nerve that lies well in front of the chiasm (*prechiasmal;* see Chapter 2). If the field defect is of the nerve fiber bundle type, it has less than a 3% chance of being a mass lesion.[19] That is, in at least 97% of cases, the responsible disease will be congenital, inflammatory, ischemic, or traumatic. For the most part, such lesions do not appear even on the highest quality imaging studies.

On the other hand, if a temporal hemianopic defect is present in one or both eyes, the disease process is located either at the junction of the optic nerve and chiasm, at the chiasm, or at the optic tract. The probability of a compressive lesion is nearly 100%, and proper imaging should reveal it. Most such lesions are eminently treatable, especially if they are diagnosed before they have infiltrated or massively displaced vital structures.

In diagnosing the cause of unexplained visual acuity loss, distinguish between *hemianopic* visual field defects and *nonhemianopic* (nerve fiber bundle) defects.

## ☐ Hemianopic defect present

### ☐ Compressive optic nerve or tract lesion

In a patient who has subnormal acuity and an RAPD, the finding of a hemianopic field defect means that a lesion is present at the optic chiasm or optic tract.

Defined as any field defect with a border aligned to the vertical fixation meridian, a hemianopic defect need not represent loss of the entire hemifield. Although the classic pattern of visual field defects produced by compressive disease at the optic chiasm is the bitemporal hemianopia (Fig. 1-7), rarely is the visual loss total or even symmetrically depressed in the two temporal fields. Indeed, the disease process usually affects one optic nerve, as well as the chiasm, and sometimes both optic nerves (usually asymmetrically). The result is that the patient often has subnormal acuity in at least one eye and an RAPD in that eye.

Some patients who have chiasmal lesions manifest a temporal hemianopia in the field of *one eye only*. The monocular temporal hemianopia may be plotted either ipsilateral or, more commonly, contralateral to the eye with the RAPD. The causative lesion will be found on the side of the RAPD at the junction of the optic nerve and chiasm. When it is contralateral to the eye with the RAPD, the temporal hemianopia is often limited to the superior field. The explanation most often given for this phenomenon is that axons deriving from inferior nasal retina cross in the optic chiasm and loop forward in the contralateral optic nerve before proceeding on to the optic tract. Conduction in these anteriorly looping fibers ("Wilbrand's knee") is presumably compromised by lesions compressing the optic nerve–chiasm junction on that side (Fig. 1-8).

On rare occasions patients with RAPD have homonymous hemianopias (Fig. 1-9). If the RAPD and the field defect are related, then the lesion lies at the optic tract. Two possibilities exist. If the RAPD is on the side ipsilateral to the tract lesion, the lesion must be a mass (extrinsic or intrinsic) that extends forward to impair function of the ipsilateral optic nerve, hence producing an RAPD.[20] Alternatively, if the RAPD is on the side contralateral to the tract lesion, the lesion is confined to the tract and may be a mass lesion, an infarct, or a demyelinating plaque.[21] The RAPD is believed to develop because the optic tract contains more crossed than uncrossed fibers (52:48) and a lesion will therefore affect the contralateral pupil more than the ipsilateral pupil.

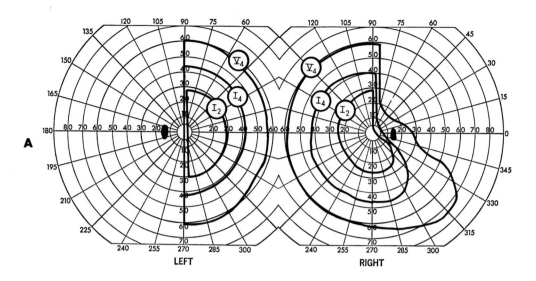

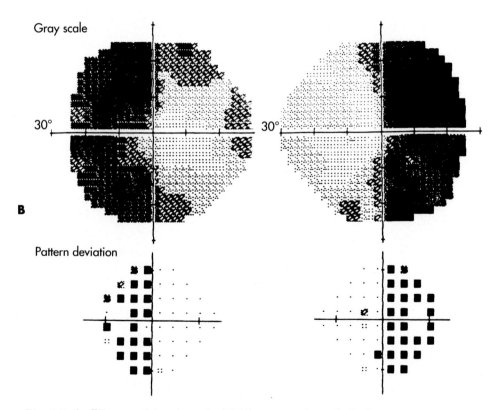

*Fig. 1-7.* **A,** Bitemporal hemianopia (Goldmann perimeter). **B,** Bitemporal hemianopia (Humphrey perimeter).

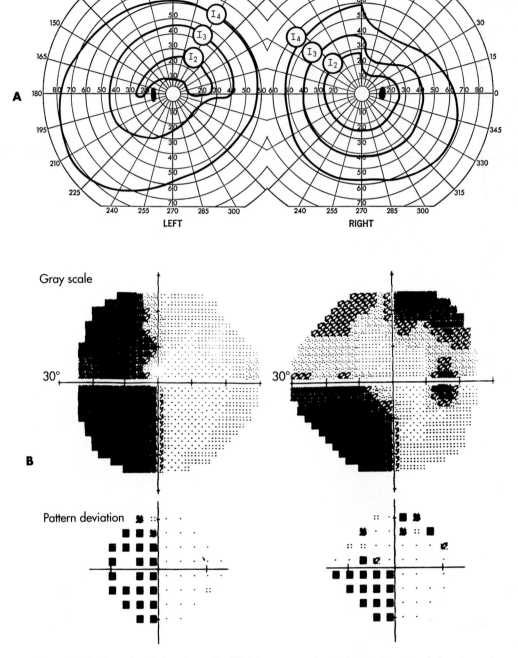

*Fig. 1-8.* **A,** Junctional hemianopia (Goldmann perimeter). **B,** Junctional hemianopia (Humphrey perimeter).

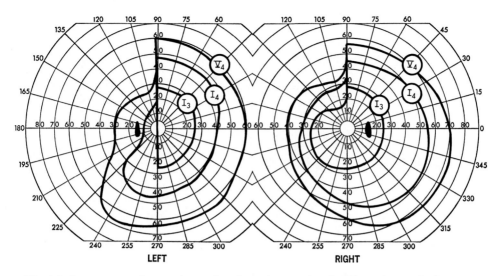

*Fig. 1-9.* Incongruous homonymous hemianopia associated with optic tract lesion.

In our experience, over 90% of perichiasmal lesions are tumors, and all should be found with imaging studies that highlight the area of suspicion. If tailored imaging studies are negative, visual field testing should be repeated to determine if an error has been made. If not, one must consider nonchiasmal lesions (optic nerve, retinal, and factitious disorders) that produce field defects that "look hemianopic."

## ☐ Nonhemianopic defect present or normal

### ☐ Retrobulbar optic nerve lesion

The nonhemianopic field defect is caused by lesions of the optic nerve and retinal nerve fiber layer. The configuration of these lesions corresponds to the organization of the nerve fiber layer of the retina:

**Central scotoma,** affecting those papillomacular fibers coming from the macular region (Fig. 1-10)

**Centrocecal scotoma,** affecting those fibers entering the optic nerve from the macula and the zone between the macula and the optic disc (Fig. 1-11)

**Arcuate scotoma,** affecting temporal retinal fibers that bend around the papillomacular bundle and course into the optic nerve (Fig. 1-12)

**Wedge-shaped scotoma,** with the apex at the blind spot, affecting nasal retinal fibers as they enter the optic nerve (Fig. 1-13)

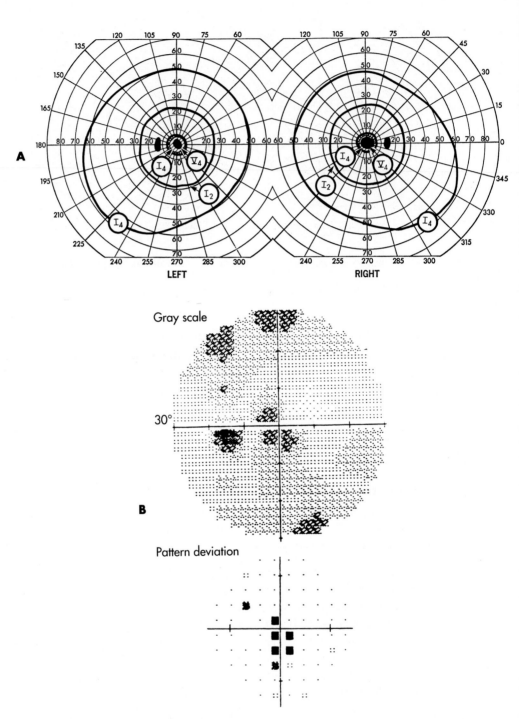

*Fig. 1-10.* **A,** Central scotomas (Goldmann perimeter). **B,** Central scotoma (Humphrey perimeter).

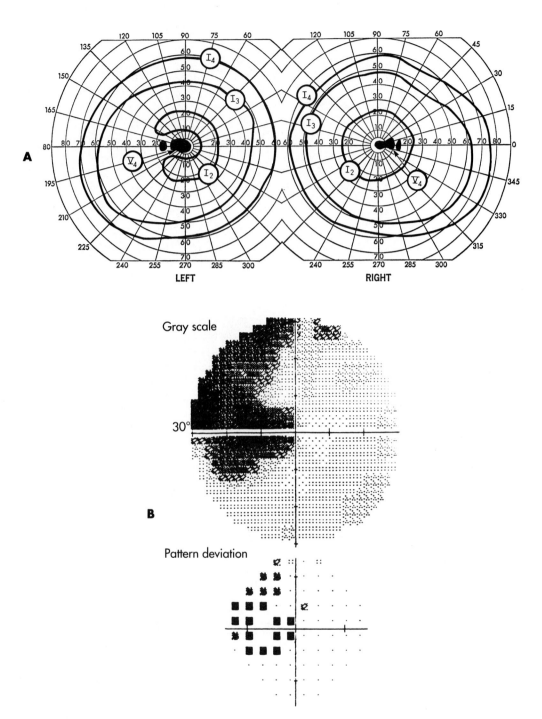

*Fig. 1-11.* **A,** Centrocecal scotomas (Goldmann perimeter). **B,** Centrocecal scotoma (Humphrey perimeter).

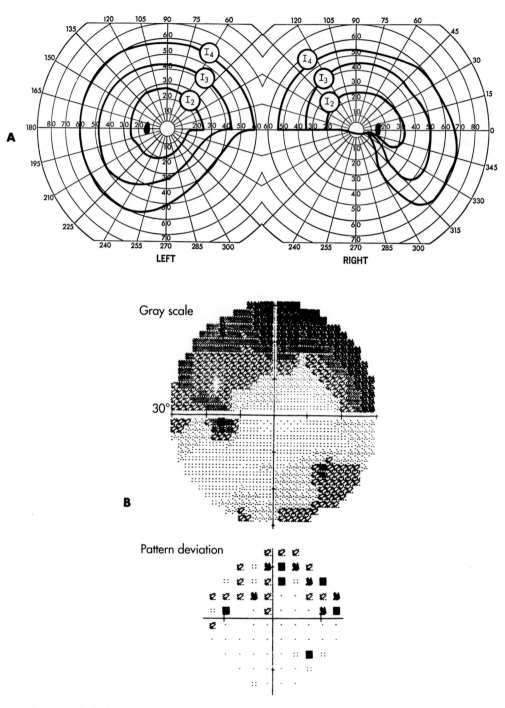

*Fig. 1-12.* **A,** Inferior arcuate scotomas with nasal steps (Goldmann perimeter). **B,** Superior arcuate scotoma (Humphrey perimeter).

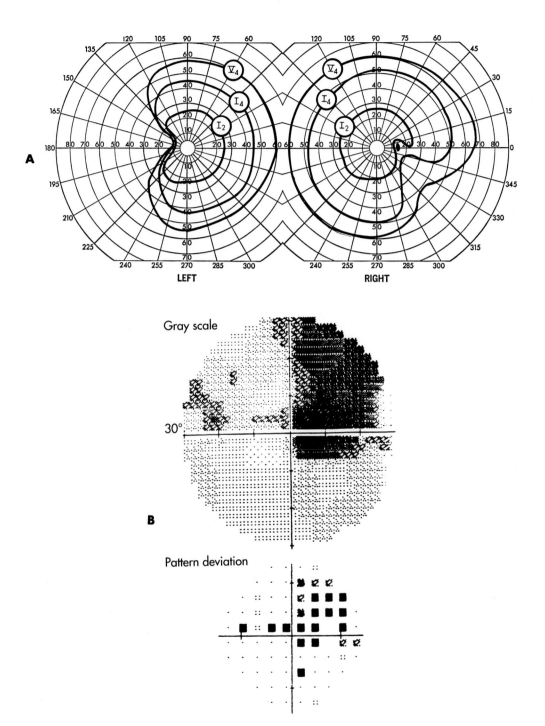

*Fig. 1-13.* **A,** Temporal wedge defects (Goldmann perimeter). **B,** Temporal wedge defect (Humphrey perimeter).

Most nonhemianopic defects consist of one or a combination of these configurations. At times the defect is so small that its shape has none of these localizing features. In such cases it is usually called a *nonspecific focal depression*. Visual field examination may also show no focal defects, but rather a general elevation of all static thresholds or an inward displacement of central isopters. Such a finding is called a *nonspecific generalized depression* and may be caused by an optic neuropathy.

In a patient with an RAPD and a nonhemianopic field defect, nonspecific focal or generalized depression, and no obvious fundus abnormalities, one may assume that the lesion lies in the retrobulbar optic nerve. *If the clinical characteristics of the illness permit a likely diagnosis of retrobulbar neuritis (see Chapter 2), we believe that imaging studies may be deferred initially.* On the other hand, if retrobulbar neuritis appears unlikely, then one must exclude a compressive lesion with appropriate imaging studies. Most compressive prechiasmal lesions can be imaged, provided the study clearly defines the intraorbital, intracanalicular, and intracranial optic nerve.

■ Relative afferent pupillary defect not present (Chart 1-1, *B*)

If no RAPD accompanies visual loss, the next step is to exclude amblyopia by looking for historical or current evidence of strabismus, markedly asymmetric refractive errors between the two eyes, or a long-standing monocular media opacity.

■ Evidence for amblyopia present

*Amblyopia* is defined as subnormal vision that results from persistently unfocused imagery at the retina, or suppression of the fovea in a deviating eye. Because it produces no objective signs of visual disturbance, amblyopia remains a presumptive cause of visual acuity loss and should be diagnosed only if the precipitating circumstances are present and after other causes of visual loss have been eliminated.

▢ Amblyopia

Amblyopia usually arises in the setting of *strabismus* (ocular misalignment) but may also be seen in association with *anisometropia* (unequal refractive error in the two eyes) and with profound *media opacities* in early childhood. If amblyopia is to develop, it will do so well within the first decade of life, when the developing visual system is still vulnerable to deprivation.

Strabismus is the most frequent setting for amblyopia. The diagnostic challenge in this circumstance is that the degree of amblyopia bears little relation to the degree of misalignment. In other words, tiny prismatic deviations (10 prism

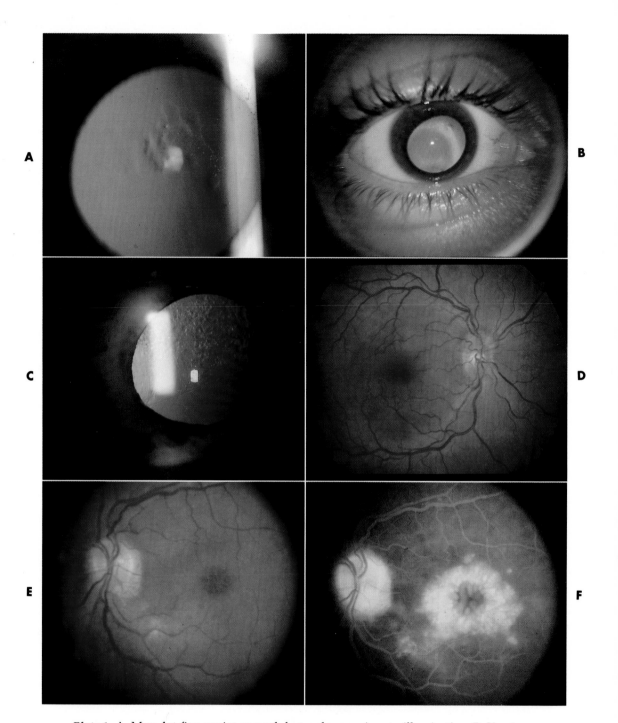

*Plate 1.* **A,** Map-dot-fingerprint corneal dystrophy seen in retroillumination. **B,** Keratoconus in retroillumination. **C,** After cataract. Pearl-like opacities of posterior lens capsule remnants in retroillumination. **D,** Central serous chorioretinopathy. Note blisterlike elevation in macular region. **E,** Cystoid macular edema. **F,** Cystoid macular edema after fluorescein angiography. Petaloid edema is now evident.

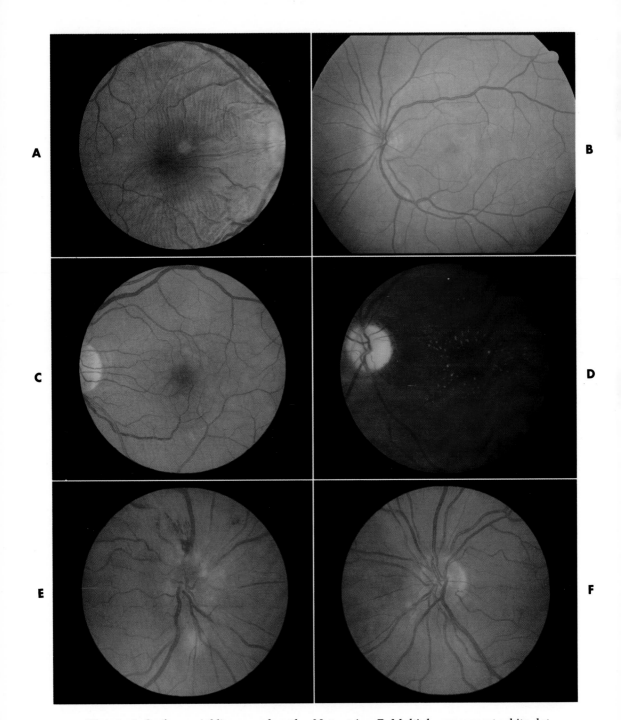

*Plate 2.* **A,** Surface-wrinkling maculopathy. Note striae. **B,** Multiple evanescent white dot syndrome (MEWDS) showing subtle deep grayish spots in macular area. **C,** Acute multifocal placoid pigment epitheliopathy (AMPPE) showing extramacular cream-colored deep retinal lesions. **D,** Macular star figure (Leber's stellate neuroretinopathy). **E,** Nonarteritic ischemic optic neuropathy, affected eye. **F,** Fellow eye of patient with nonarteritic ischemic optic neuropathy. Note crowded, hyperemic disc.

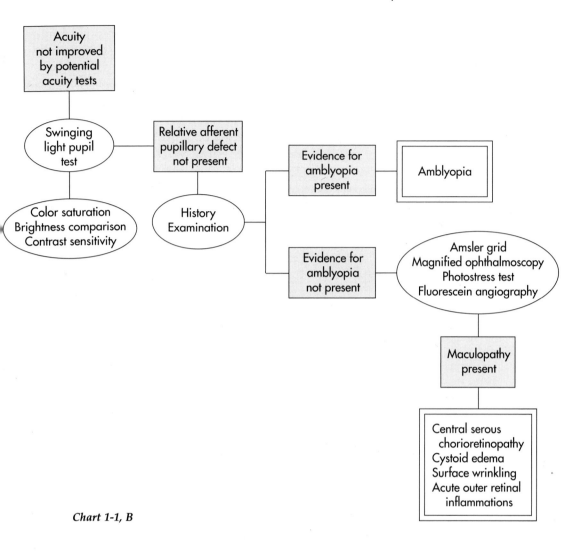

*Chart 1-1, B*

diopters or less) may be associated with dense amblyopia (visual acuity of 20/200 or worse). A history of childhood strabismus is helpful, but one should not accept a diagnosis of strabismic amblyopia unless a misalignment can be demonstrated and other causes have been excluded. Furthermore, visual acuity loss cannot be ascribed to amblyopia in the fixing eye, or in cases of obvious alternate fixation.

Anisometropic amblyopia is usually found only in patients whose refractive error in the two eyes differs by 2 diopters or more (sphere or cylinder). Moreover, amblyopia is more commonly associated with unilateral hypermetropia or astigmatism than with unilateral myopia, since the myopic eye is used preferentially for reading. Binocular amblyopia associated with refractive errors is exceedingly rare but may occur in infants with high hypermetropia.

Amblyopia associated with media opacities arises most commonly within the first years of life, the result of congenital or traumatic cataract, or corneal or vitreal disease. When the disorder is congenital, even very early surgical intervention with restoration of clear media may not eliminate a deep-seated amblyopia.

Even in the presence of long-standing strabismus, amblyopia remains a presumptive cause of subnormal acuity. No means exist to verify its presence directly. Observers have described some clinical features that appear to be characteristic of, but not specific to, amblyopia. First, patients with amblyopia are said to have a higher acuity when they are asked to read single letters rather than an entire line of optotypes ("crowding phenomenon"). Second, introducing a 2–log unit neutral density filter over an amblyopic eye does not degrade acuity nearly as much as introducing it before a nonamblyopic eye. Unfortunately, we have found too many exceptions to these two rules to rely on them. Third, when a 4-diopter prism is introduced before an amblyopic eye, the eye will not make a refixational movement, whereas a nonamblyopic eye will always move appropriately to fix the target. While this test is reliable, *it is merely diagnostic of a central scotoma of any type.* We have seen the results of the *4-diopter prism test* misinterpreted as indicating amblyopia when a child had a compressive optic neuropathy caused by a craniopharyngioma.

Finally, a confusing point about amblyopia and RAPD is worthy of reemphasis. We have deliberately entered amblyopia as a cause of unexplained visual loss in that part of the decision tree where no RAPD is present despite reports that amblyopia may cause an RAPD. In our view, the RAPD of amblyopia barely reaches the clinical threshold, and patient care is best served by considering other causes of RAPD first.

### Evidence for amblyopia not present

If no indirect evidence for amblyopia exists, the examiner must exclude the possibility of a subtle retinal (macular) lesion.

○ *Tests for maculopathy.* The diagnosis of maculopathy depends principally on careful testing with the Amsler grid and a magnified view of the posterior pole of the retina. Photostress testing and fluorescein angiography are sometimes of value.

**AMSLER GRID.** The report of *metamorphopsia* (warped or distorted vision) on testing with the Amsler grid is diagnostic of a macular disturbance. The patient views a grid of black lines presented on a white background at reading distance. Ask if he or she notes any bending of the lines (Fig. 1-14) and if the squares all appear equal in size. The report that some are smaller indicates *micropsia*. Interpreting these observations is much easier if disease is monocular and a control eye is available. Monocular metamorphopsia and micropsia, presumably the result of distortion and separation of foveal cones by edema, occur only with macular disease; unfortunately, significant macular disease can occur without either symptom.

**MAGNIFIED OPHTHALMOSCOPY.** An area of the retina far smaller than 1 disc diameter is responsible for visual acuity. Disturbances within this region are eas-

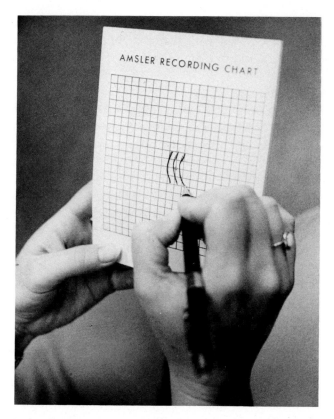

*Fig. 1-14.* Amsler grid. Patient draws bending of vertical lines, indicating metamorphopsia, a sign of macular disease.

ily overlooked unless one examines the fovea with instruments that permit a highly magnified view. Direct and indirect ophthalmoscopy are generally inadequate; the Goldmann contact lens, the Hruby lens, and the high spherical (90-diopter) hand-held lens are optimal.

**PHOTOSTRESS TEST.** In the photostress test, obtain a baseline visual acuity and then direct a bright light for 10 seconds at the eye in order to bleach it. Time the latency between bleaching and recovery to within one Snellen line of prebleaching visual acuity. If the "affected" eye has a visual recovery time substantially greater than that of the unaffected eye, the retinal pigment epithelial-receptor axis is probably disrupted.[22] The crippling drawback of this test is that the end point is highly subjective. The photostress test therefore makes only a marginal contribution to clinical diagnosis.

**FLUORESCEIN ANGIOGRAPHY.** Ocular fluorescein angiography is used to demonstrate retinochoroidal vascular occlusion, leakage, gaps in the retinal pigment epithelium, and neovascularization. Whereas this test is useful in highlighting subtle ophthalmoscopic abnormalities, we rarely encounter patients with unexplained visual acuity loss in whom fluorescein angiography reveals lesions that we had not discovered with high-magnification ophthalmoscopy. Possible exceptions are cone-rod dystrophy and acute macular retinitides.

## Maculopathy present

The retinal diseases most easily overlooked are **macular serous detachment** (Plate 1, *D*), **cystoid macular edema** (Plate 1, *E* and *F*), **macular surface wrinkling** (Plate 2, *A*), and **acute outer retinal inflammations,** including multiple evanescent white dot syndrome (MEWDS)[22-24] (Plate 2, *B*), acute macular neuroretinopathy (AMN),[25] acute retinal pigment epitheliitis,[26] and acute multifocal placoid pigment epitheliopathy (AMPPE)[27-29] (Plate 2, *C*). By the time visual acuity is degraded, age-related macular degeneration will usually disturb fundus color enough to be easily diagnosed. However, unless the macula is examined with high magnification, one can easily miss the detachment of the sensory macula in central serous chorioretinopathy, the spokelike edema of cystoid macular edema, the internal limiting membrane irregularities of surface-wrinkling maculopathy, and the delicate focal discolorations of the outer retina in the acute macular retinitides.

The acute inflammatory retinitides are particularly important to diagnose because symptoms are often acute. **MEWDS**[22] is a condition predominantly affecting women in the second and third decades, who complain of scotomas (often "flickering") in one eye and subnormal acuity. Careful fundus examination reveals grayish white dots at the level of the retinal pigment epithelium primarily in the macular and peripapillary regions. Fluorescein angiography shows early punctate fluorescence and late staining of the lesions. Electroretinogram (ERG) a-wave amplitudes are often depressed. A flulike illness may precede the ocular condition, but no pertinent systemic illness is found concurrently. Visual function and ophthalmoscopic abnormalities generally resolve within 2 months, although some recurrences have been documented several years later.[23] Some patients may complain of a temporal scotoma (blind spot enlargement) and photopsias long after the retinal lesions have disappeared.[24]

Two other acute retinopathies may be confused with MEWDS: **acute macular neuroretinopathy**[25] (reddish orange lesions confined to the macula) and **acute retinal pigment epitheliitis**[26] (dark spot in the macula surrounded by a halo of depigmentation). **AMPPE**[27] appears to be distinctive in manifesting much larger cream-colored lesions, which are mostly extramacular. Like MEWDS, all of these retinitides are acute in onset and are often preceded by a viral illness. These disorders typically manifest many outer retinal focal lesions that are self-limited and generally unassociated with nonocular symptomatology. However, cerebral vasculitis with stroke has been documented during[28] and following[29] resolution of the ocular manifestations of AMPPE. We regard all of these retinitides as postviral (possibly autoimmune) conditions that constitute underdiagnosed causes of unexplained visual acuity loss. At least in cases of AMPPE, and perhaps in its variants, the physician must rule out ongoing systemic components, particularly in the nervous system.

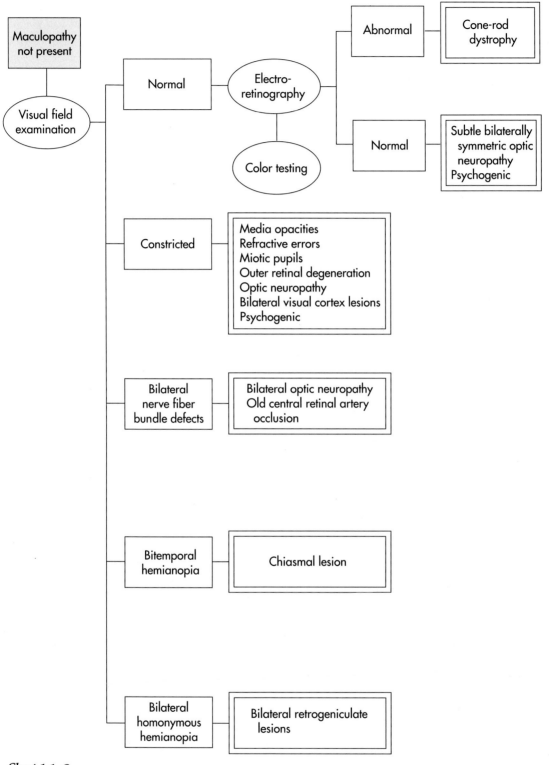

*Chart 1-1, C*

■ Maculopathy not present

If subtle foveomacular disease has been excluded as an explanation for visual loss in a patient without RAPD (Chart 1-1, C), information must be sought from visual field examination.

○ *Visual field examination.* This examination (see Appendix) will show five possible results:

1. Normal visual fields
2. Constricted fields
3. Bilateral nerve fiber bundle defects
4. Bitemporal hemianopia
5. Homonymous hemianopia

☐ Normal visual fields

If no visual field defects are found, either the testing methods are inadequate or the patient has a **cone-rod dystrophy, subtle bilaterally symmetric optic neuropathy,** or **psychogenic (factitious) visual loss.**

Distinguishing between these three conditions may be difficult. Even the most experienced perimetrists have trouble finding shallow central field defects that degrade acuity. Current automated static programs are much better here, but they still fail, especially if patient cooperation is suboptimal.

○ *Electroretinography.* Among patients with normal or nondiagnostic visual field results, abnormal color vision, and a normal fundus examination, the ERG is the most useful test in separating cone-rod dystrophy from subtle optic neuropathy or psychogenic visual loss (Fig. 1-15).

○ *Color testing.* Color vision tests may also help differentiate psychogenic visual loss (no deficit or unreasonable deficit) from subtle optic neuropathy (mild deficit) and cone-rod dystrophy (severe deficit). We caution, however, against relying too heavily on color vision tests because of their inherent subjectivity. No solid data are available on the correlation between deficits in visual acuity, visual field, and color vision, but most optic neuropathies that depress acuity below 20/30 manifest deficits on the standard (Hardy-Rand-Rittler or Ishihara) color plates.[30] The Farnsworth D-15 or D-100 tests may be more sensitive[31,32] (also more time consuming), but wide experience in formal trials is lacking. In cone-rod dystrophies color vision will be degraded even further than in optic neuropathies with equivalent visual acuity levels.

☐ Abnormal ERG

▣ Cone-rod dystrophy

The term *cone-rod dystrophy* has been applied to a condition in which cone dysfunction predominates over rod dysfunction.[33] Whereas dark adaptation and peripheral field loss are the chief findings in the typical hereditary retinal receptor

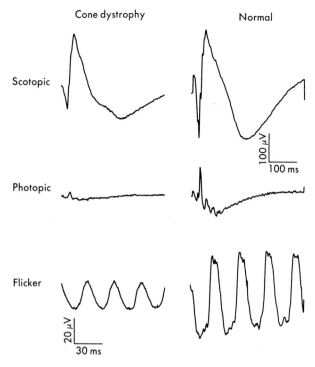

*Fig. 1-15.* Electroretinogram (ERG) in cone dystrophy. Note reduced B-wave amplitude to single-flash photopic and 30 Hz flicker stimuli.

dystrophies, failing central vision, reduced sight in bright light ("day blindness"), and poor color vision are the principal problems of those afflicted with cone-rod dystrophy. Most patients are diagnosed before adulthood, but a substantial minority become symptomatic later in life. Visual acuity may be minimally degraded, and visual fields are often normal. Fundus examination may be entirely normal. In other cases speckled depigmentation of the perifoveal retina is visible; this often subtle finding may be enhanced by fluorescein angiography. The diagnosis is suggested by color vision deficits disproportionate to visual acuity deficits and is made definitively by finding depressed cone function in the ERG.

Although no reliable prevalence information exists, we believe that cone-rod dystrophy represents one of the common causes of unexplained, slowly progressive binocular visual loss at any age. The diagnosis is missed or delayed for three reasons: (1) the entity is not considered, (2) poor color vision is falsely attributed to congenital color deficiency, or (3) the ERG has not included a stimulus battery to elicit cone (as opposed to rod) responses. Although no treatment is available, timely recognition of this condition may be helpful in family planning and in avoiding unnecessary diagnostic tangents.

### ☐ Normal ERG

If a complete ERG is normal, the diagnostic possibilities are **subtle bilaterally symmetric optic neuropathy** or **psychogenic visual loss.** If behavioral features do not allow a clear distinction between these entities (see Psychogenic Visual Loss), then one may choose among three courses: (1) no studies, reexamine after a short interval; (2) brain imaging; and (3) visual evoked potentials (VEPs) (see The Role of Visual Evoked Potentials in Evaluating Unexplained Visual Loss).

### ☐ Constricted visual fields

Constricted visual fields are characterized by inward displacement of the isopters in kinetic perimetry and elevation of edge thresholds in static perimetry (Fig. 1-16). When these changes are not the result of testing artifact, they are caused by (1) unfocused imagery or reduced illumination (media opacities, uncorrected refractive errors, miotic pupils), (2) outer retinal degeneration, (3) optic neuropathy, (4) bilateral visual cortex lesions, or (5) psychogenic visual loss.

### ☐ Media opacities, refractive errors, miotic pupils

Any of these conditions will degrade the quality of the image presented to the retina and result in depression of the visual field. The greatest depression will occur in the central, not the peripheral, field, where discriminative vision is poor anyway.

### ☐ Outer retinal degeneration

Degeneration of the retinal photoreceptors and retinal pigment epithelium occurs slowly with advancing age and prematurely in the hereditary conditions categorized as *retinitis pigmentosa.* Patients who have retinitis pigmentosa usually become symptomatic in youth, although more indolent adult-onset disease is common. They usually complain of night blindness and notice constriction of the visual field only later. Their visual fields tend to reveal most marked depression in the midperiphery, corresponding to the equatorial band of photoreceptor degeneration. Ophthalmoscopy generally shows retinal pigment clumping along blood vessels ("bone corpuscles"), particularly in this equatorial region, and retinal arterioles are attenuated. The low-amplitude ERG is diagnostic. Problems in diagnosis arise in those cases where ophthalmoscopy fails to reveal any pigmentary changes (*sine pigmento* form) and in an unusual paraneoplastic condition in which photoreceptor degeneration proceeds over months in patients with visceral (usually oat cell) carcinoma *(cancer-associated retinopathy).*[34] Ophthalmoscopy tends to be negative, except for narrowed retinal arterioles; the ERG is of low amplitude. Antibodies against retinal and optic nerve antigens have been detected.

### ☐ Optic neuropathy

Although most optic neuropathies produce focal depressions *(scotomas)* within the visual field, in some cases only the edges are depressed, giving rise to a constricted field.

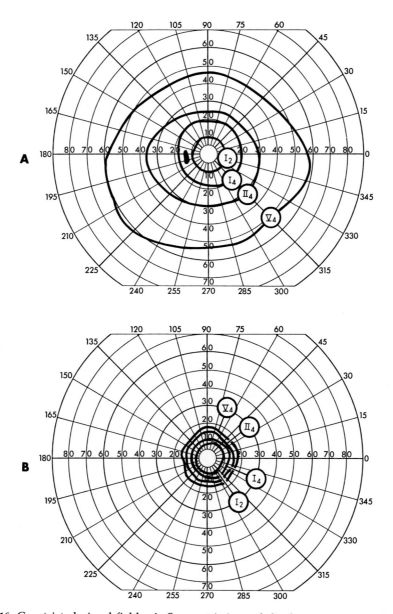

*Fig. 1-16.* Constricted visual fields. **A,** Symmetric inward displacement principally affecting inner isopters (could be caused by uncorrected refractive errors, media opacities, miotic pupils, optic neuropathy). **B,** Symmetric inward displacement of outer isopters, collapsing on inner isopter (could be caused by outer retinal degeneration, optic neuropathy, bilateral visual cortex disease, psychogenic visual loss).

*Continued.*

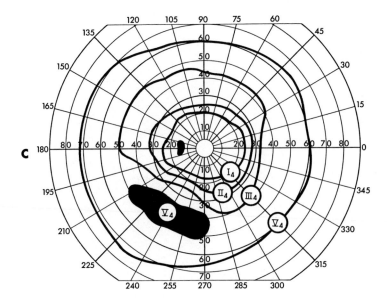

**C**

Gray scale

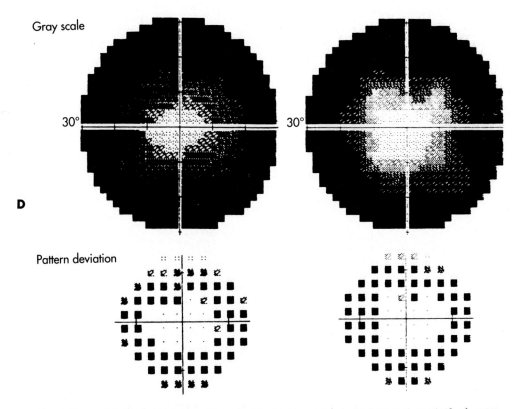

30°          30°

Pattern deviation

*Fig. 1-16, cont'd.* **C,** Asymmetric inward displacement of outer isopters, typical of outer retinal degeneration. **D,** Depression of edge static thresholds, Humphrey perimeter, caused by psychogenic visual loss.

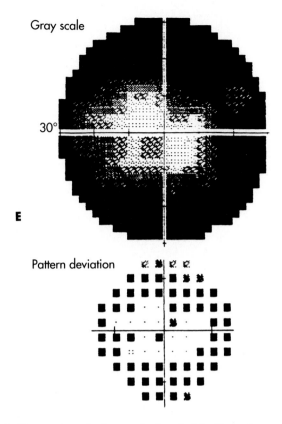

**Gray scale**

30°

**E**

**Pattern deviation**

*Fig. 1-16, cont'd.* **E,** Depression of edge static thresholds, Humphrey perimeter, caused by optic neuritis.

### ☐ Bilateral visual cortex lesions

Lesions that affect the visual cortex on both sides, especially infarcts, may spare the occipital pole, which mediates the central 5 to 10 degrees of the visual field. The visual field defects are actually showing bilateral homonymous hemianopias with macular sparing. Acuity may be normal. The differentiation of this condition from psychogenic visual loss is usually not difficult, since patients with bilateral visual cortex lesions have a history of sudden visual loss, often accompanied by other features of posterior (vertebrobasilar) circulation ischemia. Furthermore, their affect and behavior, as well as their performance in visual field testing, is unlike that of patients who have psychogenic visual loss.

### ☐ Psychogenic visual loss

The constricted field of psychogenic (as opposed to organic) origin has special features. Confrontation testing tends to reveal no expansion of the visual field at a more remote testing distance *(tunnel field)* (Fig. 1-17). Formal testing, especially kinetic perimetry, reveals marked inconsistency. For example, equivalent test objects give widely differing thresholds, and repeated presentation of the same test object elicits broad threshold fluctuations *(spiraling)*.

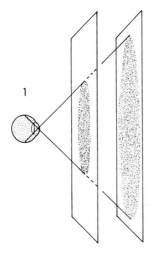

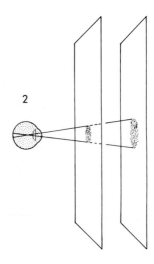

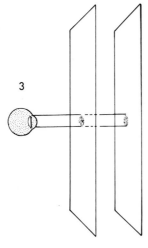

*Fig. 1-17.* Tunnel and funnel constricted visual fields. *1,* Normal. Normal-sized visual field *(shaded area)* expands as test distance is increased. *2,* Neuroretinal disease. Constricted visual field expands as test distance is increased (funnel field). *3,* Psychogenic disease. Constricted visual field does not expand as test distance is increased (tunnel field).

The diagnosis of psychogenic visual loss, often a difficult and tiresome exercise, depends on two principles: (1) excluding organic patterns of visual loss and (2) eliciting behavior incompatible with the alleged level of visual dysfunction. Few patients who allege moderate visual loss can maintain a consistent level of dissembling. We hunt for inconstancies in distance and near acuities and lack of appropriate improvement in near vision with suitable magnification devices. In testing patients who profess very poor sight (finger-counting acuity or worse), observing them walk or sign their names often gives clues to histrionic behavior. At best, these bits of evidence are circumstantial and must be combined with the exclusion of organic disease lest one overlook a layer of organic disease under an avalanche of embellishment.

We generally do not favor VEPs in the diagnosis of suspected psychogenic visual loss (see The Role of Visual Evoked Potentials in Evaluating Unexplained

Visual Loss), on the basis that patients can volitionally produce abnormal VEPs. Moreover, a normal VEP does not exclude organic visual pathway disease.

### ☐ Bilateral nerve fiber bundle defects

These defects indicate **bilateral optic neuropathy** or **old central retinal artery occlusion** (see Chapter 2). Based on the location of the nerve fiber bundle defects, three diagnostic categories should be considered:

1. Defects that affect *predominantly the papillomacular bundle.* Whereas many optic neuropathies may at times affect only this bundle, the toxic-metabolic-hereditary neuropathies selectively damage this bundle.
2. Defects that affect the *papillomacular and nonpapillomacular bundles.* Most optic neuropathies and retinal artery occlusion are included here, with the exception of the toxic-metabolic-hereditary disorders.
3. Defects that *do not affect the papillomacular bundle.* Four entities most commonly cause these defects: primary open-angle glaucoma, long-standing papilledema with secondary optic atrophy, ischemic optic neuropathy, and optic nerve dysplasia.

In many of these cases, ophthalmoscopic abnormalities are readily evident. Others may carry no observable markers. For example, the toxic and metabolic optic neuropathies typically show little optic disc pallor unless they are far advanced. The retinal opacification caused by retinal artery occlusion (see Chapter 2) disappears after 1 week, and disc pallor may not appear before 3 weeks have elapsed. Retrobulbar causes of optic neuropathy (compressive lesions, optic neuritis, carcinomatous or infectious meningitis) may never produce disc swelling and may produce atrophy only many weeks after disturbing visual function.

Compressive lesions rarely cause bilateral nerve fiber bundle defects, with the notable exception of congestive orbitopathies such as Graves' disease and orbitocranial meningioma[35] (see Chapter 2).

### ☐ Bitemporal hemianopia

The finding of bitemporal hemianopia strongly suggests a chiasmal lesion.

#### ▣ Chiasmal lesion

Proper imaging should locate the chiasmal lesion. If not, two possibilities exist: (1) the perimetry is in error—the patient has *pseudobitemporal hemianopia* (centrocecal scotomas, asymmetric retinitis pigmentosa, tilted or dysplastic optic discs), or (2) the imaging technique is inadequate.

### ☐ Bilateral homonymous hemianopia

#### ▣ Bilateral retrogeniculate lesions

Retrogeniculate lesions of the visual pathway depress visual function without producing an RAPD. Homonymous hemianopia caused by a lesion in one hemisphere *will not* reduce visual acuity. The spared optic radiations and visual cortex in the other hemisphere are sufficient to guarantee normal acuity, although

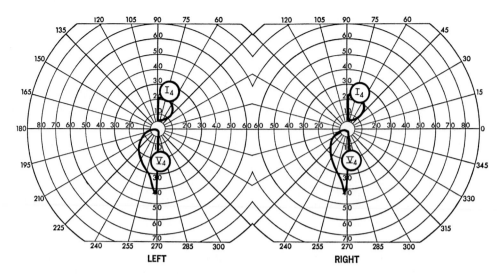

***Fig. 1-18.*** Bilateral homonymous hemianopia caused by disease of both visual cortices. Such visual field defects, affecting both fixational areas, could explain subnormal acuity.

the patient may have to struggle to place the letters in his intact hemifield. On the other hand, bilateral retrogeniculate visual pathway (usually visual cortex) lesions will degrade visual acuity if the macular projection fibers are involved (Fig. 1-18). This is most likely to occur after (1) basilar or bilateral posterior cerebral artery thromboembolism, (2) severe and sustained systemic hypotension (shock), and (3) occipital lobe contusion.

## Unexplained Visual Field Loss with Normal Visual Acuity

In analyzing the problem of visual field loss with normal visual acuity, the examiner should proceed exactly as before, bearing in mind the following facts:

1. Retinal diseases that cause visual field defects may not produce ophthalmoscopically obvious abnormalities. Retinal receptor dystrophies are the leading candidates. Peripheral retinal disorders may be difficult to detect without skilled examination.
2. Optic neuropathies may cause visual field defects without degrading visual acuity if the papillomacular bundle is spared. Many optic neuropathies characteristically spare this bundle, including primary open-angle glaucoma, ischemic optic neuropathy, pseudotumor cerebri, and optic nerve drusen.
3. Optic chiasm lesions may spare visual acuity.
4. Retrochiasmal lesions always spare visual acuity unless they are bilateral or impinge on one or both optic nerves.
5. A common cause of unexplained visual field loss is an artifact of examination. This is particularly true of automated static testing, which is demanding and highly sensitive.

# Unexplained Visual Loss with Normal Visual Acuity and Visual Fields

As we acknowledged at the outset of the chapter, many patients complain that their vision is "not normal" but their acuity and field testing appear normal. These patients fall into two groups:

1. *Subclinical optic neuropathy or maculopathy* has degraded acuity so slightly that conventional measures do not detect the deficit. These patients should be evaluated intensively if their history is convincing, or if a measurable interocular difference (such as an RAPD) is present. Color vision and contrast sensitivity testing may be useful here. We are not convinced that VEP is of value.
2. *Acuity and fields are truly normal; the complaint relates to some other aspect of vision.* These patients may be describing color deficits; floaters; glare; photophobia; metamorphopsia; micropsia; hallucinations; scintillations; reading, attentional, perceptual, or visuospatial difficulties; poor stereopsis; double vision; or oscillopsia. Proper diagnosis depends less on procedures and decision trees than on skilled interviewing.

Patients with visuospatial, visuoperceptual, and attentional disorders of vision represent a particularly vexing group. For the most part, they have Alzheimer's disease but have not been diagnosed, because their verbal and memory deficits are not as profound as their visual deficits. They typically complain of blurred vision, having objects "pop out of sight," and difficulty in reading and judging distances, especially when driving or picking up objects.[36,37] Screening mental status tests tend not to emphasize vision-related tasks and may therefore miss the diagnosis. Visual acuity is generally normal or nearly normal. Color vision is generally quite poor if tested with color confusion plates (which depend on intact visuospatial function) but normal with pure hue discrimination tests. Visual field examination may yield uninterpretable results because patients become confused and inattentive. Contrast sensitivity tests may elicit subnormal performance. Generally no structural abnormalities of the globe are observable, although mild optic disc pallor has been described.

Electrophysiologic and pathologic evidence indicates that damage to large retinal ganglion cells and their axons occurs in Alzheimer's disease,[38] but these changes probably do not account for the patients' symptoms. Instead, their symptoms probably derive from deficits in relating one piece of visual information to another, and to personal and extrapersonal space. Tests involving line cancellation, paragraph reading, picture interpretation, and puzzle assembly tend to bring out these deficits. Visual rehabilitative efforts have not been very effective, inasmuch as their dementing illness is progressive. Nevertheless, a timely identification of the cause of their vision problems helps to avoid unnecessary testing.

# The Role of Visual Evoked Potentials in Evaluating Unexplained Visual Loss

In the workup of unexplained visual loss, VEPs are traditionally used in three circumstances: (1) to confirm or deny the presence of optic neuropathy in a patient whose other findings are not, by themselves, diagnostic; (2) to buttress a diagnosis of multiple sclerosis (MS) by finding prolonged latency in the asymptomatic eye of a patient with possible optic neuritis in the other eye; and (3) to confirm suspected psychogenic visual loss by demonstrating a normal VEP in the face of alleged subnormal acuity.

## CONFIRMING THE DIAGNOSIS OF EQUIVOCAL OPTIC NEUROPATHY

When optic neuropathy is asymmetric, the RAPD is a sufficient diagnostic test. However, when optic neuropathy is symmetric in the two eyes and is too mild to cause reliable field or fundus abnormalities, knowing if conduction velocity is normal would be helpful. The VEP has demonstrably high sensitivity to subclinical optic neuropathy in MS and has been used to follow the course of ethambutol optic neuropathy.[39] We acknowledge its utility in these situations but are troubled by the poor correlation of VEP latency and other threshold measurements of optic nerve function.[40]

## BUTTRESSING A DIAGNOSIS OF MULTIPLE SCLEROSIS IN A CASE OF SUSPECTED MONOCULAR OPTIC NEURITIS

The VEP will, of course, demonstrate a prolonged latency in the affected eye of patients with fresh and clinically isolated optic neuritis. However, it is the finding of a prolonged latency *in the unaffected eye* that is important to establish dissemination of disease in space ("the second lesion"). One report describes a 27% prevalence of prolonged latencies in the unaffected eyes of patients with clinically isolated optic neuritis.[41] By comparison, magnetic resonance imaging (MRI) scans show disseminated plaquelike lesions in up to 66% of patients with isolated optic neuritis,[42] and the presence of these abnormalities appears to help predict the future likelihood of developing clinical MS.[43] At this time, then, VEP may be a less expensive test than MRI, but it is clearly less helpful.

## CONFIRMING A DIAGNOSIS OF PSYCHOGENIC VISUAL LOSS

The principal drawback of VEP in confirming a diagnosis of psychogenic visual loss is that deliberate inattention to the stimuli may produce a false-positive delay in the response signal.[44] Careful monitoring and appropriate technique may overcome these pitfalls,[45] but because a skillful examination will identify most cases, we have not often found a need to use the VEP.

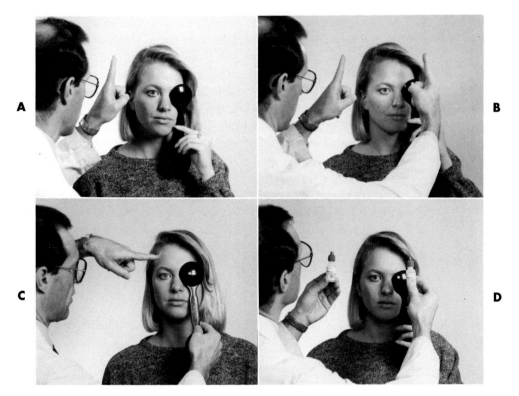

*Fig. 1-19.* Confrontation visual field examination. **A,** Patient is asked to count a single stationary finger presented in one quadrant of visual field. **B,** Patient is asked to count two stationary fingers presented simultaneously, one in nasal, the other in temporal quadrant of field. **C,** If one of the two fingers is consistently ignored, patient is asked to signal appearance of finger moved from "nonseeing" quadrant into "seeing" quadrant. **D,** Patient is asked if there is a difference in color between two red bottle caps presented in nasal and temporal quadrants.

# Appendix

## PERFORMING THE VISUAL FIELD EXAMINATION

**CONFRONTATION TESTING** (Fig. 1-19). The ideal confrontation technique is one that reveals areas of differential visual sensitivity across a well-defined line. Instead of comparing the two eyes, as in the swinging light, brightness, and color saturation tests, one compares the two halves of the visual field in each eye, with the vertical fixation meridian serving as the dividing line. Each hemifield is tested sequentially or simultaneously for sensitivity to brightness and color saturation.

1. Present stationary fingers on either side of the vertical fixational meridian well within 30 degrees of fixation, and ask the patient to count them. (In examining children and illiterate, demented, or very poorly sighted adults, ask them to mimic the number of fingers presented, or look for eye movements elicited by the stimulus.)

2. If all the fingers are counted correctly and yet the index of suspicion of a chiasmal lesion is high, present the two hands simultaneously and ask the patient to total up the number of fingers seen.
3. Ask the patient to compare the brightness of single fingers or whole hands presented simultaneously on each side of the vertical fixation meridian.
4. To increase sensitivity further, present large static red stimuli in both hemifields and ask the patient to compare saturation.
5. If the patient notes consistent differences, try to confirm that a border lies at the vertical fixation meridian by moving the target from the relatively defective field perpendicularly toward the vertical fixational meridian and asking the patient if he or she notes a change in its appearance. If a true hemianopic defect exists, the patient will announce that an abrupt change in brightness or color saturation has occurred at the vertical fixation meridian.

Performed correctly, these confrontation tests are helpful predictors of the results of formal perimetry. Although they seem crude, they may sometimes detect hemianopic defects not found even with the most precise formal methods. Even if they are applied by the most experienced examiners, however, these techniques are subject to so many false-positives and false-negatives that we do not use them as substitutes for formal testing.

**FORMAL TESTING.** Two options are available: automated (static) testing or manual (kinetic) testing. Automated perimetry can detect visual field defects with greater sensitivity and reproducibility than even the most skilled manual perimetry.[19,46] It is therefore the preferred modality in patients expected to have minimal defects, and for whom quantitative information is needed for following disease progression. Automated perimetry is, however, much more fatiguing and requires more endurance and cooperation from patients. Thus we prefer manual, kinetic perimetry for patients whose cooperation will be limited. Otherwise, we believe that automated perimetry is the method of choice.

## REFERENCES

1. Rubin ML. Optics for clinicians. Gainesville, FL: Triad, 1971:185.
2. Minkowski JS, Palese M, Guyton DL. Potential acuity meter using a minute aerial pinhole aperture. Ophthalmology 1983;90:1360-8.
3. Spurny RC, Zaldivar R, Belcher CD III, et al. Instruments for predicting visual acuity: a clinical comparison. Arch Ophthalmol 1986;104:196-200.
4. Guyton DL. Misleading predictions of postoperative visual acuity [Editorial]. Arch Ophthalmol 1986;104:189-90.
5. Waring GO III, Rodrigues MM, Laibson PR. Corneal dystrophies. I. Dystrophies of the epithelium, Bowman's layer and stroma. Surv Ophthalmol 1978;23:71-122.
6. Waring GO III, Rodrigues MM, Laibson PR. Corneal dystrophies. II. Endothelial dystrophies. Surv Ophthalmol 1978 1978;23:147-68.
7. Krachmer JH, Feder RS, Belin MW. Keratoconus and related noninflammatory corneal thinning disorders. Surv Ophthalmol 1984;28:293-322.
8. Levatin P. Pupillary escape in disease of the retina or optic nerve. Arch Ophthalmol 1959;62:768-79.
9. Miller NR. Walsh and Hoyt's clinical neuro-ophthalmology, vol 2. 4th ed. Baltimore: Williams & Wilkins, 1985:476-9.

10. Borchert M, Sadun AA. Bright light stimuli as a mask of relative afferent pupillary defects. Am J Ophthalmol 1988;106:98-9.
11. Fineberg E, Thompson HS. Quantitation of the afferent pupillary defect. In: Smith JL, ed. Neuro-ophthalmology focus. New York: Masson, 1979:25-30.
12. Thompson HS, Montague P, Cox TA, et al. The relationship between visual acuity, pupillary defect, and visual field loss. Am J Ophthalmol 1982;93: 681-6.
13. Johnson LN, Hill RA, Bartholomew MJ. Correlation of afferent pupillary defect with visual loss on automated perimetry. Ophthalmology 1988;95: 1649-55.
14. Newsome DA, Milton RC, Gass JDM. Afferent pupillary defect in macular degeneration. Am J Ophthalmol 1981; 92:396-402.
15. Portnoy JZ, Thompson HS, Lennarson L, et al. Pupillary defects in amblyopia. Am J Ophthalmol 1983;96:609-14.
16. Anderson DR, Trobe JD, Hood TW, et al. Optic tract injury after anterior temporal lobectomy. Ophthalmology 1989; 96:1065-70.
17. Lorance RW, Kaufman D, Wray SH, et al. Contrast visual testing in neurovisual diagnosis. Neurology 1987;37:923-9.
18. Rubin GS. Reliability and sensitivity of clinical contrast sensitivity tests. Clin Vis Sci 1988;2:169-77.
19. Acosta PC, Trobe JD, Shuster JJ, et al. Diagnostic strategies in the management of unexplained visual loss: a cost-benefit analysis. Med Decis Making 1981;1:125-44.
20. Savino PJ, Paris M, Schatz NJ, et al. Optic tract syndrome: a review of 21 patients. Arch Ophthalmol 1978;96:656-63.
21. Newman SA, Miller NR. Optic tract syndrome: neuro-ophthalmologic considerations. Arch Ophthalmol 1983;101: 1241-50.
22. Glaser JS, Savino PJ, Sumers KD, et al. The photostress recovery test in the clinical assessment of visual function. Am J Ophthalmol 1977;83:255-60.
23. Jampol LM, Sieving PA, Pugh D, et al. Multiple evanescent white dot syndrome. I. Clinical findings. Arch Ophthalmol 1984;102:671-4.
24. Aaberg TM, Campo RV, Joffe L. Recurrences and bilaterality in the multiple evanescent white-dot syndrome. Am J Ophthalmol 1985;100:29-37.
25. Hamed LM, Glaser JS, Gass JDM, et al. Protracted enlargement of the blind spot in multiple evanescent white dot syndrome. Arch Ophthalmol 1989;107: 194-8.
26. Bos PJM, Deutman AF. Acute macular neuroretinopathy. Am J Ophthalmol 1975;80:573-84.
27. Krill AE, Deutman AF. Acute retinal pigment epitheliitis. Am J Ophthalmol 1972;74:193-205.
28. Gass JDM. Acute posterior multifocal placoid pigment epitheliopathy. Arch Ophthalmol 1968;80:177-85.
29. Wilson CA, Choromokos EA, Sheppard R. Acute posterior multifocal placoid pigment epitheliopathy and cerebral asculitis. Arch Ophthalmol 1988;106: 796-800.
30. Lynn BH. Retrobulbar neuritis: a survey of the present condition of cases occurring over the last fifty-six years. Trans Ophthalmol Soc UK 1959;79:701-16.
31. Burde RM, Gallin PF. Visual parameters associated with recovered retrobulbar optic neuritis. Am J Ophthalmol 1975;79:1034-7.
32. Griffin JF, Wray SH. Acquired color vision defects in retrobulbar neuritis. Am J Ophthalmol 1978;86:193-201.
33. Krill AE, Deutman AF, Fishman G. The cone degenerations. Doc Ophthalmol 1973;35:1-80.
34. Thirkill CE, Roth AM, Keltner JL. Cancer-associated retinopathy. Arch Ophthalmol 1987;105:372-5.
35. Gutman I, Behrens M, Odel J. Bilateral central and centrocaecal scotomata due to mass lesions. Br J Ophthalmol 1984;68:336-42.
36. Cogan DG. Visual disturbances with focal progressive dementing disease. Am J Ophthalmol 1985;100:68-72.
37. Trobe JD. Visual distress in patients with Alzheimer's disease. In: Smith JL, Katz RS, eds. Neuro-ophthalmology

enters the nineties. Miami: Dutton Press, 1989:277-83.

38. Sadun AA, Bassi CJ. Optic nerve damage in Alzheimer's disease. Ophthalmology 1990;97:9-17.

39. Kakisu Y, Adachi-Usami E, Mizota A. Pattern electroretinogram and visual evoked cortical potential in ethambutol optic neuropathy. Doc Ophthalmol 1987;67:327-34.

40. Sanders EACM, Volkers ACW, van der Poel JC, et al. Visual function and pattern visual evoked response in optic neuritis. Br J Ophthalmol 1987;71:602-8.

41. Miller DH, Newton MR, van der Poel JC, et al. Magnetic resonance imaging of the optic nerve in optic neuritis. Neurology 1988;38:175-9.

42. Paty DW, Oger JJF, Kastrukoff LF, et al. MRI in the diagnosis of MS: a prospective study with comparison of clinical evaluation, evoked potentials, oligoclonal banding and CT. Neurology 1988;38:180-5.

43. Miller DH, Ormerod IEC, McDonald WI, et al. The early risk of multiple sclerosis after optic neuritis. J Neurol Neurosurg Psychiatry 1988;51:1569-71.

44. Howard JE, Dorfman LJ. Evoked potentials in hysteria and malingering. J Clin Neurophysiol 1986;3:39-49.

45. Kupersmith MJ. Visual evoked potential: enhancing its utility. Semin Neurol 1986;6:2117-230.

46. Keltner JL, Johnson CA. Current status of automated perimetry: is the ideal automated perimeter available? [Editorial]. Arch Ophthalmol 1986;104:347-9.

# CHAPTER 2

# *Prechiasmal Visual Loss*

• • • • • • • • • • • • • • • • • •

Diseases that cause prechiasmal visual loss include those that damage the retina and optic nerve. Chapter 1 reviews the diagnosis of conditions that *do not* cause readily observable ocular abnormalities. This chapter presents more detailed management considerations of those entities and of entities that *do* cause observable changes in the globe.

A convenient way to approach prechiasmal visual loss is to consider it an extension of the evaluation of optic neuritis.

## A Decision Tree Approach to the Management of Optic Neuritis (Chart 2-1)

Optic neuritis is best defined as visual loss caused by *primary* demyelination of the optic nerve. In primary demyelination the myelin sheath appears to be the direct target of attack, with the axon relatively spared. Many diseases produce *secondary* demyelination, in which the loss of myelin is believed to be a casualty of compression, ischemia, or metabolic dysfunction.

Using this definition, we encounter two forms of optic neuritis: *typical* and *atypical*. Management is based on this distinction.

### ▧ Typical clinical features of optic neuritis

The typical form of optic neuritis[1] consists of acute monocular visual loss in a patient between 20 and 50 years of age. Pain is felt about the involved eye and is exacerbated by eye movement. The patient may have a past history or present evidence of multiple sclerosis (MS).

Examination reveals subnormal visual function in the affected eye (and sometimes in the other eye as well), measurable by a depression in visual acuity, color vision, contrast sensitivity, or visual fields. One or more of these tests may be normal, but not all of them. Unless the patient has equivalent neural visual loss in both eyes, a relative afferent pupillary defect (RAPD) must be present to make the diagnosis. Ophthalmoscopy is often normal but may show a swollen

**41**

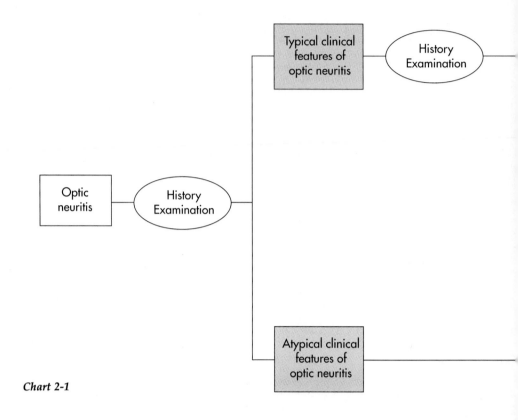

*Chart 2-1*

nerve head (see Plate 8), rarely with papillary hemorrhages. The presence of retinal exudates centered around the macula (Plate 2, *D*) ("macular star figure") *is incompatible with the diagnosis of typical optic neuritis.*[2] The presence of optic disc pallor does not invalidate the diagnosis, but it does indicate that optic neuropathy of some type antedated the present complaint.

To establish the diagnosis of typical optic neuritis, two more elements are necessary: (1) the systemic history and examination must not reveal anything that could cause optic neuropathy other than MS, and (2) the visual dysfunction must stabilize within about 14 days of onset. If the patient's illness conforms to these criteria, the diagnosis of typical optic neuritis is likely.

☐ Symptoms or signs of multiple sclerosis present

The next question that confronts the physician is whether the optic neuritis is part of MS. We believe that a reasonable *clinical* effort should be made to diagnose MS, but that *paraclinical* testing (magnetic resonance imaging [MRI], lumbar puncture, evoked potentials) is an option best exercised through consultation with a neurologist.

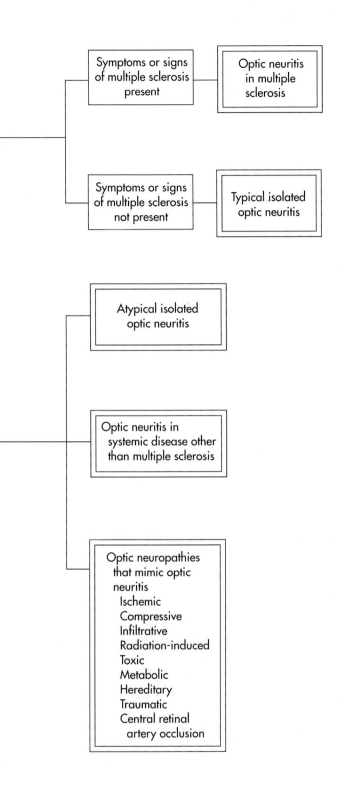

☐ Optic neuritis in multiple sclerosis

**DIAGNOSING MS WITH PARACLINICAL TESTS IN PATIENTS WITH OPTIC NEURITIS.** In the past, the visual evoked potential (VEP) was the test most often used to search for evidence of disseminated white matter involvement, as in MS. In a recent study of 30 patients presenting with clinically isolated optic neuritis,[3] all had prolonged signal latency in the symptomatic eye, as expected, and 8 (27%) had prolonged latency in the asymptomatic eye. However, in another study of 38 patients with isolated optic neuritis,[4] MRI was "strongly suggestive of MS" in 25 (66%). Although VEP is currently a less expensive test, its sensitivity *to disseminated disease* appears to be much lower than that of MRI, and we do not advocate its use. The other evoked potential studies (auditory, somatosensory) have also been found to be abnormal in about one third of patients with isolated optic neuritis.[5]

We again emphasize that prolonged latency in the VEP *is not specific for primary demyelinating disease.* Prolonged latency may be seen in any type of optic neuropathy, including that caused by compression.[6]

Spinal fluid examination enhances the diagnosis of MS by showing elevated immunoglobulins and oligoclonal bands, both of which may also be seen in such mimickers as central nervous system (CNS) infections (including neurosyphilis), systemic lupus erythematosus, progressive multifocal leukoencephalopathy, subacute sclerosing panencephalitis, and Guillain-Barré syndrome.[7] Such spinal fluid abnormalities may be expected in 30% to 60% of patients with isolated optic neuritis.[4,8,9] Evidence indicates that the presence of oligoclonal bands (at least two in the cerebrospinal fluid [CSF] and none in the serum) increases the likelihood of developing clinically definite MS.[10]

MRI scanning has emerged as the most supportive test in the diagnosis of MS in patients with optic neuritis, with 50% to 70% showing the characteristic signal aberrations[11-13] (Fig. 2-1). Like oligoclonal bands in the CSF, the MRI abnormalities appear to enhance the risk of future clinical MS.[14] However, periventricular signal aberrations resembling those seen in MS have also been identified among neurologically normal patients over 50 years of age. Thus one must be cautious about leaning too heavily on MRI in diagnosing MS in older patients.

**ASSOCIATION BETWEEN OPTIC NEURITIS AND MS.** Recent data show a consistently high association between optic neuritis and MS, provided follow-up is long enough. After 15 years 73% to 78% of patients with isolated optic neuritis will develop clinically definite MS.[15-17] This information does not controvert the old impression that most MS appears within a few years of optic neuritis. About one half of those who are to develop the disease show it within 3 years. From then on, a steady 2% to 5% per year continue to develop MS.

Do any factors help to refine this aggregate prognosis for the individual patient? Rizzo and Lessell[17] showed that men had less than half as much chance (34%) as women (74%) of developing MS. This differential gender susceptibility has been found in most series.[18] Certain HLA antigens (Dw2, B7) appear to confer greater susceptibility to MS,[19,20] but such typing is not in routine clinical use.

The MRI scan is of great value not only in assisting in the diagnosis of MS,

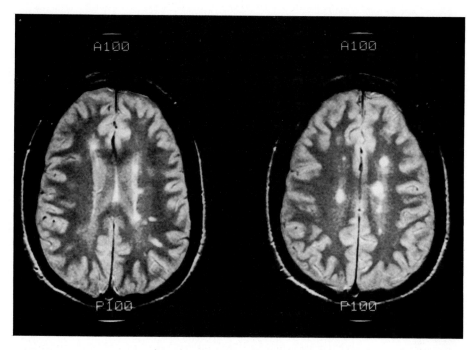

***Fig. 2-1.*** Magnetic resonance imaging (MRI) of patient with optic neuritis shows paraventricular *(left)* and supraventricular *(right)* white matter signal aberrations typical of MS.

but also in predicting further clinical events. Miller et al.[14] have reported that among 34 patients with clinically isolated typical optic neuritis and MRI brain "lesions," 12 (33%) developed definite (9) or probable (3) MS within 6 to 23 months (mean 12.3 months). In contrast, among 19 patients with similar presentation but *without* MRI brain signal abnormalities, none had clinical dissemination in the same time period.

Attacks of *recurrent* optic neuritis (same eye) or *consecutive* optic neuritis (opposite eye) separated by 2 weeks or more have been found in some[18,19] but not all[15,20] studies to constitute an increased risk of developing MS. Because of the conflicting data, we are not prepared to regard either recurrent or consecutive optic neuritis as sufficient evidence to make the diagnosis of MS without other clinical findings. Bilateral *simultaneous* optic neuritis, or involvement of both eyes *within 2 weeks,* may have a different pathogenesis and outcome and is therefore not considered part of typical optic neuritis (see Atypical Clinical Features of Optic Neuritis).

The effect of age at onset of optic neuritis on the prognosis for developing MS remains controversial. Several series have found that optic neuritis acquired between ages 20 and 40 confers a modestly worse prognosis for MS than does optic neuritis acquired later, but it is possible that "optic neuritis" with onset beyond age 40 is being overdiagnosed. When *unilateral* optic neuritis is diagnosed at or before the age of 15 years, the chance of developing MS appears to be nearly comparable to that in adults. Kennedy and Carroll[21] found MS in 5 (42%) of 12 children without specifying the length of follow-up. Kriss et al.[22] described

MS in 3 (20%) of 14 children followed for a mean of 8 years. In spite of this information, the impression that MS is a much less common aftermath of optic neuritis in children still holds *because most optic neuritis in youth is bilateral and simultaneous*, a pattern that has a much better prognosis (at least in children) than does unilateral optic neuritis.

The wide variation in the incidence of MS after optic neuritis in past reports has been partly ascribed to geographic locale, with northern latitudes reporting the highest associations. That explanation is no longer tenable, as two reports from Australia[20,23] show results comparable to those of the United Kingdom and the United States.

Spinal fluid immunoglobulin elevation and oligoclonal bands in isolated optic neuritis are significantly related to future development of clinical MS, but over 50% of patients with normal CSF studies in one report were later diagnosed as having MS.[8] Thus the absence of spinal fluid abnormalities affords little prognostic information.

**CLINICAL OUTCOME AFTER OPTIC NEURITIS AND MS.** What may the patient be told about the chances of being seriously disabled by MS? In the aggregate, the prognosis for maintaining "unrestricted activity" (ability to walk without assistance) is about 50% after 10 years of illness.[24] But if optic neuritis ushers in MS, the long-term prognosis for unrestricted activity is substantially better, measured variously at 74% after 11 to 20 years,[25] 73% after 8 years,[15] 72% after 10 years,[26] and 81% after 10 years.[27]

☐ Symptoms or signs of multiple sclerosis not present

▣ Typical isolated optic neuritis

If clinical and paraclinical tests for MS are negative, the patient has isolated optic neuritis.

The long-term visual disability after optic neuritis is not clearly documented. However, Nikoskelainen[28] found that with follow-up ranging from 6 months to 24 years (average about 6 years), the initially affected eye had an acuity of 20/30 or better in 66% of cases. Recurrences in the initially affected eye occurred in 25% of cases, and in 17% of cases the unaffected eye eventually suffered at least one attack of optic neuritis. Assuming that the visual outcome is similar in the secondarily involved eye, the patient's chances of ultimately having a visual acuity below 20/30 in both eyes are about 7%. The visual acuity may not, however, accurately reflect the patient's visual disability. In one report, 85% of patients who had recovered at least 20/30 acuity after optic neuritis complained of imperfect sight.[29] These complaints correlated with deficits in contrast sensitivity.

Although no evidence yet indicates that any form of treatment alters the ultimate course of optic neuritis, small controlled trials of adrenocorticotrophic hormone (ACTH)[30,31] and retrobulbar corticosteroids[32] accelerated recovery from a single bout. To date, no controlled trials with oral or intravenous corticosteroids have been undertaken, although at least one uncontrolled study found

*Management of Optic Neuritis*

1. Defer laboratory or imaging studies at the outset if clinical features are typical and you are not planning to treat.
2. If the patient is visually disabled, treat with prednisone, 1 mg/kg for 14 days, or intravenous methylprednisolone, 1 g/day for 3 days, followed by prednisone, 1 mg/kg for 11 days.[33,35] Before starting treatment, order a baseline complete blood count, routine chemistries, chest x-ray study, connective tissue screen, urinalysis, coagulation profile, FTA-Abs, and brain MRI.
3. Inform mentally competent adults of the association between optic neuritis and multiple sclerosis. A neurologist may be consulted to provide more information.

dramatic improvement with intravenous treatment.[33] A National Eye Institute–sponsored collaborative study began in 1988 to randomize optic neuritis patients for therapy with either intravenous methylprednisolone, oral prednisone, or oral placebo (Optic Neuritis Treatment Trial, or ONTT).[34]

## Atypical clinical features of optic neuritis

Optic neuritis qualifies as atypical if it occurs in a patient outside the 20- to 50-year age span, occurs in both eyes simultaneously, continues to show worsening beyond 14 days after onset, or is accompanied by contributory abnormalities in the patient's history or examination that cannot be attributed to MS. Three explanations are possible; the patient may have (1) isolated (demyelinating) optic neuritis with atypical features, (2) optic neuritis in the context of a systemic disease other than MS, or (3) an optic neuropathy that mimics optic neuritis but is caused by another mechanism (ischemia, compression, metabolic failure).

## Atypical isolated optic neuritis

Although optic neuritis does rarely occur in patients over 50 years of age, its development in such cases should raise serious questions about the diagnosis. Optic neuritis occurs more frequently in those under age 15, but caution is advised here as well. A reliable history or documentation of visual decline extending beyond 14 days is odd enough to warrant a full workup. We acknowledge that a slowly progressive optic neuritis (usually bilateral) exists in later stages of MS, mirroring the unremitting decline seen in that phase of the illness.

**Bilateral simultaneous optic neuritis** deserves to be singled out as atypical. Long-term outcome studies of bilateral optic neuritis in children (aged 15 or younger) show a 6% to 12% incidence of MS,[21,22,36] somewhat lower than the 20% to 48% incidence of MS after unilateral optic neuritis in the same age group. The consensus is that many children suffering bilateral optic neuritis eventually recover nearly normal visual acuity despite persistently atrophic optic discs.

Whether the reduced likelihood of developing MS after bilateral simultaneous optic neuritis also applies to adults is in dispute. Hutchinson[15] found no differences in comparison with unilateral optic neuritis, but Parkin et al.[36] found the incidence of later MS to be half that of unilateral optic neuritis. We interpret these data as follows: bilateral optic neuritis in children may often represent a postinfectious autoimmune reaction limited clinically to the optic nerves. In such cases it is a monophasic illness that does not lead to MS. Bilateral simultaneous optic neuritis in adults must still be regarded as having a risk of developing MS comparable to that of unilateral optic neuritis.

We also classify optic neuritis with **macular star figure** (Leber's stellate neuroretinopathy) (Plate 2, *D*) as atypical because, as far as we are aware, no patient with these findings has yet been reported to have or develop clinically definite MS.[2]

### ▣ Optic neuritis in systemic disease other than multiple sclerosis

Optic neuritis may be a manifestation of a **connective tissue disease; sarcoidosis; viral, bacterial,** or **fungal disease;** or, rarely, a remote **neoplasm.** Not only must the underlying disease be managed, but the optic neuritis may itself respond to treatment.

**Lupus erythematosus** may rarely cause an optic neuropathy that conforms to the clinical pattern of optic neuritis.[37] The pathology tends to be that of infarct, but some cases show pure demyelination. In some patients vision improves following intensive corticosteroid treatment,[37] a result not expected in optic nerve infarct. Three cases of optic neuropathy have also been documented in **Sjögren's syndrome.**[38] Although two cases had the features of ischemic optic neuropathy, one case appeared to be steroid responsive. Optic neuropathy is described in **Behçet's disease** but appears to be much rarer than uveitis and retinal vasculopathy.[39]

An optic neuritis–like condition has also been reported in patients with some clinical and serologic features of connective tissue diseases, but who do not fulfill the criteria for a named condition. Dubbed **autoimmune optic neuritis,** this condition evidently responds poorly to conventional oral corticosteroid regimens but may improve with intravenous ("megadose") corticosteroid treatment and cytotoxic agents.[40,41] The clinical features in these cases resemble an amalgam of MS and a connective tissue disease, including migratory CNS deficits and rheumatologic symptoms, and moderate titer autoantigens. Because patients with MS often have such modest elevations in autoantigens,[42] whether these cases are a steroid-responsive variant of MS or another hyperergic illness is not clear.

**Sarcoidosis** involves the central nervous system in about 5% of cases.[43,44] When this happens, the most common ocular manifestation is a retinal venulitis, but the optic nerve may become inflamed without other signs. Visual loss may be acute or subacute and is often very sensitive to corticosteroid treatment.[45,46] Swelling of the optic nerve head may or may not be present. Corticosteroids may be required for extended periods. Tapering should be very gradual, and cytotoxic agents may be adjunctive in cases that do not recover with corticosteroid therapy.[46]

Optic neuritis has also been reported in **syphilis,**[47] **cytomegalovirus infection** in immunocompromised patients (including AIDS),[48] **toxoplasmosis,**[49] **herpes zoster infection,**[48] and **cryptococcal**[50] and **bacterial**[51] **meningitis.** It is also seen after vaccination, flulike illnesses, as part of **acute multifocal placoid pigment epitheliopathy** (AMPPE), acute disseminated encephalomyelitis (ADEM), and **Guillain-Barré syndrome,**[52,53] in which cases it probably represents an autoimmune reaction, perhaps the clinical version of experimental allergic encephalomyelitis. A similar process may rarely occur as a paraneoplastic effect.[54,55]

In many of these conditions, optic neuritis may be accompanied by other ocular manifestations, particularly retinal vascular cuffing or occlusion and uveitis. Even though some of these features are reported in MS,[56] we view them, at least initially, as indicators of other systemic diseases.

The relationship between optic neuritis and **sinusitis** is unsettled.[57] Given that many patients with optic neuritis have imaging (and sometimes clinical) evidence of bacterial sinus infection, whether the sinusitis causes the neuritis is not clear. On the other hand, a cause-and-effect relationship is unquestioned in cases of **sinus mucocoele, Wegener's granulomatosis, aspergillosis** and **mucormycosis.** Thus we advocate vigorous evaluation and treatment of sinus disease in compromised hosts or when the optic neuritis is atypical.

Two patients have been reported to develop optic neuropathy in the setting of **Lyme neuroborreliosis,**[58,59] a disease whose prevalence has risen dramatically in recent years. The proliferation of reports on the neurologic manifestations of Lyme disease[60,61] makes it evident that optic neuropathy is exceedingly rare and may be either ischemic or inflammatory. Furthermore, the clinical and serologic diagnosis of Lyme disease is complicated because manifestations resemble those of many other diseases, including MS, and standardization and quality control of serologic testing are still poor, leading to false-negatives and false-positives. We do recommend serologic testing and neurologic evaluation of any patient with an atypical optic neuritis in an area endemic for Lyme disease. In seropositive cases a serum sample should be sent to a second laboratory for confirmation. To make the diagnosis, a lumbar puncture should show a pleiocytosis and *Borrelia burgdorferi* antibody in higher titer than in serum. Treatment with ceftriaxone, penicillin, tetracyclines, or erythromycin may reverse the symptoms and signs.

### ☐ Optic neuropathies that mimic optic neuritis

Several other conditions may clinically resemble optic neuritis but prove to have another pathogenetic mechanism. Although separating them from typical optic neuritis in the initial stages of the illness may be difficult, careful monitoring of their evolution will usually bring out their distinguishing features.

### ☐ Ischemic optic neuropathy

Ischemic optic neuropathy (ION) represents infarction of the optic nerve head. It comes in two clinical forms: **arteritic** (part of giant cell arteritis) and **nonarteritic.** The nonarteritic form is much more common, but the arteritic form is more important because it may strike both eyes within a short interval, and its progression to involve the second eye may often be prevented by prompt and intensive corticosteroid treatment.

Optic disc edema is often diffuse, but it may be segmental and accompanied by juxtapapillary nerve fiber layer hemorrhages and cotton-wool spots (Plate 2, *E*). Sometimes the edema is difficult to detect ophthalmoscopically. When optic disc edema is present, the condition is called anterior ischemic optic neuropathy (AION). When no optic disc edema has been observed in the acute phase of the illness, the condition is called posterior ischemic optic neuropathy (PION). PION may very rarely occur in patients who have arteriosclerotic vasculopathy,[62] but documentation is so sparse that we consider it a diagnosis of exclusion. On the other hand, this entity is well recognized after severe blood loss and anemia[63] or radiation therapy to the region of the optic nerve.[64]

**NONARTERITIC ISCHEMIC OPTIC NEUROPATHY.** Nonarteritic ischemic optic neuropathy is an affliction of patients aged between 45 and 80 years that is characterized by sudden, painless, mostly irreversible, and generally nonprogressive visual loss, accompanied by nerve fiber bundle field defects, an afferent pupillary defect, and, in nearly all cases, optic disc edema.[65] As such, ION shares some features of optic neuritis, and indeed this entity was formerly called "ischemic optic neuritis." That appellation has been dropped because the pathogenesis is believed to be infarction, not inflammation, although definitive pathology is not yet available. The clinical findings are explained as a manifestation of impaired axoplasmic flow at the level of the lamina cribrosa. Two risk factors have been identified: chronic (even well-regulated) hypertension[66] and a crowded optic nerve head that lacks a normal physiologic cup[67] (Plate 2, *F*).

Although abrupt and nonprogressive visual loss is the rule, a small proportion of cases of nonarteritic AION continue to worsen for as long as 6 weeks.[68] Although progression over 48 hours is common, no report has yet clearly defined how many cases worsen over a longer period. Optic nerve sheath fenestration produced substantial restoration of vision in 12 of 14 patients with this "progressive" variant of nonarteritic AION in a nonmasked, nonrandomized study.[69]

Recurrence of nonarteritic AION in the same eye has also been described,[70] but this probably occurs in 5% or fewer cases.[63] On the other hand, a 25% to 50% incidence of AION striking the *fellow* eye within 5 years has been reported.[71]

Treatment of nonprogressive nonarteritic AION has been fruitless. Because of the lack of convincing evidence of embolism, we do not advocate investigating the heart or cervical carotid artery as possible sources. Instead, we concentrate on excluding giant cell arteritis (Chart 2-2; see pp. 52-53) and on eliminating arteriosclerotic risk factors, especially hypertension, in view of one report suggesting an increased risk of stroke and myocardial infarction.[72] Yet the known association of acute hypotension and AION tempers any vigorous lowering of blood pressure in long-standing hypertension. Although no evidence supports antiplatelet aggregants to prevent AION from affecting the fellow eye, we recommend one adult aspirin tablet per day.

In those patients who demonstrate progressive visual loss over more than a few days, we recommend full evaluation for other causes. If no underlying cause is determined, we suggest they be offered the choice of optic nerve sheath fenestration. We cannot, however, support this procedure with vigor until its efficacy has been demonstrated in a large, controlled study.

**ARTERITIC ISCHEMIC OPTIC NEUROPATHY.** Infarction of the laminar disc also occurs in giant cell (cranial, temporal) arteritis (GCA),[73] as well as rarely in lupus and periarteritis nodosa.[74] Connective tissue diseases should always be excluded, but GCA so rapidly threatens both optic nerves that it rises to the top of the list of considerations.

GCA must be suspected as the cause of AION in any patient over age 50 in whom arteriosclerotic risk factors are not evident.[75,76] The index of suspicion mounts when headache, jaw claudication, scalp tenderness, proximal muscle ache or stiffness, anorexia, fever, and/or fatigue are present. Features of AION that suggest GCA are severe depression of acuity or involvement of both eyes within days or weeks. The erythrocyte sedimentation rate (ESR) is substantially above age-corrected normal in most (but not all) cases, and proper biopsy technique should provide above 90% sensitivity (see Histopathology).[77]

The incidence of GCA appears to be greatest in Caucasians in northern latitudes and has averaged 2.4/100,000 in Olmstead County, Minn.[77] In those aged 50 or older, however, it was 11.4/100,000, and in those aged 70 or older, 27/100,000.[77] Below age 50, few cases are documented. The mortality of patients with treated cranial arteritis is not greater than that of age-matched controls. No definite familial association or link to other systemic illnesses has been identified with the exception of polymyalgia rheumatica (PMR), a syndrome of uncertain cause characterized by aching and stiffness of the proximal muscles and joints of the arms and legs. Approximately half of all patients with GCA have symptoms of PMR; about 20% of patients with PMR have temporal artery biopsy results that are positive for GCA. Without a biopsy, one cannot exclude the possibility that patients with PMR symptoms, but who lack cranial symptoms, also have GCA. Although they are at risk of AION,[78] we know of no data that quantitate that risk.

The presence of headache, jaw claudication, anemia, and white race have been significantly correlated with biopsy results that are positive for GCA.[79,80] Headache, which is such a common symptom, need not be severe or localized but should be of definably recent onset and distinguishable from past headaches ("new headache"). Jaw claudication is a deep, boring pain precipitated by chewing and is not related to opening and closing the jaw or localizable to the temporomandibular joint. Scalp tenderness, while not common, is as specific for GCA as jaw claudication and is therefore important to elicit. Morning stiffness and pain in the proximal extremities, the hallmark of PMR, is also a common complaint in the elderly and should therefore be a prominent point in the history.

GCA may rarely cause AION without constitutional symptoms, a variant known as "occult GCA."[81] Although uncommon, 24% of GCA patients in one series did manifest this version.[82]

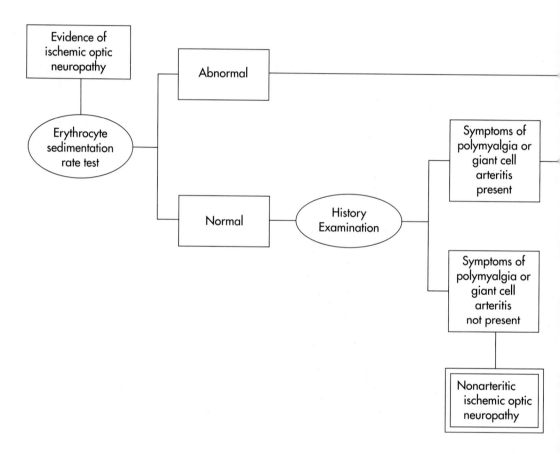

*Chart 2-2*

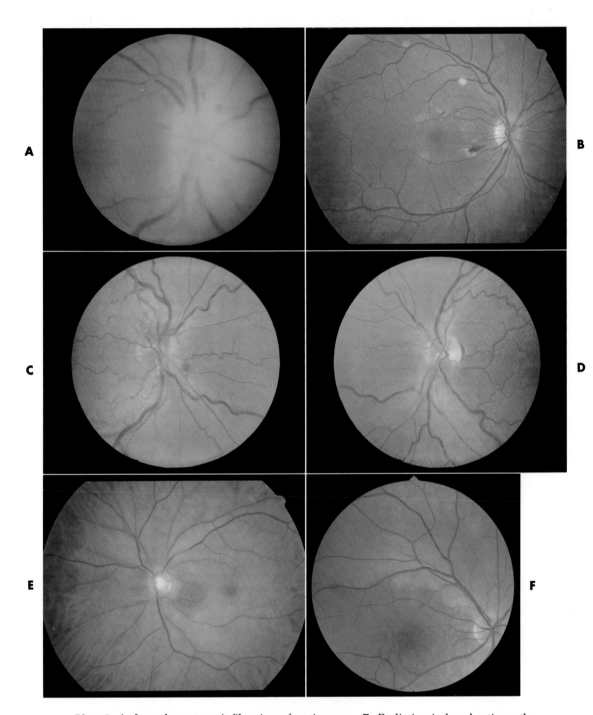

*Plate 3.* **A,** Lymphomatous infiltration of optic nerve. **B,** Radiation-induced retinopathy and optic neuropathy. Note cotton-wool spots and temporal disc pallor. **C,** Leber's optic neuropathy, acute. Note hyperemic appearance of disc and opacification of peripapillary nerve fiber layer. **D,** Leber's optic neuropathy, unaffected fellow eye of patient shown in **C.** Note mild thickening of peripapillary nerve fiber layer. **E,** Central retinal artery occlusion, acute. Note retinal turbidity, macular "cherry red spot," and sparing of small area subserved by cilioretinal artery. **F,** Branch retinal artery occlusion, acute.

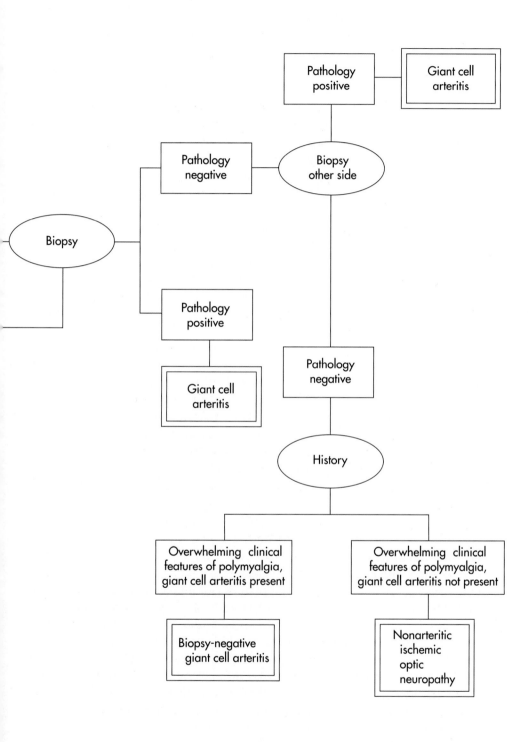

Visual loss is reported in 12% to 50% of biopsy-proven cases, depending on the source of the patient group.[83,84] A short prodrome of transient monocular visual loss is found in some 10% of cases.[85] Fixed visual loss is caused chiefly by infarct of the prelaminar optic nerve (90%) but may also be caused by central retinal artery occlusion (3%) or ischemic retinopathy (7%).[85] Although retrolaminar optic nerve infarction (PION) has been mentioned,[86] we consider it exceedingly rare. Occipital blindness is also unusual, probably because GCA tends to affect only arteries with an internal elastic lamina, a structure not present in the intradural portion of cerebral vessels.[87] Yet hemispheric and brainstem strokes are occasionally found, perhaps secondary to embolism from extradural portions of carotid and vertebral vessels involved with arteritis.[88]

Untreated GCA causes binocular visual loss in about one third of cases.[82,83] If fellow eyes are to be affected, one third will do so within 24 hours, another third within 1 week, and most of the remainder within 4 weeks.[55,82,85,89] Although visual loss has been informally reported in a single case 22 years after diagnosis of GCA,[75] we believe that the risk after 6 months is exceedingly low, whether or not the patient has been treated.

While no reports have compared untreated and treated patients with GCA and AION, anecdotal information is sufficient to state unequivocally that prompt and intensive steroid treatment reduces (but does not eliminate) involvement of the fellow eye.[88]

**Laboratory tests.** The ESR remains the single most useful laboratory test, but it is nonspecific, it is not always sensitive to the presence of GCA, and the degree of elevation is not correlated with clinical features. How often normal ESRs occur in patients with biopsy-proven GCA ("false-negatives") is not known, but enough reports exist to conclude that they certainly do occur. Using a Westergren ESR of 40 mm/hr as a cutoff for normal, Jacobson and Slamovits[90] found that 17% of biopsy-proven GCA cases had normal ESRs. The elevated ESRs appeared to occur primarily in those GCA patients who were also anemic (hematocrit <35%). They pointed out that the Westergren system contains no method to adjust for hematocrit. By comparison, the zeta method does correct for hematocrit. The Wintrobe method is now considered inaccurate.[91]

False-positive elevation of the ESR in biopsy-negative patients with AION or complaints suggestive of PMR or GCA is common. A false-negative elevation is associated with arthritis, neoplasm, connective tissue disease, and occult infections. Often, however, the only abnormality is arteriosclerosis or diabetes.[80] Because the Westergren ESR rises normally with age, a formula has been devised to optimally separate normal from abnormal scores: for men—divide the age in years by 2; for women—divide the age in years plus 10 by 2.[92] We subscribe to this rule but continue to note unexplained elevations of ESR. Since laboratory error is not infrequent in this delicate test, repeating the ESR if it is not consonant with the clinical impression is worthwhile. Other markers of vascular damage, such as C-reactive protein and von Willebrand factor, may offer advantages over the ESR but have not been sufficiently tested.

**Histopathology.** The temporal artery is the most accessible vessel with a high chance of pathologic involvement in GCA. Other branches of the external carotid would be the next choice. The selection of biopsy site should not be overly influenced by whether the vessel is tender, nodular, or on the side of visual involvement. After some controversy, the issue of whether affected vessels may show intervals of normal histology ("skip areas") is settled: they do occur in as many as 28% of biopsies,[93] and false-negatives can be minimized by removing at least a 2 cm length of artery and performing multiple-step cross sections at 0.25 to 0.5 mm intervals.[79] Since at least 5% of GCA cases involve only one temporal artery,[93] negative biopsy results and high clinical suspicion warrant a biopsy on the other side. Some centers perform frozen sections on the specimen and, if it is negative, perform a biopsy on the other side at the same sitting if clinical suspicion is high. We prefer to await the formal interpretation before performing a biopsy on the other side.

The histopathology of GCA need not include giant cells. McDonnell et al.[79] suggest that two forms be distinguished: active and healed. Active disease consists of thickening of the intima (and perhaps media and adventitia), disruption of the internal elastic lamina, and infiltration by lymphocytes, macrophages, or giant cells. Healed disease has the same features, except that fibrosis replaces cellular inflammation. In their series of 42 patients with biopsy results positive for GCA, 10 (24%) were "healed." The healed arteritis occurred in patients whose biopsies were done after a mean of 7 weeks of steroid treatment. Thus steroid treatment may not eliminate the traces of GCA but may make pathologic diagnosis more difficult. Hence, we advocate biopsy within 1 week of starting steroids. If these guidelines are followed, a normal temporal artery biopsy has a 90% to 95% chance of excluding GCA.[94,95]

---

### Management of Ischemic Optic Neuropathy

1. Draw a Westergren ESR on all patients with AION, regardless of age or symptomatology.
2. If the ESR is elevated or if symptoms or signs of PMR or GCA are present, make a presumptive diagnosis of GCA, begin treating the patient promptly with intravenous methylprednisolone, 1 to 2 g/day in divided doses, and schedule a temporal artery biopsy.
3. If the results of the biopsy are negative and the clinical history is strong for GCA or the ESR is markedly elevated (or both), perform a biopsy on the other temporal artery. If the results of that biopsy are also negative, abandon the diagnosis of GCA *unless the clinical features are persuasive.* The patient should be fully evaluated for other causes of an elevated ESR.
4. If the ESR is normal but symptoms or signs of PMR or GCA are persuasive, treat with steroids and perform a biopsy. If the results of one biopsy are negative, perform a biopsy on the other side. If the results of both biopsies are negative, maintain the diagnosis of GCA only if the clinical syndrome is convincing.
5. If the diagnosis of GCA-AION is established, maintain treatment with prednisone, 1.5 mg/kg for 2 weeks. Taper the dose at 10% per week if the ESR and symptoms normalize. Continue treatment to maintain a normal ESR and absence of symptoms for 6 months.

**Treatment.** Most patients who have GCA will note amelioration of constitutional symptoms within 48 hours of starting steroid treatment. After 2 weeks, the ESR should have normalized,[96] and gradual tapering of the steroid dose may begin at 10% of the total daily dose per week. If symptoms and ESR recrudesce, the daily steroid dose should be raised. Although alternate-day steroid regimens produce fewer side effects, they do not control disease activity sufficiently within the first few months.[97] In our experience, a substantial number of GCA patients maintain elevated ESRs despite clinical remission. Therefore we favor continued tapering of the steroid dose in the face of an elevated ESR, provided that no constitutional or visual symptoms are present and at least 6 months have elapsed since diagnosis.

Notwithstanding the dangers of GCA, we believe it is a mistake to commit patients to steroid treatment without pathologic proof of the diagnosis, and to carry on treatment beyond the period of vulnerability. GCA appears to be a self-limited disease with a risk of infarct dissipating rapidly within months of initial symptoms—even in untreated patients. Approximately 40% of patients treated for more than a few months with moderate doses of prednisone (20 to 60 mg/day) develop complications, including cushingoid features, fluid retention, vertebral collapse, hypertension, peptic ulcer disease, myopathy, cataract, osteoporosis, and psychosis.[98]

### Compressive optic neuropathy*

Compressive optic neuropathy, as with cyst, tumor (Fig. 2-2), sinus mucocoele, or aneurysm, usually progresses slowly but may have an explosive onset. Vision generally continues to worsen beyond the 14-day limit we have set for typical optic neuritis. Pain is a variable accompaniment. High-resolution imaging is essential in diagnosis. Corticosteroid treatment often results in rapid improvement in visual function, leading to a misimpression of optic neuritis.

**Graves' disease** may cause a compressive optic neuropathy if the extraocular muscles become large enough to impede axoplasmic flow at the orbital apex.[99,100] The optic nerve head may appear entirely normal. Patients usually manifest congestive adnexal features, including chemosis, conjunctival injection, lid retraction and lag, and ocular ductional deficits, but proptosis need not be marked (see Chapter 15).

### Infiltrative optic neuropathy

Infiltration of the optic nerve, at or behind its junction with the globe, may occur in **sarcoidosis,**[101] **lymphoma,**[102] (Plate 3, *A*), **leukemia,**[103] **plasmacytoma,**[104] or **carcinoma.**[105]

Retrobulbar infiltrative optic neuropathy is an excellent imitator of optic neuritis, except that visual loss is *painless.* Sudden loss of vision (usually monocular) occurs with a normal or swollen nerve head. Some evidence of a primary malignancy usually turns up, but it may be remote in time and unappreciated. Parenchymal CNS metastases need not be present, so that brain imaging is often negative (although enhanced computed tomography [CT] and MRI scans may "light up" the meninges; Fig. 2-3). Cancer cells may be difficult to harvest even

*For remaining diagnoses refer to Chart 2-1.

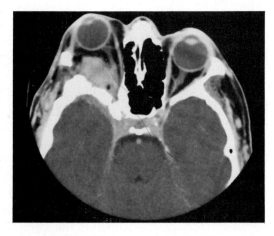

*Fig.* 2-2. Computed tomography (CT) shows sphenoid ridge meningioma invading right orbit and compressing optic nerve.

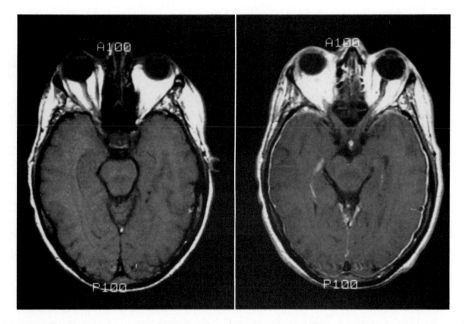

*Fig.* 2-3. Carcinomatous optic neuropathy and meningitis. Pre–gadolinium contrast axial MRI *(left)* is normal. Post–gadolinium contrast MRI *(right)* shows abnormally increased signal intensity ("brightening") of meninges around cerebral hemispheres and optic nerves, reflecting breakdown of blood-brain barrier.

after several lumbar punctures. The mechanism of visual loss is unclear, especially when cancer cells are limited on pathologic examination to the perioptic meninges or pial septae.

Vision often improves dramatically in response to systemic steroid therapy and local irradiation. In fact, our experience has been that infiltrative optic neuropathy is always more steroid responsive than is typical (demyelinating) optic neuritis. Thus a rapid improvement (within 48 hours) in vision following treatment onset is, by itself, considered evidence *against* typical optic neuritis and demands an appropriate workup.

### ☐ Radiation-induced optic neuropathy

Optic nerve toxicity from megavoltage irradiation is well documented.[106-110] In patients with malignancies of the ethmoid and sphenoid sinuses, especially when the orbit has been invaded, neither the eyes nor the optic nerves can be shielded if the proper therapeutic radiation levels are to reach the tumor. In nasopharyngeal tumors that have extended to the cranial base, the eyes are not included in the treatment field, but the optic nerves are. At standard total dosage schedules of 5500 to 6000 cGy, a majority of patients whose eyes are not shielded develop ischemic retinopathy (Plate 3, *B*). Those whose eyes are shielded but whose intracranial optic nerves are exposed develop ischemic retrobulbar optic neuropathy. After a latency period of 1 to 5 years (peak 18 months), vision may be lost abruptly or in a gradual stepwise progression. Final visual outcome is frequently blindness in both eyes, because lateral fields include both optic nerves. Two distinct manifestations appear, depending on whether the optic disc and retina or the retrobulbar optic nerve and chiasm are the principal sites of damage.

If radiation doses of more than 4000 cGy reach the retina and optic nerve, the fundus may show microaneurysms, hemorrhages, exudates, and neovascularization, a picture similar to that seen in diabetes. However, one may also see telangiectatic vessels, venous stasis, cotton-wool spots, pallid disc swelling, arteriolar narrowing, and focal retinal pigment epithelial loss, indicating compromise of retinal, ciliary, and choroidal vessels (Plate 3, *B*). The clinical course may be static but tends to be slowly progressive, leading to severe, if not total, visual loss and to intractable neovascular glaucoma (see Chapter 5).

If the optic nerves, rather than the eyes, lie within the radiated field, then optic neuropathy without retinopathy typically occurs at total tumor doses above 6000 cGy and daily dose fractions above 180 cGy. The patient has acute loss of sight, and the only abnormal findings are a relative afferent pupillary defect and visual fields that show either a prechiasmal (nerve fiber bundle) defect limited to the symptomatic eye or a junctional or bitemporal pattern indicating a lesion at the chiasm. The patient is usually misdiagnosed as having optic neuritis, ischemic or carcinomatous (meningeal) optic neuropathy, or a recurrence of tumor. Imaging shows no new masses but may be difficult to interpret because of postoperative changes. Contrast MRI will sometimes "light up" the damaged anterior visual pathway (Fig. 2-4). Spinal fluid is generally normal.

Radiation-induced retinopathy and optic neuropathy are acknowledged

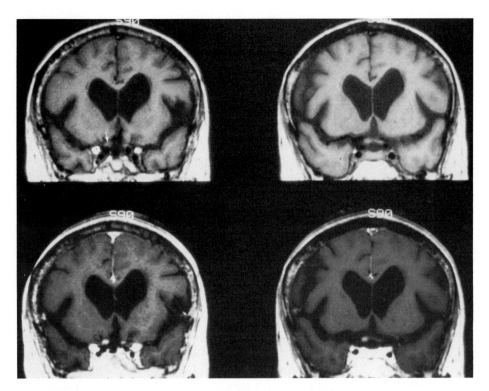

***Fig. 2-4.*** Radiation-induced optic nerve and chiasm damage. Pre–gadolinium contrast coronal MRI reveals no abnormal signal in optic nerves *(arrow, upper left)* or chiasm *(upper right)*. Post–gadolinium contrast MRI reveals abnormally increased signal intensity in right optic nerve *(lower left)* and right optic nerve-chiasm junction *(lower right).* Patient had corresponding right anterior junction visual field defects.

risks of potentially life-saving irradiation of ocular, orbital, sinus, and nasopharyngeal neoplasms. They are not expected, but have rarely occurred, after irradiation of tumors of the sellar area.[111,112] Harris and Levene[111] reported an 18% prevalence of radiation-induced visual loss in 55 patients treated for pituitary adenomas and craniopharyngiomas. All cases occurred in patients treated with dose fractions of 250 cGy/day; none occurred at lower fractions. Schatz et al.[109] described three cases of visual loss after treatment for middle fossa masses at 5000 cGy in 200 cGy daily fractions. The clinical syndrome was stereotypic: visual loss occurred suddenly in one eye between 6 months and 2 years after completion of treatment. No fundus abnormalities were present at first. Visual fields disclosed either nerve fiber bundle or hemianopic defects. Later, visual acuity and field continued to deteriorate, often in a stepwise fashion, and optic pallor appeared.

Our clinical impression, unsupported by published information, is that the risk of radiation toxicity is especially high when the optic nerve has already been compromised by previous tumor compression. Patients with diabetes and hypertension are also particularly vulnerable, probably because of underlying vascular disease.[113]

Pathologic studies of optic nerve and chiasm in all autopsied cases of radiation toxicity to the anterior visual pathway show changes similar to those encountered in delayed radiation effects on the spinal cord and brain: vascular endothelial proliferation and fibrinoid necrosis, necrosis of white and gray matter, and reactive astrocytosis.[114] Although direct toxicity to neuronal tissue is a possibility, more likely the principal target is the vascular endothelium, with brain tissue damaged by an ischemic mechanism.

Although corticosteroids have been used to reduce cerebral edema in delayed radionecrosis, no evidence indicates their efficacy in treating visual loss. Hyperbaric oxygen treatment has been similarly unhelpful.[115]

### ☐ Toxic optic neuropathy

Toxicity to the retina and optic nerves from chemicals or metabolic disorders differs from radiation damage in that the deficits tend to be symmetric. Thus these conditions are rarely confused with the foregoing entities and are instead more appropriately considered together with hereditary (dystrophic) conditions (see Metabolic Optic Neuropathy).

The relatively uniform clinical picture that toxic agents produce consists of painless bilateral loss of acuity and color vision with central scotomas. The tempo of visual loss varies according to the causative agent. Generally, the more rapid the decline in vision, the more likely it is that the optic disc will show swelling. In late phases some temporal disc pallor is usually evident. The degree of reversibility on discontinuing the drug depends on both the total dose consumed and the nature of the drug. Among the many agents that have commonly produced this syndrome (methanol, chloramphenicol, toluene, penicillamine, lead, streptomycin, isoniazid, quinine, thallium, halogenated hydroquinones),[116] one that is frequently implicated in current clinical practice is ethambutol, an antituberculosis drug.

Since the initial description by Carr and Henkind in 1962,[117] ethambutol optic nerve toxicity has been recognized as a dose-related retrobulbar neuropathy primarily but not exclusively involving papillomacular fibers. Leibold[118] reported that optic neuropathy was seen in 11 (18%) of 59 patients treated at 35 mg/kg/day. At 25 mg/kg/day the incidence of toxicity dropped to 2.25%. Others have confirmed this low risk, and present recommendations call for a dosage of 15 mg/kg/day.

The fundus is typically normal, although some hyperemia of the nerve head may rarely be seen. Visual acuity may be markedly reduced (hand movements) but is usually better than 20/100. Central and paracentral scotomas are the rule. Recovery occurs in the vast majority within 2 months of discontinuing the drug. What predisposes those rare individuals who develop ethambutol optic neuropathy at doses of 15 mg/kg/day is unknown. Most authorities agree that the risk of irreversible toxicity at these dosages is very low. Early manifestations of toxicity are exceedingly difficult to detect. The physician's principal role is to be aware of the entity, to encourage safe dosage limits, and to recommend withdrawal of the agent at the first suggestion of unexplained visual loss.

Isoniazid and streptomycin are also optic nerve toxins, and use of either of these agents with ethambutol may lower the threshold for damage.[119] While the toxicity of ethambutol is limited to the optic nerve, isoniazid is a general neurotoxin, causing peripheral neuropathy, seizures, and diffuse encephalopathy. Alcoholics and those with hepatic or renal disease are at special risk.[120] Recommended daily dosages for isoniazid are 300 mg/day in adults. Optic neuropathy clinically similar to that of ethambutol toxicity has been reported at isoniazid doses ranging from 200 to 900 mg/day. The documentation of streptomycin optic nerve toxicity is too imprecise to offer helpful guidelines.

### ◻ Metabolic optic neuropathy

The pathogenesis of the optic neuropathies associated with severe alcoholism and tobacco smoking remains unsettled. Evidence exists both for direct toxicity and for deprivation of critical nutrient factors. We will therefore hedge and consider them under the category of metabolic optic neuropathies.

The optic neuropathy of **chronic alcoholism** is characterized by painless, progressive, bilateral, and symmetric involvement of papillomacular bundles to produce centrocecal scotomas (Fig. 2-5) and subnormal acuity at the level of 20/50 to 20/200. Although the development of visual loss is slow, patients may report a relatively sudden onset when it reaches unmanageable levels. At that point they describe a fog or smudge in the center of their field of vision and note that colors look "washed out."

In advanced stages diagnosis will be straightforward if the examiner is attune to the disease and reasonably adept at performing visual field tests. Aside from the acuity and field changes, the only other ophthalmologic abnormality is temporal disc pallor. In the early stages diagnosis is difficult. At an acuity level of 20/50 or better, central or centrocecal scotomas are elusive, to be found only

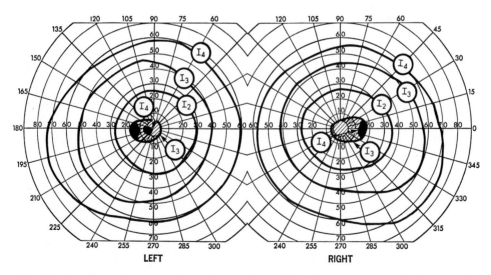

*Fig. 2-5.* Cecocentral scotomas in patient with nutritional optic neuropathy. Similar defects are noted in patients with toxic and metabolic optic neuropathies.

with small targets in very cooperative patients. The examiner will be tempted to conclude that the patient is malingering or to order imaging studies in search of intracranial disease. The diagnostic yield can be improved by applying detailed central visual field techniques, including kinetic color (red) and static perimetry techniques. The earliest field changes will be elevated thresholds in the area between fixation and the blind spot. Patients often make many errors on conventional color vision tests. Neurologic examination may reveal a peripheral neuropathy. CNS effects of alcohol, such as gait ataxia and recent memory loss, are generally not evident.

The optic neuropathy and the peripheral neuropathy of alcohol abuse are precisely mimicked by **severe malnutrition.** In both conditions solid evidence supports the notion that the critical missing dietary substance is vitamin $B_1$, or thiamine.[121] Carroll[122] found that the optic neuropathy of alcoholics could be reversed either by a well-balanced diet or by thiamine supplements (while subjects continued their drinking and poor diet). Many alcoholics do not avow a poor diet. However, even in the presence of adequate intake they absorb vitamins poorly, and because of liver disease they may not be able to convert them to bioactive forms.[123] Furthermore, the increased carbohydrate load from alcohol ingestion consumes added amounts of thiamine, reducing the available stores.

Many alcoholics also smoke heavily, raising the question of whether **tobacco** is making a toxic contribution. Indeed, the medical literature of the late nineteenth and early twentieth centuries is filled with admonitions about the pernicious effects of tobacco on the optic nerves ("tobacco amblyopia").[124] The neuro-ophthalmic syndrome described is exactly the same as that seen in alcoholics and the severely malnourished and appears to occur primarily in pipe smokers, to a lesser degree in cigar smokers, snuff users, and tobacco chewers, and not at all in cigarette smokers. The severity of optic neuropathy appears to be independent of the amount of tobacco consumed; rather, it tends to occur in patients who drink heavily and may improve if they stop drinking but continue smoking.[125]

The principal scientific support for the idea that tobacco is a separate optic nerve toxin has come from the repeated evidence that smokers with optic neuropathy have significantly lower levels of thiocyanate in their plasma and urine than do smokers without optic neuropathy.[126] The postulate is that the relatively few smokers who develop optic neuropathy have an inherent defect in their ability to detoxify the cyanide of smoke and that the free cyanide damages the optic nerves. Experimental evidence shows that high doses of cyanide produce axonal destruction in the optic nerves of animals.[127]

Foulds et al.[128] have shown that "tobacco amblyopia" patients have low or borderline levels of vitamin $B_{12}$, which is capable of binding cyanide ions. They claim to have restored vision by using the hydroxycobalamin form of $B_{12}$, a more effective acceptor of cyanate than $B_{12}$ itself. Their work implies that the rare optic neuropathy in smokers is conditioned by relative $B_{12}$ deficiency, linking this disorder mechanistically to the optic neuropathy found in patients with pernicious anemia.

Deficiency of vitamin $B_{12}$ is rarely a factor in alcoholics and the severely

> ### Management of Bilateral Progressive Painless Loss of Central Vision
>
> 1. Because bilateral optic nerve compression may cause this condition,[130-132] we recommend CT/MRI in all such patients, despite the low yield.
> 2. Screen all patients for pernicious anemia by ordering a complete blood count and indices and a serum $B_{12}$ level.
> 3. If no adequate history of familial vision loss or severe alcoholism exists, perform a thorough workup for noncompressive causes of optic neuropathy, which may include a lumbar puncture and a 24-hour urine collection to screen for lead or thallium intoxication.
> 4. Where evidence of smoking and alcohol abuse is present and other causes have been reasonably excluded, we presume that toxic and nutritional factors are pathogenic. We then recommend that the patient stop smoking and drinking, eat a balanced diet, and take multivitamins and thiamine, 25 mg three times a day.

malnourished because the ample reserves of $B_{12}$ are repleted for a month with a single meal containing meat. Thus $B_{12}$ deficiency is restricted to those patients who are unable to absorb it, either because of gastrointestinal disease or, more commonly, because of lack of a transport substance called gastric intrinsic factor. Intrinsic factor is secreted by stomach parietal cells; in pernicious anemia autoantibodies against these cells impair their function. The lack of $B_{12}$ interferes with red blood cell maturation, producing a megaloblastic anemia, and damages the posterior and lateral columns of the spinal cord, producing distal extremity paresthesias, loss of vibratory sense, weakness, and spasticity (subacute combined degeneration).

Although not a consistent feature of **pernicious anemia,** optic neuropathy is reported frequently and rarely may be the presenting sign.[129] Its clinical characteristics are similar to those of alcoholic optic neuropathy. The diagnosis is made by having a high index of suspicion when confronted with bilateral subnormal acuity and central or centrocecal scotomas in nonalcoholic elderly (age >50 years) persons of northern European extraction who have a fair complexion and no family history of visual loss. Hematologic evaluation will reveal mild anemia with peripheral or bone marrow megaloblasts. Neurologic examination may be normal or reveal the subtle findings described above. Serum $B_{12}$ levels, available by radioimmunoassay, will be below normal, and a Schilling test will reveal a significant increase in $B_{12}$ absorption with the addition of intrinsic factor. Treatment is with monthly intramuscular $B_{12}$ injections in 1000 µg doses in perpetuity. Hematologic signs are reversible; neurologic signs will remit if the condition is not far advanced.

### 🔲 Hereditary optic neuropathy

So rarely are cases of hereditary optic neuropathy seen in clinical practice that they are usually misdiagnosed. No treatment is available for the afflicted, but they deserve to be given a sage prognosis and to be spared unnecessary studies.

Similar in ophthalmologic manifestations to toxic and metabolic optic neuropathies, hereditary optic neuropathies occur both as isolated conditions and as part of degenerative CNS diseases.

ISOLATED HEREDITARY OPTIC NEUROPATHY. Glaser[133] has divided the isolated hereditary optic neuropathies into the rare, recessively inherited type, the relatively more common dominantly inherited type, and Leber's optic neuropathy.

**Recessive optic atrophy,** which is probably congenital, produces severe and stable central visual loss (20/200, hand movements) with nystagmus, achromatopsia, and optic disc pallor. The normal caliber of the retinal arterioles and a normal electroretinogram (ERG) distinguish it from Leber's amaurosis.

**Dominant optic atrophy,** which becomes symptomatic between the ages of 4 and 8 years, produces moderate visual impairment (20/40 to 20/200), slow progression, no nystagmus, moderate disc pallor, centrocecal scotomas, and a tritanopic color defect.

**Leber's optic neuropathy**[134] was described in 1871 as a hereditary optic neuropathy affecting first one eye and then the other within an interval of weeks to months. Nearly all cases involve men in their second or third decade and result in rapid, unremitting, painless visual loss. Visual acuity generally falls no lower than 20/200 and may rarely improve. Visual field examination tends to manifest central or cecocentral scotomas. Ophthalmoscopic examination during the phase of visual loss reveals dilated retinal surface vessels on and around the nerve head and a glistening, opaque peripapillary nerve fiber layer (Plate 3, C and D). Fluorescein angiography at this time reveals arteriovenous shunting around the disc *without leakage.*[135] Within weeks of the attack, these changes gradually give way to attenuation of the retinal arterioles and nerve fiber layer, and pallor of the nerve head. Nikoskelainen et al.[136] found that papillary telangiectasia and mild disc elevation were present *even in the asymptomatic state* in 61% of "at risk" males in families with Leber's disease. Whether these abnormalities presage an increased chance of developing visual loss is not clear.

Although visual loss is frequently an isolated clinical manifestation of Leber's optic neuropathy, cardiac conduction defects and dystonia have been reported.[137]

Because of matrilineal inheritance, Leber's disease has been suspected of being a disorder of mitochondrial DNA. Wallace et al.[138] have reported a mutation of mitochondrial DNA resulting in a single nucleotide change (arginine to histidine) that disturbs the function of a respiratory enzyme (NADH dehydrogenase). The reliability of this enzyme assay (performed on blood) for the diagnosis of Leber's optic neuropathy is yet unknown; only 50% of affected families have had the mutation.[139]

Leber's disease is most likely to be confused with optic neuritis. In a young male patient with painless and rapid monocular visual loss, one should look carefully for the classic fundus signs, *paying particular attention to the asymptomatic eye.* If these features are not recognized, one should ask to examine "at risk" family members. When findings are inconclusive, we apply the thorough diagnostic workup recommended in atypical optic neuritis. Unfortunately, no known treatment is effective, but we advise all patients with Leber's disease whose first eye becomes involved to stop smoking because of its potentially toxic effects on respiratory metabolism.

**COMPLICATED HEREDITARY OPTIC ATROPHY.** Optic atrophy with central or centrocecal scotomas is a manifestation of a wide variety of neurodegenerative states. The **familial eponymic spinocerebellar degenerations** such as Friedreich's, Marie's, and Behr's, as well as the polyneuropathy of Charcot-Marie-Tooth, may include optic atrophy.[140] Optic atrophy may also be seen in the neurologic diseases of **inborn metabolic errors** that manifest retinal pigmentary degeneration, maculopathy, and cherry red spots. In most of these conditions, visual loss and optic neuropathy occur either concomitantly or follow other neurologic signs. No treatment is available.

### ▣ Traumatic optic neuropathy

Traumatic damage to the optic nerve occurs most commonly during closed head injury. Based on a thorough review, Kline et al.[141] and Lessell[142] have delineated the following profile of this entity:

1. The injury usually consists of a blow to the ipsilateral forehead. The blow may only stun the patient briefly, or it may cause prolonged loss of consciousness. Curiously, the degree of optic nerve injury is only weakly correlated with the degree to which consciousness is lost or with other neurologic deficits. Perhaps, then, *the position rather than the degree of impact may be the critical determinant of optic nerve trauma.*[143]

2. Imaging evidence of structural abnormalities adjacent to the intracanalicular optic nerve (fractures, hematomas) is common but not constant. Moreover, the degree of visual loss and visual outcome are not correlated with the presence or absence of such findings.

3. In most cases no ophthalmoscopic abnormalities occur in the acute phase. Visual acuity loss, which may be mild or profound, is accompanied by nerve fiber bundle visual field defects and an afferent pupillary defect. These findings suggest that the damage generally occurs well behind the globe, sparing the retinal and ciliary circulations.

4. Autopsy examinations have confirmed that the site of injury is usually the intracanalicular optic nerve, which generally shows evidence of infarction. Some cases show no evidence of infarction, but only shearing injury of axons. Current belief is that the intracanalicular nerve is vulnerable because it is tightly adherent to periosteum, lies in a crowded, nondistensible space, and has a fragile pial circulation, especially in its superior portion. Presumably, shearing forces cause edema, as well as tear and collapse vessels, and infarction occurs secondarily. The contribution of hematomas and fractures is uncertain.

5. Visual loss usually remains static from the initial to subsequent examinations, but a substantial minority of patients show a decline. Reports[141,142]

### Management of Traumatic Optic Neuropathy

1. Assess visual function as accurately as possible. Review imaging studies of the posterior orbit for obvious structural abnormalities. CT is preferable to MRI because of its superior imaging of acute blood and bone.
2. Treat with intravenous methylprednisolone, 1 g/day for 3 days, if visual acuity is 20/100 or worse and the contralateral eye has normal acuity; treat any degree of acuity loss if the contralateral eye does not have normal acuity.
3. Consider transethmoidal optic nerve decompression if acuity declines substantially under observation and visual acuity recovers with corticosteroids and then falls when corticosteroids are withdrawn. The presence of an intracanalicular fracture or hematoma fortifies the decision to perform surgical decompression but is not a sufficient criterion by itself.
4. Consider transfrontal optic nerve decompression for the above indications if the patient requires surgery by this route for other reasons.

have now amply documented that *visual acuity improves without treatment,* even when no light perception existed initially. This spontaneous recovery complicates any assessment of the effects of treatment.

6. Treatment has consisted of corticosteroids[143] and/or surgical decompression of the optic canal, either transcranially[144] or, most commonly, transethmoidally.[145,146] Although spectacular results have been claimed by all methods, none of the studies has been controlled.

### Central retinal artery occlusion

**ACUTE PHASE.** The diagnosis of acute central retinal artery occlusion (CRAO) (Plate 3, *E*) or branch retinal artery occlusion (BRAO) (Plate 3, *F*) is usually straightforward. Patients have sudden painless loss of vision. The extent of visual loss depends on the segment of retina that has been infarcted. The event is termed a CRAO if most of the retina has been affected, and a BRAO if only a small portion is involved. BRAO infarctions often do not extend to the optic disc, originating instead at the point of termination of an embolus or the crossing of the affected arteriole and a vein. The infarcted retina has lost its transparency and appears milky white, especially in its thickest region around the macula. The transmission of the normal orange-red choroidal color in the macular area contrasts with the surrounding milky retinal pallor and gives the appearance of a cherry red spot.

The retinal turbidity is gradually lost after an interval of 10 to 14 days, and the diagnosis may be difficult to make on ophthalmoscopic grounds for the next 2 months until the retinal arterioles have become attenuated, the nerve fiber layer atrophic, and the disc pale. Visual field defects are nerve fiber bundle in configuration and typically involve the fixation area unless a cilioretinal artery has been spared.

Treatment of the acute event is based on the principle of reducing external pressure and dilating the retinal vasculature. Pressure is lowered by means of digital massage of the globe, anterior chamber paracentesis, and agents that block aqueous secretion. Ocular massage is advised especially if an embolus is visible, in hopes of dislodging it and promoting distal migration.

Only anecdotal evidence points to the efficacy of these maneuvers, and most experienced clinicians consider them hopeless if more than 6 hours have elapsed from the onset of the fixed deficit. Still, we would support the traditional heroic measures, even if 24 hours have elapsed, acknowledging that reversal of visual loss is rare. Little rationale appears to support using systemic vasodilators, since they only tend to shunt blood to healthier, more responsive vessels.

**CHRONIC PHASE.** The workup of patients with CRAO or BRAO after the acute treatment period is problematic. The considerations are similar to those involved in managing patients with transient visual loss (TVL) (see Chapter 5). One must first determine if the pathogenesis is atherosclerosis, vasculitis, or hypercoagulable state. If atherosclerosis is likely, is it local or remote with embolization? Finally, what is the risk of cerebral stroke?

Appen et al.[147] found that of 44 patients over 40 years of age, retinal stroke could be reasonably ascribed to atherosclerosis in 20 (46%). Nonatherosclerotic causes were diagnosed in 11 (25%): 5 with rheumatic heart disease, 2 with GCA, 1 with lupus erythematosus, 1 with unspecified vasculitis, 1 with syphilis, and 1 with sickle cell anemia. The rest remained idiopathic. In this elderly group 18% developed strokes within 6 years. By contrast, among 10 patients under 40 years of age, retinal stroke was ascribed to nonarteriosclerotic disease in 3 (30%), including atrial myxoma, Marfan's syndrome with mitral valve insufficiency, and orbital compression. In the remaining patients the cause was never ascertained. In all 10 young patients, carotid angiography was normal, no risk factors or signs of arteriosclerosis were present, and no retinal emboli were visible. With the exception of the patient with the atrial myxoma, no subsequent strokes occurred in the average follow-up period of 6 years.

Two retrospective series[148,149] devoted to retinal stroke in young patients disclosed that a substantial number have clinical evidence of migraine. Retrospective studies of patients with retinal infarct suggest that the risk of cerebral stroke is about 3% per year,[150-152] four times that of an age-matched population, slightly greater than that for patients with monocular TVL, but considerably less than that of patients with hemispheric transient ischemic attacks (TIAs). Patients with both CRAO and BRAO have reduced survival relative to age-matched controls. As with hemispheric TIA and stroke, the principal cause of death is myocardial infarction, not stroke.[152,153]

Thus three patient groups are apparent: an elderly population with a high likelihood of atherosclerosis, a small population with nonatherosclerotic disease, and a youthful population that probably has a variant of migraine. In this sense, patients with CRAO and BRAO so resemble patients with monocular TVL that after the acute phase has been managed, they should be evaluated in the same way as TVL patients (see Chapter 5).

## REFERENCES

1. Perkin GD, Rose FC. Optic neuritis and its differential diagnosis. Oxford: Oxford University Press, 1979.
2. Parmley VC, Schiffman JS, Maitland CG, et al. Does neuroretinitis rule out multiple sclerosis? Arch Neurol 1987; 44:1045-8.
3. Miller DH, Newton MR, Van der Poel JC, et al. Magnetic resonance imaging of the optic nerve in optic neuritis. Neurology 1988;38:175-9.
4. Paty DW, Oger JJF, Kastrukoff LF, et al. MRI in the diagnosis of MS: a prospective study with comparison of clinical evaluation, evoked potentials, oligoclonal banding, and CT. Neurology 1988;38:180-5.
5. Tackman W, Ettlin T, Strenge H. Multimodality evoked potentials and electrically elicited blink reflex in optic neuritis. J Neurol 1982;227:157-63.
6. Clifford-Jones RE, McDonald WI, Landon DN. Chronic optic nerve compression: an experimental study. Brain 1985;108:241-62.
7. Hershey LA, Trotter JL. The use and abuse of the cerebrospinal fluid IgG profile in the adult: a practical evaluation. Ann Neurol 1980;8:426-34.
8. Nikoskelainen E, Frey H, Salmi A. Prognosis of optic neuritis with special reference to cerebrospinal immunoglobulins and measles virus antibodies. Ann Neurol 1981;9:545-50.
9. Sandberg M, Bynke H. Cerebrospinal fluid in 25 cases of optic neuritis. Acta Neurol Scand 1973;49:443-52.
10. Moulin D, Paty DW, Ebers GC. The predictive value of cerebrospinal fluid electrophoresis in possible multiple sclerosis. Brain 1983;106:809-16.
11. Ormerod IEC, McDonald WI, du Boulay GH, et al. Disseminated lesions at presentation in patients with optic neuritis. J Neurol Neurosurg Psychiatry 1986;49:124-7.
12. Jacobs L, Kinkel PR, Kinkel WR. Silent brain lesions in patients with isolated idiopathic optic neuritis: a clinical and nuclear magnetic resonance imaging study. Arch Neurol 1986;43: 452-5.
13. Johns K, Lavin P, Elliott JH, et al. Magnetic resonance imaging of the brain in isolated optic neuritis. Arch Ophthalmol 1986;104:1486-8.
14. Miller DH, Ormerod IEC, McDonald WI, et al. The early risk of multiple sclerosis after optic neuritis. J Neurol Neurosurg Psychiatry 1988; 51:1569-71.
15. Hutchinson WM. Acute optic neuritis and the prognosis for multiple sclerosis. J Neurol Neurosurg Psychiatry 1976;39:283-9.
16. Francis DA, Compston DAS, Batchelor JR, et al. A reassessment of the risk of multiple sclerosis developing in patients with optic neuritis after extended follow-up. J Neurol Neurosurg Psychiatry 1987;50:758-65.
17. Rizzo JF III, Lessell S. Risk of developing multiple sclerosis after uncomplicated optic neuritis: a long-term prospective study. Neurology 1988; 38:185-90.
18. Cohen MM, Lessell S, Wolf PA. A prospective study of the risk of developing multiple sclerosis in uncomplicated optic neuritis. Neurology 1979; 29:208-13.
19. Compston DAS, Batchelor JR, Earl CJ, et al. Factors influencing the risk of multiple sclerosis developing in patients with optic neuritis. Brain 1978; 101:495-511.
20. Hely MA, McManis PG, Doran TJ, et al. Acute optic neuritis: a prospective study of risk factors for multiple sclerosis. J Neurol Neurosurg Psychiatry 1986;49:1125-30.
21. Kennedy C, Carroll FD. Optic neuritis in children. Arch Ophthalmol 1960; 63:747-55.
22. Kriss A, Francis DA, Cuendet F, et al. Recovery after optic neuritis in childhood. J Neurol Neurosurg Psychiatry 1988;51:1253-8.
23. Landy PJ. A prospective study of the risk of developing multiple sclerosis in optic neuritis in a tropical and subtropical area. J Neurol Neurosurg Psychiatry 1983;46:659-61.
24. Bauer HJ, Firnhaber W, Winkler W. Prognostic criteria in multiple sclerosis. Ann NY Acad Sci 1965;122:542-51.
25. Nikoskelainen E, Riekkinen P. Optic

neuritis—a sign of multiple sclerosis or other diseases of the central nervous system. Acta Neurol Scand 1974;50:690-718.

26. McAlpine D. The benign form of multiple sclerosis: a study based on 241 cases seen within three years of onset and followed up until the tenth year or more of the disease. Brain 1961;84:186-203.

27. Bradley WG, Whitty CMW. Acute optic neuritis: its clinical features and their relation to prognosis for recovery of vision. J Neurol Neurosurg Psychiatry 1967;30:531-8.

28. Nikoskelainen E. Later course and prognosis of optic neuritis. Acta Ophthalmol 1975;53:273-91.

29. Fleishman JA, Beck RW, Linares OA, et al. Deficits in visual function after resolution of optic neuritis. Ophthalmology 1987;94:1029-35.

30. Rawson MD, Liversedge LA, Goldfarb G, et al. Treatment of acute retrobulbar neuritis with corticotrophin. Lancet 1966;2:1044-6.

31. Bowden AN, Bowden PMA, Friedmann AI, et al. A trial of corticotrophin gelatin injection in acute optic neuritis. J Neurol Neurosurg Psychiatry 1974;37:869-73.

32. Gould ES, Bird AC, Leaver PK, et al. Treatment of optic neuritis by retrobulbar injection of triamcinolone. Br Med J 1977;1:1495-7.

33. Spoor TC, Rockwell DL. Treatment of optic neuritis with intravenous megadose corticosteroids: a consecutive series. Ophthalmology 1988;95:131-4.

34. Beck RW. The Optic Neuritis Treatment Trial [Editorial]. Arch Ophthalmol 1988;106:1051-3.

35. Milligan NM, Newcombe R, Compston DAS. A double-blind controlled trial of high dose methylprednisolone in patients with multiple sclerosis: I. Clinical effects. J Neurol Neurosurg Psychiatry 1987;50:511-6.

36. Parkin PJ, Hierons R, McDonald WI. Bilateral optic neuritis: a long-term follow-up. Brain 1984;107:951-64.

37. Jabs DA, Miller NR, Newman SA, et al. Optic neuropathy in systemic lupus erythematosus. Arch Ophthalmol 1986;104:564-8.

38. Wise CM, Agudelo CA. Optic neuropathy as an initial manifestation of Sjogren's syndrome. J Rheumatol 1988; 15:799-802.

39. Colvard DM, Robertson DM, O'Duffy JD. The ocular manifestations of Behcet's disease. Arch Ophthalmol 1977; 95:1813-7.

40. Dutton JJ, Burde RM, Klingele TG. Autoimmune retrobulbar optic neuritis. Am J Ophthalmol 1982;94:11-7.

41. Kupersmith MJ, Burde RM, Warren FA, et al. Autoimmune optic neuropathy: evaluation and treatment. J Neurol Neurosurg Psychiatry 1988; 51:1381-6.

42. De Keyser J. Autoimmunity in multiple sclerosis. Neurology 1988;38:371-4.

43. Delaney P. Neurologic manifestations in sarcoidosis: review of the literature, with a report of 23 cases. Ann Intern Med 1977;87:336-45.

44. Stern BJ, Krumholz A, Johns C, et al. Sarcoidosis and its neurological manifestations. Arch Neurol 1985;42:909-17.

45. Graham EM, Ellis CJK, Sanders MD, et al. Optic neuropathy in sarcoidosis. J Neurol Neurosurg Psychiatry 1986; 49:756-63.

46. Gelwan MJ, Kellen RI, Burde RM, et al. Sarcoidosis of the anterior visual pathway: successes and failures. J Neurol Neurosurg Psychiatry 1988; 51:1473-80.

47. Weinstein JM, Lexow SS, Ho P, et al. Acute syphilitic optic neuritis. Arch Ophthalmol 1981;99:1392-5.

48. Winward KE, Hamed LM, Glaser JS. The spectrum of optic nerve disease in human immunodeficiency virus infection. Am J Ophthalmol 1989;107: 373-80.

49. Willerson D Jr, Aaberg TM, Reeser F, et al. Unusual ocular presentation of acute toxoplasmosis. Br J Ophthalmol 1977;61:693-8.

50. Kupfer C, McCrane E. A possible cause of decreased vision in cryptococcal meningitis. Invest Ophthalmol 1974;13:801-4.

51. Hanna LS, Girgis NI, Yassin MMW, et al. Incidence of papilloedema and optic atrophy in meningitis. Jpn J Ophthalmol 1981;25:69-73.

52. Miller NR. Walsh and Hoyt's clinical neuro-ophthalmology, vol 1. 4th ed. Baltimore: Williams & Wilkins, 1982: 240-2.

53. Phanthumchinda K, Intragumtornchai T, Kasantikul V. Guillain-Barré syndrome and optic neuropathy in acute leukemia. Neurology 1988;38:1324-6.

54. Pillay N, Gilbert JJ, Ebers GC, et al. Internuclear ophthalmoplegia and "optic neuritis": paraneoplastic effects of bronchial carcinoma. Neurology 1984;34:788-91.

55. Boghen D, Sebag M, Michaud J. Paraneoplastic optic neuritis and encephalomyelitis: report of a case. Arch Neurol 1988;45:353-6.

56. Lightman S, McDonald WI, Bird AC, et al. Retinal venous sheathing in optic neuritis: its significance for the pathogenesis of multiple sclerosis. Brain 1987;110:405-14.

57. Miller NR. Walsh and Hoyt's clinical neuro-ophthalmology, vol 1. 4th ed. Baltimore: Williams & Wilkins, 1982: 238-9.

58. Schechter SL. Lyme disease associated with optic neuropathy. Am J Med 1986;81:143-5.

59. Farris BK, Webb RM. Lyme disease and optic neuritis. J Clin Neuro Ophthalmol 1988;8:73-8.

60. Halperin JJ, Luft BJ, Anand AK, et al. Lyme neuroborreliosis: central nervous system manifestations. Neurology 1989;39:753-9.

61. Pachner AP, Duray P, Steere AC. Central nervous manifestations of Lyme disease. Arch Neurol 1989; 46:790-5.

62. Miller NR. Walsh and Hoyt's clinical neuro-ophthalmology, vol 1. 4th ed. Baltimore: Williams & Wilkins, 1982: 279-80.

63. Johnson MW, Kincaid MC, Trobe JD. Bilateral retrobulbar optic nerve infarctions after blood loss and hypotension: a clinicopathologic case study. Ophthalmology 1987;94:1577-84.

64. Ross HS, Rosenberg S, Friedman AH. Delayed radiation necrosis of the optic nerve. Am J Ophthalmol 1973; 76:683-6.

65. Boghen DR, Glaser JS. Ischaemic optic neuropathy: the clinical profile and history. Brain 1975;98:689-708.

66. Repka MX, Savino PJ, Schatz NJ, et al. Clinical profile and long-term implications of anterior ischemic optic neuropathy. Am J Ophthalmol 1983; 96:478-83.

67. Beck RW, Servais GE, Hayreh SS, et al. Anterior ischemic optic neuropathy. IX. Cup-to-disc ratio and its role in pathogenesis. Ophthalmology 1987; 94:1503-8.

68. Kline LB. Progression of visual defects in ischemic optic neuropathy. Am J Ophthalmol 1988;106:199-203.

69. Sergott RC, Cohen MS, Bosley TM, et al. Optic nerve decompression may improve the progressive form of nonarteritic ischemic optic neuropathy. Arch Ophthalmol 1989;107:1743-54.

70. Borchert M, Lessell S. Progressive and recurrent nonarteritic anterior ischemic optic neuropathy. Am J Ophthalmol 1988;106:443-9.

71. Beri M, Klugman MR, Kohler JA, et al. Anterior ischemic optic neuropathy. VII. Incidence of bilaterality and various influencing factors. Ophthalmology 1987;94:1020-8.

72. Guyer DR, Miller NR, Auer CL, et al. The risk of cerebrovascular and cardiovascular disease in patients with anterior ischemic optic neuropathy. Arch Ophthalmol 1985;103:1136-42.

73. Henkind P, Charles NC, Pearson J. Histopathology of ischemic optic neuropathy. Am J Ophthalmol 1970; 69:78-90.

74. Miller NR. Walsh and Hoyt's clinical neuro-ophthalmology, vol 1. 4th ed. Baltimore: Williams & Wilkins, 1982: 219.

75. Cullen JF, Coleiro JA. Ophthalmic complications of giant cell arteritis. Surv Ophthalmol 1976;20:247-60.

76. Keltner JL. Giant-cell arteritis: signs and symptoms. Ophthalmology 1982; 89:1101-10.

77. Hunder GG, Michet CJ. Giant cell arteritis and polymyalgia rheumatica. Clin Rheum Dis 1985;11:471-83.

78. Fessel WJ and Pearson CM. Polymyalgia rheumatica and blindness. N Engl J Med 1967;276:1403-5.

79. McDonnell PJ, Moore W, Miller NR. Temporal arteritis: a clinicopathologic study. Ophthalmol 1986;93:518-30.

80. Roth AM, Milsow L, Keltner JL. The ultimate diagnoses of patients undergoing temporal artery biopsies. Arch Ophthalmol 1984;102:901-3.

81. Simmons RJ and Cogan DG. Occult temporal arteritis. Arch Ophthalmol 1962;68:8-13.

82. Jonasson F, Cullen JF, Elton RA. Temporal arteritis: a 14 year epidemiological, clinical and prognostic study. Scott Med J 1979;11:111-9.

83. Goodman BW. Temporal arteritis. Am J Med 1979;67:839-52.

84. Huston KA, Hunder GG, Lie JT et al. Temporal arteritis: a 25 year epidemiologic, clinical and pathologic study. Ann Intern Med 1978;188:162-7.

85. Wagener HP, Hollenhorst RW. The ocular lesions of temporal arteritis. Am J Ophthalmol 1958;45:617-630.

86. Crompton MR. The visual changes in temporal (giant cell) arteritis. Brain 1959;82:377-90.

87. Wilkinson IMS, Russell RWR. Arteries of the head and neck in giant cell arteritis: a pathological study to show the pattern of arterial involvement. Arch Neurol 1972;27:378-98.

88. Goodwin JA. Temporal arteritis. In: Vinken PJ, Bruyn GW, eds. Handbook of clinical neurology. Vol 39. Neurological manifestations of systemic diseases, pt II. Amsterdam: Elsevier–North Holland, 1980:chap 15.

89. Hollenhorst RW, Brown JR, Wagener HP, et al. Neurologic aspects of temporal arteritis. Neurology 1960;10:490-8.

90. Jacobson DM, Slamovits TL. Erythrocyte sedimentation rate and its relationship to hematocrit in giant cell arteritis. Arch Ophthalmol 1987;105:965-7.

91. Bull BS, Brecher G. An evaluation of the relative merits of the Wintrobe and Westergren sedimentation methods, including hematocrit correction. Am J Clin Pathol 1974;62:502-10.

92. Miller A, Green M, Robinson D. Simple rule for calculating normal erythrocyte sedimentation rate. Br Med J 1983;286:266.

93. Klein RG, Campbell RJ, Hunder GG, et al. Skip lesions in temporal arteritis. Mayo Clin Proc 1976;51:504-10.

94. Hall S, Persellin S, Lie JT, et al. The therapeutic impact of temporal artery biopsy. Lancet 1983;2:1217-20.

95. Hedges TR III, Gieger GL, Albert DM. The clinical value of negative temporal artery biopsy specimens. Arch Ophthalmol 1983;101:1251-4.

96. Hamilton CR Jr, Shelley WM, Tumulty PA. Giant cell arteritis: including temporal arteritis and polymyalgia rheumatica. Medicine 1971;50:1-27.

97. Hunder GG, Sheps SG, Allen GL, et al. Daily and alternate-day corticosteroid regimens in treatment of giant cell arteritis: comparison in a prospective study. Ann Intern Med 1975;82:613-8.

98. Nadeau SE. Temporal arteritis: a decision-analytic approach to temporal artery biopsy. Acta Neurol Scand 1988;78:90-100.

99. Trobe JD, Glaser JS, Laflamme P. Dysthyroid optic neuropathy: clinical profile and rationale for management. Arch Ophthalmol 1978;96:1199-209.

100. Feldon SE, Weiner JM. Clinical significance of extraocular muscle volumes in Graves' ophthalmopathy: a quantitative computed tomography study. Arch Ophthalmol 1982;100:1266-9.

101. Jampol LM, Woodfin W, McLean EB. Optic nerve sarcoidosis: report of a case. Arch Ophthalmol 1972;87:355-60.

102. Kraus AM, O'Rourke JO. Lymphomatous optic neuritis. Arch Ophthalmol 1963;70:173-5.

103. Ellis W, Little HL. Leukemic infiltration of the optic nerve head. Am J Ophthalmol 1973;75:867-71.

104. Gudas PP Jr. Optic nerve myeloma. Am J Ophthalmol 1971;71:1085-9.

105. Altrocchi PA, Reinhardt PH, Eckman PB. Blindness and meningeal carcinomatosis. Arch Ophthalmol 1972;88:508-12.

106. Kline LB, Kim JY, Ceballos R. Radiation optic neuropathy. Ophthalmology 1985;92:1118-26.

107. Nakissa N, Rubin P, Strohl R, et al. Ocular and orbital complications following radiation therapy of paranasal

sinus malignancies and review of the literature. Cancer 1983;51:980-6.

108. MacDonald DR, Rottenberg DA, Schultz JS, et al. Radiation-induced optic neuropathy [Abstract]. Neurology 1981;31:43-4.

109. Schatz NJ, Lichtenstein S, Corbett JJ. Delayed radiation necrosis of the optic nerves and chiasm. In: Glaser JS, Smith JL, eds. Neuro-ophthalmology: symposium of the University of Miami and the Bascom Palmer Eye Institute, vol 8. St Louis: Mosby–Year Book 1975:131-9.

110. Shukovsky LJ, Fletcher GH. Retinal and optic nerve complications in a high dose irradiation technique of ethmoid sinus and nasal cavity. Radiology 1972;104:629-34.

111. Harris JR, Levene MB. Visual complications following irradiation for pituitary adenomas and craniopharyngiomas. Radiology 1976;120:167-71.

112. Bagan SM, Hollenhorst RW. Radiation retinopathy after irradiation of intracranial lesions. Am J Ophthalmol 1979;88:694-7.

113. Chacko DC. Considerations in the diagnosis of radiation injury. JAMA 1981;245:1255-8.

114. Crompton MR, Layton DD. Delayed radionecrosis of the brain following therapeutic x-radiation of the pituitary. Brain 1961;84:85-101.

115. Roden D, Bosley TM, Fowble B, et al. Delayed radiation injury to the retrobulbar optic nerves and chiasm: clinical syndrome and treatment with hyperbaric oxygen and corticosteroids. Ophthalmology 1990;97:346-51.

116. Miller NR. Walsh and Hoyt's clinical neuro-ophthalmology, vol 1. 4th ed. Baltimore: Williams & Wilkins, 1982: 254-60, 289-307.

117. Carr RE, Henkind P. Ocular manifestations of ethambutol: toxic amblyopia after administration of an experimental antituberculous drug. Arch Opththalmol 1962;67:566-71.

118. Leibold JE. The ocular toxicity of ethambutol and its relation to dose. Ann NY Acad Sci 1966;135:904-9.

119. Karmon G, Savir H, Zevin D, et al. Bilateral optic neuropathy due to combined ethambutol and isoniazid treatment. Ann Ophthalmol 1979;11:1013-7.

120. Leibold JE. Drugs having a toxic effect on the optic nerve. Int Ophthalmol Clin 1971;11(2):137-57.

121. Victor M, Adams RD. On the etiology of the alcoholic neurologic diseases: with special reference to the role of nutrition. Am J Clin Nutr 1961;9:379-97.

122. Carroll FD. The etiology and treatment of tobacco-alcohol amblyopia. Am J Ophthalmol 1944;27:713-25.

123. Victor M. Tobacco-alcohol amblyopia: a critique of current concepts of this disorder, with special reference to the role of nutritional deficiency in its causation. Arch Ophthalmol 1963; 70:313-8.

124. Potts AM. Tobacco amblyopia. Surv Ophthalmol 1973;17:313-39.

125. Krumsiek J, Kruger C, Patzold U. Tobacco-alcohol amblyopia:neuro-ophthalmological findings and clinical course. Acta Neurol Scand 1985; 72:180-7.

126. Foulds WS, Bronte-Stewart JM, Chisholm IA. Serum thiocyanate concentrations in tobacco amblyopia. Nature 1968;218:586.

127. Lessell S. Experimental cyanide optic neuropathy. Arch Ophthalmol 1971; 86:194-204.

128. Foulds WS, Chisholm IA, Bronte-Stewart J, et al. Vitamin $B_{12}$ absorption in tobacco amblyopia. Br J Ophthalmol 1969;53:393-7.

129. Hamilton HE, Ellis PE, Sheets RF. Visual impairment due to optic neuropathy in pernicious anemia: report of a case and review of the literature. Blood 1959;14:378-85.

130. Gutman I, Behrens M, Odel J. Bilateral central and centrocaecal scotomata due to mass lesions. Br J Ophthalmol 1984;68:336-42.

131. Page NGR, Sanders MD. Bilateral central scotomata due to intracranial tumor. Br J Ophthalmol 1984;68:449-57.

132. Spector RT, Smith JL, Parker JC Jr. Cecocentral scotomas in gliomatosis cerebri. J Clin Neuro Ophthalmol 1984;4:229-38.

133. Glaser JS. Heredofamilial disorders of

the optic nerve. In: Renie WA, ed. Goldberg's genetic and metabolic eye disease. 2nd ed. Boston: Little, Brown, 1986:465-88.

134. Leber T. Ueber hereditäre und congenital-angelegte Sehnervenleiden. Graefes Arch Ophthal 1871;17(2): 249-91.

135. Smith JL, Hoyt WF, Susac JO. Ocular fundus in acute Leber optic neuropathy. Arch Ophthalmol 1973;90:349-54.

136. Nikoskelainen E, Hoyt WF, Nummelin K. Ophthalmoscopic findings in Leber's hereditary optic neuropathy. I. Fundus findings in asymptomatic family members. Arch Ophthalmol 1982;100:1597-602.

137. Nikoskelainen EK, Savontaus ML, Wanne OP, et al. Leber's hereditary optic neuroretinopathy, a maternally inherited disease: a geneologic study in four pedigrees. Arch Ophthalmol 1987;105:665-71.

138. Wallace DC, Singh G, Lott MT, et al. Mitochondrial DNA mutation associated with Leber's hereditary optic neuropathy. Science 1988;242:1427-30.

139. Vilkki J, Savontaus ML, Nikoskelainen EK. Genetic heterogeneity in Leber hereditary optic neuroretinopathy revealed by mitochondrial DNA polymorphism. Am J Hum Genet 1989;45:205-11.

140. Greenfield JG. The spinocerebellar degenerations. Oxford: Blackwell Scientific Publications, 1954.

141. Kline LB, Morawetz RB, Swaid SN. Indirect injury of the optic nerve. Neurosurgery 1984;14:756-64.

142. Lessell S. Indirect optic nerve trauma. Arch Ophthalmol 1989;107:382-6.

143. Gross CE, DeKock JR, Panje WR, et al. Evidence for orbital deformation that may contribute to monocular blindness following minor frontal head trauma. J Neurosurg 1981;55:963-6.

144. Waga S, Kubo Y, Sakakura M. Transfrontal intradural microsurgical decompression for traumatic optic nerve injury. Acta Neurochir 1988;91:42-6.

145. Niho S, Yasuda K, Sato T, et al. Decompression of the optic canal by the transethmoidal route. Am J Ophthalmol 1961;51:659-65.

146. Joseph MP, Lessell S, Rizzo J, et al. Extracranial optic nerve decompression for traumatic optic neuropathy. Arch Ophthalmol 1990;108:1091-3.

147. Appen RE, Wray SH, Cogan DG. Central retinal artery occlusion. Am J Ophthalmol 1975;79:374-81.

148. Tippin J, Corbett JJ, Kerber RE et al. Amaurosis and ocular infarction in adolescents and young adults. Ann Neurol 1989;26:69-77.

149. Brown GC, Magargal LE, Shields JA et al. Retinal arterial obstruction in children and young adults. Ophthalmology 1981;88:18-25.

150. Liversedge LA, Smith YH. Neuromedical and ophthalmic aspects of central retinal artery occlusion. Trans Ophthalmol Soc UK 1962;82:571-591.

151. Lorentzen SE. Occlusion of the central retinal artery: a follow-up. Acta Ophthalmol 1969;47:690-709.

152. Savino PJ, Glaser JS, Cassidy J. Retinal stroke: is the patient at risk? Arch Ophthalmol 1977;95:1185-1189.

153. Pfaffenbach DD, Hollenhorst RW. Morbidity and survivorship of patients with embolic cholesterol crystalization in the ocular fundus. Am J Ophthalmol 1973;75:66-75.

# CHAPTER 3

# Chiasmal Visual Loss

• • • • • • • • • • • • • • •

It has been estimated that 25% of all brain tumors occur in the chiasmal area, and of these almost one half produce an initial complaint of visual loss. Of the lesions causing chiasmal compression, pituitary tumors are the most frequent (50% to 55%), followed by craniopharyngiomas (20% to 25%), meningiomas (10%), and gliomas (7%).[1] The other causes of chiasmal compression, including aneurysm, are relatively rare. The major, and sometimes only, symptom produced by these gradually enlarging masses is progressive visual loss.

## Diagnosis of Chiasmal Syndrome

### SYMPTOMS OF CHIASMAL SYNDROME

**VISUAL LOSS.** Decreased vision is the primary symptom of chiasmal compression. Slowly growing neoplasms produce a gradual, insidious, painless visual loss that may progress for months or years before being discovered by the patient. It is decreased acuity and not the realization of a peripheral field constriction that usually prompts the patient with chiasmal compression to seek medical care. The pattern of visual field loss depends on the portion of the anterior visual pathway that is compromised by the mass lesion (see Signs of Chiasmal Syndrome). However, this pattern of visual field loss may not exactly correspond to the position of the mass in relation to the visual system (e.g., suprachiasmal mass lesions do not invariably produce inferior bitemporal visual field defects).

Rarely, visual loss may be rapidly progressive or even apoplectic in onset. An apoplectic loss of vision is highly suggestive of rapid expansion of a pituitary tumor because of infarction or hemorrhage (see Pituitary Apoplexy).

**DIPLOPIA.** Perichiasmal lesions may cause diplopia by two mechanisms. Double vision may result from ocular misalignment caused by lateral extension of the parachiasmal lesion into the cavernous sinus, producing dysfunction of the third, fourth, or sixth cranial nerve. A second form of diplopia is said to occur without obvious muscle paresis (nonparetic diplopia).[2] This has been dubbed the *hemifield slide phenomenon*.[3]

**HEADACHE.** Headache is a prominent complaint in patients with perichiasmal mass lesions. Hollenhorst and Younge[1] report that 13% of 1000 patients with pituitary tumors had headache as a presenting complaint. Elkington[4] recorded severe headache ·in one third of his 260 patients (11 had pituitary apoplexy), whereas another òne third complained of slight headache. The headache is usually frontal in location and attributed to stretching of the diaphragma sellae.

**ENDOCRINE DYSFUNCTION.** The endocrine abnormalities associated with chiasmal mass lesions are discussed under each individual entity.

## SIGNS OF CHIASMAL SYNDROME

Perimetry is the cornerstone on which rests the clinical diagnosis of chiasmal disorders. To understand the localizing value and clinical implications of chiasmal visual field defects, certain aspects of gross and microscopic fiber anatomy of the chiasm must be kept in mind.

The optic chiasm is formed by the confluence of the optic nerves. An average vertical distance of 10 mm separates the chiasm from the dorsum sellae and the pituitary fossa. Since chiasmal visual loss is observed only when the chiasm and its vascular supply are greatly compressed and distorted, pituitary lesions must have a substantial suprasellar extension before visual field defects are produced (Fig. 3-1). Small intrasellar lesions never produce visual field defects.

The chiasm does not bear a constant relationship to the pituitary gland. The body of the chiasm is situated over the pituitary in 80% of patients, over the tuberculum sellae (prefixed) in 9%, and over the dorsum sellae (postfixed) in

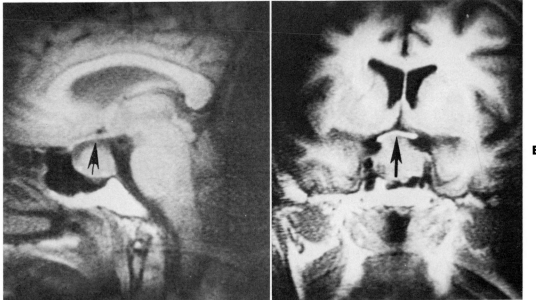

*Fig. 3-1.* Magnetic resonance imaging (MRI) of large pituitary tumor. Note how tumor compresses optic chiasm *(arrow)* in both the sagittal, **A,** and coronal, **B,** sections.

11%. Pituitary tumors are likely to produce a homonymous hemianopia in prefixed chiasms and a nerve fiber bundle defect in postfixed chiasms.[5] In a study of 1000 pituitary tumors, bitemporal defects were the most common (67%), whereas junction scotoma (29%), homonymous hemianopia (7%), and prechiasmal visual field loss (2%) occurred with less regularity.[1]

Trobe et al.[6] retrospectively reviewed 49 patients with parachiasmal mass lesions and found that all patients had either a relative afferent pupillary defect or a hemianopic defect in at least one eye. The junctional pattern of visual field loss was nearly as common (39%) as the classic bitemporal pattern (46%).

The chiasm is bordered laterally by the supraclinoid portion of the carotid arteries, superiorly by the anterior cerebral and anterior communicating arteries, and below by the posterior cerebral, basilar, and posterior communicating arteries.[5] Although these arteries (especially the carotid artery) can produce grooving of the chiasm, the production of visual field defects corresponding to these grooves is difficult to document.

The inferior nasal (crossed) retinal fibers are the first to decussate in the chiasm. A few fibers actually course forward to occupy a portion of the contralateral optic nerve (Wilbrand's knee). The superior nasal fibers cross mainly in the superoposterior portion of the chiasm. Almost the entire median portion of the chiasm is occupied by macular crossing fibers. No discrete macular bundle exists within the chiasm, although these fibers are mostly concentrated centrally and dorsally.[7]

Using the knowledge of chiasmal fiber anatomy, we can understand that essentially four types of visual field defects are possible with parachiasmal mass lesions. All of these visual field defects localize lesions to the optic chiasm. When any of them are encountered, directed imaging is required to establish the precise localization of the mass lesion.

**CENTRAL SCOTOMA (PRECHIASMAL COMPRESSION).** Visual loss is usually slowly progressive and manifests an optic neuropathy, but the visual field in the contralateral eye is full. This implies compression of the intracranial prechiasmal portion of the optic nerve. The causes are identical to the causes of a chiasmal syndrome, but the visual field differs either because the chiasm is postfixed or because the lesion is located anteriorly. The central scotoma is the most consistent perimetric finding in prechiasmal compressive lesions. The time course of the development of the optic neuropathy is as critical to diagnosis as the pattern of the visual field loss. In any patient with a slowly progressive optic neuropathy, a compressive etiology must be sought.

**JUNCTION SCOTOMA** (Fig. 3-2, *A*). Lesions that involve the intracranial optic nerve frequently extend backward toward the chiasm. Since the nasal crossing fibers from the fellow eye course anteriorly and inferiorly into the opposite optic nerve, the ipsilateral central scotoma may be accompanied by a contralateral, superotemporal visual field depression (junction syndrome). The detection of such a combination of visual field defects exquisitely localizes the lesion to the junction of the involved optic nerve and chiasm and should prompt investigation identical to that for a bitemporal hemianopia.

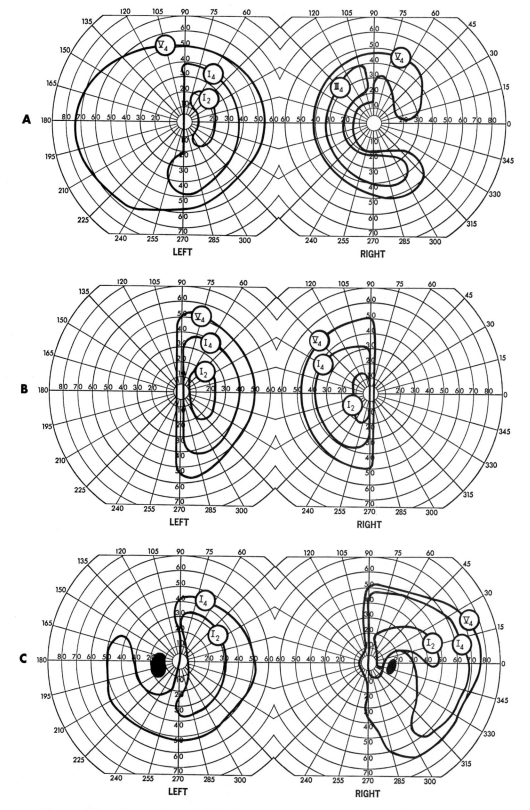

*Fig.* 3-2. Three forms of visual field loss with chiasmal compression. **A,** Junctional defect: right central scotoma with left temporal hemianopia due to lesion at junction of right optic nerve and chiasm. **B,** Bitemporal hemianopia: complete defect to largest isopters. **C,** Incongruous homonymous hemianopia: from involvement of right optic tract.

**BITEMPORAL HEMIANOPIA** (Fig. 3-2, *B*). The most obvious pattern of visual field loss involving the chiasm is a form of bitemporal hemianopia. In practice, however, an isolated bitemporal defect with no loss of central acuity in at least one eye is unusual. Visual loss occurs because the causative mass lesions are large and tend to distort the entire chiasm and compromise the optic nerves as well. Thus central acuity depression in one or both eyes is the rule; a pure bitemporal hemianopia with intact acuity is the exception.

Bitemporal hemianopias may be complete or incomplete, symmetric or asymmetric. At times the hemianopia may be exclusively paracentral and will be overlooked unless the central field is explored carefully, using small white or large red test objects. The examiner should not predict the mass lesion from the character of the hemianopia. For example, hemianopias that are denser inferiorly do not invariably imply compression by a suprachiasmal lesion.

**INCONGRUOUS HOMONYMOUS HEMIANOPIA** (Fig. 3-2, *C*). Extending posteriorly from the optic chiasm are the optic tracts. Lesions of the optic tracts most frequently are due to mass lesions, but demyelination or stroke may occur in this region.[8] Gross incongruity of an incomplete homonymous hemianopia is the hallmark of a tract lesion.[8,9]

The optic tract syndrome is most often produced by mass lesions,[8,9] which result in incomplete homonymous hemianopias and decreased vision ipsilateral to the mass lesion due to optic nerve or chiasmal compression. A relative afferent pupillary defect is detectable in the eye with poor vision. Nonmass lesions (trauma, infarct, demyelinating disease) affecting the optic tracts may produce hemianopia with normal acuity. In this instance the afferent pupillary defect will be ipsilateral to the temporal hemianopic defect (contralateral to the tract lesion) (see Chapter 1).[8,10-12]

**NYSTAGMUS.** A peculiar type of dissociated nystagmus termed *seesaw nystagmus* occasionally accompanies mass lesions in the chiasmal area. When seesaw nystagmus is present, a bitemporal hemianopia should be sought[13] (see Chapter 12).

# Imaging Recommendations for Parachiasmal Lesions

All patients with lesions considered to be located in the parachiasmal area must have imaging performed. We suggest that computed tomography (CT) scanning be performed only on high-resolution scanners, with views obtained in the axial and coronal planes with and without intravenous contrast administration. Magnetic resonance imaging (MRI) should be performed with a high–field strength superconducting system, preferably of 1.5 T. Views should be obtained in the axial, coronal, and sagittal planes. Gadolinium-DTPA, a paramagnetic substance, does not normally cross the intact brain barrier, but in pathologic lesions (e.g., ischemia or demyelination) the barrier becomes permeable and gadolinium accumulates in extravascular areas. The intravenous injection of gadolinium will enhance solid adenomas or meningiomas and facilitate documentation of cavernous sinus invasion.[14]

CT and MRI are equivalent in detecting the presence of lesions in the parachiasmal area, but MRI appears to better define anatomic relationships with surrounding structures.[15,16] CT appears to be superior to MRI in detecting bony abnormalities of the sellar floor and the presence of calcium in craniopharyngiomas or meningiomas. Vascular lesions are visualized more specifically with MRI, which can sometimes obviate the need for arteriography. Neuroradiologists now favor high-resolution MRI as the primary test for mass lesions in this region. We are in agreement with this and strongly favor high-resolution MRI as the first study in patients with suspected parachiasmal signs or symptoms.

Arteriography is largely unnecessary in the workup of patients with parachiasmal lesions. Transsphenoidal removal of a pituitary tumor may be accomplished safely without prior cerebral angiography. Those who still prefer to perform arteriography preoperatively do so for these reasons:

1. To be absolutely certain that the lesion is a pituitary tumor and not an aneurysm
2. To ascertain the position of the carotid arteries in relation to the planned operative field

## Specific Causes of Chiasmal Syndrome

### PITUITARY TUMORS

The prevalence of visual compromise with pituitary tumors varies from 30% to 96%,[1,17-19] depending on the primary orientation of the subspecialist studying the tumors. Endocrine abnormalities often occur before extrasellar extension produces visual loss. Thus reports from endocrine and neurosurgical sources show a lower prevalence of visual loss than series reported by ophthalmologists. The more liberal use of imaging has also contributed to the detection of pituitary tumors before they become visually symptomatic.

Visual loss typically progresses slowly. Frequently the patient has only vague complaints of visual difficulty whose true nature goes undetected until perimetry is performed. Although the progression of visual field defects is usually slow, a rather dramatic form of chiasmal syndrome is associated with apoplectic visual loss (called *pituitary apoplexy*).

**PITUITARY APOPLEXY.** Pituitary apoplexy is precipitated by the rapid expansion of a pituitary tumor due either to infarction or to hemorrhage in the tumor (Fig. 3-3). The exact mechanism for this event remains unknown. Rapid tumor growth outstripping its blood supply or compression of the tumor's vascular supply by the mass itself may cause ischemic necrosis of the tumor.[20,21]

In one series of 560 consecutive cases of pituitary adenoma, 51 (9.1%) patients had symptoms of pituitary apoplexy, with 38 of the events being classified as major (disturbances of consciousness, hemiparesis, loss of vision, or ocular motor palsy). Forty-two patients (7.5%) were verified at surgery to have hemor-

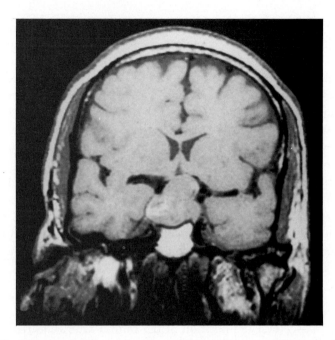

*Fig. 3-3.* MRI without gadolinium of patient with rapid onset of bilateral visual loss and right ophthalmoplegia. Large pituitary tumor compresses optic chiasm. Blood is seen as white area where tumor extends into right cavernous sinus.

rhaged into their tumors but had manifested no clinical symptoms of pituitary apoplexy.[22] With the use of modern imaging techniques, hemorrhage may be detected more frequently without a preceding dramatic clinical event. Ostrov et al.[23] diagnosed apoplexy clinically in only 3 of 12 patients with pituitary hemorrhage confirmed by imaging and at surgery. Yousem et al.[24] found the new onset of headache, visual field defects, or oculomotor cranial nerve dysfunction—the signs of pituitary apoplexy—in only 8 (44%) of 18 patients who had hemorrhage within a pituitary tumor demonstrated with MRI. Therefore pituitary apoplexy is an unusual clinical phenomenon, but its imaging characteristics are encountered more frequently.

**Symptoms of pituitary apoplexy.** *Headache* is usually of sudden onset and severe enough to be frequently mistaken for a ruptured aneurysm. Pain may be generalized or retrobulbar in location. *Double vision* may be due to unilateral or bilateral ophthalmoplegia. The third, fourth, and sixth cranial nerves are usually compromised in the cavernous sinus. *Subarachnoid hemorrhage* is not present in all patients with pituitary apoplexy. While grossly bloody cerebrospinal fluid (CSF) is the rule, xanthochromia, pleocytosis, or a normal CSF finding may be encountered. Headache, double vision, and subarachnoid hemorrhage should strongly suggest pituitary apoplexy especially in the setting of visual acuity or visual field loss.[25]

*Visual loss* does not occur in every patient with pituitary apoplexy. However, when vision is compromised, the patient may be blind bilaterally or manifest any of the patterns of chiasmal visual loss (see Fig. 3-2).

*Coma* was an almost constant finding in earlier publications dealing with pituitary apoplexy. It is now recognized that some patients may have a relative paucity of symptoms and still have undergone apoplexy.

**Diagnosis.** Patients whose presenting symptoms are headache, ophthalmoplegia, and signs of meningeal irritation are usually diagnosed as having a ruptured intracranial aneurysm. However, any patient with a preexisting pituitary tumor who develops these rapidly evolving symptoms must be considered to have pituitary apoplexy. While imaging almost invariably permits diagnosis of a pituitary tumor, even with high-resolution imaging no recognized pathognomonic signs of pituitary apoplexy have been identified.[26] Areas of hemorrhage within a pituitary tumor are best visualized with MRI, although hemorrhage may be unrecognized in the first few hours after apoplexy.[23] MRI is the diagnostic procedure of choice in suspected pituitary apoplexy.

**Contributing factors.** Several factors have been clearly implicated in precipitating pituitary apoplexy: radiation therapy,[27] trauma,[28] pregnancy,[25,29] and dynamic testing of anterior pituitary function.[30] The prevalence of apoplexy during hormonal therapy remains unknown. Magyar and Marshall[31] found that with the use of various ovulation-stimulating agents to induce pregnancy, 22 (30%) of their patients required surgery, radiation therapy, or both, for an enlarging pituitary tumor during the induced pregnancy or in the puerperium. Since their study predates high-resolution imaging of the chiasm, the data should be regarded as less than definitive.

**Treatment.** Corticosteroid replacement therapy is the first therapeutic maneuver in pituitary apoplexy. This is especially important if the patient is to be subjected to a variety of stressful neurodiagnostic procedures. Neurosurgical decompression of the anterior visual pathways should be performed expeditiously if vision is decreased. The transsphenoidal approach has become the procedure of choice in most centers.[32,33]

**ENDOCRINOLOGIC SIGNS AND SYMPTOMS OF PITUITARY TUMORS.** While visual symptoms are more common with endocrinologically inactive pituitary tumors, visual loss may be an initial complaint in all adenomas.[1,17] The endocrine changes of Cushing's disease usually prompt investigation long before the tumor achieves significant suprasellar extension, but about 37% of patients with acromegaly in one series had visual field defects.[1] About 70% of tumors in children and adolescents are endocrinologically active and are therefore usually detected prior to the onset of visual loss.[34]

The traditional cellular classification of pituitary tumors was based on light microscopic characteristics of the tumor's chief cellular component. Newer classifications of these cell types and tumors have been constructed using clinical hormonal criteria, as well as immunocytochemical and electromicroscopic techniques.

Pituitary tumors are now classified as being hormonally active or inactive. Four studies reviewed the relative prevalence of these tumor types[35-38] (Table 3-1). Extensive endocrine evaluation should be performed in the presence of all pituitary tumors. Deficiencies in thyroid and adrenocorticoid secretion must be

| TABLE 3-1 | *Relative Prevalence of Pituitary Tumors* | | | |
|---|---|---|---|---|
| Tumor type | Mukai[35] No. (%) | Challa et al.[36] No. (%) | Wilson[37] No. (%) | Scheithauer et al.[38] No. (%) |
| Secreting | | | | |
| Prolactin | 60 (40) | 7 (11.2) | 410 (41.0) | 24 (6.6) |
| Growth hormone | 13 (8.7) | 13 (20.9) | 195 (19.5) | 23 (6.6) |
| ACTH | 9 (6.0) | 15 (24.2) | 167 (16.7) | 91 (24.9) |
| Gonadotropin | 7 (4.7) | — | — | 32 (8.7) |
| TSH | — | — | 2 (0.2) | 4 (1.0) |
| Combined | 9 (6.0) | — | | 98 (26.8) |
| Nonsecreting | 52 (34.6) | 27 (43.5) | 226 (22.6) | 93 (25.4) |
| TOTAL | 150 | 62 | 1000 | 365 |

corrected before the patient has neurosurgical intervention. Those with prolactin-secreting tumors may be treated with dopaminergic agents (bromocriptine) (see Medical Treatment under Treatment of Pituitary Tumors).

**SPECIAL FORMS OF PITUITARY TUMORS**

**Nelson's syndrome.** Nelson's syndrome is characterized by acquired cutaneous hyperpigmentation, increased concentration of adrenocorticotropic hormone (ACTH), and pituitary tumor growth following total adrenalectomy for Cushing's disease.[39] The frequency with which these ACTH-producing tumors enlarge following adrenalectomy varies from approximately 10%[40] to 38% or higher[41] in adults and 25% in children.[42]

Any patient with Cushing's disease should have a high-resolution MRI scan of the sella turcica prior to adrenalectomy. Sequential visual field testing and MRI are recommended in these patients.

**"Malignant" pituitary adenomas.** Controversy continues as to the existence of a truly malignant pituitary adenoma. The presence of mitosis or abnormal-appearing cells does not necessarily imply malignancy. "Invasive pituitary adenoma" is said to be a more appropriate term.[43] These tumors destroy bone, escape from their capsule, invade the cavernous sinus and brain (causing cranial nerve palsies and seizures), and frequently produce elevated serum prolactin levels. True carcinomas of the pituitary, which are characterized by blood-borne metastases, are rare.

**Prolactin-secreting tumors.** Prolactin-secreting tumors account for approximately 35% of all pituitary adenomas.[37] Most of these tumors arise in lactotroph cells in the anterior lobe of the pituitary gland. Elevated prolactin levels that remain under 100 ng/ml are almost always produced by intrasellar microadenomas, which cause no neuro-ophthalmic signs or symptoms. When the prolactin exceeds 100 ng/ml, the serum levels tend to directly correspond to tumor size, with larger tumors producing higher serum prolactin levels. Levels over 1000 ng/ml almost always signify extrasellar extension of the tumor. All prolactin-secreting tumors, irrespective of size, may produce impotence in men and an amenorrhea-galactorrhea syndrome in women.

Prolactinomas may increase in size during pregnancy, causing at times a rapidly progressive chiasmal syndrome. Postpartum spontaneous recovery of visual function appears to be the rule,[44,45] but permanent visual loss may occur. Pregnancy does not necessarily adversely affect prolactinomas. Enlargement of microadenomas during pregnancy occurs in 1.6% to 5.5% of patients.[46-48] Symptomatic enlargment of macroadenomas is more frequent, being observed in approximately 15% of patients.[46,48] Therefore pregnant women with prolactinomas should be observed closely for visual loss that could signal tumor enlargement.

## TREATMENT OF PITUITARY TUMORS

**Surgery.** Transsphenoidal microsurgical removal of pituitary tumors has become the procedure of choice. This approach has significantly decreased the morbidity and mortality rates in patients with pituitary tumors.[37,49]

The relative and absolute indications and contraindications for transfrontal craniotomy or transsphenoidal surgery vary from surgeon to surgeon and need not be enumerated here. Large pituitary tumors, as well as smaller ones, may be removed via the transsphenoidal route with excellent results.[50]

Tumors with extensive extrasellar extension are difficult (or impossible) to excise totally, since 40% show microscopic dural invasion independent of the tumor type.[51] The goal of surgery in this situation should be to decompress the anterior visual pathways. Residual tumor may then be treated with radiation.

**Radiation therapy.** The role of routine adjunctive radiation in the treatment of pituitary tumors remains controversial. Modern imaging now permits sequential visualization of the original tumor bed to detect recurrence or regrowth of tumor. However, radiotherapy following incomplete transsphenoidal tumor removal is often used, since the recurrence rate of nonradiated tumors is higher than that of radiated tumors.[52-54] Ciric et al.[49] reported that incompletely removed tumor recurred in 9 (28%) of 32 patients not radiated postoperatively, but in only 4 (6%) of 67 patients who received postoperative radiation for pituitary macroadenomas.

The use of radiation as the *primary* treatment modality for pituitary tumors has certain disadvantages:

1. The beneficial effects of radiation are delayed; surgery results in immediate decompression of the anterior visual pathways.
2. The tissue type of the tumor and thus its radiosensitivity can only be ascertained by histologic examination. Epidermoid tumors or craniopharyngiomas can at times be indistinguishable from pituitary adenomas by imaging criteria.
3. Even radiosensitive tumors may have cystic components that are relatively radioresistant.
4. Deficiencies of pituitary hormone secretion develop in the years following radiotherapy especially when the radiotherapy is preceded by surgery, even if these hormones were secreted normally prior to radiation.[55] By contrast, selective adenomectomy may permit improvement of hypopituitarism in a substantial number of patients.[56]

5. Tumors, especially gliomas and sarcomas, may occur in the area irradiated.[57,58]

6. Radiation may produce delayed vasculopathy of the optic nerves or chiasm with subsequent visual loss and has been implicated as a contributing factor in pituitary apoplexy. Yet radiation does not appear to increase the incidence of cerebral infarction.[59]

To compare meaningfully the efficacy of surgery and radiation is difficult. Many patients treated with radiation alone are in poorer medical condition, and frequently their tumors have little to no suprasellar extension. Without doubt, the morbidity and mortality rate with radiation is lower than that with surgery. However, when visual loss is present, the rapid decompression of the optic nerves and chiasm achieved by surgery seems more reasonable. Visual improvement with radiation alone appears to be more likely in patients without severely impaired acuity, complete hemianopias, and diffuse optic atrophy.[60]

Because radiation therapy is not without complications, we do not advocate it when gross total removal of tumor has been accomplished. However, adjunctive radiation is given routinely when gross tumor remains on postoperative imaging studies.

**Medical treatment.** Bromocriptine is a welcome alternative to surgery and radiation in the therapy of the 35% of pituitary tumors that secrete prolactin. These tumors are susceptible to shrinkage with bromocriptine, an ergot derivative and dopamine agonist. The mechanism by which bromocriptine lowers prolactin levels and reduces tumor size remains unknown. Dopamine receptors are present on pituitary lactotrophs, and their stimulation (by ergot derivatives) probably causes decreased synthesis and release of prolactin. In addition, a direct (but yet unknown) effect on the hypothalamus likely occurs. In animals dopamine agents reduce mitotic activity of pituitary cells that are stimulated by estrogen.[61] Pathologic investigation of prolactinomas from 95 patients suggests that bromocriptine produces a reduction in size of individual tumor cells and cell loss secondary to necrosis.[62] A long-acting nonergot dopamine agonist (CV 205-502) has been effective, in initial clinical trials, in reducing serum prolactin levels and tumor size in 26 patients treated.[63]

Moster et al.[64] documented the progressive improvement of visual acuity and sustained resolution of visual field defects in 9 of 10 patients with macroprolactinomas treated only with bromocriptine. Visual improvement began within days of institution of therapy and was accompanied by a corresponding shrinkage of the tumor on CT scanning. This report agrees with MRI findings that maximum shrinkage of tumor volume appears to occur within 3 weeks of insitution of bromocriptine.[24] Unfortunately, not all prolactinomas respond to therapeutic doses of bromocriptine. Eight (15%) of 55 patients in one series proved to be refractory to this treatment.[65]

One difficulty with bromocriptine therapy is that it must be prolonged. The dose may be tapered without producing prolactin elevation or an increase in tumor size,[66] but only rare patients may have the drug withdrawn without tumor recurrence. A rarer but important complication during bromocriptine therapy is CSF rhinorrhea.[67,68]

## Management of Prolactinomas

1. Treat intrasellar microprolactinomas with prolactin levels <200 ng/ml primarily with either bromocriptine or transsphenoidal hypophysectomy.
2. Treat prolactinomas with levels >200 ng/ml primarily with bromocriptine. Surgical removal may be attempted when the tumor has decreased in size.
3. If postoperative prolactin levels do not return to normal, treat further with either radiotherapy or bromocriptine.

Primary transsphenoidal surgical removal of prolactinomas, instead of medical therapy, has its advocates.[37,69,70] The success rates, however, depend largely on tumor size and initial prolactin levels. Wilson[37] reported successful long-term remission of hyperprolactinoma by surgery alone in 30 (86%) of 35 patients with initial prolactin levels under 154 ng/ml and in tumors without suprasellar extension (microadenomas). This difference in the prolactin response to surgery according to tumor size and the initial level of serum prolactin was confirmed by Barrow et al.,[70] who found that postoperative tumor control rates decreased with serum prolactin levels over 200 ng/ml. Control became progressively poorer with higher initial serum prolactin levels.

Pretreatment with bromocriptine does not appear to affect surgical results. Hubbard et al.[71] found no difference in the surgical cure rate between patients whose serum prolactin normalized with bromocriptine and hyporesponders. Likewise, no increased incidence or extent of fibrosis or calcification was found at surgery in the treated patients.

Medical treatment of other hormonally active pituitary tumors remains investigational. Acromegaly has been treated with a somatostatin analog producing improvement of serum endocrinologic disturbances.[72,73] However, visible shrinkage of the mass lesion on CT scanning was appreciated in only 6 of 16 patients who had a therapeutic endocrinologic result. Unfortunately no visual information was provided in either report.[74,75]

**CAUSES OF RECURRENT VISUAL LOSS AFTER TREATMENT.** Irrespective of the treatment used, deterioration of vision or a worsening of the visual field defects may occur following the apparently successful treatment of a parachiasmal tumor. In this instance the following conditions should be considered.

**Tumor recurrence.** Recurrence or continued growth of treated pituitary adenoma must be considered as a cause of progressive visual loss. Hollenhorst and Younge[1] reported 213 recurrences in 781 patients following treatment of pituitary tumors.

In the pre-CT era diagnosis of tumor recurrence was dependent largely on the reappearance or progression of visual signs or symptoms. Muhr et al.[76] examined the CT scans of 25 asymptomatic patients 10 to 15 years after surgical treatment of pituitary tumors. Recurrence with suprasellar extension was found in six patients (25%). Interestingly, only three of the six patients had progressive visual field defects. This suggests that reliance on perimetry alone may result in drastic underestimation of tumor recurrence rates. Conversely, the tissue seen on CT scanning may represent residual tumor and not regrowth, since the patients reported had no immediate postoperative CT scans. In a second communication Muhr et al.[77] reported clinical recurrence or regrowth of pituitary adenomas up to 9 years following treatment. Therefore it appears that patients treated for pituitary tumors should have repeat perimetry and sequential imaging in perpetuity.

**Empty sella syndrome with chiasmal prolapse.** Successful treatment of pituitary tumors leaves the sella enlarged but now devoid of tumor and therefore "empty." Although it is often stated that the chiasm may prolapse into the enlarged empty sella with resultant visual field loss, documentation of improvement with surgery is thin. Some reported cases lack enough ophthalmologic documentation to be convincing, or other causes of visual loss (e.g., radionecrosis) are possible.[78] On the other hand, Decker and Carras[79] reported an isolated instance of chiasmal prolapse with preoperative and postoperative visual field documentation, showing dramatic visual improvement following elevation of the chiasm from within the sella.

Kaufman et al.[80] reviewed the visual findings in 3 of 24 patients with a primary and 8 patients with a secondary empty sella and MRI demonstration of intrasellar herniation of the suprasellar visual system (optic nerve, optic chiasm, optic tract). They found that the herniation was well seen with MRI but that progression of visual acuity or visual field loss was not inevitable. In fact, visual disturbances proved to be an unreliable indicator of herniation.

**Radiation injury to anterior visual pathways.** The onset of radiation damage typically occurs 12 to 24 months after radiation therapy has been completed (see Chapter 2) and may be signaled by a rather sudden and dramatic loss of visual function following months of sustained improvement.

Cumulative chiasmal radiation doses of 4500 to 5000 cGy per day do not produce this syndrome; however, chiasmal radionecrosis may occur even in this dose range if the daily fractions exceed 200 cGy.[81,82] Patients with acromegaly are said to be more likely to develop anterior visual pathway damage even with these otherwise well-tolerated doses.[83] However, a review of 25 acromegalic patients treated with radiotherapy did not reveal these patients to be at increased risk.[84]

The mechanism by which the visual defect is produced remains speculative. Direct radiation necrosis of the chiasm or necrosis secondary to an obliterative vasculopathy are the two theories most frequently advanced.

The patient who has the reappearance of chiasmal or prechiasmal visual loss months after radiation therapy must have an MRI scan. If no evidence of tumor recurrence or cyst formation in the suprasellar cistern is found, the diagnosis of optic nerve or chiasmal radiation necrosis should be entertained. High-resolution MRI with gadolinium-DTPA may demonstrate intrinsic enhancement of the optic nerves and chiasm caused by radiation. This radiation effect is distinguishable from residual tumor.[85] Corticosteroids alone or in combination with hyperbaric oxygen therapy may be beneficial in these patients.[86] However, a review of 13 patients treated in this mode showed no improvement of acuity or visual field.[87]

| TABLE 3-2 | *A Proposed Schedule for Follow-up Visual Field Testing in Patients with Pituitary Tumors* |
|---|---|

| Treatment | Visual field examination |
|---|---|
| Surgery alone | Immediately postoperatively |
| | At 3 months |
| | At 6-month intervals for 2 years |
| | Yearly up to 5 years |
| | Then every 2 years |
| Radiation alone | At the end of radiotherapy |
| | At 3-month intervals for 1 year |
| | Yearly up to 5 years |
| | Then every 2 years |
| Surgery and radiation | Immediately postoperatively |
| | At completion of radiotherapy |
| | At 6-month intervals for 1 year |
| | Yearly for 5 years |
| | Then every 2 years |
| Medical (bromocriptine) | Monthly in patients with visual field loss until visual field stabilizes |
| | During pregnancy, monthly for tumors of any size |
| | At 6-month intervals for 1 year |
| | Then yearly if bromocriptine dose is unchanged |

**FOLLOW-UP CARE IN PITUITARY TUMOR.** The ophthalmologist should determine the amount of change in visual function that has occurred as a result of treatment (Table 3-2). Return of vision following surgical decompression usually is rapid. In a small series Kayan and Earl[88] document return of acuity and visual field within 48 hours of decompression. However, the bulk of vision probably returns even earlier. Therefore, if possible, vision should be evaluated in the recovery room as soon as the patient can respond. If vision is poorer than the preoperative level, imaging should be obtained to rule out hematoma, air, or a migrated pituitary fossa muscle pack that may be compressing the chiasm. The first postoperative visual field may be done within days of surgery. If postoperative radiation is administered, perimetry should be repeated at the end of radiation. It is unusual for vision to deteriorate during postsurgical radiation therapy.

If, however, the original treatment is radiation alone, the visual field should be monitored at the completion of radiation therapy. Monitoring is needed because of the unlikely but real possibility of a radiation-induced tumor swelling, producing further visual loss or, on rare occasions, pituitary apoplexy.[27] Should apoplexy occur, immediate surgical evacuation of the tumor is required.

Bromocriptine is an accepted treatment for prolactin-secreting tumors (see Medical Treatment under Treatment of Pituitary Tumors). The optimal interval of visual field examination in these patients is unknown.

## CRANIOPHARYNGIOMA

Craniopharyngiomas arise from nests of squamous epithelial cells that are the remnants of Rathke's pouch that lie between the anterior and posterior lobes of the pituitary gland. They are found in children (13% of all intracranial tumors) more frequently than in adults (3% of all intracranial tumors). Craniopharyngiomas may be solid, cystic, or a combination of the two. The cysts are frequently filled with a thick viscous fluid and glistening cholesterol-like material.

The clinical manifestations of craniopharyngioma vary according to the time of life in which the tumor presents[89-93] (Table 3-3). In children under 15, visual difficulty and headache are the most frequent findings, with growth retardation or other endocrinologic disturbances also frequently recorded. Papilledema occurs in at least one half of the patients in this age group. In older patients visual loss is still of paramount importance, but papilledema is uncommon. Endocrinologic abnormalities occur as well, and about one third of patients in the older age group are demented or confused.

Visual field abnormalities are found in the majority of patients with craniopharyngioma. This slowly expanding, at times cystic, tumor produces compression and distortion of the chiasm and surrounding structures. Some form of a bitemporal hemianopia is the single most frequently detected abnormality; however, incongruous homonymous hemianopia of optic tract origin may be plotted as well.[8]

The diagnosis of craniopharyngioma is made on the basis of the clinical findings, the plotting of chiasmal or optic tract visual field defects, and imaging. CT is superior at revealing calcifications in the tumor, whereas MRI better delineates involvement of surrounding structures. CT and MRI both may be needed to diagnose craniopharyngioma[94] (Fig. 3-4), although most neuroradiologists favor MRI.

| TABLE 3-3 | *Clinical Signs and Symptoms in Craniopharyngioma* | | | | |
|---|---|---|---|---|---|
| | Banna et al.[89] | Matson and Crigler[92] | Kennedy and Smith[91] | Bartlett[90] | Stahnke et al.[93] |
| Children under age 15 | N = 57 | N = 57 | N = 19 | N = 30 | N = 28 |
|   Visual defects | 64% | 64% | 50% | 76% | 87% |
|   Papilledema | 31% | 31% | 45% | 73% | 13% |
|   Endocrine abnormalities | 94% | 47% | 43% | 46% | 40% |
|   Headache | 66% | 80% | 100% | — | 56% |
|   Vomiting | 50% | 34% | 65 | — | |
| Adults | N = 85 | | N = 26 | N = 55 | |
|   Visual defects | 80% | — | 94% | 74% | |
|   Endocrine abnormalities | 57% | — | 75% | 32% | |
| Dementia | 10% | — | 35% | 32% | |
|   Papilledema | 15% | — | 15% | 5% | |
|   Headache | 39% | — | 60% | — | |

The preferred treatment of craniopharyngioma still provokes debate. Although total excision alone results in a cure, most authorities believe it is rare to obtain total removal of these tumors, at least in adults,[95] and that it is dangerous to attempt it. Extensive subtotal surgery also has complications, with a mortality of 22.2% being reported in a series of 20 patients.[96]

Adjunctive postoperative radiation therapy reduces the recurrence rate after subtotal removal of craniopharyngioma. Manaka et al.[97] used extensive subtotal surgical removal plus radiotherapy to treat 45 of 125 patients; the other 80 patients had surgery alone. Median survival of the radiated group was greater than 10 years, compared with only 3.1 years for the nonradiated group. Five- and 10-year survival rates were 88.9% and 76% for the radiated group, and 34.9% and 27.1% for the nonradiated group, respectively.

Extensive subtotal excision followed by radiation therapy produced a remission rate of 91% in 74 patients reviewed by Baskin and Wilson.[95] In another study of 52 patients,[98] surgery and radiation also achieved the best local control.

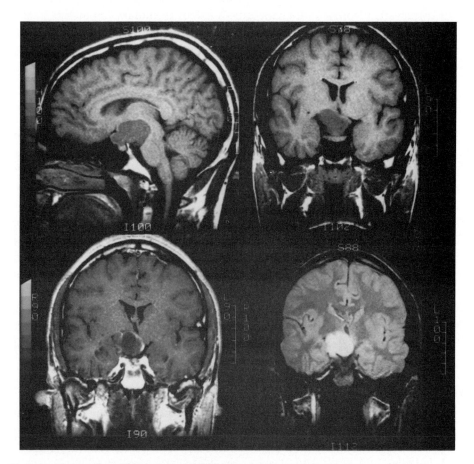

*Fig. 3-4.* Craniopharyngioma. Sagittal *(upper left)* and coronal *(upper right)* precontrast MRI show mass elevating and flattening optic chiasm. Gadolinium contrast MRI *(lower left)* shows some signal enhancement on borders of mass, and T2-weighted MRI *(lower right)* shows diffuse increase in signal intensity.

## Management of Craniopharyngioma

1. During surgery, attempt to remove as much tumor as possible while sparing vital structures.
2. If total tumor removal is accomplished, observe the patient with regular visual field examinations and sequential imaging, without postoperative radiation.
3. If subtotal removal of the tumor is performed, administer postoperative radiation to all patients over age 5.
4. If cyst formation is a prominent feature of a recurrence, consider intracavitary instillation therapy.

Cystic craniopharyngioma is notoriously difficult to treat. Therefore placing radioactive agents within the tumor cyst cavities has been attempted. Phosphorus-32 colloidal chromic phosphate and yttrium-90 silicate colloid[99] have improved vision or halted progressive visual loss in several small series.[100,101] Intracystic bleomycin appears to be a useful secondary adjunctive treatment of recurrent craniopharyngioma. This anticancer antibiotic has also been effective in preventing recurrences when used in patients with cystic tumors. However, patients with either solid or mixed craniopharyngiomas treated with intracavitary bleomycin have demonstrated tumor recurrence.[102]

Visual recovery following surgical treatment of craniopharyngioma appears less extensive than it is with pituitary tumors or meningiomas. Repka et al.[103] reviewed preoperative and immediate (within 1 month) postoperative visual function in 30 patients undergoing surgery for craniopharyngioma. Only 50% of patients with decreased vision improved postoperatively. The authors note that lost visual acuity or visual field defects did not improve after the first postoperative month.

Like pituitary tumors, craniopharyngiomas also may recur or regrow following surgery, even after so-called total excision.[104] Sequential perimetry therefore should be performed following treatment of craniopharyngiomas, although imaging has the distinct advantage of detecting recurrence before it becomes visually symptomatic. Rapid deterioration of visual function in the postoperative period may reflect reformation of a cyst within a craniopharyngioma or the shifting of residual tumor into the chiasmal area. This sudden loss of vision requires immediate imaging and further surgical decompression or cyst drainage if indicated.

## MENINGIOMA

Meningiomas of the suprasellar area (tuberculum sellae and planum sphenoidale) (Fig. 3-5) are slow-growing tumors that frequently remain undiagnosed before significant visual loss is sustained.[105] The visual loss may initially be monocular and is usually slowly progressive. Pregnancy rarely may stimulate the rapid growth of these tumors and accelerate the tempo of visual loss.[106,107]

The pattern of visual field deficit is dependent on the site of the tumor and the position of the chiasm (see Signs of Chiasmal Syndrome). Tumors involving

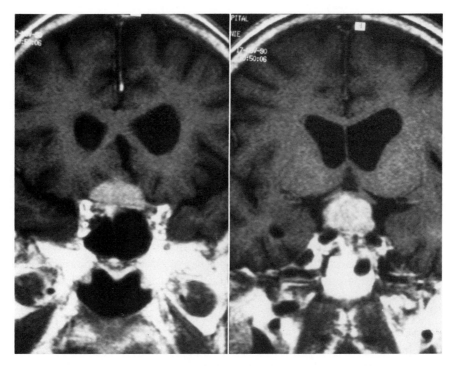

***Fig. 3-5.*** Meningioma. T1-weighted MRI coronal scan with gadolinium-DTPA shows *(left)* meningioma on tuberculum sellae. Meningioma on planum sphenoidale *(right)* elevates and compresses optic chiasm.

the optic foramen or medial sphenoid wing produce unilateral visual loss, whereas those of tuberculum sellae and diaphragma sellae tend to cause bilateral visual loss.[108] The optic disc is usually pale. Rarely, however, one disc may be elevated while its fellow is atrophic, a combination of findings that constitutes part of the Foster-Kennedy syndrome (which also includes anosmia and dementia).[109] The Foster-Kennedy syndrome is classically said to be due to a compressive optic neuropathy causing unilateral optic atrophy and hydrocephalus, which produces contralateral papilledema due to increased intracranial pressure. An alternate proposal implicates bilateral compressive optic neuropathy as the cause of all fundus findings in this syndrome.[110]

Imaging may reveal alteration in surrounding bone. Although not pathognomonic,[111] hyperostosis is a rather sensitive indicator of meningioma. CT scanning will reveal a mass lesion with various degrees of contrast enhancement depending on the vascularity of the tumor. Since meningiomas are frequently vascular, arteriography and preoperative embolization may be a prudent step prior to attempting neurosurgical extirpation of a highly vascular tumor.

The preferred treatment of meningioma is surgical removal. However, total removal may not always be possible or advisable if critical structures are densely encased by tumor. Andrews and Wilson[108] found the location of the tumor to be the most important predictor of visual outcome in 38 patients treated with microsurgical removal of meningioma. Tumors of the tuberculum sellae

### Management of Parachiasmal Meningiomas

1. Perform total resection when technically feasible.
2. If surrounding vital structures would have to be sacrificed for total resection, perform subtotal excision.
3. Perform sequential neuro-ophthalmic evaluation to detect postoperative progression.
4. Use postoperative radiation therapy for residual nonresectable tumor if signs or symptoms progress.

were most often resected completely, and postoperative visual recovery occurred most frequently in this group (8 of 11). Apparently, then, patients with meningiomas of the tuberculum sellae and those in whom the visual loss is diagnosed earliest have the best chance of visual return with microsurgery. Meningiomas of the medial sphenoid wing or diaphragma sellae in three patients could not be completely removed and did not show postoperative visual improvement. In this series 42% of patients had visual improvement postoperatively, 30% were unchanged, and 28% had worse visual function.

Rosenberg and Miller[112] found the duration of visual symptoms (and not tumor size or preoperative visual function) to be the most important determinant of visual outcome in a series of 20 patients with meningiomas. Unlike the study of Andrews and Wilson,[108] this series did not consider tumor location as a prognostic factor; therefore which factor is most important is not clear.

After reviewing the literature up to 1988, Salazar[113] concluded that radiation therapy was effective in the treatment of meningioma. CT evidence of meningioma necrosis after radiation therapy and pathologic verification in one case is also available.[114] In a group of 132 patients, a local 10-year control rate was highest in the patients who received a combination of surgery and irradiation as compared with either modality alone.[115]

Total surgical removal of meningioma is not always possible, and overly aggressive attempts may result in visual and neurologic morbidity or mortality.

We do not recommend radiation following subtotal excision of meningioma unless progression occurs. Meningiomas are typically slow-growing tumors that often take years to regrow. Under these circumstances we believe the potential risks of radiation vasculopathy outweigh the benefit of any retardation of the meningioma's growth.

## GLIOMA

*Optic glioma* is a term that has been applied to gliomatous (grade I or II astrocytoma) infiltration of one or both optic nerves and to involvement of the optic chiasm, hypothalamus, optic tract, and third-ventricle and periventricular structures. These tumors occur in children below age 10. Since the natural history of the disorder is far from clear, the efficacy of treatment remains debatable.

Patients with gliomas of the optic nerve alone seem to have a much better prognosis for life and lack of disease progression than patients with chiasmal involvement. The mortality rate associated with optic nerve glioma is estimated at 14%; the mortality rate associated with chiasmal glioma varies from 47% in uncomplicated glioma to 77% when glioma is accompanied by hydrocephalus, to 91% when hypothalamic involvement occurs.[116] In essence it is the location rather than the cytologic characteristics that affects prognosis.[117,118] These histologically benign tumors become functionally "malignant" when vital structures are involved.

Miller et al.[119] have suggested a topographic division into three groups: (1) glioma of only one optic nerve, (2) glioma of the optic chiasm, and (3) glioma with involvement of the hypothalamus and third-ventricle structures. The first two groups (anterior tumors) are associated with a favorable prognosis, whereas the latter group (posterior tumors) has a poorer but not invariably fatal outcome.

Optic glioma is frequently associated with neurofibromatosis. The exact prevalence of neurofibromatosis in patients with optic glioma is unknown. Also, the information that is available does not use MRI. Despite this limitation, the risk of a patient with glioma having neurofibromatosis is from 10% to 50%.[120] However, among patients with neurofibromatosis as many as 32% have gliomas of the anterior visual pathways on imaging.[121] CT scanning alone underestimates the prevalance of glioma. In one study CT showed only a 15% prevalence of glioma in 65 children with neurofibromatosis type I.[122] Therefore an imaging diagnosis of glioma should be made only by using MRI with gadolinium[121] (Fig. 3-6). CT scanning alone is not adequate to exclude the presence of glioma. Imaging appearance does not correlate with the degree of visual dysfunction.

The treatment of chiasmal gliomas is a controversial issue. Hoyt and Baghdassarian[123] described these lesions as benign and nonprogressive. An update of these same 28 patients 25 years later[124] showed that 16 patients had died, 5 from chiasmal glioma. The authors state that "the prognosis for survival in patients with chiasmal glioma is not as good as it was thought to be in 1969."

Radiation appears to be an effective treatment for chiasmal gliomas, although no controlled data are available. Seven of 14 radiated patients with chiasmal glioma had prolongation of life and maintenance of visual function with a follow-up of up to 20 years.[125] In a study of 25 biopsy-proven chiasmal gliomas treated with radiation therapy, survival was 96%, 90%, and 90% at 5, 10, and 15 years, respectively. The progression-free survival was 87% at 5, 10, and 15 years. Vision stabilized or improved in 86% of patients.[126] In another study, however, 62 similar patients had a long-term survival rate of only 50%[127] with a 13-year mean follow-up. Pierce et al.[128] reported 100% survival and 88% freedom from disease progression with a median follow-up of 6 years in 24 irradiated children who all presented with visual, other clinical, or radiologic evidence of disease progression.

Packer et al.[129] documented progressive neurologic or visual deterioration in 10 of 18 patients treated with radiation after a median follow-up of 6 years. Actuarial survival for this group was 89% and 60% at 5 and 10 years, respec-

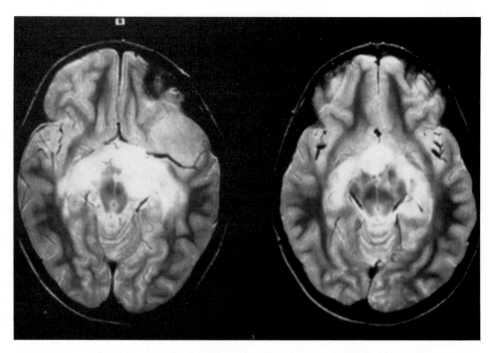

*Fig.* *3-6.* Two patients with chiasmal gliomas. Axial T2-weighted MRI without contrast shows mass lesion in chiasmal area. White streaming extends into optic tracts bilaterally.

tively. A major concern raised in this study was the intellectual deficits noted in 5 of 17 survivors and presumed to be due to radiation to the young brain. Radiotherapy therefore appears to temporarily stabilize visual and neurologic progression in about 50% of patients. However, the high incidence of intellectual impairment in patients who receive radiation in the first years of life may limit its usefulness.

Chemotherapy for chiasmal gliomas shows promise.[130] Packer et al.[131] treated 24 children with actinomycin D and vincristine without radiotherapy. All were alive, and 15 (62.5%) of the 24 had remained free of progressive disease and had received no other therapy after a median of 4.3 years. Intelligence testing showed no deterioration, indicating that chemotherapy may offer a safe alternative to radiotherapy in these children.[131]

A more aggressive form of glioma is found in adults. The syndrome occurs in middle-aged patients with a possible male predominance and is characterized by rapid visual loss mimicking optic neuritis. The visual loss progresses to total blindness within 5 to 6 weeks and is invariably fatal if untreated. Funduscopic examination shows disc edema, which may progress to complete arterial and venous occlusion.

Histopathologically the tumor involves the entire anterior optic pathway and appears to spread via the subpial and dural routes. Imaging revealing thickened optic nerves or chiasm has allowed antemortem diagnosis of these tumors, which previously were rarely diagnosed before death.[132,133] Of two such patients

*Management of Optic Gliomas*

Acknowledging that there is no good comparative randomized series evaluating these treatment options, we make the following recommendations in the management of gliomas of the anterior visual pathways:

1. Use MRI with gadolinium to define the extent of tumor.
2. No biopsy is needed if imaging features are typical, the tumor is intraaxial, or the patient has neurofibromatosis.
3. If the tumor is confined to the optic nerve, no treatment is indicated regardless of visual signs. Surgery may be considered for unsightly proptosis or exposure keratitis.
4. Provide radiation therapy for chiasmal/hypothalamic tumor in children over 5 years of age if clinical or MRI evidence of progression is present. If the effects on vision cannot be adequately assessed, we favor treating the patient.
5. Give chemotherapy in lieu of radiation to children under 5 years of age.
6. Surgery is recommended for any chiasmal lesion with an exophytic component.
7. Perform shunting procedures in the presence of obstructive hydrocephalus.

so diagnosed, one has survived for 18 months with visible shrinkage of the tumor on CT scanning following radiotherapy and chemotherapy.[134]

## ANEURYSM

Aneurysmal dilatation of the vessels of the circle of Willis is an infrequent cause of chiasmal syndrome.[135] The combination of imaging and cerebral arteriography serves to establish the origin of the aneurysm, as well as the extent of its mass effect.

## INFECTION

Infection of the sphenoid sinus or pituitary abscess may mimic pituitary tumors.

*Mucoceles* in the posterior ethmoid and sphenoid sinuses may produce slowly progressive visual loss or, even less frequently, sudden visual loss similar to pituitary apoplexy. Chiasmal syndromes from sphenoid mucoceles, while they do exist, are rare. Mucoceles more often produce unilateral or bilateral optic nerve involvement.[136]

*Pituitary abscess* is uncommon but of importance because it is curable if promptly diagnosed and treated. Clinical presentation may be signs of a chiasmal syndrome or meningitis. In almost all instances the sellar area is abnormal on imaging. Interestingly, abscess formation may occur in a preexisting tumor in the area.[137]

The source of the infection is not always easily identified. Cultures are said to be "sterile" in more than half of the patients.[138] It has been proposed, however, that this may be due to involvement by anaerobic organisms.[137]

Transsphenoidal drainage of the abscess combined with the appropriate antibiotic coverage is the treatment of choice. The prognosis is guarded, since the overall mortality is 28%, increasing to 45% if meningitis develops.[137]

## MISCELLANEOUS LESIONS

Rarer lesions in the parachiasmal area that may produce a chiasmal syndrome include dermoid and epidermoid tumors, ectopic pinealomas, chordoma, inflammatory masses, metastatic tumors, or vascular malformations.

## OTHER, NONTUMOROUS CAUSES

When a chiasmal visual field abnormality is noted, the physician should go to all reasonable lengths to exclude a mass lesion. Rarely, however, a mass is not present, and the visual defect is due to one of the following causes.

**TRAUMA.** Traumatic chiasmal syndrome is an uncommon occurrence seen following severe frontal head trauma. This condition is usually accompanied by skull fracture and associated neurologic signs and symptoms, including diabetes insipidus.[139]

**INFLAMMATION.** Inflammatory optic neuropathies rarely may be associated with a superior temporal visual depression in the fellow eye (junction scotoma). Bitemporal hemianopias have been reported with demyelinating disease,[140,141] sarcoidosis,[142] and viral infection.[143] MRI may reveal an enlarged chiasm, but extrinsic tumors are readily excluded.

**CHIASMAL ARACHNOIDITIS.** Chiasmal arachnoiditis is characterized by inflammatory changes in the arachnoid of the chiasm, producing chiasmal visual field defects. This entity enjoyed wide acceptance in the early part of this century, but with more sophisticated neuroradiologic techniques and a better understanding of optic nerve dysfunction, the significance of this disorder as a frequent cause of visual loss is questionable. Nonetheless, chiasmal adhesions rarely can follow tuberculous meningitis[144] and subarachnoid hemorrhage.[145]

Several reports[146,147] have proposed that chiasmal arachnoiditis occurs frequently but is often overlooked. However, the authenticity of the diagnosis of this disorder is questionable in many of the reported cases. Close review suggests alternative explanations for the visual loss in many of these patients.

**TRACTION.** Prolapse of the chiasm into a primary empty sella has been implicated as a cause of chiasmal visual loss, but we are not convinced of a cause-and-effect relationship. The primary empty sella syndrome (ESS) probably results from extension of the subarachnoid space into the sella through a congenitally incompetent diaphragma sellae.

Isolated reports of visual loss due to herniation of the suprasellar visual apparatus into a primary empty sella have been recorded.[148,149] Mortara and Norrell[150] state that visual loss with a primary deficient sellar diaphragm produced by the pushing down or kinking of an optic nerve or chiasm was found in 5 of their 10 patients. However, MRI with neuro-ophthalmologic correlation suggests that this cause-and-effect relationship is much less frequent, being seen in only 3 (12.5%) of 24 patients.[80]

An association does exist between ESS and pseudotumor cerebri. In one report, four of eight patients with both entities had visual field loss. However, all patients with visual field defects had papilledema. One patient was said to have a "bitemporal hemianopia," but no visual fields were shown. The other field defects could all be attributed to the disc edema and not to ESS with chiasmal prolapse. No patient with ESS without papilledema had a visual field defect.[151]

Buckman et al.[152] described an alcoholic patient who had a subtle bitemporal hemianopia attributed to an empty sella. Craniotomy was not performed; therefore proof of chiasmal prolapse is lacking.

The prevalence of ESS as determined at autopsy is approximately 5%.[153] If ESS is a significant cause of visual loss, we would expect to see visual loss more frequently. Thus diagnosis of an empty sella as the cause of chiasmal visual field loss should be made with great caution. In most instances the true etiology is an undetected mass lesion.

## REFERENCES

1. Hollenhorst RW, Younge BR. Ocular manifestations produced by adenomas of the pituitary gland: analysis of 1000 cases. In: Kohler PO, Ross GT, eds. Diagnosis and treatment of pituitary tumors. Amsterdam: Excerpta Medica, 1973:53-68.
2. Nachtigäller H, Hoyt WF. Störungen des Seheindruckes bei bitemporaler Hemianopsie und Verschiebung der Sehachsen. Klin Monatsbl Augenheilkd 1970;156:821-36.
3. Kirkham TH. The ocular symptomatology of pituitary tumours. Proc R Soc Med 1972;65:517-8.
4. Elkington SG. Pituitary adenoma: preoperative symptomatology in a series of 260 patients. Br J Ophthalmol 1968;52:322-8.
5. Bergland RM, Ray BS, Torack RM. Anatomical variations in the pituitary gland and adjacent structures in 225 human autopsy cases. J Neurosurg 1968;28:93-9.
6. Trobe JD, Tao AH, Schuster JJ. Perichiasmal tumors: diagnostic and prognostic features. Neurosurgery 1984;15:391-9.
7. Hoyt WF, Luis O. The primate chiasm. Arch Ophthalmol 1963;70:69.
8. Savino PJ, Paris M, Schatz NJ et al. Optic tract syndrome: a review of 21 patients. Arch Ophthalmol 1978;96:656-63.
9. Newman SA, Miller NR. Optic tract syndrome: neuro-ophthalmologic considerations. Arch Ophthalmol 1983;101:1241-50.
10. Bell RA, Thompson HS. Relative afferent pupillary defect in optic tract hemianopias. Am J Ophthalmol 1978;85:538-40.
11. O'Connor PS, Kasdon D, Tredici TJ, et al. The Marcus Gunn pupil in experimental tract lesions. Ophthalmology 1982;89:160-4.
12. Anderson DR, Trobe JD, Hood TW, et al. Optic tract injury after anterior temporal lobectomy. Ophthalmology 1989;96:1065-70.
13. Druckman R, Ellis P, Kleinfeld J, et al. Seesaw nystagmus. Arch Ophthalmol 1966;76:668-75.
14. Nakamura T, Schörner W, Bittner RC, et al. The value of paramagnetic contrast agent gadolinium-DTPA in the diagnosis of pituitary adenomas. Neuroradiology 1988;30:481-6.
15. Nicholas DA, Laws ER, Houser OW, et al. Comparison of magnetic resonance imaging and computed tomography in the preoperative evaluation of pituitary adenomas. Neurosurgery 1988;22:380-5.
16. Karnaze MG, Sartor K, Winthrop JD, et al. Suprasellar lesions: evaluation with MR imaging. Radiology 1986;161:77-82.
17. Chamlin M, Davidoff LM, Feiring EH.

Ophthalmologic changes produced by pituitary tumors. Am J Ophthalmol 1955;40:353-68.

18. Miller NR. Walsh and Hoyt's clinical neuro-ophthalmology, vol 3. 4th ed. Baltimore: Williams & Wilkins, 1988: 1447.

19. Anderson D, Faber P, Marcovitz S, et al. Pituitary tumors and the ophthalmologist. Ophthalmology 1983; 90:1265-70.

20. Brougham M, Heusner AP, Adams RD. Acute degenerative changes in adenomas of the pituitary body—with special reference to pituitary apoplexy. J Neurosurg 1950;7:421-39.

21. Rovit RL, Fein JM. Pituitary apoplexy: a review and reappraisal. J Neurosurg 1972;37:280-8.

22. Wakai S, Fukushima T, Teramoto A, et al. Pituitary apoplexy: its incidence and clinical significance. J Neurosurg 1981;55:187-93.

23. Ostrov SG, Quencer RM, Hoffman JC, et al. Hemorrhage within pituitary adenomas: how often associated with pituitary apoplexy syndrome? Am J Neuroradiol 1989;10:503-10.

24. Yousem DM, Arrington JA, Zinreich SJ, et al. Pituitary adenomas: possible role of bromocriptine in intratumoral hemorrhage. Radiology 1989; 170:239-43.

25. David NJ, Gargano FP, Glaser JS. Pituitary apoplexy in clinical perspective. In: Glaser JS, Smith JL, eds. Neuro-ophthalmology: symposium of the University of Miami and the Bascom Palmer Eye Institute, vol 8. St Louis: Mosby–Year Book, 1975:140-65.

26. Post MJD, David NJ, Glaser JS, et al. Pituitary apoplexy: diagnosis by computed tomography. Radiology 1980; 134:665-70.

27. Weisberg LA. Pituitary apoplexy: association of degenerative change in pituitary adenoma with radiotherapy and detection by cerebral computed tomography. Am J Med 1977;63:109-15.

28. Holness RO, Ogundimu FA, Langille RA. Pituitary apoplexy following closed head trauma: case report. J Neurosurg 1983;59:677-9.

29. Van Wagenen WP. Haemorrhage into a pituitary tumor following trauma. Ann Surg 1932;95:625-8.

30. Arafah BM, Taylor HC, Salazar R, et al. Apoplexy of a pituitary adenoma after dynamic testing with gonadotropin-releasing hormone. Am J Med 1989;87:103-5.

31. Magyar DM, Marshall JR. Pituitary tumors and pregnancy. Am J Obstet Gynecol 1978;132:739-51.

32. Conomy JP, Ferguson JH, Brodkey JS, et al. Spontaneous infarction in pituitary tumors: neurologic and therapeutic aspects. Neurology 1975;25: 580-7.

33. Kosary IZ, Braham J, Tadmor R, et al. Trans-sphenoidal surgical approach in pituitary apoplexy. Neurochirurgia 1976;19:55-8.

34. Richmond IL, Wilson CB. Pituitary adenomas in childhood and adolescence. J Neurosurg 1978;49:163-8.

35. Mukai K. Pituitary adenomas: immunocytochemical study of 150 tumors with clinicopathologic correlation. Cancer 1983;52:648-53.

36. Challa VR, Marshall RB, Hopkins MB III, et al. Pathobiologic study of pituitary tumors: report of 62 cases with a review of the recent literature. Hum Pathol 1985;16:873-84.

37. Wilson CB. A decade of pituitary microsurgery: the Herbert Olivecrona lecture. J Neurosurg 1984;61:814-33.

38. Scheithauer BW, Kovacs KT, Laws ER Jr, et al. Pathology of invasive pituitary tumors with special reference to functional classification. J Neurosurg 1986;65:733-44.

39. Nelson DH, Meakin JW, Dealy JB Jr, et al. ACTH-producing tumor of the pituitary gland. N Engl J Med 1958; 259:161-4.

40. Moore TJ, Dluhy RG, Williams GH, et al. Nelson's syndrome: frequency, prognosis, and effect of prior pituitary irradiation. Ann Intern Med 1976;85: 731-4.

41. Cohen KL, Noth RH, Pechinski T. Incidence of pituitary tumors following adrenalectomy: a long-term follow-up of patients treated for Cushing's disease. Arch Intern Med 1978;138:575-9.

42. Hopwood NJ, Kenny FM. Incidence of Nelson's syndrome after adrenalectomy for Cushing's disease in children: results of a nationwide survey. Am J Dis Child 1977;131:1353-6.

43. Lundberg PO, Drettner B, Hemmingsson A, et al. The invasive pituitary adenoma: a prolactin-producing tumor. Arch Neurol 1977;34:742-9.

44. Fujimoto M, Yoshino E, Mizukawa N, et al. Spontaneous reduction in size of prolactin-producing adenoma after delivery: case report. J Neurosurg 1985;63:973-4.

45. Miller NR. Walsh and Hoyt's clinical neuro-ophthalmology, vol 3. 4th ed. Baltimore: Williams & Wilkins, 1988: 1468.

46. Molitch ME. Pregnancy and the hyperprolactinemic woman. N Engl J Med 1985;312:1364-70.

47. Gemzell C, Wang CF. Outcome of pregnancy in women with pituitary adenoma. Fertil Steril 1979;31:363-72.

48. Melmed S, Braunstein GD, Chang RJ, et al. Pituitary tumors secreting growth hormone and prolactin. Ann Intern Med 1986;105:238-53.

49. Ciric I, Mikhael M, Stafford T, et al. Transsphenoidal microsurgery of pituitary macroadenomas with long-term follow-up results. J Neurosurg 1983;59:395-401.

50. Orr LS, Schatz NJ, Savino PJ, et al. Transsphenoidal surgery for large pituitary tumors. In: Glaser JS, ed: Neuro-ophthalmology: symposium of the University of Miami and the Bascom Palmer Eye Institute, vol 9. St Louis: Mosby–Year Book, 1977:128-39.

51. Selman WR, Laws ER Jr, Scheithauer BW, et al. The occurrence of dural invasion of pituitary adenomas. J Neurosurg 1986; 64:402-7.

52. Sheline GE. Treatment of chromophobe adenomas of the pituitary gland and acromegaly. In: Kohler PO, Ross GT, eds. Diagnosis and treatment of pituitary tumors. Amsterdam: Excerpta Medica, 1973:201-16.

53. Ray BS, Patterson RH Jr. Surgical experience with chromophobe adenomas of the pituitary gland. J Neurosurg 1971;34:726-9.

54. Grigsby PW, Simpson JR, Fineberg B. Late regrowth of pituitary adenomas after irradiation and/or surgery. Cancer 1989;63:1308-12.

55. Snyder PJ, Fowble BF, Schatz NJ, et al. Hypopituitarism following radiation therapy of pituitary adenomas. Am J Med 1986;81:457-62.

56. Arafah BM. Reversible hypopituitarism in patients with large nonfunctioning pituitary adenomas. J Clin Endocrinol Metab 1986;62:1173-9.

57. Hufnagel TJ, Kim JH, Lesser R, et al. Malignant glioma of the optic chiasm eight years after radiotherapy for prolactinoma. Arch Ophthalmol 1988;106: 1701-5.

58. Liwnicz BH, Berger TS, Liwnicz RG, et al. Radiation-associated gliomas: a report of four cases and analysis of postradiation tumors of the central nervous system. Neurosurgery 1985; 17:436-45.

59. Flickinger JC, Nelson PB, Taylor FH, et al. Incidence of cerebral infarction after radiotherapy for pituitary adenoma. Cancer 1989;63:2404-8.

60. Rush SC, Kupersmith MJ, Lerch I, et al. Neuro-ophthalmological assessment of vision before and after radiation therapy alone for pituitary macroadenomas. J Neurosurg 1990;72:594-9.

61. Thorner MO, Martin WH, Rogol AD, et al. Rapid regression of pituitary prolactinomas during bromocriptine treatment. J Clin Endocrinol Metab 1980;51:438-45.

62. Mori H, Mori S, Saitoh Y, et al. Effects of bromocriptine on prolactin-secreting pituitary adenomas. Cancer 1985; 56:230-8.

63. Vance ML, Lipper M, Kilbanski A, et al. Treatment of prolactin-secreting pituitary macroadenomas with the long-acting non-ergot dopamine agonist CV 205-502. Ann Intern Med 1990;112:668-73.

64. Moster ML, Savino PJ, Schatz NJ, et al. Visual function in prolactinoma patients treated with bromocriptine. Ophthalmology 1985;92:1332-41.

65. Pellegrini I, Rasolonjanahary R, Gunz G, et al. Resistance to bromocriptine

in prolactinomas. J Clin Endocrinol Metab 1989;69:500-9.

66. Liuzzi A, Dallabonzana D, Oppizzi G, et al. Low doses of dopamine agonists in the long-term treatment of macro-prolactinomas. N Engl J Med 1985; 313:656-9.

67. Holness RO, Shlossberg AH, Heffernan LPM. Cerebrospinal fluid rhinorrhea caused by bromocriptine therapy of prolactinoma. Neurology 1984; 34:111-3.

68. Kok JG, Bartelink AKM, Schulte BPM, et al. Cerebrospinal fluid rhinorrhea during treatment with bromocriptine for prolactinoma. Neurology 1985; 35:1193-5.

69. Parl FF, Cruz VE, Cobb CA, et al. Late recurrence of surgically removed prolactinomas. Cancer 1986;57:2422-6.

70. Barrow DL, Mizuno J, Tindall GT. Management of prolactinomas associated with very high serum prolactin levels. J Neurosurg 1988;68:554-8.

71. Hubbard JL, Scheithauer BW, Abboud CF, et al. Prolactin-secreting adenomas: the preoperative response to bromocriptine treatment and surgical outcome. J Neurosurg 1987;67:816-21.

72. Lamberts SWJ, Uitterlinden P, Verschoor L, et al. Long-term treatment of acromegaly with the somatostatin analogue SMS. N Engl J Med 1985; 313:1576-80.

73. Pieters GFFM, van Liessum PA, Smals AGH, et al. Long-term treatment of acromegaly with Sandostatin (SMS 201-995): normalization of most anomalous growth hormone responses. Acta Endocrinol Suppl 1987;286:9-18.

74. Chiodini PG, Cozzi R, Dallabonzana D, et al. Medical treatment of acromegaly with SMS 201-995, a somatostatin analog: a comparison with bromocriptine. J Clin Endocrinol Metab 1987;64:447-53.

75. Lamberts SWJ, Uitterlinden P, del Pozo E. SMS 201-995 induces a continuous decline in circulating growth hormone and somatomedin-C levels during therapy of acromegalic patients for over two years. J Clin Endocrinol Metab 1987;65:703-10.

76. Muhr C, Bergström K, Hugosson R, et al. Pituitary adenomas: computed tomography and clinical evaluation in a follow-up after surgical treatment. Eur Neurol 1980;19:171-9.

77. Muhr C, Bergström K, Enoksson P, et al. Follow-up study with computerized tomography and clinical evaluation 5 to 10 years after surgery for pituitary adenoma. J Neurosurg 1980; 53:144-8.

78. Olson DR, Guiot G, Derome P. The symptomatic empty sella: prevention and correction via the transsphenoidal approach. J Neurosurg 1972;37: 533-7.

79. Decker RE, Carras R. Transsphenoidal chiasmapexy for correction of posthypophysectomy traction syndrome of the optic chiasm: case report. J Neurosurg 1977;46:527-9.

80. Kaufman B, Tomsak RL, Kaufman BA, et al. Herniation of the suprasellar visual system and third ventricle into empty sellae: morphologic and clinical considerations. AJR Am J Roentgenol 1989;152:597-608.

81. Harris JR, Levene MB. Visual complications following irradiation for pituitary adenomas and craniopharyngiomas. Radiology 1976;120:167-71.

82. Aristizabal S, Caldwell WL, Avila J. The relationship of time-dose fractionation factors to complications in the treatment of pituitary tumors by irradiation. Int J Radiat Oncol Biol Phys 1977;2:667-73.

83. Atkinson AB, Allen IV, Gorden DS, et al. Progressive visual failure in acromegaly following external pituitary irradiation. Clin Endocrinol 1979;10: 469-79.

84. Dowsett RJ, Fowble B, Sergott RC, et al. Results of radiotherapy in the treatment of acromegaly: lack of ophthalmologic complications. Int J Radiat Oncol Biol Phys 1990;19:453-9.

85. Guy J, Mancuso A, Beck R, et al. Radiation-induced optic neuropathy: a magnetic resonance imaging study. J Neurosurg 1991;74:426-32.

86. Guy J, Schatz NJ. Hyperbaric oxygen in the treatment of radiation-induced optic neuropathy. Ophthalmology 1986;93:1083-8.

87. Roden D, Bosley TM, Fowble B, et al. Delayed radiation injury to the retrobulbar optic nerves and chiasm: clinical syndrome and treatment with hyperbaric oxygen and corticosteroids. Ophthalmology 1990;97:346-51.

88. Kayan A, Earl CJ: Compressive lesions of the optic nerves and chiasm: pattern of recovery of vision following surgical treatment. Brain 1975;98:13.

89. Banna M, Hoare RD, Stanley P, et al. Craniopharyngioma in children. J Pediatr 1973;83:781-5.

90. Bartlett JR. Craniopharyngiomas—a summary of 85 cases. J Neurol Neurosurg Psychiatry 1971;34:37-41.

91. Kennedy HB, Smith RJS. Eye signs in craniopharyngioma. Br J Ophthalmol 1975;59:689-95.

92. Matson DD, Crigler JF Jr. Management of craniopharyngioma in childhood. J Neurosurg 1969;30:377-90.

93. Stahnke N, Grubel G, Lagenstein I, et al. Long-term follow-up of children with craniopharyngioma. Eur J Pediatr 1984;142:179-85.

94. Freeman MP, Kessler RM, Allen JH, et al. Craniopharyngioma: CT and MR imaging in nine cases. J Comput Assist Tomogr 1987;11:810-4.

95. Baskin DS, Wilson CB. Surgical management of craniopharyngiomas: a review of 74 cases. J Neurosurg 1986;65:22-7.

96. Symon L, Sprich W. Radical excision of craniopharyngioma: results in 20 patients. J Neurosurg 1985;62:174-81.

97. Manaka S, Teramoto A, Takakura K. The efficacy of radiotherapy for craniopharyngioma. J Neurosurg 1985;62:648-56.

98. Wen BC, Hussey DH, Staples J, et al. A comparison of the roles of surgery and radiation therapy in the management of craniopharyngiomas. Int J Radiat Oncol Biol Phys 1989;16:17-24.

99. Julow J, Lanyi F, Hajda M, et al. The radiotherapy of cystic craniopharyngioma with intracystic installation of $^{90}$Y silicate colloid. Acta Neurochir 1985;74:94-9.

100. Pollack IF, Lunsford LD, Slamovits TL, et al. Stereotaxic intracavitary irradiation for cystic craniopharyngiomas. J Neurosurg 1988;68:227-33.

101. Anderson DR, Trobe JD, Taren JA, et al. Visual outcome in cystic craniopharyngiomas treated with intracavitary phosphorus-32. Ophthalmology 1989;96:1786-92.

102. Takahashi H, Nakazawa S, Shimura T. Evaluation of postoperative intratumoral injection of bleomycin for craniopharyngiomas in children. J Neurosurg 1985;62:120-7.

103. Repka MX, Miller NR, Miller M. Visual outcome after surgical removal of craniopharyngiomas. Ophthalmology 1989;96:195-9.

104. Amacher AL. Craniopharyngioma: the controversy regarding radiotherapy. Childs Brain 1980;6:57-64.

105. Finn JE, Mount LA. Meningiomas of the tuberculum sellae and planum sphenoidale: a review of 83 cases. Arch Ophthalmol 1974;92:23-7.

106. Ehlers N, Malmros R. The suprasellar meningioma: a review of the literature and presentation of a series of 31 cases. Acta Ophthalmol Suppl 1973;121:1-74.

107. Wan WL, Geller J, Feldon SE, et al. Visual loss caused by rapidly progressive intracranial meningiomas during pregnancy. Ophthalmology 1990;97:18-21.

108. Andrews BT, Wilson CB. Suprasellar meningiomas: the effect of tumor location on postoperative visual outcome. J Neurosurg 1988;69:523-8.

109. Kennedy F. Retrobulbar neuritis as an exact diagnostic sign of certain tumors and abscesses in the frontal lobes. Am J Med Sci 1911;142:355-68.

110. Watnick RL, Trobe JD. Bilateral optic nerve compression as a mechanism for the Foster-Kennedy syndrome. Ophthalmology 1989;96:1793-8.

111. Lee KF, Whiteley WH III, Schatz NJ, et al. Juxtasellar hyperostosis of nonmeningiomatous origin. J Neurosurg 1976;44:571-9.

112. Rosenberg LF, Miller NR. Visual results after microsurgical removal of meningiomas involving the anterior visual system. Arch Ophthalmol 1984;102:1019-23.

113. Salazar OM. Ensuring local control in meningiomas. Int J Radiat Oncol Biol Phys 1988;15:501-4.

114. Carella RJ, Ransohoff J, Newall J. Role of radiation therapy in the management of meningioma. Neurosurgery 1982;10:332-9.

115. Taylor BW Jr, Marcus RB Jr, Friedman WA, et al. The meningioma controversy: postoperative radiation therapy. Int J Radiat Oncol Biol Phys 1988;15:299-304.

116. Alvord EC Jr, Lofton S. Gliomas of the optic nerve or chiasm: outcome by patient's age, tumor site, and treatment. J Neurosurg 1988;68:85-98.

117. Heiskanen O, Raitta C, Torsti R. The management and prognosis of gliomas of the optic pathways in children. Acta Neurochir 1978;43:193-9.

118. Oxenhandler DC, Sayers MP. The dilemma of childhood optic gliomas. J Neurosurg 1978;48:34-41.

119. Miller NR, Iliff WJ, Green WR. Evaluation and management of gliomas of the anterior visual pathways. Brain 1974;97:743-54.

120. Lewis RA, Gerson LP, Axelson KA, et al. von Recklinghausen neurofibromatosis. II. Incidence of optic gliomata. Ophthalmology 1984;91:929-35.

121. Aoki S, Barkovich AJ, Nishimura K, et al. Neurofibromatosis types 1 and 2: cranial MR findings. Radiology 1989;172:527-34.

122. Listernick R, Charrow J, Greenwald MJ, et al. Optic gliomas in children with neurofibromatosis type 1. J Pediatr 1989;114:788-92.

123. Hoyt WF, Baghdassarian SA: Optic glioma of childhood: natural history and rationale for consecutive management. Br J Ophthalmol 1969;53:793-8.

124. Imes RK, Hoyt WF. Childhood chiasmal gliomas: update on the fate of patients in the 1969 San Francisco Study. Br J Ophthalmol 1986;70:179-82.

125. Weiss L, Sagerman RH, King GA, et al. Controversy in the management of optic nerve glioma. Cancer 1987;59:1000-4.

126. Flickinger JC, Torres C, Deutsch M. Management of low-grade gliomas of the optic nerve and chiasm. Cancer 1988;61:635-42.

127. Tenny RT, Laws ER Jr, Younge BR, et al. The neurosurgical management of optic glioma: results in 104 patients. J Neurosurg 1982;57:452-8.

128. Pierce SM, Barnes PD, Loeffler JS, et al. Definitive radiation therapy in the management of symptomatic patients with optic glioma: survival and long-term effects. Cancer 1990;65:45-52.

129. Packer RJ, Savino PJ, Bilaniuk LT, et al. Chiasmatic gliomas of childhood: a reappraisal of natural history and effectiveness of cranial irradiation. Childs Brain 1983;10:393-403.

130. Rosenstock JG, Packer RJ, Bilaniuk LT, et al. Chiasmatic optic glioma treated with chemotherapy: a preliminary report. J Neurosurg 1985;63:862-6.

131. Packer RJ, Sutton LN, Bilaniuk LT, et al. Treatment of chiasmatic/hypothalamic gliomas of childhood with chemotherapy: an update. Ann Neurol 1988;23:79-85.

132. Harper CG, Stewart-Wynne EG. Malignant optic gliomas in adults. Arch Neurol 1978;35:731-5.

133. Hoyt WF, Meshel LG, Lessell S, et al. Malignant optic glioma of adulthood. Brain 1973;96:121-32.

134. Albers GW, Hoyt WF, Forno LS, et al. Treatment response in malignant optic glioma of adulthood. Neurology 1988;38:1071-4.

135. Walsh FB. Visual field defects due to aneurysms at the circle of Willis. Arch Ophthalmol 1964;71:15-27.

136. Goodwin JA, Glaser JS. Chiasmal syndrome in sphenoid sinus mucocele. Ann Neurol 1978;4:440-4.

137. Domingue JN, Wilson CB. Pituitary abscesses: report of seven cases and review of the literature. J Neurosurg 1977;46:601-8.

138. Lindholm J, Rasmussen P, Korsgaard O. Intrasellar or pituitary abscess. J Neurosurg 1973;38:616-9.

139. Savino PJ, Glaser JS, Schatz NJ. Traumatic chiasmal syndrome. Neurology 1980;30:963-70.

140. Sacks JG, Melen O. Bitemporal visual field defects in presumed multiple sclerosis. JAMA 1975;234:69-72.

141. Spector RH, Glaser JS, Schatz, NJ. Demyelinative chiasmal lesions. Arch Neurol 1980;37:757-62.

142. Gudeman SK, Selhorst JB, Susac JO, et al. Sarcoid optic neuropathy. Neurology 1982;32:597-603.

143. Purvin V, Herr GJ, De Myer W. Chiasmal neuritis as a complication of Epstein-Barr virus infection. Arch Neurol 1988;45:458-60.

144. Navarro IM, Peralta VHR, Leon JAM, et al. Tuberculous optochiasmatic arachnoiditis. Neurosurgery 1981;9:654-60.

145. Marcus AO, Demakas JJ, Ross HA, et al. Optochiasmatic arachnoiditis with treatment by surgical lysis of adhesions, corticosteroids, and cyclophosphamide: report of a case. Neurosurgery 1986;19:101-103.

146. Iraci G, Gerosa LT, Gerosa M, et al. Opto-chiasmatic arachnoiditis in brothers. Ann Ophthalmol 1979;11:479-87.

147. Iraci G, Secchi AG, Gerosa M, et al. Opto-chiasmatic "phlogosis" (82 cases). In: Deutman AF, Cruysberg IRM, eds. Neurogenetics and neuro-ophthalmology: 5th International Congress. The Hague: Dr W Junk, 1978: 261-81. (Doc Ophthalmol Proc Ser;17.)

148. Jordan RM, Kendall JW, Kerber CW. The primary empty sella syndrome: analysis of the clinical characteristics, radiographic features, pituitary function and cerebrospinal fluid adenohypophysial hormone concentrations. Am J Med 1977;62:569-80.

149. Cupps TR, Woolf PD. Primary empty sella syndrome with panhypopituitarism, diabetes insipidus, and visual field defects. Acta Endocrinol 1978;89:445-60.

150. Mortara R, Norrell H. Consequences of a deficient sellar diaphragm. J Neurosurg 1990;32:565-73.

151. Foley KM, Posner JB. Does pseudotumor cerebri cause the empty sella syndrome? Neurology 1975;25:565-9.

152. Buckman MT, Husain M, Carlow TJ, et al. Primary empty sella syndrome with visual field defects. Am J Med 1976;61:124-8.

153. Busch W. Die Morphologie der Sella turcica und ihre Beziehungen zur Hypophyse. Arch Pathol Anat 1951;320:437.

# CHAPTER 4

# Postchiasmal Visual Loss

• • • • • • • • • • • • • •

The visual field defect produced by lesions posterior to the optic chiasm is a homonymous hemianopia. Patients with retrochiasmal lesions also may have a variety of visual symptoms or signs, thereby producing different clinical pictures.

## Clinical Presentations

### DECREASED VISUAL ACUITY AND HOMONYMOUS HEMIANOPIA

Decreased visual acuity in a patient with homonymous hemianopia may be seen in two circumstances: (1) a mass lesion that involves the area of the optic tract or (2) a lesion that involves both occipital lobes.

**OPTIC TRACT SYNDROME.** Mass lesions of the optic tract are usually large enough to compromise the optic nerve and chiasm. Therefore it is more appropriate to speak of an *optic tract syndrome* than an optic tract lesion. This syndrome is characterized by a complete or incongruous homonymous hemianopia, a relative afferent pupillary defect in the eye with reduced central acuity or greater visual field loss, or both, and "hemioptic" optic atrophy. Associated neurologic signs and symptoms are not essential to the diagnosis. The lesions most frequently causing this syndrome are craniopharyngiomas, aneurysms, and pituitary tumors. A mass lesion must be excluded when an optic tract syndrome is encountered.[1] Smaller lesions of the lateral geniculate nucleus (LGN) may produce visual field defects that may be confused with those produced by the optic tract syndrome. These lesions in the optic tract region occur infrequently and may result from tumors,[2] demyelination,[3] or infarction.[4]

**BILATERAL HOMONYMOUS HEMIANOPIA.** The second circumstance in which patients may have reduced central acuity with homonymous hemianopia is when bilateral occipital lobe lesions occur. These patients have decreased acuity that is bilateral and symmetric. No relative afferent pupillary defect is present. Sometimes the dysfunction in one occipital lobe is only temporary and the patient will be left with a unilateral homonymous hemianopia.

## REDUCED VISUAL PERCEPTION ON ONE SIDE OF VISUAL SPACE

Patients may notice difficulty with peripheral vision, such as in parking their cars. The presence of the visual field defect may be brought to their attention dramatically when a large object suddenly appears out of a previously unrecognized hemianopic field. More frequently, however, patients have vague visual complaints, which they may localize to one eye, usually ipsilateral to the temporal hemianopic defect, not realizing that the true difficulty is a homonymous visual field loss. Some complain of difficulty reading. Patients with a right homonymous hemianopia have difficulty finding the next word and continually lose their place reading across the page; patients with a left hemianopia cannot accurately locate the next line of print. If the homonymous hemianopia is paracentral and not complete, it may go undetected with Goldmann perimetry. A tangent screen examination that magnifies small paracentral scotomas may be needed to plot the defect. This type of scotoma is said to be relatively infrequent, having been found in only 3 of 230 patients with homonymous visual field defects at one institution,[5] and in 3 of 104 patients at another.[6] When a patient with normal acuity has difficulty reading, visual field examination may reveal hemianopic defects.

## HALLUCINATIONS IN A HOMONYMOUS FIELD

The most frequent cause of homonymous visual field loss is migraine, but these visual field defects are almost always transient. In addition, migraineurs often experience visual hallucinatory phenomena in a homonymous distribution. The visual abnormality is usually a small scotoma surrounded by sharp-edged lines (fortification scotoma). This small paracentral defect gradually expands to involve the entire homonymous field over a period of approximately 20 to 30 minutes and then disappears. If a headache occurs on resolution of the scotoma, the term *migraine with aura* is applied. The scotoma is not followed by headache in acephalgic migraine. Migraine without aura, which is the most frequent form, does not have an associated visual phenomenon (see Chapter 16).

Occipital tumors or arteriovenous malformations (AVMs) may cause migrainelike visual symptoms. These symptoms are usually brief and not associated with the fortification spectra of migraine.[7] Rarely, hallucinatory phenomena indistinguishable from migraine may be caused by occipital AVMs. Monotonous unilaterality of the hallucinatory phenomenon or a headache that precedes the visual phase suggests a structural lesion.[8] Under these circumstances we suggest an imaging study (Fig. 4-1). (See also Chapter 6.)

Although the hemianopia of migraine is usually fleeting, in rare instances a fixed neurologic deficit may be produced.[9,10] In these instances imaging usually demonstrates the area(s) of infarction,[11] which are typically in the occipital lobe.

A time-honored concept is that the migraineur is more likely to experience complications with arteriography.[12] In a retrospective review of 149 arteriograms performed on 142 migraineurs, Shuaib and Hachinski[13] reported focal cerebral events in 2.6% of patients. This was essentially the complication rate for all arteriograms at the same institution (2.8%), indicating that migraineurs may safely undergo arteriography.

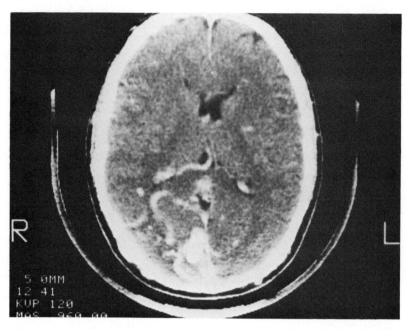

*Fig. 4-1.* Patient with symptoms of fortification scotoma lasting 20 minutes followed by headache always in same location. Computed tomography (CT) shows extensive arterio-venous malformation (AVM) involving right occipital lobe.

Oral contraceptives may precipitate or aggravate preexisting migraine.[14] Women who have migraines should avoid these drugs.

## HOMONYMOUS HEMIANOPIA ASSOCIATED WITH OTHER NEUROLOGIC SIGNS OR SYMPTOMS

Lesions of the temporal and parietal lobes produce homonymous hemianopias. However, for these patients to have a chief or exclusive complaint of a visual disturbance would be distinctly unusual, since their neurologic deficits tend to outweigh any visual abnormality.

## HOMONYMOUS HEMIANOPIA FOLLOWING ARTERIOGRAPHY

Visual field defects of the transient or permanent variety may occur as a complication of arteriography. A permanent homonymous hemianopia due to occipital lobe damage is rare, having been recorded in only 4 of 30,000 cardiac catheterizations over a 5-year period.[15]

The mechanism of homonymous hemianopia following angiography is thought to be an alteration of the blood-brain barrier causing a toxic effect of the contrast material on the occipital lobe. Imaging performed immediately in four patients who developed cortical blindness during cerebral angiography revealed contrast enhancement in the occipital area in all patients.[16]

Nevertheless, competently performed arteriography remains a safe procedure. Dion et al.[17] prospectively studied 1001 cerebral angiograms. The incidence of ischemic events occurring within the first 24 hours of the angiogram was 1.3% (0.1% permanent). The incidence did increase when the procedure lasted longer than 60 minutes, when increased amounts of contrast were used, and when more than three catheters were involved, again showing the need for a high level of expertise in performing angiography.

## HOMONYMOUS HEMIANOPIA DETECTED ON ROUTINE EXAMINATION

Patients with homonymous hemianopias may be asymptomatic, with the hemianopia being discovered on routine examination. A lack of other symptoms almost assuredly represents a silent occipital lobe infarction.[6] However, an imaging study in all patients with homonymous hemianopias is warranted, since tumors may present in an identical fashion.

# Diagnosis

The patient with predominantly visual symptoms who proves to have a homonymous hemianopia usually has a lesion of the optic tract or occipital lobe. The location of a lesion may be inferred from the character of the visual field loss (see below). The visual fibers in the anterior portion of the optic radiations are less highly segregated than they are posteriorly. Therefore a visual field defect from an anterior lesion is less congruous than a defect from a posterior lesion. However, completely unilateral destruction of the visual pathway at any point posterior to the chiasm produces a total homonymous hemianopia. Therefore a total hemianopia is not localizing. While sudden onset implies a vascular etiology, and while a progressive course suggests a mass lesion, enough variability exists in the presentation of any lesion to make imaging the initial investigation of choice in any patient with a homonymous hemianopia.

# Specific Lesions of the Optic Tract and Radiations

## OPTIC TRACT

Isolated lesions of the optic tract or lateral geniculate body are rare. Large mass lesions that also involve the optic chiasm will produce the optic tract syndrome[1] (see earlier under Optic Tract Syndrome)

## LATERAL GENICULATE NUCLEUS

The fibers that originate in the retina synapse in the LGN, which is a triangular structure composed of six layers. Visual fibers enter the LGN anteriorly on its convex surface. Fibers from the ipsilateral eye terminate in layers 2, 3, and 5, whereas the contralateral fibers synapse in layers 1, 4, and 6. The superoposterior aspect of the LGN gives rise to the optic radiations. The hallmark of LGN disease is the wedge-shaped homonymous visual field defect.

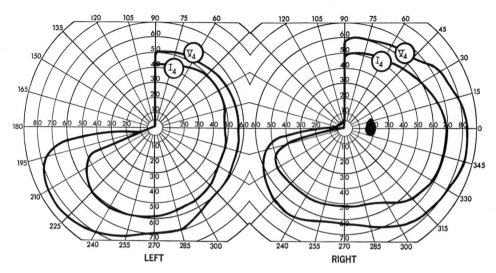

*Fig. 4-2.* Congruous left superior homonymous quadrantanopia following right temporal lobectomy for epilepsy.

## TEMPORAL LOBE

As visual fibers leave the LGN, the inferior fibers (subserving the superior visual field) course anteriorly around the temporal horn to form Meyer's loop. These inferior fibers lie also in close proximity to the internal capsule and the temporal isthmus (the region just posterior and lateral to the internal capsule). Blood supply to the temporal isthmus is provided by the anterior choroidal artery. Vascular episodes (or tumors) in this region produce the syndrome of the temporal isthmus. If the dominant temporal lobe is affected, the patient is hemianopic, hemiparetic, hemianesthetic, and aphasic. A nondominant lesion produces contralateral hemianopia, hemiparesis, hemianesthesia, and neglect.[18]

The typical temporal lobe visual field defect is a homonymous hemianopia that is often denser in the superior quadrants (Fig. 4-2). Some disagreement exists concerning the congruity of the visual field loss with temporal lobe lesions. Perhaps the best evidence is to be found in patients who have undergone temporal lobectomy for epilepsy. Van Buren and Baldwin[19] encountered incongruous field defects in 23 of 33 patients subjected to temporal lobectomy for relief of epilepsy. Walker and Walsh[20] also studied field defects in patients who had undergone temporal lobectomy. They concluded that characteristic temporal lobe visual field defects were pie-shaped sectors that extended from the vertical meridian with a sharp, congruous, straight vertical border and an irregular, ill-defined, sloping horizontal margin. They emphasized that the criteria for congruity of each examiner, as well as the results obtained with various perimetric techniques, may be different. Scrutiny of the visual field defects in both of these series shows incongruity, but the magnitude of incongruity is usually minimal.

In the examination of the visual fields of 69 patients following temporal lobectomy, Jensen and Seedorff[21] detected visual field incongruity in 20 of 51 patients who had field defects. It should be noted that these authors considered a 5-degree discrepancy between corresponding isopters as the maximum allowable difference between "congruous" fields. Furthermore, temporal lobectomy may compromise the blood supply to the ipsilateral optic tract.[22] The postoperative field defect in such a case would be incongruous, but on the basis of optic tract rather than temporal lobe involvement.

Temporal lobe dysfunction may produce a variety of neurologic disturbances. Seizures may be generalized or localized. They are often preceded by an aura of an unpleasant odor or taste (uncinate fit). Dreamlike states with a feeling of déjà-vu and visual hallucinations that are usually vivid and formed are important signs of temporal lobe disease.

## PARIETAL LOBE

As the visual fibers course toward the calcarine area, their topographic organization becomes more highly segregated and a lesion should produce a more congruous hemianopia. However, patients with extensive parietal lobe lesions usually have neurologic signs and symptoms that overshadow their homonymous visual field defect. Lesions of the nondominant parietal lobe produce neglect of the contralateral part of the patient's visual and nonvisual environment. Formal visual fields are frequently unrewarding ventures and are frustrating for both the patient and the perimetrist.

Two neuro-ophthalmic signs have been described in patients with parietal lesions. We find these signs to be only of historical and not diagnostic interest in this age of sophisticated imaging technology.

**SPASTICITY OF CONJUGATE GAZE.** Cogan[18] suggests that tonic deviation of the eyes to the side opposite parietal lesions during an attempt at producing Bell's phenomenon is a useful sign of parietal lobe localization.

**OPTOKINETIC ASYMMETRY.** A specific sign of parietal lobe disease, described by Cogan,[18] is diminished or absent response with rotation of optokinetic objects toward the side of the lesion. Rotation of objects toward the intact parietal lobe provokes a normal optokinetic response. This phenomenon appears to be a deficit of ipsilateral pursuit,[23] although proponents of an abnormality of the saccadic system exist.[24]

## OCCIPITAL LOBE

Optic radiation fibers become totally segregated when the visual cortex is reached. Therefore the hallmark of occipital lobe disease is exquisite congruity whether the visual field defects are quadrantic or involve a lesser area of field (homonymous scotoma) (Fig. 4-3). Total hemianopias occur, but these cannot be considered congruous. Two perimetric peculiarities are observed with occipital lobe disease.

**PRESERVATION OF THE TEMPORAL CRESCENT.** An area of visual cortex lying anteriorly in the interhemispheric fissure receives input only from the nasal ret-

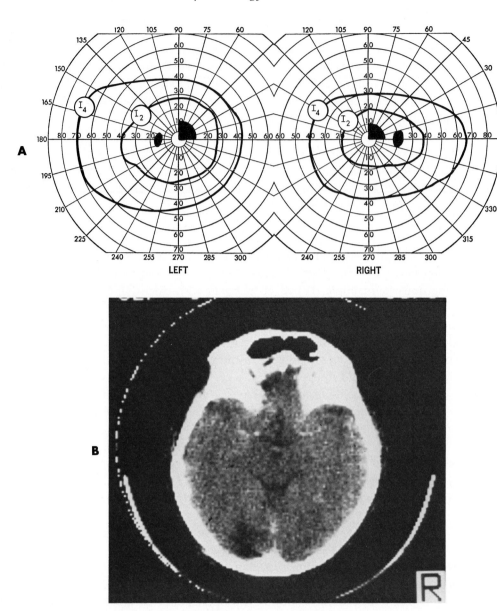

*Fig. 4-3.* **A,** Small exquisitely congruous right homonymous quadrantic scotomas. **B,** CT scan shows hypodense area of infarction at left occipital pole.

ina of the contralateral eye. There is no contribution from the ipsilateral eye.[25] At times the portion of cortex subserving this area of retina will be spared in occipital strokes[26] (Fig. 4-4). The area of the temporal crescent theoretically may be the only portion of the visual cortex that is abnormal, resulting in loss of the temporal portion of only one field but not in a hemianopic pattern. We have never seen a convincing example of this phenomenon.

Monocular hemianopic defects with otherwise normal visual function are most likely due to retinal disease[27] or psychogenic visual loss.[28]

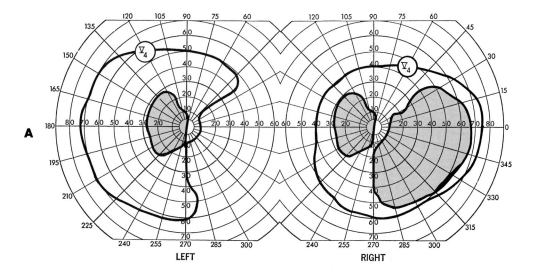

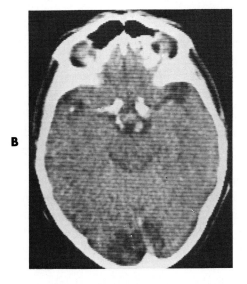

*Fig. 4-4.* Temporal crescent sparing with bilateral occipital infarction. **A,** Highly congruous left homonymous scotoma is present. Right homonymous defect appears incongruous until it is realized that intact peripheral rim of vision in right temporal field is preserved crescent. **B,** CT scan shows bilateral occipital infarcts.

**MACULAR SPARING.** Some occipital hemianopias appear to preserve or retain a small area around fixation (macular sparing), in contrast to the more typical respecting of the vertical meridian through fixation (macular splitting) (Fig. 4-5). Sparing may be due to the dual vascular supply of the occipital pole by branches of either the posterior cerebral or middle cerebral artery.[29] However, by injecting horseradish peroxidase into one lateral geniculate nucleus of monkeys, Bunt and Minckler[30] have shown that retinal ganglion cells projecting ipsilaterally and contralaterally are intermixed (although they make no statement concerning the receptive fields of these cells). This finding appears to reestablish bilateral macular representation as an explanation of some instances of macular sparing. It now appears that either mechanism may be involved in producing this phenomenon.[31]

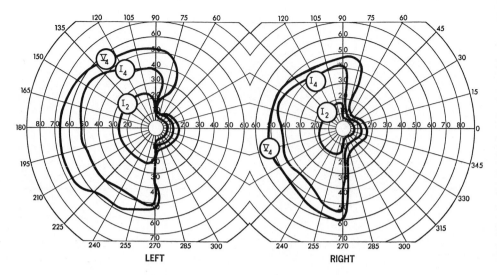

*Fig. 4-5.* Macular sparing. Right homonymous hemianopia with sparing of macular area in right homonymous field.

**SPECIAL MANIFESTATIONS OF OCCIPITAL LOBE DISEASE.** Several occipital lobe syndromes should be recognized.

**Cortical blindness.** This syndrome consists of total blindness due to bilateral occipital lobe lesions. The pupillary reactions are intact, and the funduscopic examination is normal. These two findings frequently lead to the misdiagnosis of functional blindness. This impression may be fortified, since these patients may deny their blindness and fabricate an imaginary visual environment (Anton's syndrome).

The most frequent cause of cortical blindness is bilateral simultaneous infarction of the occipital lobes, presumably from basilar artery thromboembolic disease.[32] The infarcts may occur simultaneously during severe blood loss or hypotensive shock,[33] following arteriography,[16,34] or in the postpartum period in toxemia of pregnancy syndrome.[35] The syndrome of cortical blindness also may result from sequential occipital infarctions.

Other, rarer causes of cortical blindness include occipital lobe epilepsy,[36] chiropractic cervical manipulation,[37] carbon monoxide poisoning,[38] cyclosporine A toxicity,[39] head trauma,[40] and sarcoidosis.[41]

**Riddoch phenomenon.** The perception of movement without the perception of form (statokinetic dissociation) was originally thought to be a specific indicator of occipital lobe disease. It is now apparent that this phenomenon may be detected in lesions at any point along the visual system and is not a pathognomonic sign of occipital lobe disease.[42]

**Cerebral dyschromatopsia.** Although acquired alteration of color vision is predominantly a sign of anterior visual pathway disease, an unusual form of dyschromatopsia is associated with occipital lobe disease. These patients have bilateral occipital lesions but may not have extensive visual field defects. When they have defects, they are usually superior, indicating a lesion inferiorly in the occipital area. *Prosopagnosia* (inability to recognize faces) is a frequent associated finding.[43]

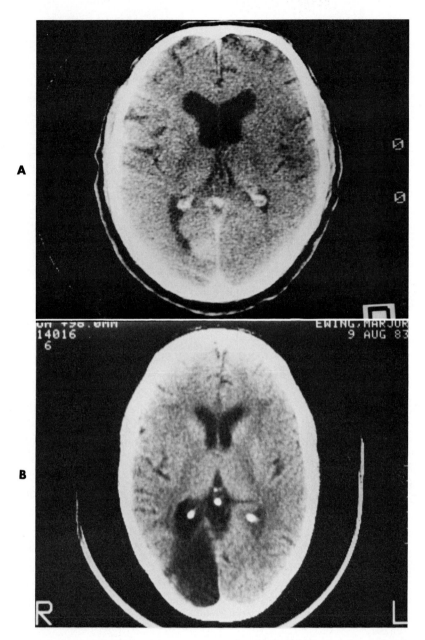

*Fig. 4-6.* Occipital infarction. **A,** Acute occipital infarct with brain edema that is contrast enhancing. Surrounding structures are not displaced, as they would be with mass lesion. **B,** Long-standing occipital infarct with areas of lucency in territory of posterior cerebral artery.                                                          *Continued.*

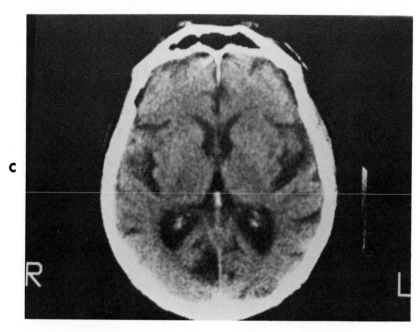

*Fig. 4-6, cont'd.* **C,** Partial occipital infarct involving only a portion of right occipital lobe.

**Disconnection syndromes.** A variety of other higher cortical dysfunctions are associated with primary and associational visual cortex.[44]

**Alexia without agraphia.** Patients who cannot read but who can write and speak, and in whom language is unimpaired, have lesions of the left occipital lobe and the splenium of the corpus callosum. The occipital lesion produces a right homonymous defect, depriving the left hemisphere of visual input. The information from the right hemisphere cannot be transmitted to the left side because of the splenium lesion.

**Palinopsia.** The persistence or recurrence of visual images after the stimulus has been removed is referred to as palinopsia. The patient usually, but not invariably, experiences these false images in an area of homonymous hemianopic defect. The causative lesion is occipital in location[45] (see Chapters 9 and 16).

**Hallucinations.** Although unformed visual hallucinations are classically ascribed to occipital lobe disease, formed images may also be experienced with occipital lesions. Unformed hallucinations rarely may indicate temporal lobe malfunction, although in this area formed images are the rule.[46,47] (see also Chapter 6).

The lesions that produce occipital lobe dysfunction may be vascular (infarction), neoplastic (meningioma, metastatic disease, glioma), congenital (porencephaly, arteriovenous malformations), traumatic, or toxic. The single most important test in differentiating among these various etiologies is imaging (Fig. 4-6). Any patient with a fixed homonymous hemianopia must undergo imaging.

Postchiasmal Visual Loss **115**

# REFERENCES

1. Savino PJ, Paris M, Schatz NJ, et al. Optic tract syndrome: a review of 21 patients. Arch Ophthalmol 1978;96:656-63.
2. Gunderson CH, Hoyt WF. Geniculate hemianopia: incongruous homonymous field defects in two patients with partial lesions of the lateral geniculate nucleus. J Neurol Neurosurg Psychiatry 1971;34:1-6.
3. Vedel-Jensen N. Optic tract neuritis in multiple sclerosis. Acta Ophthalmol 1959;37:537-45.
4. Frisén L, Holmegaard L, Rosencrantz M. Sectorial optic atrophy and homonymous, horizontal sectoranopia: a lateral choroidal artery syndrome? J Neurol Neurosurg Psychiatry 1978;41:374-80.
5. Kölmel HW. Homonymous paracentral scotomas. J Neurol 1987;235:22-5.
6. Trobe JD, Lorber ML, Schlezinger NS. Isolated homonymous hemianopias: a review of 104 cases. Arch Ophthalmol 1973;89:377-81.
7. Troost BT, Newton TH. Occipital lobe arteriovenous malformation: clinical and radiologic features in 26 cases with comments on differentiation from migraine. Arch Ophthalmol 1975;93:250-6.
8. Troost BT, Mark LE, Maroon JC. Resolution of classic migraine after removal of an occipital lobe AVM. Ann Neurol 1979;5:199-201.
9. Rothrock JF, Walicke P, Swenson MR, et al. Migrainous stroke. Arch Neurol 1988;45:63-7.
10. Bogousslavsky J, Regli F, Van Melle G, et al. Migraine stroke. Neurology 1988;38:223-7.
11. Bousser MG, Baron JC, Iba-Zizen MT, et al. Migrainous cerebral infarction: a tomographic study of cerebral blood flow and oxygen extraction fraction with the oxygen-15 inhalation technique. Stroke 1980;11:145-53.
12. Patterson RH Jr, Goodoll H, Dunning HS. Complications of carotid arteriography. Arch Neurol 1964;20:513-20.
13. Shuaib A, Hachinski VC. Migraine and the risks from angiography. Arch Neurol 1988;45:911-2.
14. Dalton K. Migraine and oral contraceptives. Headache 1976;15:247-51.
15. Kosmorsky G, Hanson MR, Tomsak RL. Neuro-ophthalmologic complications of cardiac catheterization. Neurology 1988;38:483-5.
16. Lantos G. Cortical blindness due to osmotic disruption of the blood-brain barrier by angiographic contrast material: CT and MRI studies. Neurology 1989;39:567-71.
17. Dion JE, Gates PC, Fox AJ, et al. Clinical events following neuroangiography: a prospective study. Stroke 1987;18:997-1004.
18. Cogan DG. Neurology of the visual system. Springfield, IL: Charles C Thomas, 1966:254.
19. Van Buren JM, Baldwin M. The architecture of the optic radiation in the temporal lobe of man. Brain 1958;81:15-40.
20. Walker AE, Walsh FB. The visual disturbances in temporal lobectomized patients. In: Smith JL, ed. Neuro-ophthalmology: symposium of the University of Miami and the Bascom Palmer Eye Institute, vol 4. St Louis: Mosby–Year Book, 1968:230-48.
21. Jensen I, Seedorff HH. Temporal lobe epilepsy and neuro-ophthalmology: ophthalmological findings in 74 temporal lobe resected patients. Acta Ophthalmol 1976;54:827-41.
22. Lindenberg R, Walsh FB, Sacks JG. Neuropathology of vision: an atlas. Philadelphia: Lea & Febiger, 1973:332.
23. Baloh RW, Yee RD, Honrubia V. Optokinetic nystagmus and parietal lobe lesions. Ann Neurol 1980;7:269-76.
24. Gay AJ, Newman NM, Keltner JL, et al. Eye movement disorders. St Louis: Mosby–Year Book, 1974:50.
25. Stensaas SS, Eddington KD, Dobelle WH. The topography and variability of the primary visual cortex in man. J Neurosurg 1974;40:747-55.
26. Benton S, Levy I, Swash M. Vision in the temporal crescent in occipital infarction. Brain 1980;103:83-97.
27. Johnson LN, Rabinowitz YS, Hepler RS. Hemianopia respecting the vertical meridian and with foveal sparing from

retinal degeneration. Neurology 1989;
39:872-3.

28. Gittinger JW JR. Functional monocular temporal hemianopsia. Am J Ophthalmol 1986;101:226-31.

29. Marinkovic SV, Milisavljevic MM, Lolic-Draganic V, et al. Distribution of the occipital branches of the posterior cerebral artery: correlation with occipital lobe infarcts. Stroke 1987;18:728-32.

30. Bunt AH, Minckler DS. Foveal sparing: new anatomical evidence for bilateral representation of the central retina. Arch Ophthalmol 1977;95:1445-7.

31. Miller NR, ed. Walsh and Hoyt's clinical neuro-ophthalmology, vol 1. 4th ed. Baltimore: Williams & Wilkins, 1982: 147.

32. Mehler MF. The neuro-ophthalmologic spectum of the rostral basilar artery syndrome. Arch Neurol 1988;45:966-71.

33. Nepple EW, Appen RE, Sackett JF. Bilateral homonymous hemianopia. Am J Ophthalmol 1978;86:536-43.

34. Studdard WE, Davis DO, Young SW. Cortical blindness after cerebral angiography: case report. J Neurosurg 1981;54:240-4.

35. Coughlin WF, McMurdo SK, Reeves T. MR imaging of postpartum cortical blindness. J Comput Assist Tomogr 1989;13:572-6.

36. Jaffe SJ, Roach ES. Transient cortical blindness with occipital lobe epilepsy. J Clin Neuro Ophthalmol 1988;8:221-4.

37. Gittinger JW Jr. Occipital infarction following chiropractic cervical manipulation. J Clin Neuro Ophthalmol 1986; 6:11-3.

38. Katafuchi Y, Nishimi T, Yamaguchi Y, et al. Cortical blindness in acute carbon monoxide poisoning. Brain Dev 1985; 7:516-19.

39. Wilson SE, de Groen PC, Aksamit AJ, et al. Cyclosporine A–induced reversible cortical blindness. J Clin Neuro Ophthalmol 1988:8:215-20.

40. Eldridge PR, Punt JAG. Transient traumatic cortical blindness in children. Lancet 1988;1:815-6.

41. Powers JM. Sarcoidosis of the tentorium with cortical blindness. J Clin Neuro Ophthalmol 1985;5:112-5.

42. Safran AB, Glaser JS. Statokinetic dissociation in lesions of the anterior visual pathways: a reappraisal of the Riddoch phenomenon. Arch Ophthalmol 1980;98:291-5.

43. Green GJ, Lessell S. Acquired cerebral dyschromatopsia. Arch Ophthalmol 1977;95:121-8.

44. Lessell S. Higher disorders of visual function: negative phenomena. In: Glaser JS, Smith JL, eds. Neuro-ophthalmology: symposium of the University of Miami and the Bascom Palmer Eye Institute, vol 8. St Louis: Mosby–Year Book, 1975:1-26.

45. Michel EM, Troost BT. Palinopsia: cerebral localization with computed tomography. Neurology 1980;30:887-9.

46. Cogan DG. Visual hallucinations as release phenomena: Albrecht Von Graefes Arch Klin Exp Ophthalmol 1973; 188:139-50.

47. Weinberger LM, Grant FC. Visual hallucinations and their neuro-optical correlates. Arch Ophthalmol 1940;23:166-99.

# CHAPTER 5

# Transient Visual Loss

• • • • • • • • • • • • • • • • • • •

Transient visual loss (TVL), or amaurosis fugax, is a reversible deficit in visual function that lasts less than 24 hours. The term should be reserved for discrete events in which patients describe an *abrupt* loss of all or a portion of their field of vision in *one or both eyes*. It is the suddenness of onset that distinguishes TVL from the fluctuations in visual clarity that occur in corneal endothelial dysfunction, diabetes, and multiple sclerosis (MS).

## Mechanisms of TVL

The above definition of TVL makes it a subtype of transient ischemic attack (TIA), a reversible focal neurologic deficit of 24 hours' duration or less. In fact, the principal mechanism for TVL is ischemia. The other accepted mechanism is neuronal depression after a seizure or a migraine attack. Seizures within the visual cortex, generally caused by neoplasms, arteriovenous malformations, meningoencephalitis, ischemia, and trauma, may rarely cause loss of vision alone,[1] but they more typically have an excitatory component as well. That is, the patient experiences hallucinations, usually of unformed images, at some time during the abnormal discharge. The hallucinations tend to consist of flickering lights that do not move across the visual field (see Chapter 6). The visual loss associated with migraine is often associated with scintillations; it is distinctive in that it spreads across the field of vision like a wave, leaving dim, blurred, or absent sight behind it (see Chapter 16).

Ischemia produces TVL by temporary vascular occlusion or reduced blood flow through nonoccluded vessels.

### OCCLUSION

TVL results from temporary vascular occlusion in three circumstances: thromboembolism, vasospasm, and compression.

**THROMBOEMBOLISM.** The circulation to the eye or visual cortex may be temporarily blocked by an embolus originating from a diseased vessel, cardiac wall or valve, or from injection of particulate matter. A common source of embolism is atheromatous ulceration of large arteries, which collects fibrin and platelets, forming a thrombus that may or may not totally occlude the vessel lumen. Parts of the thrombus break off and drift downstream to plug distal vessels. Whether transient arterial thrombosis or embolism should be blamed for TIAs and strokes in patients with atheromatous extracranial disease is unsettled. Embolism is considered the mechanism in patients with cardiac valve or wall abnormalities, although even here, it may be difficult to exclude other mechanisms.[2]

TVL may also occur from temporary thrombosis of a feeder vessel close to the eye or visual cortex. The processes that affect these smaller vessels include lipohyalinosis, vasculitis, and hypercoagulable states. Lipohyalinosis, the hyperplastic process associated with systemic hypertension that obliterates the lumen of small arterioles, is responsible for subcortical lacunar infarcts and perhaps for the nonarteritic form of ischemic optic neuropathy (see Chapter 2). TVL is associated with vasculitis most commonly in giant cell arteritis and less commonly in Takayasu's (pulseless) disease, lupus erythematosus, rheumatoid arthritis, and polyarteritis nodosa. Hypercoagulable states causing TVL include sickle cell anemia, macroglobulinemia, multiple myeloma, and the primary antiphospholipid syndrome.[3,4]

Atherosclerosis of the internal carotid system is found primarily at the origin of the internal carotid and to a lesser extent in its intracavernous (siphon) portion and proximal middle and anterior cerebral branches. The vertebrobasilar system is affected by atheroma at the origin of the vertebral arteries, at the junction of the vertebral and basilar arteries, and at the junction of the basilar and superior cerebellar arteries. Atheromatous involvement of these vessels is believed to produce cerebral ischemia either by generating emboli or by temporarily occluding them and reducing perfusion to vulnerable distal territories.

**Visual symptoms.** The TVL associated with carotid atheromatous disease consists of brief monocular attacks lasting up to 15 minutes, but usually less than 5 minutes. Patients may describe a shade or veil descending or ascending over a portion of their field, a wedge defect or central scotoma, peripheral loss with central sparing, or a "Swiss cheese" pattern of irregularly spared areas. Some describe a blackout, others a brownout or grayout, but many patients simply report that vision was diffusely blurred. Patients may describe momentary flashes or spots of light *(photopsias)*. Usually no coincident nonvisual symptoms occur.

Visual cortical ischemia caused by vertebrobasilar atheroma produces binocular visual loss. Attacks are typically even briefer than those associated with carotid disease, lasting less than a minute. Visual loss may be an isolated symptom[5] or may be accompanied by brainstem ischemic symptoms, which include disequilibrium, diplopia, dysarthria, dysphagia, sudden weakness of the legs (drop attack), and perioral and extremity numbness. Patients may describe seeing flashing lights during an attack, but they rarely report that the lights progress across the visual field (as in migraine). Loss of vision may be total. If the loss is partial, it will be homonymous, but the patient is frequently unaware of its binocularity, localizing it to the eye with the temporal field loss.

**Thromboembolic TVL as an isolated symptom.** Several cogent theories have been advanced to explain why TVL is often an isolated symptom of carotid and vertebrobasilar thromboembolism:

1. Fleeting visual loss is a symptom more readily noticed than fleeting weakness or numbness.
2. The visual system is topographically organized, with little functional reduplication, so that ischemia of a small area will be clinically expressed.
3. The retinal circulation is poorly collateralized, and the parieto-occipital cortex is a circulatory watershed zone, so that both regions are vulnerable to reduced blood flow.
4. Laminar flow favors the ocular circulation, so that emboli are preferentially carried to the eye.

**Embolic theory.** Emboli from extracranial vessels are believed to account for most episodes of TVL, based on several lines of evidence. In 1959 Fisher[6] described a patient with multiple attacks of monocular TVL and ipsilateral internal carotid stenosis in whom he observed "strikingly white and glistening" particles coursing through the retinal arterioles during an episode of visual loss. He suggested that these particles were emboli from the carotid artery. In 1961 Hollenhorst[7] observed "orange, yellow, or copper-colored plaques at bifurcations of retinal arterioles." In some cases these plaques appeared during carotid endarterectomy. He postulated that they were "cholesterol crystals or liquid cholesterol dislodged from eroded atheromatous lesions in the aorta or the innominate, carotid, or opthalmic arteries." In 1963 David et al.[8] reported that bright intraluminal plaques observed in the retina after cervical carotid exploration proved at autopsy to be composed of cholesterol esters identical to those found in the carotid atheroma. Similar emboli were found in an occluded middle cerebral artery. McBrien et al.[9] noted whitish particles in the retinal arterioles after endarterectomy and pathologic examination disclosed platelet aggregates.

Further indirect support for the theory that the cervical carotid was the seat of cerebral emboli came from the observations of Gunning et al.[10] They reported that patients with recent attacks of monocular blindness or hemispheric ischemia were found at endarterectomy to have carotid atheromas covered with a loose network of fibrin and platelets. In contrast, those whose TIAs had occurred at least 7 weeks prior to surgery had smooth atheromas.

The embolic theory does *not* adequately explain several clinical facts. Emboli are not always observed in the retinal vessels during monocular TVL attacks. Dyll et al.[11] have observed the fundus of patients suffering transient monocular blindness and noted circulatory arrest with segmentation of venous blood without emboli. Hollenhorst[12] has described a perfectly normal fundus and an amaurotic pupil during an episode of monocular TVL. Furthermore, recurrent embolization does not easily account for the fact that TVL (and other TIA) symptoms are frequently identical from episode to episode. Fisher[13] has noted that cardiac emboli do not cause stereotyped TIAs. Instead, they produce varying symptoms corresponding to the different central nervous system (CNS) areas to which they travel.

The embolic theory of TVL must also consider that a substantial number of patients with TVL do not have atheromatous carotid artery disease. Chawluk et al.[14] found that only 16% of patients with monocular TVL or retinal arterial occlusions had greater than 60% ipsilateral carotid stenosis. Pessin et al.[15] reported that of 33 patients who underwent angiography for monocular TVL, only 19 (57%) had hemodynamically significant carotid stenosis, and 8 (25%) patients had completely normal carotid arteries. The description of the attacks of TVL was the same whether or not patients had stenosing carotid atheroma.

The fact that angiographically normal carotid arteries occur in the presence of monocular TVL has led to the postulation that even when carotid atheroma is found in patients with TVL, it may not be the cause of the symptom, but merely a bystander. In fact, before the thromboembolic theory of TIAs gained preeminence, the conventional explanation for many of these episodes was vasospasm.[16] Vasospasm lost favor because structural damage to cerebral vessels from arteriosclerosis was believed to impair their reactivity. Angiographic studies of the coronary arteries in patients with variant (Prinzmetal) angina pectoris have now disclosed vasospasm temporally linked to symptoms.[17] The vasospasm occurs both in normal and in arteriosclerotic vessels. These facts have revived the notion that vasospasm is contributory in the TVL suffered by patients with (or without) arteriosclerotic vascular disease.

**Temporary in situ thrombosis.** An alternative explanation for TVL in patients bearing arteriosclerotic or prothrombotic risk factors is that temporary vascular occlusion results from platelet-fibrin thrombi in the distal circulatory bed (ophthalmic or retinal arteries, or branches of the posterior cerebral arteries). As the thrombi are dissolved or washed away, and adequate circulation restored, the symptoms disappear. Because deciding from a postmortem pathologic examination whether the occluded vessel contains an embolus or an in situ thrombus is often difficult, the pathogenesis of TVL remains unsettled.

**VASOSPASM.** Formerly invoked as the most likely mechanism for all TIAs, vasospasm is now implicated only in subarachnoid hemorrhage and hypertensive crisis, and perhaps in some forms of migraine. Although definite evidence is lacking, vasospasm of retinal arterioles may account for the monocular TVL described by otherwise healthy young adults.

**COMPRESSION.** A relatively rare cause of TVL is external compression of blood vessels that nourish the visual pathway. This mechanism is involved in papilledema, in which pressure on vessels in the swollen nerve head causes blackout of vision over the entire field of one or both eyes, lasting a second or two (transient obscurations of vision).[18] The episodes, which are so brief that the patient is apt to ignore them at first, may be precipitated by standing up or by the Valsalva maneuver. Fundus examination shows markedly swollen discs, and the intracranial pressure is generally above 200 mm $H_2O$. Normalization of the pressure eliminates the symptom, although the disc swelling may take weeks to dissipate.

Compression of a part of the visual pathway by an adjacent or intrinsic tumor generally causes slowly progressive visual loss but may rarely produce TVL as well. For example, an intraorbital tumor may intermittently compress the optic nerve as the eye is rotated into eccentric gaze positions (gaze-evoked amaurosis).[19]

## REDUCED FLOW THROUGH NONOCCLUDED VESSELS

The visual pathway may become ischemic in the presence of patent blood vessels if cerebral perfusion is reduced as a result of subnormal cardiac output or hyperviscosity. Binocular TVL caused by reduced perfusion is generally accompanied by dizziness, light-headedness, confusion, nausea, headache, and occasionally photopsias. Clinical and experimental evidence[20] suggests that cardiogenic hypoperfusion rarely produces TVL as an isolated symptom.

Hyperviscosity states may produce ischemia not only by sluggish blood flow but also by an increased propensity to thrombosis. In patients with such disorders, TVL may be a prominent symptom. A study of 511 polycythemia patients found that 11% complained of TVL that was relieved by phlebotomy.[21]

The symptoms of TVL are not specific enough to attribute them to a given mechanism in a great many cases. Largely on the basis of circumstantial evidence, atheromatous thromboembolism is considered responsible for the vast majority of TVL episodes in those over 40 years of age. Among patients aged 40 years or less, most cases of TVL remain unexplained, although migraine and cardioembolism are often invoked. In both age groups nonatheromatous vasculopathies and papilledema must always be excluded.

# A Decision Tree Approach to the Evaluation of Transient Visual Loss (Chart 5-1)

### ▨ Scintillations present

The first step in history taking is to determine if the patient is experiencing scintillations. If these are present, especially with fortification, the diagnosis is likely to be migraine.

### ☐ Other features of classic migraine present

If the symptom complex consists of a stereotyped scintillating scotoma lasting approximately 15 to 20 minutes and the patient has no evidence of a systemic or neurologic illness, then the diagnosis of migraine becomes virtually certain.

### ▣ Migraine

An atypical form of migraine affects only one eye. Whereas the form of migraine that causes binocular TVL (classic migraine) usually produces scintillations, monocular TVL usually produces no scintillations, and often no headache. Sometimes called *ocular migraine* or *retinociliary migraine,* this condition is best diagnosed after excluding other causes. Visual loss rarely lasts longer than a few minutes. In cases in which the fundus has been observed during an attack, retinal arteriolar and venous narrowing, retinal edema, venous dilatation, and de-

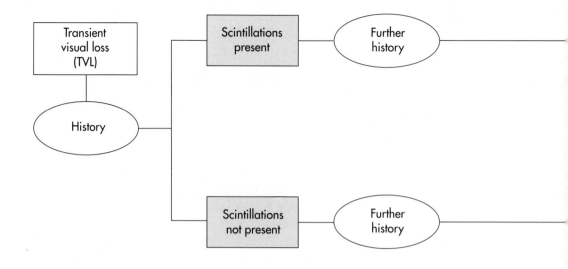

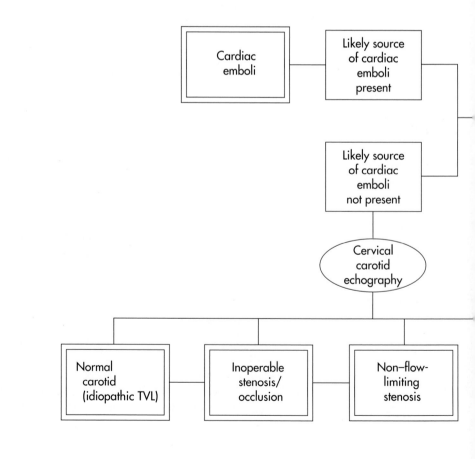

*Chart 5-1*

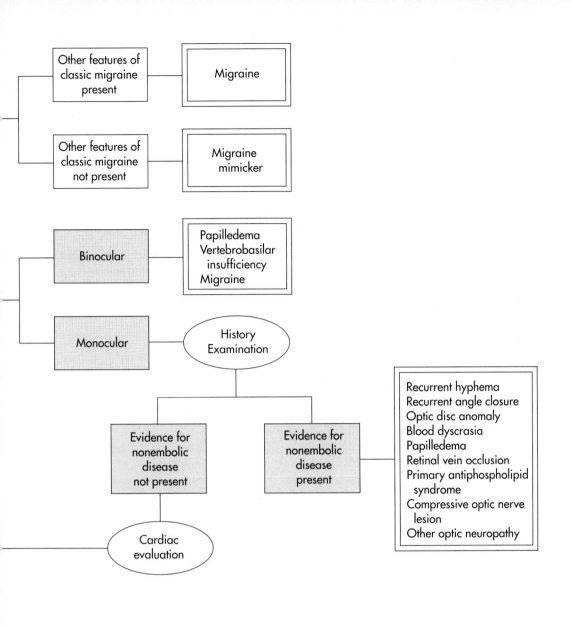

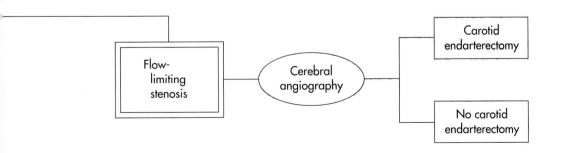

layed fluorescein filling of retinal vessels have been noted.[22,23] If retinal ischemia is severe, infarction of the inner retina may occur.

Migraine patients may also rarely suffer ischemic papillopathy and central serous chorioretinopathy. The underlying abnormality is considered to be vasospasm of retinal and/or choroidociliary circulations.

☐ Other features of classic migraine not present

▣ Migraine mimicker

Migraine should be considered a "reaction" pattern within the CNS, rather than as a disease. Many pathologic states, such as **lupus erythematosus, occipital lobe masses,** or **chronic meningitis,** can trigger this reaction pattern and thus mimic migraine. The examiner should be prepared to look for underlying causes if atypical features turn up (see Chapters 6 and 16).

▨ Scintillations not present

If scintillations are not present, the diagnosis of migraine is weakened but not excluded, since migraine can be nonscintillatory. However, one must also consider other mechanisms, and the next step is to decide if the TVL is monocular or binocular. This judgment must be made early, since *management does not include endarterectomy if the TVL is binocular.*

▨ Binocular TVL without scintillations

Binocular TVL without scintillations is caused by **papilledema, vertebrobasilar insufficiency** (occipital cortex ischemia),[24] or **migraine.** After an ophthalmologic examination to rule out papilledema, patients should have a thorough medical evaluation to identify and treat risk factors for arteriosclerosis. Angiography is generally not indicated, because reconstruction of atherosclerotic vessels of the posterior cerebral circulation is currently too risky. Patients who do not have evidence of arteriosclerosis should be evaluated for other causes of TIA.

▨ Monocular TVL without scintillations

If the TVL is monocular, the examiner must discover if it has an embolic or nonembolic cause. Clues come both from the history and from ophthalmologic examination (Chart 5-1, *A*).

◯ History and examination

**OTHER CONCURRENT CEREBRAL ISCHEMIC SYMPTOMS.** Dizziness, confusion, seizures, or syncope accompanying the TVL suggest global cerebral is-

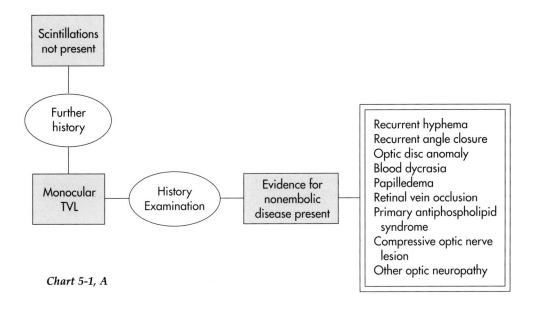

*Chart 5-1, A*

chemia, possibly caused by cardiogenic hypotension. If the episode was precipitated by assuming an upright posture, then orthostatic hypotension must be considered. If diplopia, dysarthria, vertigo, or disequilibrium accompanied the TVL, the diagnosis is probably brainstem ischemia from cardiac or vertebrobasilar atheromatous thromboembolism. In those rare instances when ipsilateral hemispheric ischemic symptoms coincide with monocular TVL, then cardiac or carotid emboli are likely.

**ARTERIOSCLEROTIC RISK FACTORS.** Hypertension, diabetes, familial arteriosclerotic disease, and a personal history of heavy smoking are risk factors associated not only with extracranial atheromatous thromboembolism but also with cardiac disease.

**HEART DISEASE.** The finding of prosthetic or rheumatic valves, abnormal cardiac rhythm (especially atrial fibrillation or sick sinus syndrome), reduced wall motion, or septal defects establishes a special risk for cardiac emboli.

**CONSTITUTIONAL SYMPTOMS.** Fever, chills, headache, malaise, and lethargy suggest the possibility of endocarditis, cardiac myxoma, giant cell (or non–giant cell) arteritis, or hyperviscous states. Transient blurred vision is a complaint in patients with increased serum viscosity, as in polycythemia vera, thrombocytosis, leukemia, multiple myeloma, macroglobulinemia, cryoglobulinemia, sickle cell anemia, and primary antiphospholipid syndrome.[3,4]

**RHEUMATOLOGIC DISEASE.** The finding of serositis, arthritis, alopecia, photosensitivity, Raynaud's phenomenon, xerostomia, or keratitis sicca suggests a possibility of connective tissue disease.

**MIGRAINE.** Even if no scintillations are present and TVL is monocular, a strong history of migraine fortifies a suspicion of ocular migraine, especially in young people.

**BIRTH CONTROL PILL INGESTION, PREGNANCY, AND POSTPARTUM OR DE-HYDRATED STATES.** These conditions may produce a hypercoagulable state. Although strokes often occur in these settings, they are rarely preceded by TIAs. It is not yet possible to predict which of these patients is at risk for stroke.

**HEAD OR NECK TRAUMA.** If head or neck trauma has occurred, it invites the possibility of bony compression or a dissecting aneurysm of neck vessels.

**ANTERIOR SEGMENT AND ADNEXAL SIGNS.** An anatomically narrow angle with anterior synechiae introduces a consideration of recurrent angle closure. The history of recent intraocular surgery (especially a lens implant) gives rise to the possibility of TVL from recurrent hyphema.[25] Conjunctivitis, uveitis, and scleritis may be part of a picture of vasculitis or of anterior segment ischemia. Although often associated with proximal (carotid artery) atherosclerosis, anterior segment ischemia reflects, in our view, atheromatous compromise of distal (ophthalmic artery) circulation to the eye.

**POSTERIOR SEGMENT SIGNS.** The presence of bilaterally swollen discs suggests increased intracranial pressure as a possible cause of TVL and directs the investigation away from the more common extracranial sources. If, however, only one disc shows acquired swelling and it is on the side of the TVL, one must consider ischemic, infiltrative, or inflammatory optic neuropathy. Anomalous discs, especially those containing visible drusen, have been reported in patients suffering TVL and who have no vascular risk factors.[26,27] Retinal intraluminal plaques suggest embolism, but the appearance of the plaques (Plate 4, *A*) is rarely distinctive enough to betray their source. Venous tortuosity, peripheral perivenous hemorrhages, and microaneurysms suggest reduced flow (Plate 4, *B*). Cotton-wool and Roth spots (Plate 4, *C* and *D*) suggest arteritis, hypertension, blood dyscrasia, or embolism. Attenuated arterioles are usually evidence of hypertension; peripheral sea fans (Plate 4, *E*) and sunbursts suggest sickle cell anemia, and pallid disc swelling implies ischemic optic neuropathy (vasculitis or lipohyalinosis).

**VISUAL FIELD DEFECTS .** Patients with TVL caused by compressive visual pathway disease will generally also have a fixed deficit apparent in the visual field examination.

### Evidence for nonembolic disease present

The principal nonembolic conditions causing TVL are **recurrent hyphema, recurrent angle closure, optic disc anomaly, blood dyscrasia, papilledema,** impending **retinal vein occlusion, primary antiphospholipid syndrome,** and **compressive optic nerve lesion.**

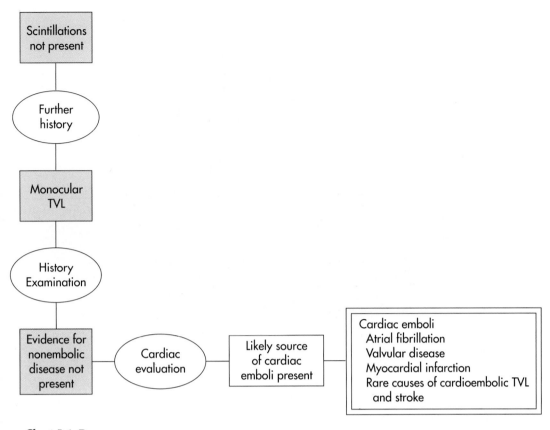

**Chart 5-1, B**

▓ Evidence for nonembolic disease not present

If nonembolic causes of TVL have been excluded, one must turn to the consideration of emboli (Chart 5-1, *B*). The heart should first be excluded as a source.

⭕ *Cardiac evaluation.* The purpose of cardiac evaluation in patients with TVL is to discover a likely—or presumptive—source of embolism.

▢ Likely source of cardiac emboli present

▣ Cardiac emboli

Cardioembolic causes are believed to account for about 15% of all ischemic strokes.[28] Although emboli are an established cause of retinal and occipital infarction,[29] no adequate data on how frequently they cause TVL are available. Such data are usually collected retrospectively, as in a series of 54 patients with rheumatic heart disease, in which 33% of patients had TVL but none mentioned the symptoms spontaneously, none had coincident TIAs, and none had retinal strokes.[30] The frequency of TVL episodes was unrelated to anticoagulation.

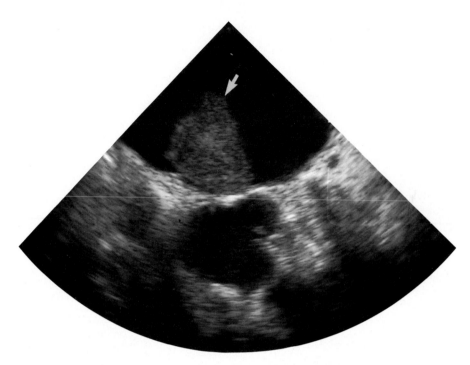

*Fig. 5-1.* Echocardiogram shows atrial thrombus *(arrow)* in patient with atrial fibrillation.

The diagnosis of a cardiac source for TVL is difficult because patients often have coexisting hypertensive or atheromatous arterial disease. Also, visual symptoms and signs of cardiac emboli are indistinguishable from those caused by artery-to-artery emboli. Traditional teaching holds that the orange-yellow reflective cholesterol (Hollenhorst) plaque derives from a carotid atheromatous source, whereas the large white retinal arteriolar calcific plaque comes from a cardiac valve or wall lesion, and the platelet-fibrin plaque originates from either source.[31] We find it hard to differentiate ophthalmoscopically between these three types of retinal emboli.

Strong suspicion of a cardiac source of embolus comes into play when clinical findings of cardiac disease are present in a patient who has no evidence of or risk factors for vascular disease. When evidence of recent infarction in multiple parts of the brain or body is also found, the diagnosis becomes more likely, although vasculitis and hypercoagulable states must still be considered. Cardiac emboli must be considered likely in the following disorders.

**ATRIAL FIBRILLATION.** Population studies[32,33] have established that nonrheumatic atrial fibrillation (AF) increases the risk of stroke at least fivefold in patients aged over 60 years. Most of these strokes are believed to be embolic (Fig. 5-1), since cervical carotid stenosis is unusual in these patients. Although nonrheumatic AF is implicated in nearly half of all cardioembolic strokes, the frequency with which it affects the visual system is unknown. The risk of stroke appears to be aggravated by congestive heart failure, coexisting rheumatic valvular disease, recent onset of fibrillation, and echocardiographic wall motion abnormalities.[34] A prospective controlled study has established the efficacy of warfarin anticoagulation and aspirin in reducing stroke.[35] The relative efficacy of warfarin and aspirin is still to be determined. Pending further information, low-intensity coumadin (prothrombin times = 1.3 to 1.6 times normal) is favored for high-risk subgroups, including patients who have already had a presumed cardioembolic TIA or mild stroke.[34]

**VALVULAR DISEASE.** The valvular causes of emboli are rheumatic heart disease; prosthetic valves; bacterial, marantic, and Libman-Sacks (lupus) endocarditis; mitral valve prolapse; and calcific aortic stenosis.

**Rheumatic heart disease** is a source of cerebral emboli both from platelet-fibrin vegetations on mitral valve leaflets and from associated atrial fibrillation, which causes stagnation of blood flow and secondary mural thrombus formation. About 20% of patients with rheumatic mitral stenosis suffer cerebral TIAs or strokes at a rate of 4% per year.[36] Coexisting atrial fibrillation worsens that risk to eighteenfold as compared with age-mached controls.[33] Recurrent embolism occurs in 30% to 75% of patients who have rheumatic mitral valve disease.[34]

Embolization remains one of the principal long-term risks of **prosthetic heart valves.** Mechanical valves have such a high propensity to trigger emboli that all patients bearing them are anticoagulated. Even so, patients still suffer cerebral TIAs or strokes at a yearly rate of 1.5% (aortic) to 3% (mitral).[37] Bioprosthetic heart valves are less likely to cause embolization (2% to 4% per year), so that routine anticoagulation is not advised, unless they are in atrial fibrillation.[38] The value of adding dipyridamole (Persantine) to aspirin treatment is unsettled.

**Infective endocarditis** causes cerebral emboli in an estimated 10% to 50% of cases[39,40] (Fig. 5-2). It should be suspected whenever the patient has fever, chills, night sweats, or retinal nerve fiber layer hemorrhages with white centers (Roth spots, nonspecific indicators of retinal infarction) (Plate 4, *D*). Acute endocarditis usually occurs in individuals with normal hearts whose valves are infected with *Staphylococcus aureus.* Subacute endocarditis usually affects patients with rheumatic or congenital valvular disease or prosthetic valves; *Streptococcus viridans* is the major causative organism. Physical findings include cardiac murmurs, skin petechiae, nail bed splinter hemorrhages, and splenomegaly. The valvular vegetations are usually very difficult to detect by echocardiography. Fortunately, early intensive antibiotic therapy is often effective in preventing serious complications, including a reduction in the rate of reembolization to near zero, so that anticoagulation is not recommended.[41]

**Nonbacterial thrombotic (marantic) endocarditis** occurs in cancer patients (particularly those with mucinous adenocarcinomas) and in other chronic debilitating conditions, including acquired immunodeficiency syndrome (AIDS). Considered a previously underrecognized cause of clinical embolization, nonbacteric thrombotic endocarditis is now believed to account for 27% of strokes in cancer patients.[42] These patients may develop vegetations of the mitral (60%) or aortic (40%) valves, perhaps because of endothelial disruption and a prothrom-

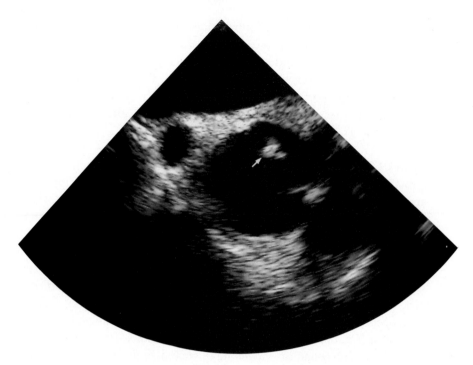

*Fig. 5-2.* Echocardiogram shows vegetation *(arrow)* on aortic valve in patient with subacute bacterial endocarditis.

botic tendency. Similar noninfective vegetations may occur in lupus erythematosus (Libman-Sacks endocarditis) and embolize to the brain.[43]

Fibromyxomatous **degeneration of the mitral valve** (mitral valve prolapse, or MVP) may give rise to cerebral emboli and TVL (Fig. 5-3). In 1963 Barlow et al.[44] associated a typical midsystolic cardiac clicking sound with evidence of a prolapsing motion of the mitral valve leaflets. It has since been noted as an incidental finding in 5% of healthy young women.[45] However, MVP was the only abnormality found in a group of young women with stroke,[46] and pathologic examination has shown vegetations adherent to the deformed valves in cases of MVP. Thus MVP became causally linked to TIA and stroke in young people on a presumed embolic basis.

Evidence now exists that MVP has two forms: (1) a common type, found in young women, where aberrant valve motion is the only abnormality and the risk of stroke is very low,[47] and (2) an uncommon type, found mostly in older men, where thickened leaflets and annulus abnormalities are associated with regurgitation, and the risk of TIA, stroke, angina, endocarditis, and sudden death is greater.[48] Separating these two groups echocardiographically may be difficult. The precise risks in the older patients are not well known. Among 32 young patients followed for a mean of 8 years after an initial TIA, no strokes occurred, and only 16% had recurrent TIAs.[49] Accordingly, these young patients are either

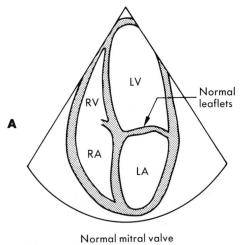

Normal mitral valve

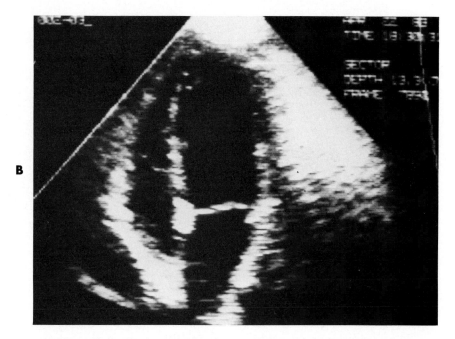

*Fig. 5-3.* Echocardiogram of normal heart, **A** and **B,** and of mitral valve prolapse, **C** and **D.**                                                   *Continued.*

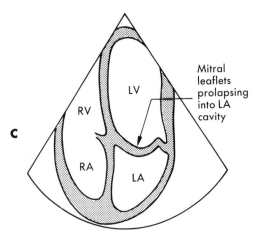

Prolapsed mitral valve

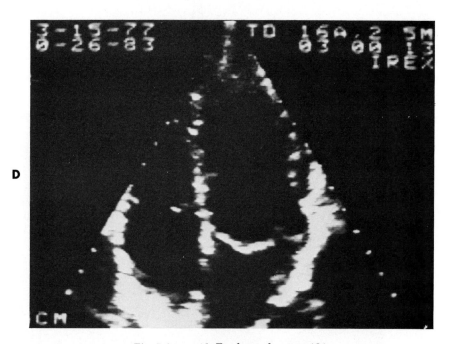

*Fig. 5-3, cont'd.* For legend see p. 131.

not treated or are given aspirin. Considering that MVP is a relatively common finding in young adults, we agree with Adams et al.[50] that ocular and cerebral TIA and stroke should not be ascribed to this entity until other causes have been ruled out.

In **calcific aortic stenosis** the risk of stroke is low, but monocular TVL is reported frequently, sometimes in association with the finding of a white intraluminal retinal plaque.[51] Ischemic events apparently occur most frequently during catheterization or valvuloplasty.

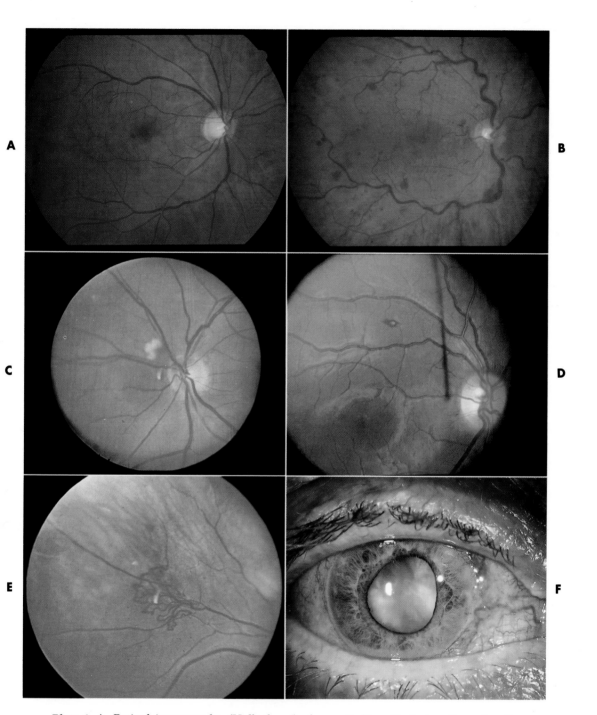

*Plate 4.* **A,** Retinal intravascular (Hollenhorst) plaque. **B,** Venous stasis retinopathy. **C,** Cotton-wool spot. **D,** Roth spot. Note white-centered flame hemorrhage superior to macula. **E,** Retinal sea fan typical of sickle cell retinopathy. **F,** Ischemic ocular syndrome. Note conjunctival injection, iris new vessels, irregular pupil, and cataract.

**MYOCARDIAL INFARCTION.** Cerebral emboli may arise from the mural thrombi associated with myocardial infarction. Most common after anterior infarction, left ventricular thrombi usually appear within the first 8 weeks, and cause embolic stroke in about 6% of cases.[52] However, ventricular wall segments rendered akinetic by infarction may allow thrombi to form many months after the acute event. In patients who have suffered TIAs or strokes and have mural thrombi detectable by two-dimensional echocardiography, we recommend long-term warfarin anticoagulation.

**RARE CAUSES OF CARDIOEMBOLIC TVL AND STROKE.** In unexplained CNS ischemic events, some thought should be given to the following unusual cardioembolic conditions because they may be treatable.

**Atrial myxomas** are rare tumors (1 in 4000 autopsies) that account for about 1% of strokes in young adults.[53] Most myxomas occur in the left atrium, appearing in individuals between the ages of 30 and 60 years.[54] About 50% of patients with these tumors develop emboli, chiefly to the brain. Patients often have unexplained malaise, weight loss, fever, petechiae, and abdominal pain. The myxoma generally has little effect on cardiac function but may give rise to subtle, changing murmurs and rarely to signs of mitral insufficiency. Whenever the diagnosis of endocarditis is entertained, atrial myxoma should be on the list. The diagnosis is made by echocardiography and cardiac computed tomography (CT). Treatment is surgical removal.

**Cardiomyopathies** have an estimated 4% per year incidence of clinical embolization,[55] probably as a result of reduced ventricular contractility and the formation of mural thrombi. Even in the absence of demonstrable thrombi, the mere documentation of ventricular dysfunction warrants long-term anticoagulation.

**Paradoxical emboli** occur when material travels from the venous to the arterial circulation through a communication between the right and left parts of the heart or by way of pulmonary vascular shunts. Cerebral and retinal ischemic events have been ascribed to such emboli, coming from occult venous sites and passing through a patent foramen ovale during a Valsalva-induced sudden increase in right ventricular pressure.[56] Diagnosis is made with contrast echocardiography. Patients have been treated with short-term anticoagulation followed by aspirin, with a low rate of recurrent ischemic events.[56] TVL may also occur in intravenous drug abusers, in whom talc emboli may sometimes be found in the retinal arterioles. The emboli are believed to pass from the venous to the arterial circulation through pulmonary vascular shunts.

In the evaluation of patients suspected of having a cardiac source of emboli whose clinical and electrocardiographic studies are normal, echocardiography (two-dimensional, M mode) and arrhythmia monitoring have at best a 6% chance of discovering a pertinent abnormality.[57] Hence, we place greater importance on a careful cardiologic evaluation than on the ordering of these tests. Still, in youthful patients with recurrent monocular TVL and no history of migraine, these noninvasive tests may be worthwhile in spite of the low yield.

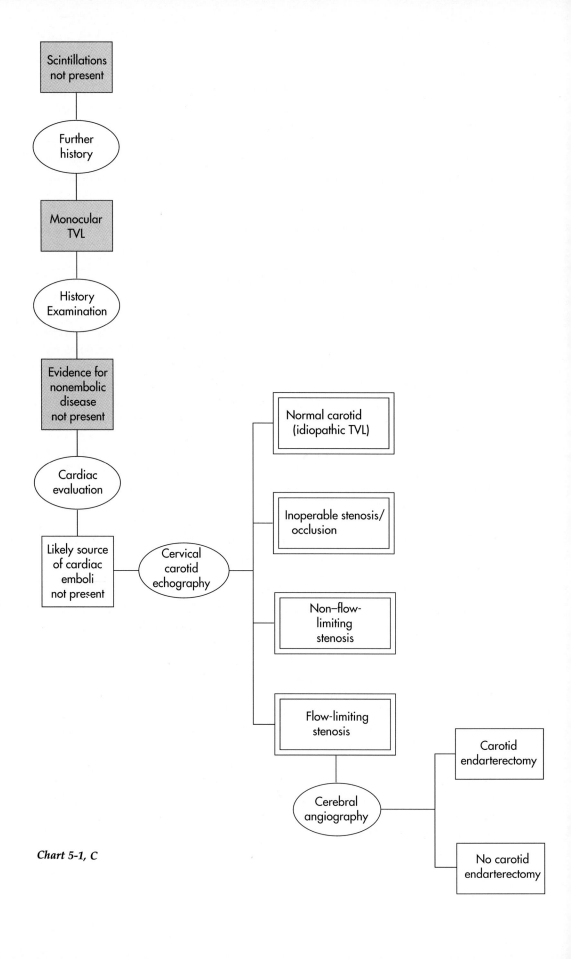

*Chart 5-1, C*

☐ Likely source of cardiac emboli not present

Once the cardiologic examination has ruled out a cardiac source of cerebral emboli, then the examiner must turn to the consideration of cervical atheromatous thromboembolism as a cause of TVL (Chart 5-1, C).

○ *Cervical carotid echography.* Whereas retinal intraluminal plaques and carotid bruits are strong predictors of angiographically proven carotid stenosis, their absence does not exclude such a lesion. The finding of a cholesterol (Hollenhorst) plaque indicates a greater than 50% chance of finding ipsilateral carotid high-grade stenosis (high specificity).[14,58] However, plaques are present in only 10% to 20% of patients with angiographically proven carotid stenosis (low sensitivity).[59,60] Carotid bruits are more specific (90%) for carotid stenosis and more sensitive (60%) than are retinal plaques.[59,60]

The noninvasive carotid studies (in contrast to the invasive study: cerebral arteriography) are designed to measure cervical carotid contour and blood flow and are currently used whenever a reasonable doubt exists that atheromatous carotid lesions will be found. The value of these studies is based on their reliability in excluding carotid wall lesions so that the morbidity and expense of cerebral angiography may be avoided. Of the noninvasive studies in widespread use, the majority depend on finding locally turbulent flow as measured by Doppler and anatomic narrowing noted on B-mode ultrasound. Reliable results with this combined mode (Duplex) scanning depend on considerable examiner skill and experience. Under ideal conditions Duplex carotid scanning is about 95% sensitive to carotid stenosis equivalent to 70% or greater compromise of the luminal diameter (*hemodynamically significant stenosis*)[61] (Fig. 5-4).

Because the search is for flow-limiting and accessible carotid stenosis, we believe that Duplex scanning is a useful screening tool in patients with monocular TVL in whom nonembolic and cardiogenic causes have been excluded. Duplex scanning may provide one of four results.

▢ Normal carotid

If the examination is normal, the cause of TVL remains **idiopathic.** We recommend that such patients be evaluated carefully for nonembolic causes; they may be placed on a regimen of aspirin.

▢ Inoperable stenosis/occlusion

Inoperable stenosis (complete cervical occlusion, inaccessible high cervical occlusion) requires risk factor management and perhaps aspirin therapy.

▢ Non–flow-limiting stenosis

Patients with non–flow-limiting (less than 70% reduction in luminal diameter) cervical stenosis are managed as if they had inoperable stenosis, except that repeat echography may be considered in the future.

▢ Flow-limiting stenosis

Patients with flow-limiting (70% to 90% reduction in luminal diameter) cervical stenosis should be considered for cerebral angiography *only if they are deemed candidates for endarterectomy.*

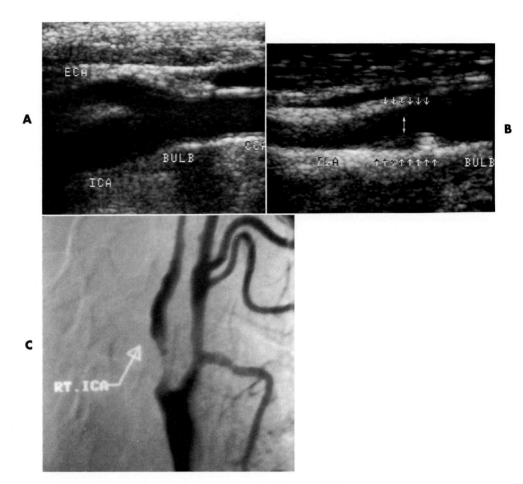

*Fig. 5-4.* Duplex carotid scan of normal cervical carotid bifurcation, **A,** and hemodynamically significant internal carotid stenosis, **B.** Multiple arrows indicate normal position of endothelium. Single arrows indicate actual position of endothelium. Angiography confirms stenosis, **C.** *ECA,* External carotid artery; *ICA,* internal carotid artery; *CCA,* common carotid artery.

○ *Cerebral angiography and carotid endarterectomy.* Before recommending cerebral angiography and carotid endarterectomy, one must take into account the natural history of presumed thromboembolic TVL, the risks of angiography and surgery, and the efficacy of surgery as compared with medical therapy.

**NATURAL HISTORY.** No entirely satisfactory data on the natural (untreated) history of TVL are available. One prospective study[62] showed that of 80 patients with monocular TVL followed for an average of 4.5 years, only 6% suffered a cerebral stroke and 11% a retinal infarction. This is a relatively low stroke rate compared with the 20% stroke rate reported for patients with hemispheric TIAs within the same follow-up period.[63] However, the results of this seminal TVL study may be misleading. Only 27 of the patients had undergone cerebral angiography, and 11 of these showed no abnormalities. Evidently patients with and those without underlying atheromatous disease were mixed together. Since the two groups probably have vastly different stroke prognoses,[64] the aggregate data are not meaningful. A more recent study[65] did include 35 patients with monocular TVL and angiographically verified ipsilateral carotid stenosis. Followed for an average of 7 years without endarterectomy (some were treated with aspirin), only 4 (14%) patients developed stroke, at a yearly rate of 2%. Another study[66] found that of 21 patients with TVL and angiographic carotid stenosis, 8 (38%) developed stroke over an average 8-year follow-up period; of 35 patients with angiographically normal cervical carotid arteries, none developed stroke in the same period.

These studies imply that at least two groups of patients with TVL exist: (1) those with atheromatous carotid disease, who are generally aged over 40 years and who have a risk of stroke slightly below that for hemispheric TIA, and (2) those without atheromatous carotid disease, who are generally aged under 40 years and who have a negligible risk of stroke.

Retrospective data on the course of untreated patients with retinal infarcts[67-69] and plaques[70,71] disclose a stroke rate comparable to that of patients who have TVL and atheromatous carotid disease—about 3% per year. This is somewhat below the stroke risk of 5% per year that is associated with hemispheric TIAs, a discrepancy that may reflect the fact that ischemic events sufficient to interrupt vision are not as severe as those that interrupt other cerebral functions.

Yet, patients with ocular and hemispheric ischemic events have an equal prevalence of carotid atherostenosis and a distressing 30% 5-year expectancy of myocardial infarction.[72] In fact, most patients in either group die of myocardial infarction, not of stroke. The survival of patients with TVL appears to be comparable to that of patients with other types of TIAs. Pfaffenbach and Hollenhorst[73] found a 54% death rate after 7 years in patients with retinal intraluminal plaques, and Savino et al.[71] noted a 49% death rate after 7 years as compared with a 20% expected age-corrected death rate in a control population.

No information is available as to whether the threat of stroke in TVL is greatest within the first few months after the first event. This phenomenon has been observed in other types of TIAs, where 20% of strokes will occur within 1 month and 50% within 1 year.[74] After that, the stroke rate falls to 5% per year, still about five times greater than that for a control population. The duration and frequency of TIAs have no prognostic value, except that some authors consider a sudden increase in frequency an ominous sign of impending stroke.[75]

As noninvasive carotid studies have improved, they have revealed that flow-limiting carotid stenosis is more likely to cause stroke than is non–flow-limiting carotid stenosis.[76,77] This information has led to a sense, though not a consensus, that endarterectomy should be limited to carotid stenosis of 70% or greater.[78,79] Whether carotid ulceration is a separate risk factor is debatable.

**RISKS AND BENEFITS OF INTERVENTION.** Therapy in patients with presumed atheromatous thromboembolism consists of endarterectomy, warfarin anticoagulants, and platelet antiaggregants.

**Endarterectomy.** The risks of endarterectomy begin with those associated with cerebral angiography. In a prospective series of 637 consecutive studies for suspected cerebrovascular disease, angiography produced a 4.2% rate of neurologic complications, of which 0.6% were permanent.[80] Among large retrospective reviews of cerebral angiography, neurologic complications range from 0% [81,82] to 5.4%.[83]

The operative risks of endarterectomy are generally divided into neurologic complications (stroke) and death (myocardial infarction). The combined stroke and death rates have been reported to be between 2.5% and 24.4%.[84] Although the skill and experience of the surgeon would be expected to influence these figures, that has not been conclusively shown.[85,86] More important may be the fact that these patients have widespread arteriosclerosis and are therefore poor surgical risks. Coronary artery disease, hypertension, obstructive pulmonary disease, obesity, and age greater than 70 years all adversely affect outcome.[87] Neurologic risk factors include recent, evolving, or multiple strokes. The principal imaging risk factor is stenosis involving the distal ipsilateral carotid artery or the contralateral carotid artery.[88]

To justify these "up front" risks, endarterectomy must provide a significant reduction in disabling stroke. From 1961 to 1968 a multiinstitutional prospective trial randomized 316 TIA patients to undergo carotid endarterectomy (169) or receive anticoagulant treatment (147).[88] In an average follow-up of 42 months, only 6 (4%) of the surgical patients had strokes after hospital discharge, whereas 20 (14%) of the medical patients had strokes. However, 13 patients (7%) had perioperative strokes, and 6 (4%) of these died. Thus, if the perioperative outcomes are counted, the surgical patients actually fared slightly worse. Careful statistical review indicates that endarterectomy would have had to yield a postoperative stroke-mortality rate of 2.9% or less to provide greater benefit than anticoagulation.[89]

**Anticoagulation.** Even if strictly monitored, warfarin anticoagulation predisposes patients to a dangerously high rate of bleeding, much of it intracerebral, some of it fatal.[90] Low-intensity warfarin, which raises the prothrombin level to 1.2 to 1.6 times control (rather than 2 times control) may be safer, but experience is lacking.[91] Unfortunately, randomized studies of heparin and warfarin reveal no definitive evidence that standard anticoagulation reduces strokes.[92] Because of these dismal statistics, we limit our use of warfarin to patients whose TVL "breaks through" aspirin. Even then, we recommend a low-intensity regimen for a maximum of 4 months.

**Platelet antiaggregation.** Agents that interfere with platelet aggregation have been used for the past decade to prevent stroke. They are of variable efficacy. In controlled studies neither dipyridamole nor sulfinpyrazone (Anturane), when added to aspirin, has proved to be any better in preventing stroke than aspirin alone.[93,94]

Aspirin has been used to prevent stroke in at least 25 controlled trials, with an average reduction of nonfatal stroke of 30%.[95] The initial large-scale Canadian study[94] had reported no stroke-preventing effect of aspirin for women. In subsequent trials no such clear sex difference has emerged, but women have constituted too small a fraction of the study population to be analyzed sepa-

## Management of Transient Visual Loss

1. Try to elicit a history of scintillations. If they are not classic for migraine and the patient lacks a past or family history of migraine, evaluate for "migraine mimickers" such as lupus erythematosus, chronic meningitis, or an occipital lobe lesion causing epilepsy.
2. If scintillatons are not present, determine if symptoms are definitely binocular. If so, the patient may have either vertebrobasilar ischemia or nonscintillatory migraine. When other arteriosclerotic risk factors are present and the patient is elderly and has no clinical evidence of other pertinent disease, attend to arteriosclerotic risk factors. Imaging of the cervical or cerebral circulation is generally not indicated, because vascular surgery in this region is considered too risky. Youthful patients and those without arteriosclerotic risk factors should have a thorough medical evaluation for nonarteriosclerotic vasculopathy and blood dyscrasias.
3. If monocular TVL seems a likely possibility, try to exclude such nonthromboembolic conditions as recurrent hyphema, recurrent angle closure, optic disc anomaly, blood dyscrasia, papilledema, impending retinal vein occlusion, antiphospholipid syndrome, or optic neuropathy.
4. If these nonthromboembolic conditions are excluded, presume that extracranial thromboembolism is causative—with either the heart or the cervical carotid artery as the likely source. Refer the patient for cardiac evaluation.
5. If the heart is not a likely source of embolism, study the cervical carotid vessels with echographic (Duplex) scanning. If this study reveals an operable lesion and the patient is deemed suitable for endarterectomy, perform cerebral angiography to confirm the lesion, and carotid endarterectomy if the appropriate lesion is found.
6. The operative risks of carotid endarterectomy are too high to justify its performance except under ideal circumstances[98] (i.e., no significant cardiovascular or pulmonary disease or obesity, and age below 75 years). Patients with binocular TVL are not suitable for carotid endarterectomy. These patients and patients with monocular TVL who are not candidates for endarterectomy should take one adult aspirin tablet (325 mg) per day. If a history of gastroduodenal ulceration is present, enteric-coated aspirin or ticlopidine are alternatives.

rately with confidence. Thus the efficacy of aspirin in reducing stroke in women remains uncertain. The UK-TIA Study Group[96] found that aspirin doses of 300 mg/day were as effective as higher doses, and much less gastrotoxic.

Ticlopidine hydrochloride, a new platelet antiaggregant, has been shown to be slightly more effective than aspirin in preventing stroke in both men and women who have suffered recent TIAs or mild cerebral or retinal strokes.[97] Side effects, including diarrhea (20%) and skin rash (14%), were mild and self-limited, but severe neutropenia occurred in 0.9%, with one fatality.

# Chronic Ocular Ischemia

Although we have assumed that TVL is a manifestation of acute ischemia, it may rarely occur in a setting of acute-on-chronic ischemia. In such cases the findings and management may be quite different.

The examination of patients with TVL may rarely reveal the findings of persistently marginal circulation to the posterior and anterior segments of the globe. When the posterior segment is chronically deprived of blood, the retinal veins often become dilated and incompetent, scattering round and flame-shaped hemorrhages throughout the fundus, but most densely in the retinal periphery. Cotton-wool spots may also be seen (reflecting nerve fiber layer infarction), as well as retinal surface microaneurysms and neovascularization (reflecting chronic hypoxia). Fluorescein angiography can be used to document areas of capillary closure and nonperfusion of inner retina.

These signs constitute *venous stasis retinopathy*[99] (VSR) (Plate 4, *B*) (see Chapter 7), a condition that may eventually lead to thrombosis of the central retinal vein with attendant massive nerve fiber layer hemorrhage. Some patients with VSR also manifest signs of diminished blood supply to the anterior segment (Plate 4, *F*): aqueous cells and flare, cataract, iris neovascularization, and eventually angle-closure glaucoma. The combination of posterior and anterior ocular ischemia is called ischemic ocular inflammation,[100] or ischemic oculopathy, and reflects inadequate ophthalmic artery perfusion.

Anecdotal reports without long-term documentation have described resolution of the posterior segment findings, and in some cases visual function, after carotid endarterectomy[101] and superficial temporal-middle cerebral artery bypass surgery.[102-104] We have observed improvement in peripheral venous hemorrhages in untreated patients, and we await more solid clinical information in support of the efficacy of any vascular procedure in reversing the ocular ischemic syndrome. Because venous stasis retinopathy is rare even in patients who have complete ipsilateral carotid occlusion,[105] we presume that it signifies compromise of arterial supply much closer to the eye. Thus the opening of proximal large channels would not be expected to be of enduring benefit.

We acknowledge the proven ability of panretinal photocoagulation (PRP) to induce regression of iris neovascularization in diabetes and in nondiabetic ischemic oculopathy, particularly following ischemic central retinal vein occlusion (CRVO).[106] We consider a CRVO ischemic if it is accompanied by a relative afferent pupillary defect or by fluorescein angiographic perfusion defects. Whether to perform PRP prophylactically following ischemic CRVO is controversial, considering that panretinal photocoagulation will inevitably compromise the peripheral visual field. However, neovascular glaucoma follows ischemic CRVO in 20% to 50% of patients.[187] Pending further information, we therefore recommend that PRP be performed prophylactically unless close patient follow-up can be maintained.

## REFERENCES

1. Aldrich MS, Vanderzant CW, Alessi AG, et al. Ictal cortical blindness with permanent visual loss. Epilepsia 1989; 30:116-20.
2. Helgason CM, Sherman DG. Neurologic manifestations of cardiac disease. Neurol Clin 1989;7:469-88.
3. Schafer AI. The hypercoagulable states. Ann Intern Med 1985;102:814-28.
4. Asherson RA, Khamashta MA, Gil A, et al. Cerebrovascular disease and antiphospholipid antibodies in systemic lupus erythematosus, lupuslike disease, and the primary antiphospho-

lipid syndrome. Am J Med 1989; 86:391-9.

5. Dennis MS, Bamford JM, Sandercock PA, et al. Lone bilateral blindness: a transient ischaemic attack. Lancet 1989;1:185-8.

6. Fisher CM. Observations of the fundus oculi in transient monocular blindness. Neurology 1959;9:333-47.

7. Hollenhorst RW. Significance of bright plaques in the retinal arterioles. JAMA 1961;178:23-9.

8. David NJ, Klintworth GK, Friedberg SJ, et al. Fatal atheromatous cerebral embolism associated with bright plaques in the retinal arterioles: report of a case. Neurology 1963;13:708-13.

9. McBrien DJ, Bradley RD, Ashton N. The nature of retinal emboli in stenosis of the internal carotid artery. Lancet 1963;1:697-9.

10. Gunning AJ, Pickering GW, Robb-Smith AHT, et al. Mural thrombosis of the internal carotid artery and subsequent embolism. Q J Med 1964;33:155-95.

11. Dyll L, David NJ. Amaurosis fugax: funduscopic and photographic observations during an attack. Neurology 1966;16:135-8.

12. Hollenhorst RW. The neuro-ophthalmology of strokes. In: Smith JL, ed. Neuro-ophthalmology: symposium of the University of Miami and the Bascom Palmer Eye Institute, vol 2. St Louis: Mosby–Year Book, 1965:109-21.

13. Fisher CM. Transient ischemic attacks—an update [Discussion]. In: Scheinberg P, ed. Cerebrovascular diseases: Tenth Princeton Conference. New York: Raven Press, 1976:50-3.

14. Chawluk JB, Kushner MJ, Bank WJ, et al. Atherosclerotic carotid artery disease in patients with retinal ischemic syndromes. Neurology 1988;38:858-63.

15. Pessin MS, Duncan GW, Mohr JP, et al. Clinical and angiographic features of carotid transient ischemic attacks. N Engl J Med 1977;296:358-62.

16. Fisher CM. Transient monocular blindness associated with hemiplegia. Arch Ophthalmol 1952;47:167-203.

17. Conti CR, Pepine CJ, Curry RC Jr. Coronary artery spasm: an important mechanism in the pathophysiology of ischemic heart disease. Curr Probl Cardiol 1979;4:1-70.

18. Cogan DG. Blackouts not obviously due to carotid occlusion. Arch Ophthalmol 1961;66:180-7.

19. Orcutt JC, Tucker WM, Mills RP, et al. Gaze-evoked amaurosis. Ophthalmology 1987;94:213-8.

20. Barnett HJM. Pathogenesis of transient ischemic attacks. In: Scheinberg P, ed. Cerebrovascular diseases: Tenth Princeton Conference. New York: Raven Press, 1976:1-21.

21. Silverstein A, Gilbert H, Wasserman LR. Neurologic complications of polycythemia. Ann Intern Med 1962; 57:909-16.

22. Kline LB, Kelly CL. Ocular migraine in a patient with cluster headaches. Headache 1980;20:253-7.

23. Wolter JR, Burchfield WJ. Ocular migraine in a young man resulting in unilateral transient blindness and retinal edema. J Pediatr Ophthalmol 1971;8:173-6.

24. Pessin MS, Lathi ES, Cohen MB, et al. Clinical features and mechanism of occipital infarction. Ann Neurol 1987; 21:290-9.

25. Kosmorsky GS, Rosenfeld SI, Burde RM. Transient monocular obscuration—?amaurosis fugax: a case report. Br J Ophthalmol 1985;69:688-90.

26. Lorentzen SE. Drusen of the optic disk: a clinical and genetic study. Acta Ophthalmol Suppl 1966;90:9-180.

27. Beck RW, Corbett JJ, Thompson HS, et al. Decreased visual acuity from optic disc drusen. Arch Ophthalmol 1985; 103:1155-9.

28. Foulkes MA, Wolf PA, Price TR, et al. The Stroke Data Bank: design, methods, and baseline characteristics. Stroke 1988;19:547-54.

29. Meyer JS, Charney JZ, Rivera VM, et al. Cerebral embolization: prospective clinical analysis of 42 cases. Stroke 1971;2:541-54.

30. Swash M, Earl CJ. Transient visual obscurations in chronic rheumatic heart disease. Lancet 1970;2:323-6.

31. Hoyt WF. Ocular symptoms and signs. In: Wylie EJ, Ehrenfield WK,

eds. Extracranial occlusive cerebrovascular disease: diagnosis and management. Philadelphia: WB Saunders, 1970:72.

32. Flegel KM, Shipley MJ, Rose G. Risk of stroke in non-rheumatic atrial fibrillation. Lancet 1987;1:526-9

33. Wolf PA, Dawber TR, Thomas HE Jr, et al. Epidemiologic assessment of chronic atrial fibrillation and risk of stroke: the Framingham study. Neurology 1978;28:973-7.

34. Cerebral Embolism Task Force. Cardiogenic brain embolism: the second report of the Cerebral Embolism Task Force. Arch Neurol 1989;46:727-43.

35. Preliminary report of the Stroke Prevention in Atrial Fibrillation Study. N Engl J Med 1990;322:863-8.

36. Cerebral Embolism Task Force. Cardiogenic brain embolism. Arch Neurol 1986;43:71-84.

37. Kuntze CE, Ebels T, Eijgelaar A, et al. Rates of thromboembolism with three different mechanical heart valve prostheses: randomized study. Lancet 1989;1:514-7.

38. Edmunds LH Jr. Thrombotic and bleeding complications of prosthetic heart valves. Ann Thorac Surg 1987; 44:430-45.

39. Pruitt AA, Rubin RH, Karchmer AW, et al. Neurologic complications of bacterial endocarditis. Medicine 1978; 57:329-43.

40. Aita JA. Systemic and nonarteriosclerotic causes of cerebral infarctions. In: Vinken PJ, Bruyn GW, eds. Handbook of clinical neurology, vol 11. Amsterdam: North Holland, 1972:chap 17.

41. Salgado AV, Furlan AJ, Keys TF, et al. Neurologic complications of endocarditis: a 12-year experience. Neurology 1989;39:173-8.

42. Lopez JA, Ross RS, Fishbein MC, et al. Nonbacterial thrombotic endocarditis: a review. Am Heart J 1987;113:773-84.

43. Devinsky O, Petito CK, Alonso DR. Clinical and neuropathological findings in systemic lupus erythematosus: the role of vasculitis, heart emboli, and thrombotic thrombocytopenic purpura. Ann Neurol 1988;23:380-84.

44. Barlow JB, Pocock WA, Marchand P,

et al. The significance of late systolic murmurs. Am Heart J 1963;66:443-52.

45. Barnett HJM, Boughner DR, Taylor DW, et al. Further evidence relating mitral valve prolapse to cerebral ischemic events. N Engl J Med 1980; 302:139-44.

46. Barnett HJM, Jones MW, Boughner DR, et al. Cerebral ischemic events associated with prolapsing mitral valve. Arch Neurol 1976;33:777-82.

47. Nishimura RA, McGoon MD, Shub C, et al. Echocardiographically documented mitral-valve prolapse: long-term follow-up of 237 patients. N Engl J Med 1985;313:1305-9.

48. Devereux RB, Hawkins I, Kramer-Fox R, et al. Complications of mitral valve prolapse: disproportionate occurrence in men and older patients. Am J Med 1986;81:751-8.

49. Jackson AC, Boughner DR, Barnett HJM. Mitral valve prolapse and cerebral ischemic events in young patients. Neurology 1984;34:784-7.

50. Adams HP Jr, Butler MJ, Biller J, et al. Nonhemorrhagic cerebral infarction in young adults. Arch Neurol 1986; 43:793-6.

51. Lombard JT, Selzer A. Valvular aortic stenosis: a clinical and hemodynamic profile of patients. Ann Intern Med 1987;106:292-8.

52. Arvan S, Boscha K. Prophylactic anticoagulation for left ventricular thrombi after acute myocardial infarction: a prospective randomized trial. Am Heart J 1987;113:688-93.

53. Hart RG, Miller VT. Cerebral infarction in young adults: a practical approach. Stroke 1983;14:110-4.

54. Cogan DG, Wray SH. Vascular occlusions in the eye from cardiac myxomas. Am J Ophthalmol 1975;80:396-403.

55. Gottdiener JS, Gay JA, VanVoorhees L, et al. Frequency and embolic potential of left ventricular thrombus in dilated cardiomyopathy: assessment by 2-dimensional echocardiography. Am J Cardiol 1983;52:1281-5.

56. Biller J, Johnson MR, Adams HP Jr, et al. Further observations on cerebral or retinal ischemia in patients with right-

left intracardiac shunts. Arch Neurol 1987;44:740-3.

57. Come PC, Riley MF, Bivas NK. Roles of echocardiography and arrhythmia monitoring in the evaluation of patients with suspected systemic embolism. Ann Neurol 1983;13:527-31.

58. Sandok BA, Trautmann JC, Ramirez-Lassepas M, et al. Clinical-angiographic correlations in amaurosis fugax. Am J Ophthalmol 1974;78:137-42.

59. Lemak NA, Fields WS. The reliability of clinical predictors of extracranial artery disease, Stroke 1976;7:377-8.

60. Ramirez-Lassepas M, Sandok BA, Burton RC. Clinical indicators of extracranial carotid artery disease in patients with transient symptoms. Stroke 1973;4:537-40.

61. Taylor DC, Strandness DE Jr. Carotid artery duplex scanning. JCU 1987; 15:635-44.

62. Marshall J, Meadows S. The natural history of amaurosis fugax. Brain 1968;91:419-34.

63. Easton JD, Hart RG, Sherman DG, et al. Diagnosis and management of ischemic stroke. I. Threatened stroke and its management. Curr Probl Cardiol 1983;8:1-76.

64. Tippin J, Corbett JJ, Kerber RE, et al. Amaurosis fugax and ocular infarction in adolescents and young adults. Ann Neurol 1989;26:69-77.

65. Hurwitz BJ, Heyman A, Wilkinson WE, et al. Comparison of amaurosis fugax and transient cerebral ischemia: a prospective clinical and arteriographic study. Ann Neurol 1985; 18:698-704.

66. Poole CJM, Ross Russell RW. Mortality and stroke after amaurosis fugax. J Neurol Neurosurg Psychiatry 1985; 48:902-5.

67. Appen RE, Wray SH, Cogan DG. Central retinal artery occlusion. Am J Ophthalmol 1975;79:374-81.

68. Liversedge LA, Smith VH. Neuromedical and ophthalmic aspects of central retinal artery occlusion. Trans Ophthalmol Soc UK 1962;82:571-88.

69. Lorentzen SE. Occlusion of the central retinal artery: a follow-up. Acta Ophthalmol 1969;47:690-703.

70. Howard RS, Ross Russell RW. Prognosis of patients with retinal embolism. J Neurol Neurosurg Psychiatry 1987;50:1142-7.

71. Savino PJ, Glaser JS, Cassidy J. Retinal stroke: is the patient at risk? Arch Ophthalmol 1977;95:1185-9.

72. Heyman A, Wilkinson WE, Hurwitz BJ, et al. Risk of ischemic heart disease in patients with TIA. Neurology 1984;34:626-30.

73. Pfaffenbach DD, Hollenhorst RW. Morbidity and survivorship of patients with embolic cholesterol crystals in the ocular fundus. Am J Ophthalmol 1973;75:66-72.

74. Matsumoto N, Whisnant JP, Kurland LT, et al. Natural history of stroke in Rochester, Minnesota, 1955 through 1969: an extension of a previous study, 1945 through 1954. Stroke 1973;4:20-9.

75. Sandok BA, Furlan AJ, Whisnant JP, et al. Guidelines for the management of transient ischemic attacks. Mayo Clin Proc 1978;53:665-74.

76. Meissner I, Wiebers DO, Whisnant JP, et al. The natural history of asymptomatic carotid artery occlusive lesions. JAMA 1987;258:2704-7.

77. Chambers BR, Norris JW. Outcome in patients with asymptomatic neck bruits. N Engl J Med 1986;315:860-5.

78. Winslow CM, Solomon DH, Chassin MR, et al. The appropriateness of carotid endarterectomy. N Engl J Med 1988;318:721-7.

79. Ojemann RG, Crowell RM, Roberson GH, et al. Surgical treatment of extracranial carotid occlusive disease. Clin Neurosurg 1975;22:214-63.

80. Earnest F IV, Forbes G, Sandok BA, et al. Complications of cerebral angiography: prospective assessment of risk. Am J Roentgenol 1984;142:247-53.

81. Kerber CW, Cromwell LD, Drayer BP, et al. Cerebral ischemia. I. Current angiographic techniques, complications, and safety. Am J Roentgenol 1978; 130:1097-103.

82. Eisenberg RL, Bank WO, Hedgcock MW. Neurologic complications of angiography for cerebrovascular disease. Neurology 1980;30:895-7.

83. Faught E, Trader SD, Hanna GR. Cerebral complications of angiography for transient ischemia and stroke: prediction of risk. Neurology 1979;29:4-15.

84. Warlow C. Carotid endarterectomy: does it work? Stroke 1984;15:1068-76.

85. Slavish LG, Nicholas GG, Gee W. Review of a community hospital experience with carotid endarterectomy. Stroke 1984;15:956-9.

86. Hertzer NR, Avellone JC, Farrell CJ, et al. The risk of vascular surgery in a metropolitan community, with observations on surgeon experience and hospital size. J Vasc Surg 1984;1:13-21.

87. Sundt TM, Sandok BA, Whisnant JP. Carotid endarterectomy: complications and preoperative assessment of risk. Mayo Clin Proc 1975;50:301-6.

88. Fields WS, Maslenikov V, Meyer JS, et al. Joint study of extracranial arterial occlusion. V. Progress report of prognosis following surgical or nonsurgical treatment for transient cerebral ischemic attacks and cervical carotid artery lesions. JAMA 1970;211:1993-2003.

89. Hass WK, Jonas S. Caution: falling rock zone: an analysis of the medical and surgical management of threatened stroke. Proc Inst Med Chic 1980;33:80-4.

90. Levine M, Hirsh J. Hemorrhagic complications of long-term anticoagulant therapy for ischemic cerebral vascular disease. Stroke 1986;17:111-6.

91. Hirsh J, Levine M. Therapeutic range for the control of oral anticoagulant therapy. Arch Neurol 1986;43:1162-4.

92. Grotta JC. Current medical and surgical therapy for cerebrovascular disease. N Engl J Med 1987;317:1505-16.

93. The Canadian Cooperative Study Group. A randomized trial of aspirin and sulfinpyrazone in threatened stroke. N Engl J Med 1978;299:53-9.

94. FitzGerald GA. Dipyridamole. N Engl J Med 1987;316:1247-57.

95. Antiplatelet Trialists' Collaboration. Secondary prevention of vascular disease by prolonged antiplatelet treatment. Br Med J 1988;296:320-31.

96. UK-TIA Study Group. United Kingdom transient ischaemic attack (UK-TIA) aspirin trial: interim results. Br Med J 1988;296:316-20.

97. Hass WK, Easton JD, Adams HP Jr, et al. A randomized trial comparing ticlopidine hydrochloride with aspirin for the prevention of stroke in high-risk patients. Ticlopidine Aspirin Stroke Study Group. N Engl J Med 1989;321:501-7.

98. Matchar DB, Pauker SG. Endarterectomy in carotid artery disease: a decision analysis. JAMA 1987;258:793-8.

99. Kearns TP, Hollenhorst RW. Venous-stasis retinopathy of occlusive disease of the carotid artery. Mayo Clin Proc 1963;38:304-12.

100. Knox DL. Ischemic ocular inflammation. Am J Ophthalmol 1965;60:995-1002.

101. Neupert JR, Brubaker RF, Kearns TP, et al. Rapid resolution of venous stasis retinopathy after carotid endarterectomy. Am J Ophthalmol 1976;81:600-2.

102. Kearns TP, Younge BR, Piepgras DG. Resolution of venous stasis retinopathy after carotid artery bypass surgery. Mayo Clin Proc 1980;55:342-6.

103. Johnston ME, Gonder JR, Canny CLB. Successful treatment of the ocular ischemic syndrome with panretinal photocoagulation and cerebrovascular surgery. Can J Ophthalmol 1988;23:114-9.

104. Kiser WD, Gonder J, Magargal LE, et al. Recovery of vision following treatment of the ocular ischemic syndrome. Ann Ophthalmol 1983;15:305-10.

105. Kearns TP, Siekert RG, Sundt TM. The ocular aspects of carotid artery surgery. Trans Am Ophthalmol Soc 1978;76:246-65.

106. Magargal LE, Brown GC, Augsburger JJ, et al. Efficacy of panretinal photocoagulation in preventing neovascular glaucoma following ischemic central retinal vein obstruction. Ophthalmology 1982;89:780-4.

107. Hayreh SS, Rojas P, Podhajsky P, et al. Ocular neovascularization with retinal vascular occlusion. III. Incidence of ocular neovascularization with retinal vein occlusion. Ophthalmology 1983;90:488-506.

# CHAPTER 6

# Visual Illusions and Hallucinations

• • • • • • • • • • • • • • • • • •

Most disturbances of the visual pathways give rise to "negative" symptoms such as reduced acuity or visual field defects. However, patients often report "positive" symptoms: flashing lights or alterations in the shape, size, position, and motion of viewed objects. Their descriptions may range from momentary scintillations to complex scenes, and from minor distortions to grotesque and frightening visual transformations.

Experiences of this sort may originate from many parts of the visual system, from the temporal lobe, and perhaps from the mesencephalon. In some cases of disordered spatial perception, the lesion may be within the oculomotor or vestibular systems. The nature of the visual experience, its position within the visual field, and the patient's underlying mental and visual state are our principal clues to localization and diagnosis.

## Distinguishing Illusions from Hallucinations

Two types of visual transformations are possible. *Illusions* are misperceptions of external objects. In that sense, they represent disordered processing of incoming sensory information. *Hallucinations* are sensory experiences that are *not* based on incoming sensory information. They are properly considered figments—neural activity that is not directly based on viewing external objects. A simple way to distinguish between illusions and hallucinations is to ask the patient if they disappear when the eyes are closed. If the answer is yes, they are probably illusions; if it is no, they are hallucinations.

Making this distinction may not always be so easy for either the patient or the physician. For example, the perceptions of patients who have poor vision, a clouded sensorium, or dementia may be so altered that simple objects suggest complex forms to them. A misperception may trigger a full-fledged hallucination. In some instances, how to label the experience is not clear. For example, when a patient reports that he or she is now seeing a dog crossing the road, and actually did witness such a scene 10 minutes earlier, is this an illusion or a hallucination?

Illusions and hallucinations most commonly derive either from the globe or from vision-related cortex. The intervening portions of the visual pathway appear to be relatively silent. Although micropsia has been described in chiasmal disease,[1] we have not seen it.

Illusions differ in their origins from hallucinations in that they may be caused by optical ("preneural") abnormalities, whereas hallucinations are always neural events. Illusions may be caused by improper refractive corrections (altered shape) and disorders of the lens (multiple images, altered color), outer retina (micropsia, metamorphopsia, xanthopsia), visual association and parietal cortex (altered size, shape, position, distance, motion, multiple images), and oculomotor or vestibular systems (altered position, motion).

In contrast to illusions, hallucinations always derive from endogenous activation of anterior visual pathways (retina, optic nerve), visual and temporal cortex, and, less commonly, brainstem limbic circuits. In a retrospective study of 104 consecutive patients diagnosed as having retinocalcarine lesions, Lepore[2] found that 51% complained of elementary hallucinations (flashes, simple geometric forms), whereas 21% complained of complex hallucinations (people, faces, animals, vehicles, clothing)—figures that are comparable to those of a previous study by Kolmel.[3,4] Among Lepore's patients the nature of the hallucination did not correlate with the location of the lesion. Hallucinations were often associated with a visual acuity of 20/50 or worse in at least one eye. Lepore concluded that the nature of hallucinations occurring in the context of visual pathway disease has no localizing value and that these hallucinations represent "release phenomena," that is, an emergence of endogenous neural activity normally suppressed by vision. Weinberger and Grant[5] had previously come to the same conclusion. While we generally support this point of view, we believe that the following statements are correct provided that the patient has a clear sensorium:

1. Very brief flashes of white or colored light exacerbated by eye movement are likely to represent physical deformation of retinal receptors (vitreous tug, retinal tear or detachment).
2. Sparkling lights confined to one eye are characteristic of damage to the retina or optic nerve.
3. Geometric scintillations are likely to represent visual cortex damage; a progression of scintillations across a hemianopic field over a period of 20 to 30 minutes is nearly pathognomonic of migraine.
4. Scenes with animate figures are typical of visual association cortex lesions.[6]
5. Scenes that have a sense of familiarity are derived from temporal lobe neural activity.[7]

These principles of localization are based on both clinicopathologic correlation and cortical electrode stimulation in awake patients.[7] While they are useful guidelines, they are so often violated that we place heavy diagnostic weight on the patient's background mental and visual state, the medication and drug abuse history, and the location of the altered sensation within the visual field.

The pathophysiology of illusions and hallucinations is not well understood. Illusions may result from:

1. Optical aberrations such as those imposed by astigmatic lenses or lenticular surface and refractive index inhomogeneities
2. Disordered processing within the occipital lobe or as a release of endogenous neural activity in a setting of reduced sight and altered cognition

Hallucinations, on the other hand, probably represent abnormal neural discharges generated by three possible mechanisms[8]:

1. A partial seizure
2. Imbalance in central nervous system (CNS) neurotransmitter systems caused by pharmacologic agents, toxins, or other diffuse disease processes
3. Disinhibition of "dreamlike" experiences caused by visual deprivation or an altered state of consciousness

Only if the first mechanism is operative will hallucinations be attenuated by antiepileptic medications. The second and third mechanisms are best alleviated by removing the underlying cause or treating with antipsychotic or minor tranquilizing agents.

**DELUSIONS.** Illusions and hallucinations must be distinguished from *delusions*, or thought disorders in which reality testing is defective. Patients who are having altered sensory experiences, whether illusory or hallucinatory, may also be deluded if they believe that the images they see are real. Temporary delusions are common and need not indicate ongoing psychopathology, as, for example, when vivid hallucinations are experienced by children or suggestible adults, especially in near-sleep states.

# A Decision Tree Approach to the Evaluation of Illusions and Hallucinations

The diagnosis of illusions and hallucinations demands an integration of many aspects of the clinical examination. With the usual limitations that process can be analyzed as a series of information-gathering steps (Chart 6-1).

First, the examiner should decide if the altered visual experience—whether it be an illusion or hallucination—could be caused by a psychoactive agent.

■ Psychoactive agent present

▣ Pharmacologically induced visual illusions or hallucinations

Virtually every psychoactive medication or drug has been associated with the production of visual hallucinations[9] (see box on p. 149). The medications most often implicated are those with anticholinergic and dopaminergic properties. Among hallucinogenic street drugs, mescal, psilocybin, lysergic acid, and am-

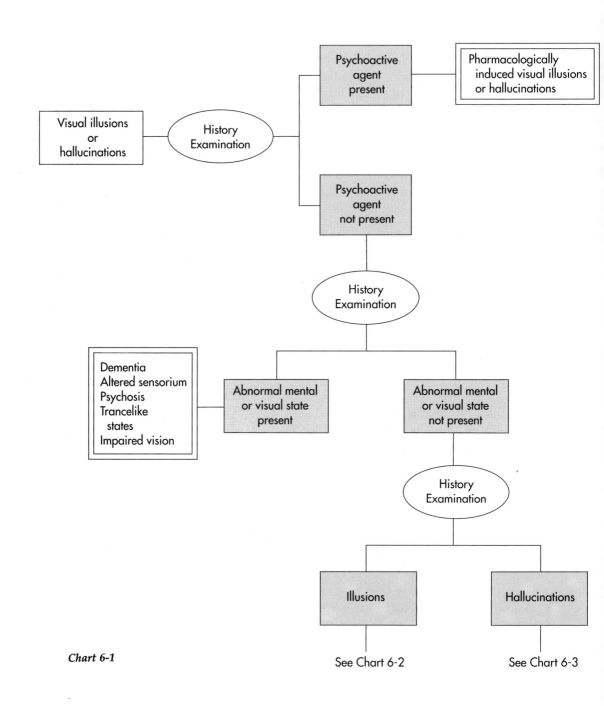

*Chart 6-1*

## Psychoactive Agents That Cause Visual Illusions and Hallucinations

**Dopaminergics**

Levodopa
Selegiline
Bromocriptine
Methyldopa

**Anticholinergics**

Trihexyphenidyl
Atropine
Cyclopentolate
Benztropine
Scopolamine

**Tricyclic antidepressants**

Amitriptyline
Nortriptyline
Doxepin
Trazodone
Imipramine

**Beta-adrenergic blockers**

Propranolol
Betaxolol
Atenolol
Timolol

**Adrenergics**

Phenylephrine
Theophylline
Pseudoephedrine
Albuterol

**Miscellaneous**

Histamine $H_2$ receptor antagonists
Narcotic analgesics
Antineoplastic agents
Nonsteroidal antiinflammatory agents
Calcium channel blockers
Antifungal agents
Antiarrhythmics
Salicylates
Intravenous and intrathecal contrast agents
Benzodiazepines
Anticonvulsants
Corticosteroids
Antibacterial agents
Antiviral agents
Nitrates
Fluoxetine
Methysergide

**Street drugs**

Amphetamines
Lysergic acid
Cocaine
Mescal
Psilocybin

phetamines are most commonly cited. Withdrawal from habitual use of some of these agents, as well as alcohol, may cause prominent illusions and hallucinations. Although drug-induced or drug-withdrawal visual hallucinations may be accompanied by auditory hallucinations, psychotic thought disorder, or delirium, it is critical to recognize that the *visual aberrations may exist as an isolated manifestation.*

### ▮ Psychoactive agent not present

If no psychoactive agent can be blamed for the altered visual experiences, then the examiner must decide if these experiences are occurring in a setting of an abnormal mental or visual state.

■ Abnormal mental or visual state present

Visual illusions and hallucinations are common manifestations of a variety of altered states of consciousness, psychosis, and impaired vision. We consider these conditions together for two reasons: (1) they do not usually result from a focal lesion, and (2) they are not abrupt in onset, tending rather to drift in and out. The altered visual experiences probably reflect a destabilization of neurotransmitter systems and not partial seizures, and respond better to antipsychotics or tranquilizers than to anticonvulsants.

▣ Dementia

Visual hallucinations are widely reported in the advancing stages of all dementing processes. They may arise spontaneously and are exacerbated when the patient is sensorially deprived (e.g., left alone in a darkened room) or treated with psychoactive medications ("sundowning").

▣ Altered sensorium

Visual hallucinations occur in many normal individuals (and in narcoleptics) as they are about to enter sleep *(hypnagogic hallucinations)* or as they emerge from sleep *(hypnopompic hallucinations).* How these relate physiologically to dreams is not clear.

Visual illusions and hallucinations are also frequent manifestations of delirium, an altered behavioral and autonomic state brought on by infection, fever, metabolic disarray, anoxia-ischemia, increased intracranial pressure, toxins, drugs, and drug withdrawal states.

▣ Psychosis

The visual hallucinations of psychosis are generally complex and often integrated with auditory hallucinations and delusional thought processes.[8] They are typically paranoid and held to be real. We have also encountered such paranoid hallucinations among demented or severely visually impaired patients.

▣ Trancelike states

Visual hallucinations are a prominent feature of trancelike states, which may be entered by suggestible individuals as a result of hypnosis, intense emotional stress, or religious ritual.[10] Children are known to have fantasies of imaginary playmates whom they sometimes regard as real.[11] Such childhood fantasizing may easily be misinterpreted as a pathologic hallucination.

▣ Impaired vision

Patients who are deprived of incoming visual stimuli report all types of visual illusions and hallucinations. The imagery may be uncommonly detailed and graphic, often reflecting past experiences. The visual creations may be threatening, particularly among the elderly, who need not be demented. More perplexing are the occasional reports of patients who describe hallucinations after visual loss in only one eye.[12] We have not seen such cases. Among patients who have visual deprivation hallucinations, we have found that low-dose haloperidol (0.5 to 1.0 mg/day) often quiets their symptoms. Anticonvulsants have been less effective, leading us to agree with Lepore[2] that the "released" visual activity is not epileptic.

### Abnormal mental or visual state not present

If the mental and visual backgrounds are intact and the patient has no psychoactive drug history, the examiner should try to ascertain whether the visual experience is an illusion or a hallucination, and then whether it is confined to one eye or one hemifield.

### Illusions (Chart 6-2)

In inquiring if the illusion is seen with one or both eyes, the examiner should always guard against the possibility that the illusion is restricted to a homonymous field and that the patient incorrectly interprets it as emanating from a single eye. A mistake here would upset the analysis.

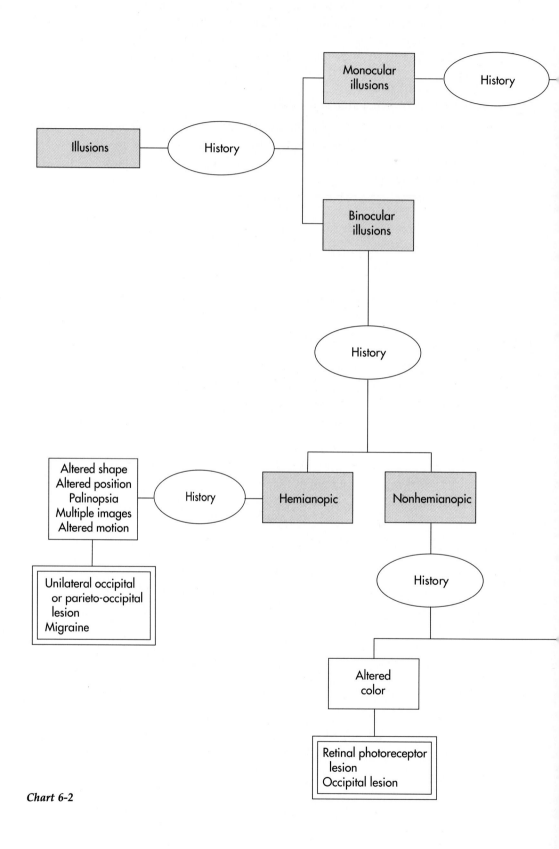

**Chart 6-2**

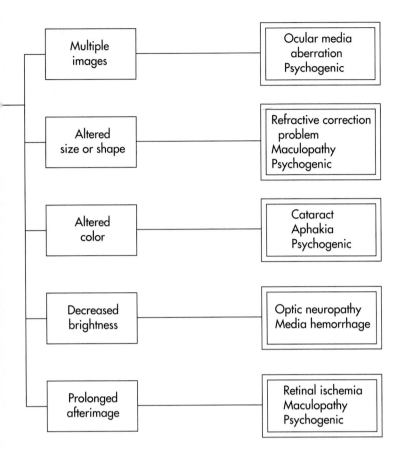

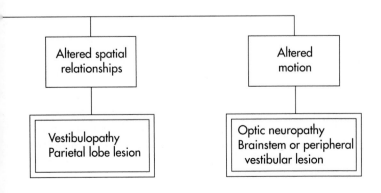

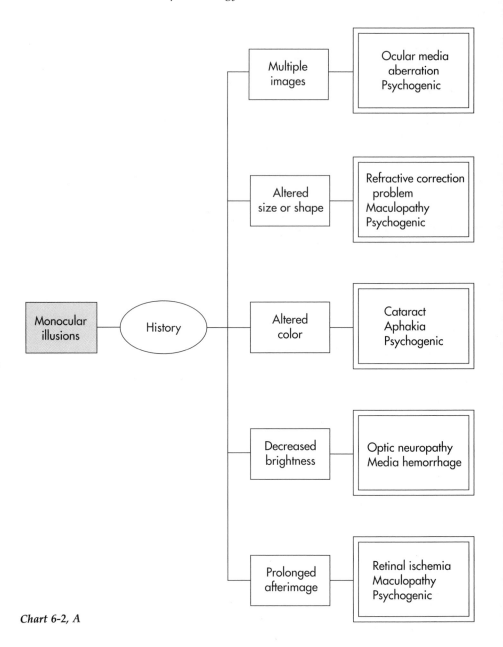

*Chart 6-2, A*

## Monocular illusions (Chart 6-2, A)

Monocular illusions derive from far forward within the visual processing chain: the refractive correction or the retina.

### Multiple images

When one eye sees two images (usually one clear image, the second a "ghost" around the first), the explanation is nearly always an **aberration within the re-**

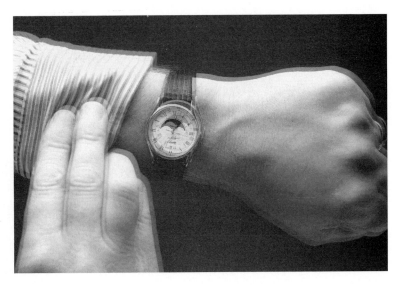

***Fig. 6-1.*** "Ghosting." Two images are slightly displaced from one another. One image is typically clear, the other faint. A monocular illusion, it is usually caused by refractive or media aberrations.

**fracting media** of the eye (Fig. 6-1; see Chapter 9). The diagnosis is made by finding that a pinhole eliminates the accessory image. Myopic astigmatism or early cataract are common causes. If refractive correction is unhelpful, a topical miotic may attenuate the diplopia.

When patients complain of continuously seeing two or more distinct images with one eye and a pinhole does not eliminate the diplopia, the problem is likely to be **psychogenic.**

### ☐ Altered size or shape

The first consideration should always be a **refractive problem**—a new corrective lens that contains a power, axis, or base curve change for one eye only.[13] The patient will say that edges of objects appear tilted or bowed and that viewing them induces a deep-seated ache about the eyes. Although patients often adapt in time, to prescribe a refraction that creates a substantial image size difference between the two eyes *(aniseikonia)* is unwise.

If the patient complains of seeing a smaller image in one eye and refractive changes are not the explanation, then **maculopathy** (macular edema or scarring) should be considered. As the cones become separated by edema, fewer of them are stimulated by the viewed object, and the object is perceived as smaller than normal *(micropsia)*. As the edema is usually not evenly distributed, the object may also appear distorted *(metamorphopsia)* (Fig. 6-2). The receptors may be drawn abnormally close together in the healing phase to produce an illusion of *macropsia*.

Here again, the problem may also be **psychogenic.**

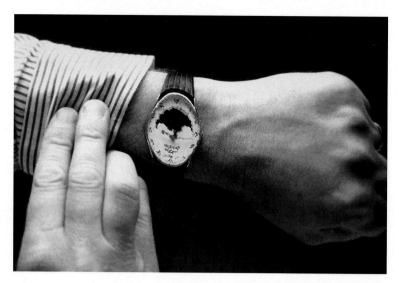

*Fig. 6-2.* Retinal metamorphopsia. Image borders have curvilinear distortion. Arising from displacement of foveal cones, illusion is confined to fixational area. Micropsia often coexists.

### ☐ Altered color

Monocular alterations in color are of three types: (1) brunescence, (2) cyanopsia, and (3) erythropsia. *Brunescence* refers to the yellowish brown tint that discolors images seen by an eye with **cataract.** *Cyanopsia* is the blue tint that discolors the vision of patients who have recently undergone cataract extraction.[14] *Erythropsia* refers to the reddish cast to the vision of **aphakic** or pseudophakic patients when they are exposed to bright sun or snow.[15] Its mechanism is unknown; fortunately, it lasts no more than 48 hours. Erythropsia may also be experienced by patients who suffer anterior chamber or vitreous hemorrhages.

    **Psychogenic** causes may also be involved.

### ☐ Decreased brightness

Many patients who have suffered damage to the retinal nerve fiber layer or optic nerve report that the image appears dimmer when viewed with the affected eye. The objective correlate of their complaint is the **afferent pupillary defect** (see Chapter 1). However, the same complaint is generated by opacification of the ocular media by anterior chamber or vitreous **hemorrhage.**

### ☐ Prolonged afterimage

Patients who report that their vision is impaired after viewing a bright light or object usually do not have an organic correlate for their complaint. However, on occasion they may be describing a pathologically prolonged afterimage, the result of delayed photopigment regeneration in **retinal ischemia**[16] or **maculopathy. Psychogenic** causes must also be considered.

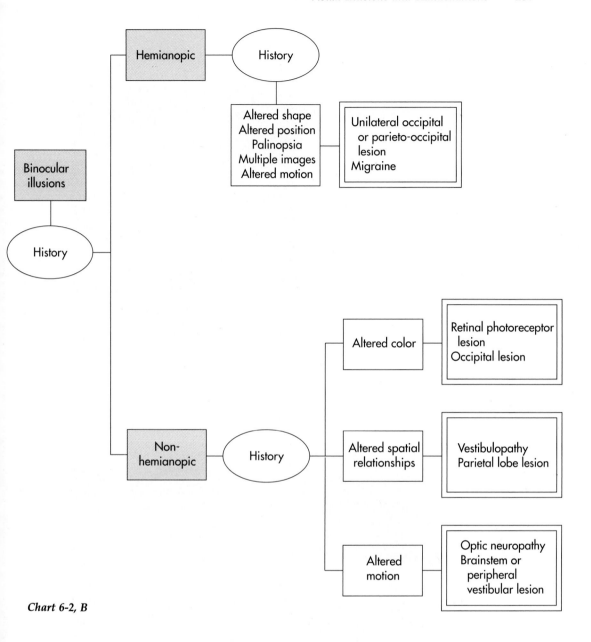

*Chart 6-2, B*

## ▨ Binocular illusions (Chart 6-2, *B*)

In contrast to monocular illusions, binocular illusions are rarely associated with refractive corrections, arising instead from injury to photoreceptors, optic nerve, visual cortex, or oculomotor or vestibular pathways. In sorting out where these illusions come from, it is wise to ask if they seem to *originate in or remain predominantly confined to one hemifield.* If so, they are likely to derive from an injured hemispheric cortex on the opposite side.

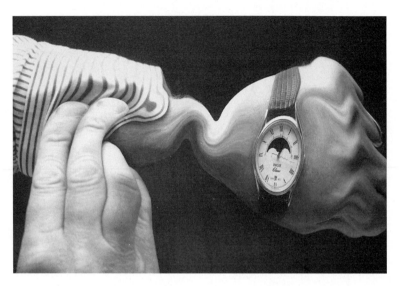

*Fig. 6-3.* Cerebral metamorphopsia (illusory spread). Components of entire scene are displaced and distorted in an often grotesque and frightening way. This illusion may be caused by psychoactive agents, other delirious states, or posterior hemispheric lesions.

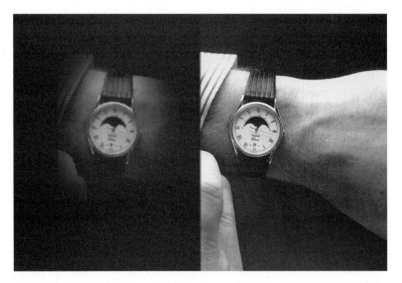

*Fig. 6-4.* Cerebral diplopia. Object viewed in intact (right) hemifield is displaced into defective (left) hemifield (visual allesthesia). If original object remains in view, patient will experience diplopia.

## Binocular hemianopic illusions

### Altered shape

Binocular distortions of shape are reported most commonly shortly after an acute occipital lobe lesion, usually an infarct, trauma, or an expanding tumor or hemorrhage. If one hemisphere has been injured, the illusion may be confined to the contralateral hemifield. Patients typically describe elongations of forms along one plane, with overlapping of one object onto another (*cerebral metamorphopsia*, or *illusory spread*[17]) (Fig. 6-3). Cone-heads may grow out of shoulders, and gigantic fingers from elbows, rather like a Cubist painting. Such illusions may be episodic or persistent, but they usually disappear spontaneously within days to weeks of onset. They often coexist with palinopsia (see below) or hallucinations.

### Altered position

Patients who have had unilateral occipital lobe injury may episodically displace the image of a previously viewed object into the opposite hemifield (*visual allesthesia*)[18] (Fig. 6-4). For example, a figure standing to the right of fixation will, a moment later, appear to be standing to the left of fixation. When the inciting visual stimulus for allesthesia is still within view, patients may think they are having double vision (*cerebral diplopia*).

All patients who experience visual allesthesia have hemianopic field defects, but the defects are rarely total. The allesthetic image is almost always "seen" in the defective hemifield. This altered visual experience appears to be an epileptic phenomenon. During the episode patients have either an altered sensorium, focal tonic-clonic movements, or a focal discharge on the electroencephalogram (EEG). Antiepileptic medications are frequently effective.

### Palinopsia

Patients may report seeing a previously viewed scene, such as a household setting or a highway signpost, suddenly "played back" before their eyes (Fig. 6-5). Critchley called this "a visual perseveration in time," or *palinopsia* ("palinopia," "paliopia").[17] The "playback" may occur immediately after the object has been viewed, or hours later. The greater the time gap, the more likely it is to be considered a hallucination rather than an illusion.

Palinopsia is most often associated with unilateral acute, enlarging, or recovering temporal-parietal-occipital junction lesions. In some patients the palinopsic experience appears to be part of a focal seizure, but in others it may not be.[19,20] Right posterior hemisphere lesions have outnumbered left hemisphere lesions. Whereas the episodes generally subside within weeks, they may persist. Anticonvulsant therapy is worth a try.

### Multiple images

Patients who have unilateral occipital lesions may say that an object moving across their path of vision appears to be broken up into many objects along that path. This "piecemealing" of motion is probably a perseverative or palinopsic disturbance. Patients interpret it as a polyopia for moving objects.[21]

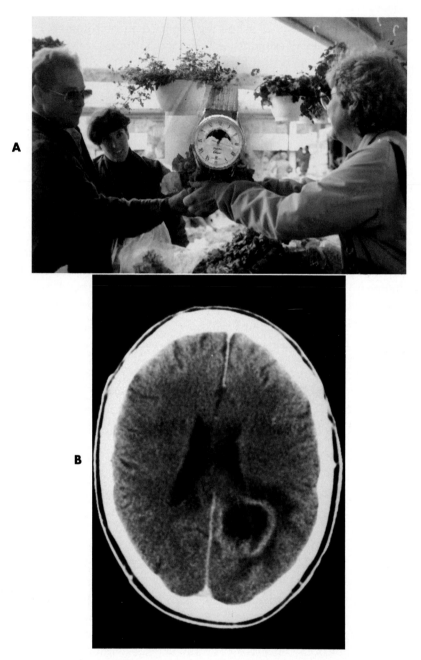

*Fig. 6-5.* Palinopsia (visual perseveration). **A,** Having first looked at his watch, viewer looks up and sees a faint image of the watch superimposed on this market scene. **B,** Later brain computed tomography (CT) scan reveals causative lesion, a left parieto-occipital glioblastoma multiforme.

☐ Altered motion

A partially damaged occipital cortex may also give rise to the sensation of continuous or episodic motion of stationary viewed objects.[22]

☐ Unilateral occipital or parieto-occipital lesion

Many of the hemianopic visual illusions (and hallucinations) occur together. They generally reflect abnormal neural activity in a subtotal unilateral posterior hemispheric lesion. If the lesion involves primary visual cortex or optic radiations, a visual field defect will be present. Because the hemianopic field defect has important localizing value, it is worth searching for. However, it may be small, shallow, or absent altogether.

☐ Migraine

Migraine may produce many of these illusory distortions in the size, position, and shape of viewed objects (the "Alice in Wonderland syndrome"[23]). We suggest, however, that the examiner actively exclude other causes before settling on migraine as the diagnosis.

■ Binocular nonhemianopic illusions

The very illusions reported by patients as emanating from one hemifield may also be described as emanating from the entire field. When the illusions are not confined to one hemifield, the examiner must consider four possibilities:

1. The lesion is confined to one posterior hemisphere but the patient's history is poor.
2. The lesion is in both posterior hemispheres.
3. The lesion is in the retinas or optic nerves of both eyes.
4. The lesion lies outside the afferent visual pathways, in the vestibular or oculomotor systems.

Clues to localization come principally from the nature of the illusion and the neuro-ophthalmologic findings.

☐ Altered color

When patients have become toxic on digitalis preparations, they may report a yellowish green tinge or frosting to their vision *(xanthopsia)*, a reflection of **retinal photoreceptor damage.**[24]

**Lesions** restricted to the inferior **occipital lobes,** affecting lingual and fusiform gyri, may cause achromatopsia *over the entire field of vision.* Such patients typically also have superior altitudinal visual field defects to achromatic stimuli.[25,26] Bilateral posterior cerebral infarctions are the most common cause.

☐ Altered spatial relationships

Infarction of the lateral medullary plate (Wallenberg's syndrome) may cause patients to see their environment as tilted or even "upside down" for days to weeks.[27] The diagnosis of this **vestibulopathy** is based on finding objective cor-

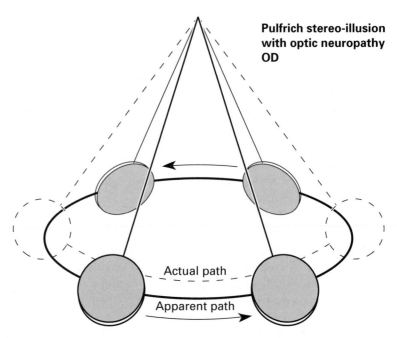

*Fig. 6-6.* Pulfrich stereo-illusion. Pendulum swinging in a line is mistakenly perceived as swinging in a counterclockwise arc by patient with optic neuropathy in right eye. Illusion results from differential conduction rates through normal and damaged optic nerves.

relates of brainstem damage (nystagmus, ataxia, faulty ocular pursuit). Brief illusions of this type may occur during vertebrobasilar transient ischemic attacks.[28]

Bilateral **parieto-occipital damage** may lead to severe difficulty in judging the relative distances of objects in space and manifest itself as misreaching under visual guidance, bumping into furniture, or getting lost.[29] Although such patients may complain that objects appear displaced, their problem is not that they are experiencing illusions, but that they cannot function within space *(topographic agnosia)*. Their deficit is believed to result from a disconnection between visual cortex and parietal cortex, where multiple sensory inputs are integrated.[30]

### Altered motion

Illusions of motion may be caused by unilateral (or markedly asymmetric) **optic nerve lesions.** When these patients are shown a pendulum oscillating in a plane, they incorrectly perceive it as describing an ellipse (counterclockwise rotation if the right optic nerve is lesioned; clockwise rotation if the left optic nerve is lesioned) (Fig. 6-6). Called the *Pulfrich stereo-illusion,* this misperception is believed to result from unequal conduction rates in the two optic nerves.[31] Some patients who demonstrate the Pulfrich stereo-illusion also complain that they can no longer tell how fast a tennis ball or baseball is moving or judge its distance from them. A ball thrown at them appears to curve as it approaches. Whether these complaints and the Pulfrich illusion are related is uncertain.

The most frequent illusions of motion do not arise from visual pathway lesions, but from oculomotor disturbances. *Oscillopsia* is the name given to the illusion of rhythmic movement of stationary objects.[32] Oscillopsia is most clearly described by patients who have large-amplitude nystagmus. If the nystagmus is pendular (both phases are slow eye movements), patients will perceive a to-and-fro movement. If the nystagmus is jerk (one phase is fast), they will perceive the objects as moving only in the direction of the fast phase (no vision occurs during the fast phase; during the slow phase the image is perceived as moving opposite to its direction of movement on the retina). Sometimes the patient does not clearly distinguish movement and instead reports a "shimmery" sensation that may be misinterpreted as a scintillation.

Oscillopsia may also be described by patients who do not have nystagmus, but who have a defective vestibulo-ocular reflex (VOR).[33] When the VOR is functioning normally, head and body movements are synchronized perfectly with eye movements in the opposite direction. When the VOR is defective, this synchrony is disturbed, and the eyes cannot be maintained immobile in space during slight head or body movements. The result is that the patient sees stationary objects as blurred or "jiggling."[34] The offending lesion lies in the **vestibular pathways,** in either the end organs, nerves, or brainstem connections. In our experience, patients with chronic lesions adapt quite well to VOR defects; the symptom is encountered more frequently in acute processes such as aminoglycoside ototoxicity and brainstem infarct, demyelination, or tumor. A simple way to verify that the VOR is the cause of the symptom is to have the patient read a Snellen near card while moving the head rapidly from side to side. Under normal circumstances the VOR compensation permits continued clear vision; if the VOR is defective, acuity will be severely degraded.

Oscillopsia is *never a complaint of patients with congenital nystagmus,* even when the ocular oscillations are very large.

## Hallucinations (Chart 6-3)

The analysis of hallucinations proceeds as it does for illusions. The pattern of the hallucination has some localizing value, but *only in a setting of normal mentation and adequate vision.*

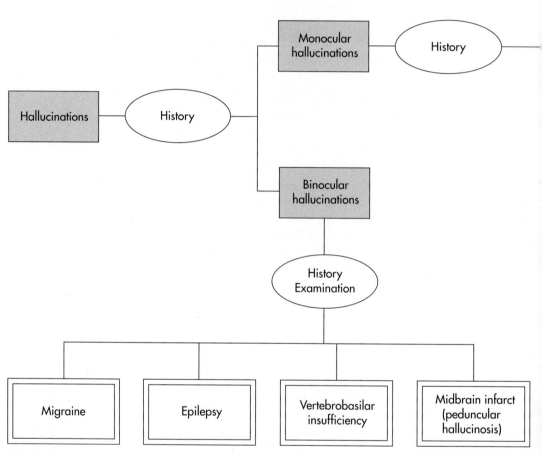

*Chart 6-3*

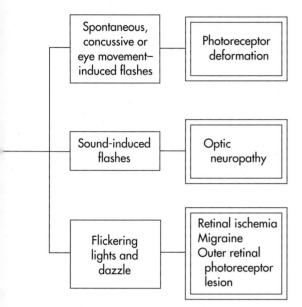

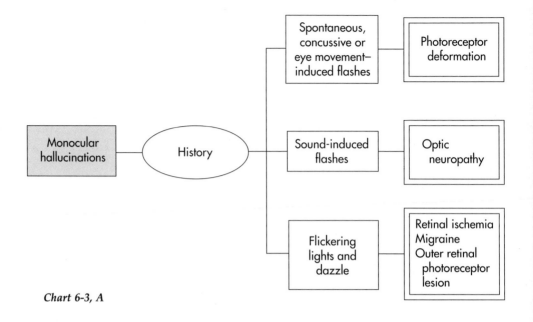

*Chart 6-3, A*

## Monocular hallucinations (Chart 6-3, A)

If hallucinations appear to come from one eye, they originate from the photoreceptors or the optic nerve.

### Spontaneous, concussive or eye movement–induced flashes

These momentary hallucinations probably derive from retinal **photoreceptor deformation.** When the flashes *(phosphenes, Moore's lightning flashes)* are spontaneous or eye movement induced, one must suspect contracting vitreous or vitreous detachment. An indirect ophthalmoscopic examination is advisable to rule out a retinal tear, detachment, or tumor.

### Sound-induced flashes

If a sudden sound triggers a flash of light (phosphene) in one eye, the patient has an **optic nerve lesion,** usually demyelinative. These sound-induced phosphenes,[35] or auditory-visual synesthetic phenomena, usually arise when the patient is in a state of repose or near sleep.

### Flickering lights and dazzle

Silvery scintillations and dazzle restricted to one eye are symptoms of **retinal ischemia** (reduced arterial flow or impaired venous drainage).[16] However, the same symptoms are often seen in young patients who have no evidence of ocular vascular insufficiency, and who may have a history of **migraine** with aura. In these cases the attacks are labeled *ocular migraine* or *cilioretinal migraine,* but the mechanism is unknown[36] (see Chapter 16).

Flickering scintillations that look like "snow" or "noise on a television screen" are also reported in patients who have **outer retinal disorders affecting photoreceptors,** especially in multiple evanescent white dot syndrome (MEWDS), presumed to be a viral or dysimmune condition affecting the outer retina.[37]

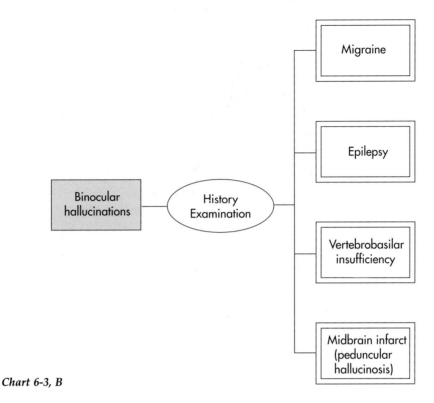

*Chart 6-3, B*

## Binocular hallucinations (Chart 6-3, *B*)

The examiner must differentiate between four processes: migraine, epilepsy, vertebrobasilar insufficiency, or, very rarely, a midbrain infarct (peduncular hallucinosis). This differentiation may not always be straightforward.

### Migraine

The visual hallucinations of migraine are distinctive in that they progress slowly across the visual field, completing their march within a period of 20 to 30 minutes (Fig. 6-7; see also Chapter 16). Although zigzag, "fortification" scintillations *(teichopsia)* are common, they need not occur. Furthermore, whereas the scintillations are usually confined to one hemifield, they may not occupy it completely, and they may spread to involve the opposite hemifield. Headache need not follow the visual hallucination *(acephalgic migraine)*.

Visual hallucinations of animate objects or scenes do rarely occur in migraine,[23] making its differentiation from partial complex epilepsy very difficult.

### Epilepsy

The nature of the visual hallucinations in epilepsy appears to depend on the origin of the initial discharge. Primary visual cortex sources tend to give rise to flashing lights or simple geometric forms. Sources closer to the temporal lobe generate more complex shapes, more complete scenes, and visual memories.[38] To complicate further the distinction between migraine and epilepsy, the scintillations of occipital seizures may be followed by headache and blindness, espe-

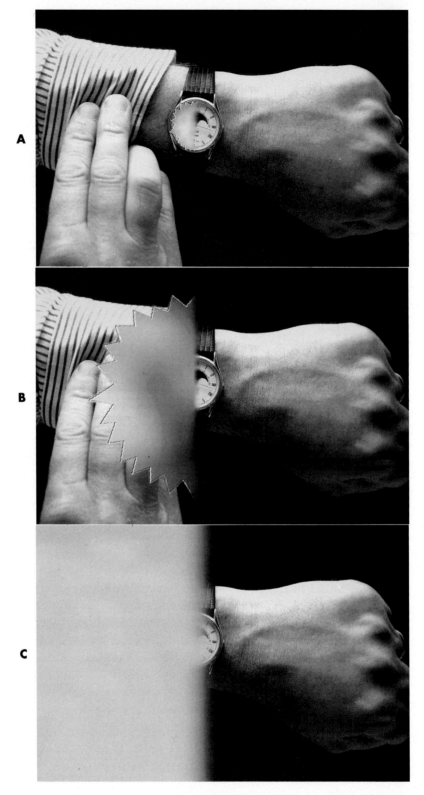

*Fig. 6-7.* Migraine with typical visual aura. **A,** Small left paracentral translucent scotoma with lateral sparkling zigzag ("fortification") border begins to intrude on vision. **B,** Scotoma spreads laterally. **C,** Within 20 to 30 minutes of onset, entire left hemifield has become obscured. Defect clears rapidly at this point.

> ### Management of Binocular Hallucinations
>
> 1. Build as robust a case for classic migraine as possible, the most reliable features being the "march" of scintillations across the hemianopic visual field, the 20 to 30-minute duration, and the sterotypy of attacks.
> 2. Perform brain imaging and electroencephalography if the clinical case for migraine is not absolutely convincing. Because small occipital and temporal lesions may escape detection with computed tomography (CT), we prefer magnetic resonance imaging (MRI).

cially in children.[39] However, marching scintillations, so typical of migraine, are very rare in epilepsy.

### ▣ Vertebrobasilar insufficiency

Transient ischemic attacks in the vertebrobasilar circuit can produce binocular scintillations. They are distinguished from migraine by the absence of a march across the visual field, and by lack of stereotypy.

### ▣ Midbrain infarct (peduncular hallucinosis)

Binocular visual hallucinations of colored lights have been elicited by electrical stimulation of the midbrain,[40] and hallucinations of brightly colored scenes including animate figures have been reported in patients who have sustained mesencephalic infarcts (peduncular hallucinosis).[41,42] The more complex experiences may be related to an altered sleep-wake cycle, or, alternatively, to coexistent injury to the occipitotemporal cortex, since many patients may also have had damage to the distal posterior circulatory bed.

# A Final Caveat

Psychogenic illness without psychosis can produce all of the symptoms described in this chapter. Because no deficit can be measured, correct diagnosis may be even more difficult than in cases of unexplained visual loss (see Chapter 1). As with unexplained visual loss, our approach is to consider visual illusions and hallucinations psychogenic only after organic entities have been reasonably ruled out.

## REFERENCES

1. Bender MB, Savitsky N. Micropsia and teleopsia limited to the temporal fields of vision. Arch Ophthalmol 1943;29:904-8.
2. Lepore FE. Spontaneous visual phenomena with visual loss: 104 patients with lesions of retinal and neural afferent pathways. Neurology 1990;40:444-7.
3. Kolmel HW. Coloured patterns in hemianopic fields. Brain 1984;107:155-67.
4. Kolmel HW. Complex visual hallucinations in the hemianopic field. J Neurol Neurosurg Psychiatry 1985;48:29-38.
5. Weinberger LM, Grant FC. Visual hallucinations and their neuro-optical correlates. Arch Ophthalmol 1940;23:166-99.
6. Lance JW. Simple formed hallucinations confined to the area of a specific visual field defect. Brain 1976;99:719-34.
7. Penfield W, Rasmussen T. The cerebral cortex of man: a clinical study of localization of function. New York: Macmillan, 1950.
8. Asaad G, Shapiro B. Hallucinations: theoretical and clinical overview. Am J Psychiatry 1986;143:1088-97.
9. Drugs that cause psychiatric symptoms. Med Lett Drugs Ther 1989 (Dec 29; issue 808).
10. Sarbin TR, Juhasz JB. The social context of hallucinations. In: Siegel RK, West LJ, eds. Hallucinations: behavior, experience, and theory. New York: John Wiley & Sons, 1975:241-56.
11. Egdell HG, Kolven I. Childhood hallucinations. J Child Psychol Psychiatry 1972;13:279-87.
12. Duke-Elder S. System of ophthalmology, vol XII. Neuro-ophthalmology. London: Kimpton, 1971:567.
13. Milder B, Rubin ML. The fine art of prescribing glasses without making a spectacle of yourself. Gainesville, FL: Traid, 1984:404-8.
14. Lepore FE. Visual obscurations: evanescent and elementary. Semin Neurol 1986;6:167-75.
15. Sternberg P Jr, Fagadau WR, Massof RW, et al. Blizzard of '83 erythropsia [Letter]. N Engl J Med 1983;308:1482-3.
16. Furlan AJ, Whisnant JP, Kearns TP. Unilateral visual loss in bright light: an unusual symptom of carotid artery occlusive disease. Arch Neurol 1979;36:675-6.
17. Critchley M. Types of visual perseveration: "palinopsia" and "illusory visual spread." Brain 1951;74:267-99.
18. Jacobs L. Visual allesthesia. Neurology 1980;30:1059-63.
19. Cummings JL, Syndulko K, Goldberg Z, et al. Palinopsia reconsidered. Neurology 1982;32:444-7.
20. Michel EM, Troost BT. Palinopsia: cerebral localization with computed tomography. Neurology 1980;30:887-9.
21. Bender MB. Polyopia and monocular diplopia of cerebral origin. Arch Neurol Psychiatry 1945;54:323-38.
22. Bender MB. Oscillopsia. Arch Neurol 1965;13:204-13.
23. Todd J. The syndrome of Alice in Wonderland. Can Med Assoc J 1955;73:701-4.
24. Robertson DM, Hollenhorst RW, Callahan JA. Ocular manifestations of digitalis toxicity: discussion and report of three cases of central scotomas. Arch Ophthalmol 1966;76:640-5.
25. Meadows JC. Disturbed perception of colours associated with localized cerebral lesions. Brain 1974;97:615-32.
26. Pearlman AL, Birch J, Meadows JC. Cerebral color blindness: an acquired defect in hue discrimination. Ann Neurol 1979;5:253-61.
27. Hörnsten G. Wallenberg's syndrome. I. General symptomatology, with special reference to visual disturbances and imbalance. Acta Neurol Scand 1974;50:434-46.
28. Steiner I, Shahin R, Melamed E. Acute "upside down" reversal of vision in transient vertebrobasilar ischemia. Neurology 1987;37:1685-6.
29. Holmes G. Disturbances of visual orientation [and continuation]. Br J Ophthalmol 1918;2:449-86, 506-16.
30. Damasio AR. Disorders of complex visual processing: agnosias, achromatopsia, Balint's syndrome, and related difficulties of orientation and construction. In: Mesulam MM, ed. Principles

of behavioral neurology. Philadelphia: FA Davis, 1985:259-88.

31. Sokol S. The Pulfrich stereo-illusion as an index of optic nerve dysfunction. Surv Ophthalmol 1976;20:432-4.

32. Brickner R. Oscillopsia: a new symptom commonly occurring in multiple sclerosis. Arch Neurol Psychiatry 1936; 36:586-9.

33. Leigh RJ. Management of oscillopsia. In: Barber HO, Sharpe JA, eds. Vestibular disorders. St Louis: Mosby–Year Book, 1988:201-11.

34. JC. Living without a balancing mechanism. N Engl J Med 1952;246:458-60.

35. Jacobs L, Karpik A, Bozian D, et al. Auditory-visual synesthesia: sound-induced photisms. Arch Neurol 1981; 38:211-6.

36. Hupp SL, Kline LB, Corbett JJ. Visual disturbances of migraine. Surv Ophthalmol 1989;33:221-36.

37. Jampol LM, Sieving PA, Pugh D, et al. Multiple evanescent white dot syndrome. I. Clinical findings. Arch Ophthalmol 1984;102:671-4.

38. Penfield W, Perot P. The brain's record of auditory and visual experience: a final summary and discussion. Brain 1963;86:595-696.

39. Panayiotopoulos CP. Difficulties in differentiating migraine and epilepsy based on clinical and EEG findings. In: Andermann F, Lugaresi E, eds. Migraine and epilepsy. Boston: Butterworths, 1987:31-46.

40. Nashold BS Jr. Phosphenes resulting from stimulation of the midbrain in man. Arch Ophthalmol 1970;84:433-5.

41. Lhermitte J. Syndrome de la calotte du pédoncule cérébral: les troubles psycho-sensoriels dans les lésions du mésocéphale. Rev Neurol 1922;38:1359-65.

42. Lessell S. Higher disorders of visual function: positive phenomena. In: Glaser JS, Smith JL, eds. Neuro-ophthalmology: symposium of the University of Miami and the Bascom Palmer Eye Institute, vol 8. St Louis: Mosby–Year Book, 1975:27-44.

# CHAPTER 7

# *Abnormal Optic Discs*

• • • • • • • • • • • • • • • • • •

The abnormal optic disc may represent acquired disease or a congenital anomaly. We have divided optic disc abnormalities into those with and those without disc elevation.

## A Decision Tree Approach to the Evaluation of Abnormal Optic Discs

When a patient has an abnormal optic disc, the first disc characteristic to be evaluated is elevation (Chart 7-1).

### ▮ Disc not elevated

When the optic disc is abnormal but not elevated, dysplastic changes are sought.

### ☐ Signs of dysplasia not present

If no signs of dysplasia are detected even on magnified stereoscopic viewing of the disc, the examiner should look for cupping.

### ☐ Cupping present

The presence of pathologic cupping (with loss of rim tissue or asymmetric cup/disc ratios between eyes) suggests glaucoma or a glaucoma mimicker. Overwhelmingly, the most frequent cause of cupping is glaucoma.

### ▣ Glaucoma

The combination of increased intraocular pressure, nerve fiber bundle visual field defects, and cupping of the optic disc is the classic triad of glaucoma. The disc cupping progresses usually in a vertical direction and later obliterates the temporal disc rim tissue. Often nasal displacement of the disc vessels and loss of nasal rim tissue are evident. Occasionally this progressive cupping may be found along with the visual field defects without an abnormally elevated intraocular pressure—an entity known as *normotensive glaucoma*.

173

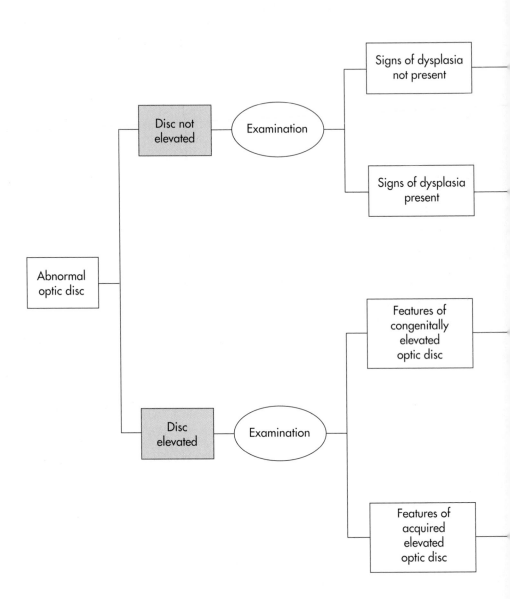

*Chart 7-1*

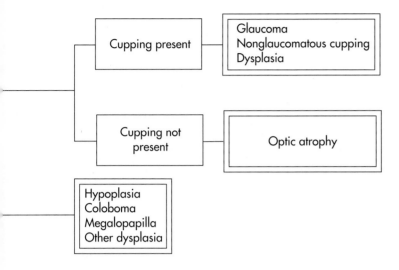

Cupping present → Glaucoma / Nonglaucomatous cupping / Dysplasia

Cupping not present → Optic atrophy

Hypoplasia
Coloboma
Megalopapilla
Other dysplasia

Congenitally elevated optic disc

Papilledema
Compressive optic neuropathy
Hypertensive retinopathy with
  disc elevation
Infiltrative optic neuropathy
Inflammatory optic neuropathy
Toxic and hereditary optic
  neuropathy
Diabetic papillopathy
Ischemic optic neuropathy
Central retinal vein occlusion
  and venous stasis retinopathy
Optic disc vasculitis
Uveitis or ocular hypotony

### ▣ Nonglaucomatous cupping

Excavation of optic disc tissue is not pathognomonic of glaucoma. Loss of optic disc tissue producing cupping may be encountered in optic atrophy following ischemia, trauma, demyelination, or infection.[1] At times distinguishing glaucomatous from nonglaucomatous cupping may be difficult. The absence of the neuroretinal rim is highly specific for glaucoma, which must remain the diagnosis of exclusion when this portion of the optic disc is altered.

### ▣ Dysplasia

Some dysplasias may resemble glaucomatous cupping and may also produce nerve fiber bundle visual field defects. The scotomas associated with dysplasia are, however, not progressive. Thus sequential perimetry and intraocular pressure determinations permit accurate diagnosis of these congenital anomalies.

### ☐ Cupping not present

### ▣ Optic atrophy

Optic atrophy with loss of color, disc vasculature, and retinal nerve fibers is the final result of various insults to the optic nerve or retina. When arteriolar narrowing occurs, an ischemic process is most likely to have occurred. We believe that the ophthalmoscopic appearance of optic atrophy is almost always nonspecific and nondiagnostic of a particular etiology. Other clinial, imaging, or laboratory data are required to discover the underlying cause of optic atrophy when the acute fundus event went unobserved.

### ☐ Signs of dysplasia present

### ▣ Hypoplasia

Complete absence of the optic disc and retinal vessels (optic disc aplasia) is rare. However, optic disc hypoplasia, where the optic nerve head is smaller than normal, is recognized as a relatively frequent cause of visual dysfunction. Optic disc hypoplasia may be unilateral or bilateral. The diagnosis is made ophthalmoscopically; the optic disc appears smaller than its fellow or smaller than normal. The diagnosis is not difficult to make when the disc is severely hypoplastic. However, a spectrum of hypoplasia exists such that ophthalmoscopically subtle hypoplasia may be associated with severe visual deficits.

Photographically measuring the optic discs may be helpful in detecting optic disc hypoplasia.[3] The small optic nerve head is often surrounded by two rings of pigmentation, which constitutes the double ring sign (Plate 5, *A*). The outer ring represents the junction between sclera and lamina cribrosa where the choroid is discontinuous, whereas the inner ring represents the termination of the retinal pigment epithelium.[4] Ophthalmoscopic evaluation of the retina usually reveals a decrease in the plushness of the nerve fiber layer.[5]

The cause of optic disc hypoplasia is not known, although several hypotheses have been advanced.[6] Hypoplasia may represent a primary failure of differentiation of retinal ganglion cells, but it may also be caused by secondary degeneration of ganglion cells and their fibers.[4] Contributing etiologic factors are a young maternal age, the use of anticonvulsants, alcohol, or hallucinogens during the gestational period,[7,8] and maternal diabetes mellitus.[9]

Children of diabetic mothers may show a specific form of disc hypoplasia called **superior segmental optic hypoplasia.**[10] This entity has four characteristic ophthalmoscopic findings: relative superior entrance of the central retinal artery, pallor of the superior disc, a superior peripapillary halo, and thinning of the superior peripapillary nerve fiber layer.

Optic nerve hypoplasia may be produced by lesions at any site of the visual system. Macular colobomas, chiasmal malformations (de Morsier syndrome), and occipital porencephaly have been associated with the anomaly.[11]

Visual acuity in patients with optic nerve hypoplasia may be normal or depressed. Even with normal acuity, visual field defects of an arcuate, altitudinal, or temporal sector variety may exist.[12,13] Recognizing the disorder is important so that unnecessarily prolonged occlusion of the contralateral eye is not undertaken because of the mistaken impression that amblyopia alone is the cause of decreased vision. However, a short trial of occlusion in the appropriate age group is indicated, since associated amblyopia may be present. If vision does not improve within 2 weeks, patching should be discontinued.

Optic disc hypoplasia often is associated with nonocular abnormalities. Skarf and Hoyt[14] found developmental delay, neuroendocrinologic abnormalities, and central nervous system (CNS) anomalies in 32 (70%) of 41 children with bilateral optic disc hypoplasia and poor vision studied prospectively. Only 11 (21%) of 52 children with unilateral hypoplasia or bilateral segmental hypoplasia had nonocular developmental anomalies.

**Septo-optic dysplasia** is a syndrome that classically includes optic disc hypoplasia, agenesis of the septum pellucidum and hypothalamus, and malformations of the optic chiasm resulting in a bitemporal hemianopia. Often these patients are too young to permit an assessment of visual function. The presence of optic disc hypoplasia and bitemporal hemianopia should prompt neuroradiologic investigation with computed tomography (CT) or magnetic resonance imaging (MRI) scanning to document fusion of the lateral ventricles anteriorly.

These findings may be subtle, however. High-resolution MRI scanning in two patients with septo-optic dysplasia revealed normal midline anatomy except for the failure to visualize the pituitary stalk, presumably because of hypoplasia.[15] This tends to support the concept that the endocrinologic abnormalities are not pituitary in origin. Neuropathologically the major anomaly appears to be in the hypothalamic nuclei, with the adenohypophysis being normal histologically and immunocytochemically.[16]

Imaging may be deferred in these patients, since the cerebral malfunctions are usually static, but investigation for growth hormone deficiency should not be delayed. Short stature is reversible if treatment with growth hormone is instituted before epiphyseal closure occurs. These children may also have deficiences or hypersecretion of other trophic hormones, including corticotropin and prolactin.[17] Therefore all these patients should be referred for endocrinologic evaluation.

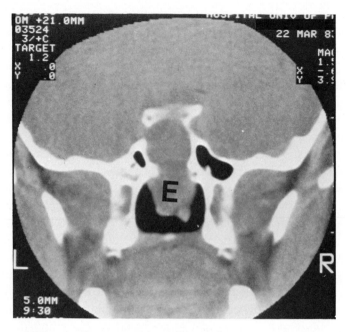

*Fig. 7-1.* Coronal CT scan of patient with midline cleft syndrome (patient's disc shown in Plate 5, *C*). Encephalocele *(E)* is seen extending through midline defect into sphenoid sinus.

### ☐ Coloboma

Colobomas are dysplastic excavations of the disc that can extend to involve the retina and choroid or be limited to the disc (optic pit). Pits are small, incomplete colobomas that routinely occupy the temporal, usually inferior, portion of the optic disc (Plate 5, *B*). These nonprogressive lesions are often associated with arcuate visual field defects that correspond to the location of the pits. Acuity remains normal unless serous detachment of the macula occurs. The origin of this serous fluid is probably the vitreous cavity.[18] A large colobomatous optic disc (Plate 5, *C*) may occur with midline facial or skull abnormalities.[19] The complete syndrome includes midline cranial defects, such as hypertelorism; a broad, flat nasal root; cleft lip; and basal encephaloceles. Patients with large colobomatous optic discs require imaging of the base of the skull to demonstrate any midline bony defects with encephaloceles (Fig. 7-1).

The **morning glory disc** is a funnel-shaped, excavated disc with a central depression, surrounded by a retinal pigment epithelial disturbance. It has been associated with encephaloceles,[19] as well as retinal detachment and retinoschisis.[20] Chorioretinal lesions surrounding a colobomatous optic disc are characteristic of Aicardi's syndrome.

### ☐ Megalopapilla

Certain optic discs are larger than normal (megalopapilla). This abnormality is encountered much less frequently than hypoplasia. Some optic discs are large but not pathologic. Others are dysplastic and may be associated with cerebral defects (see above).

## ▣ Other dysplasia

Some congenitally abnormal discs do not conveniently fit into any category. This spectrum of disc anomalies includes tilted discs, congenital crescents, situs inversus, and other oddly shaped discs that defy classification.

The **tilted optic disc** results from an oblique instead of a direct insertion of the optic nerve into the globe. As a result, the disc appears oval, with its vertical axis directed obliquely, resulting in an inferior depression and relative superior elevation of the disc margin. Often nasal sweeping of the retinal vessels (situs inversus) is present with a rim of sclera visible inferiorly **(crescent).** The inferior nasal fundus is often hypopigmented because of scleral thinning or a localized ectasia[21] (Plate 5, *D*).

These patients may be referred for neurosurgical evaluation because visual field loss may resemble bitemporal hemianopia, caused by a compressive chiasmal lesion. The scotoma, however, does not respect the vertical meridian on perimetry but tends to cross to the nasal side, thus distinguishing it from a true chiasmal visual field defect (see Chapter 3). Field loss in some of these patients may be due to an exaggerated myopic astigmatism at an oblique axis. When perimetry is performed with an appropriate astigmatic lens in place, the scotoma often disappears.

## ▮ Disc elevated

When the optic disc is found to be elevated, a critical distinction must be made between a congenital and an acquired disc elevation (Chart 7-1, *A*). This distinction may almost always be made on the basis of ophthalmoscopic criteria alone.

## ◯ *Examination.* 

Congenital disc elevations include optic disc drusen and other dysplasias, whereas acquired entities include disc edema due to increased intracranial pressure (ICP) (papilledema), compressive optic neuropathy, papillitis, hypertensive retinopathy, infiltrative optic neuropathy, toxic/hereditary optic neuropathies, diabetic papillopathy, ischemic optic neuropathy, central retinal vein occlusion, venous stasis retinopathy, optic disc vasculitis, uveitis, and hypotony.

## ▢ Features of congenitally elevated optic disc

## ▣ Congenitally elevated optic disc

The congenitally elevated disc has a monotonously consistent appearance. It has no optic cup, and the retinal vessels appear to originate at the central core of the

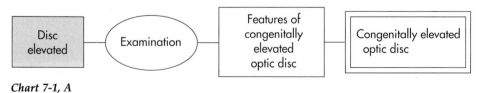

*Chart 7-1, A*

disc. In acquired disc elevation the central cup is generally preserved unless the swelling is marked, in which case other signs of acquired disc edema will be present.*

The vascular pattern of the large optic disc vessels is abnormal in one third of patients with congenital disc elevation.[22] Arterial and venous trifurcations or quadrifurcations, as well as loops or coils on the optic disc, are present (Plate 6, A). These large-vessel anomalies are distinctly different from the telangiectasia or neovascularization of acquired disc swelling. Spontaneous venous pulsations are often present in congenital disc elevation but absent in acquired disc swelling because of increased ICP. Obscuration of the nerve fiber layer is an important sign that helps distinguish acquired from congenital disc elevation. The underlying mechanism by which acquired disc elevation occurs is swelling of the nerve fiber layer axons secondary to interruption or stagnation of axoplasmic flow. Conversely, the nerve fiber remains clear in the congenitally elevated optic disc.

The ophthalmoscopic detection of glistening hyalin bodies **(drusen)** within the optic nerve head indicates a congenital cause of disc elevation. Congenitally anomalous discs due to buried hyalin bodies are usually bilateral (66%).[22] Hyalin bodies are found almost exclusively anterior to the lamina cribrosa and tend to enlarge, becoming more visible with age (Plate 6, B).

Hemorrhage on or around the disc may occur rarely with intrapapillary hyalin bodies (Plate 7, C). The hemorrhages commonly are located in the superficial nerve fiber layer or in the subretinal space. The deeper hemorrhages lie beneath the retinal pigment epithelium (RPE) or between this layer and Bruch's membrane[23] (Plate 6, D). Hemorrhages of the subretinal pigment epithelium (subRPE) can produce peripapillary pigment alterations, with areas of loss of RPE at times alternating with pigment hypertrophy. Approximately one third of patients with intrapapillary hyalin bodies show these pigment changes,[22] suggesting that subRPE hemorrhages are more frequent than presently appreciated. Subretinal neovascular membranes may develop and cause bleeding into the subretinal space. Bleeding may uncommonly extend into the vitreous.[24] Because peripapillary nerve fiber layer hemorrhages are rare with hyalin bodies of the disc, the appearance of this hemorrhage in or around an elevated optic disc suggests acquired disc elevation.

Unfortunately, no single ophthalmoscopic feature can reliably separate acquired from congenital optic disc elevation (Table 7-1). All the features of the optic disc must be examined according to an ophthalmoscopic checklist or balance sheet:

1. The optic cup: Absence of an optic cup with no other signs of florid disc edema strongly suggests a congenitally anomalous disc.
2. The optic disc vasculature: Large-vessel trifurcations, loops, or coils indicate a congenitally anomalous elevated disc, whereas abnormalities of the

*Even though some types of congenitally anomalous discs, such as intrapapillary drusen, may progress, we have elected to place them in the category of congenitally elevated discs.

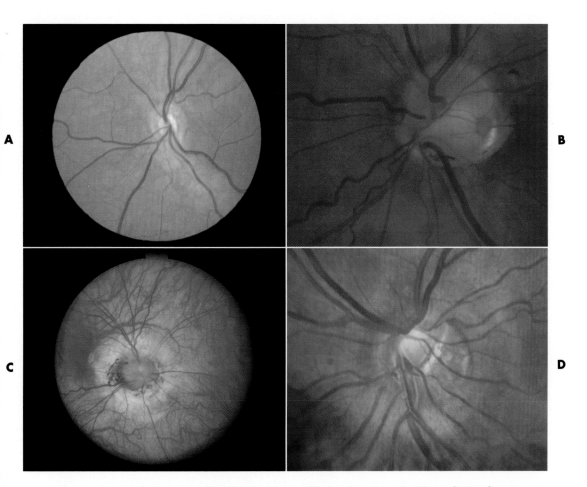

***Plate 5.*** Congenitally anomalous optic discs without elevation. **A,** Hypoplasia: disc is smaller than normal, but vessels are of normal caliber. Rim of depigmentation (double ring sign) is evident. There is attrition of retinal nerve fiber layer. **B,** Optic pit: excavation at inferotemporal portion of left disc. **C,** Dysplasia: disc is larger than normal and is dysplastic. **D,** Tilted disc: disc is obliquely inserted into globe with a crescent being present inferotemporally.

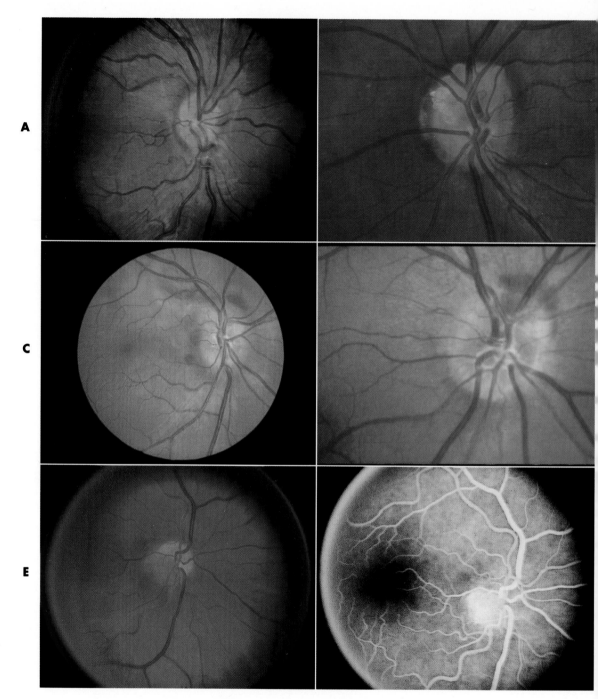

*Plate 6.* Congenitally anomalous optic discs with elevation. **A,** Without hyalin bodies: elevated disc without a cup showing abnormal branching pattern of large disc vessels. **B,** Hyalin bodies: note crystalline appearance of superior portion of disc. **C,** Subretinal hemorrhage adjacent to congenitally anomalous disc with buried intrapapillary hyalin bodies. **D,** Subretinal-subRPE hemorrhage at superior pole of congenitally anomalous disc. **E,** Hemangioma: reddish elevation may simulate sector swelling of ischemic optic neuropathy. Fluorescein angiography, **F,** delineates extent of this vascular malformation of disc.

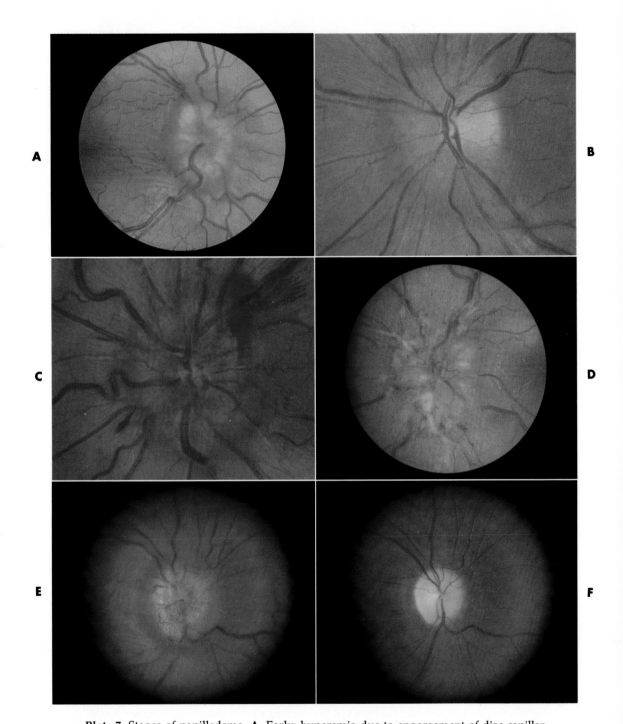

*Plate 7.* Stages of papilledema. **A,** Early: hyperemia due to engorgement of disc capillaries. **B,** Early: opacification of peripapillary nerve fiber layer obscures detail of disc margin. **C,** Fully developed: peripapillary nerve fiber layer hemorrhages appear. **D,** Well established: disc is elevated, but nerve fiber hemorrhages have disappeared. Pallor is developing at superior pole. Retinal striae are seen radiating toward macula. **E,** Chronic: disc is elevated without hemorrhages. Crystalline deposits presumably of chronically stagnant axoplasm (pseudodrusen) are evident. **F,** Atrophic: same patient as in **E** following optic nerve sheath decompression. Disc is flat and pale; pseudodrusen have disappeared.

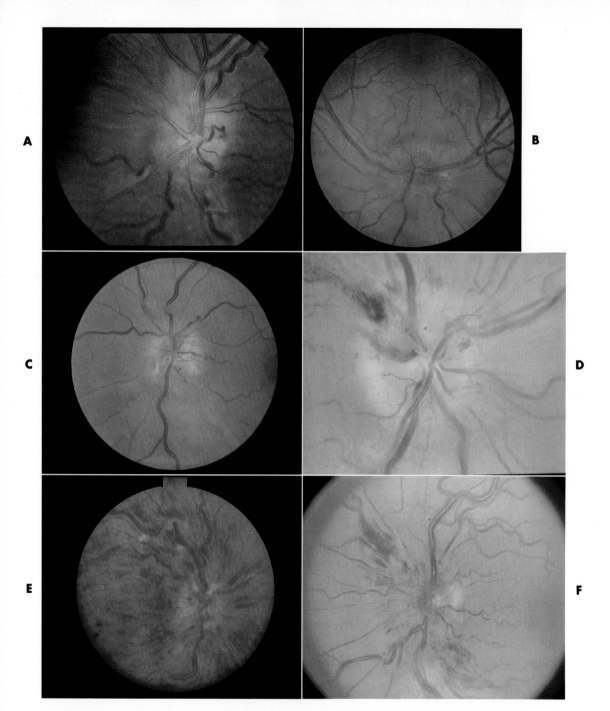

*Plate 8.* Disc elevation not secondary to increased intracranial pressure. **A,** Optociliary shunt: disc becoming atrophic in patient with optic nerve sheath meningioma. **B,** Papillitis: disc hyperemic with blurred margins. Patient had venous sheathing in retinal periphery and clinical signs consistent with multiple sclerosis. **C,** Diabetic papillopathy: swelling of left optic nerve with dilatation of disc capillary net in asymptomatic, insulin-dependent diabetic patient with 20/20 vision and normal visual field. **D,** Ischemic optic neuropathy: superior sector of disc is elevated and pale. Hemorrhage appears in this sector as well. **E,** Central retinal vein occlusion: disc margins blurred with nerve fiber layer infarcts at disc margin. Extensive nerve fiber layer hemorrhages beyond peripapillary area indicate primary retinal venous problem. **F,** Papillophlebitis: hemorrhages extend off elevated disc but not to periphery as in **E.**

smaller vessels—telangiectasia, new vessel formation, or optociliary shunt vessels—suggest acquired elevation.

3. Spontaneous venous pulsations: The presence of these pulsations is further evidence against increased ICP.[25]
4. Peripapillary hemorrhages: The presence of nerve fiber layer hemorrhages strongly suggests an acquired disc elevation, although in some patients drusen of the optic disc can produce hemorrhages indistinguishable from those of true papilledema.
5. The nerve fiber layer: Opacification due to axoplasmic damming is a sign of acquired disc elevation; a clear nerve fiber layer suggests congenital disc elevation.
6. Family occurrence: The presence of congenital disc elevation in a parent or sibling is good circumstantial evidence that the disc in question is congenitally anomalous.

Even with the use of this checklist, the distinction between congenital and acquired disc elevation may not be obvious.

Certain congenital vascular anomalies of the optic disc and retina may cause progressive visual loss and may therefore be mistaken for acquired disc

---

### Management of Congenital Disc Elevation

1. Observe the patient with a normal neurologic examination and a strong clinical suspicion of congenital disc elevation.
2. Use imaging to rule out an intracranial mass lesion or hydrocephalus. Imaging without subsequent lumbar puncture does not exclude papilledema due to increased ICP (pseudotumor cerebri).
3. For patients whose congenital disc elevation may be confused with papilledema, photograph the optic disc and give the patient a copy. If the question of the cause of disc elevation arises again, comparison with these fundus photographs should provide the answer.

---

**TABLE 7-1**  *Ophthalmoscopic Features of Congenital and Acquired Disc Elevation*

| Ophthalmoscopic features | Congenital disc elevation | Acquired disc elevation |
| --- | --- | --- |
| Color | Yellow | Hyperemic (acutely) |
| Nerve fiber layer | Clear | Opacified |
| Large disc vessels | Anomalous | Normal |
| Small disc vessels | Normal | Telangiectatic |
| Nerve fiber layer hemorrhage | Rare | Frequent |
| Physiologic cup | Small or absent | Normal |
| Spontaneous venous pulsations | Present | Absent |
| Hyalin bodies | Sometimes present | Absent |

elevation. Capillary hemangiomas are examples of such lesions. They are usually reddish, and on close inspection the vascular nature of the lesions can be appreciated (Plate 6, *E*). Fluorescein angiography will reveal early filling and late dye leakage (Plate 6, *F*). Most hemangiomas are isolated abnormalities, but they may be associated with von Hippel–Lindau disease.[26,27]

## ☐ Features of acquired elevated optic disc (Chart 7-1, *B*)

### ▣ Papilledema

Most neuro-ophthalmologists reserve the term *papilledema* for optic disc elevation due to increased ICP. However, the term *papilledema* itself is to a certain extent a misnomer. Light and electron microscopy have shown that disc elevation is due primarily to axonal swelling and degeneration. Some interstitial edema is present, but the glial cells show no sign of intracellular edema.[28] What the exact mechanism is that produces papilledema is still being debated. Increased pressure is apparently being transmitted to the optic nerves along their meningeal sheaths, since surgical opening of the perioptic meninges results in detumescence of the disc[29] without normalization of ICP.[30] This increased perineural pressure results in a damming of the slow component of axoplasmic flow at the lamina cribrosa. This process is believed to produce disc swelling and nerve fiber layer opacification. The fast component of axoplasmic flow is also involved, but this is probably a secondary phenomenon.

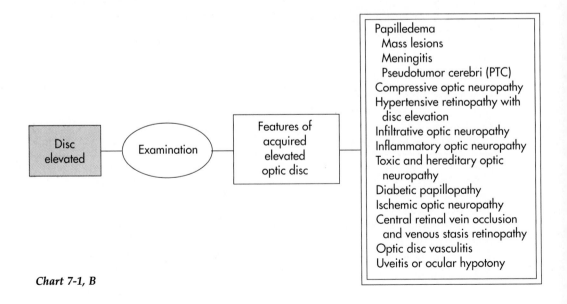

Papilledema
  Mass lesions
  Meningitis
  Pseudotumor cerebri (PTC)
Compressive optic neuropathy
Hypertensive retinopathy with
  disc elevation
Infiltrative optic neuropathy
Inflammatory optic neuropathy
Toxic and hereditary optic
  neuropathy
Diabetic papillopathy
Ischemic optic neuropathy
Central retinal vein occlusion
  and venous stasis retinopathy
Optic disc vasculitis
Uveitis or ocular hypotony

Disc elevated → Examination → Features of acquired elevated optic disc

*Chart 7-1, B*

Papilledema is almost invariably a bilateral phenomenon if both optic discs were previously normal. If one disc is atrophic, nerve fiber layer edema cannot develop. For example, the papilledema seen in Foster Kennedy's syndrome is truly unilateral, because one optic disc has become atrophic from chronic compression of the optic nerve by a subfrontal tumor.[31] On rare occasions strictly unilateral papilledema may occur with a normal-appearing contralateral optic disc. It is suggested that the increased ICP is not transmitted to the subarachnoid space around the "normal" optic nerve because of an optic nerve sheath anomaly.[32] However, the patient who has unilateral optic disc swelling with a normal-appearing fellow optic disc is unlikely to have papilledema. In this instance one should look for a local ocular or orbital process as the cause of disc elevation.

The ophthalmoscopic appearance of papilledema varies depending on the duration of the disc swelling. Hoyt and Beeston[33] described the following stages of papilledema:

1. Early papilledema: There is minimal hyperemia of the disc, early opacification of the nerve fiber layer, and the absence of spontaneous venous pulsations (Plate 7, *A* and *B*).
2. Acute (fully developed) papilledema: Hemorrhage or exudation are added to the signs of early papilledema (Plate 7, *C* and *D*).
3. Chronic papilledema: Hemorrhages and exudates are scarce, but capillary telangiectasia is evident on the disc surface. Small refractile, drusenlike bodies may appear on the disc surface, but they may disappear should the disc swelling abate[34] (Plate 7, *E*). Optociliary shunt vessels also develop at this stage.
4. Atrophic papilledema: There is optic disc pallor with nerve fiber bundle visual field defects (Plate 7, *F*). Optociliary shunt vessels also develop at this stage.

We do not advocate the use of fluorescein angiography as an aid in the diagnosis of papilledema. In fully developed papilledema, fluorescein angiography is unnecessary. In incipient papilledema, if the ophthalmoscopic diagnosis is uncertain, fluorescein angiography is likely to be equivocal as well.

The patient with papilledema may complain of transient obscurations of vision. These may occur in one or both eyes and typically last only for seconds. Obscurations frequently are associated with moving from a sitting to a standing position, or they may be independent of any postural change. Obscurations occur only with well-developed papilledema and are probably caused by compression of the blood vessels at the optic nerve itself.[35] The occurrence of obscurations does not appear to be a sign of impending infarction of the optic disc,[36] although infarction does occur rarely in papilledema.[37] Orcutt et al.[38] have cited a higher percentage of a poor visual outcome in patients who experience transient obscurations. However, they were not willing to implicate transient obscurations as a predictor of visual loss.

Visual acuity is normal in acute papilledema unless concomitant macular edema is present. Preretinal or subretinal pigment epithelium hemorrhages, exudates in a star figure, or choroidal folds extending through the macula may also decrease central acuity in acute papilledema.[39,40]

Perimetry reveals only enlargement of the blind spots in the early stages of papilledema. In the more chronic forms visual field defects will appear, the most frequent being inferior nasal nerve fiber bundle defects identical to those seen in glaucoma.[36,41] Visual acuity loss is a late finding.

The diagnosis of papilledema constitutes a medical emergency. The patient should have imaging performed immediately. If a mass lesion is discovered, hospitalization for further testing to determine its nature and appropriate treatment is indicated. If no mass is detected and the ventricles are not dilated, lumbar puncture is performed to measure the cerebrospinal fluid (CSF) pressure and to exclude meningitis. If the spinal fluid is normal, except for increased pressure, the patient probably has *pseudotumor cerebri* (PTC).

**PSEUDOTUMOR CEREBRI.** PTC is diagnosed under the following conditions:

1. Signs of increased ICP usually but not invariably[42,43] manifested by papilledema.
2. The absence of neurologic signs with the exception of sixth cranial nerve paresis.
3. No imaging evidence of ventriculomegaly or of an intracranial mass lesion. An empty sella may be seen in up to 25% of patients.[36,44,45]
4. Increased opening pressure (>200 mm $H_2O$) and normal spinal fluid formula.

**Etiology.** The syndrome of PTC may be produced by a variety of conditions or agents, or it may be idiopathic.

*Intracranial (dural) venous sinus thrombosis.* Dural sinus thrombosis may occur following head trauma, suppurative otitis media, or mastoiditis,[46] and obstruction of the superior vena cava or jugular vein. Dural sinus thrombosis decreases the pressure differential across the arachnoid villi, causing decreased absorption of CSF.[47] A CT scan may reveal a hyperdensity within the sagittal sinus with a lucent defect in the torcula Herophili. An MRI scan will show high signal on both short-TR and long-TR images (Fig. 7-2). MRI is so sensitive to dural sinus thrombosis that arteriography is usually not needed to establish the diagnosis.[48] The thrombosed sinus usually recanalizes, with resultant resolution of the PTC.

The dural sinuses need not be thrombosed to influence ICP. PTC has been described with unruptured cerebral arteriovenous malformations presumably on the basis of increased cortical venous and superior sagittal sinus pressure.[49]

*Exogenous agents.* Tetracycline,[50,51] nalidixic acid,[52] nitrofurantoin,[53] danazol,[54] corticosteroid use or withdrawal,[55] or hypervitaminosis A[56] may cause PTC. The dose of vitamin A necessary to induce PTC varies from 25,000 to 60,000 IU daily. Excessive ingestion of liver[57] may also induce these levels of vitamin A and thus produce PTC.

*Endocrinologic abnormalities.* Endocrine dysfunction is likely to play an important role in the PTC syndrome. Most patients are obese young women who

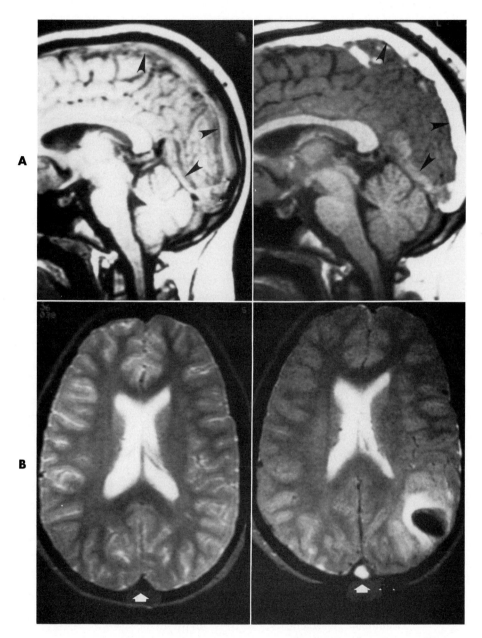

*Fig. 7-2.* Sinus thrombosis. **A,** Sagittal MRI scan of patient with pseudotumor cerebri. *Left,* Clot *(white linear structure indicated by arrowheads)* in superior sagittal and straight sinus. *Right,* MRI scan 3 days later showing a massive clot *(arrowheads)* in these structures. **B,** *Left,* Axial T2-weighted MRI scan shows deoxyhemoglobin in superior sagittal sinus of the same intensity as flowing blood *(arrowhead).* Three days later *(right)* the sinus shows obvious clot *(arrowhead)* in the sinus plus an intracerebral hemorrhage.

frequently have menstrual irregularities. Yet, no definable endocrine abnormality has been consistently detected in these patients. A mild hypothalamic-hypophyseal insufficiency was documented in five patients with PTC, but this may be an effect of chronically increased ICP and not its cause.[58] Pseudotumor cerebri has also been reported in patients with Turner's syndrome,[59] hypoparathyroidism, and adrenal adenoma.[60] Because of the infrequency of definable endocrinologic abnormalities in PTC, we recommend that no endocrinologic studies be performed in these patients unless relevant clinical signs are present.

*Systemic disorders.* Rarely, certain systemic disorders such as systemic lupus erythematosus,[61] chronic respiratory insufficiency, iron-deficiency anemia, uremia,[62] and Lyme disease[63] may be associated with PTC.

*Idiopathic PTC.* Johnston and Patterson[46] were able to identify a cause for PTC in 44% of their 110 patients. Rush,[64] however, found a cause in only 15% of his 63 patients. In our collective experience, a cause for PTC is usually identified in fewer than 5% of patients.

Most patients with the idiopathic variety of PTC are obese women in the third decade of life.[36] In this population the incidence of PTC is approximately 15/100,000.[65] Although PTC is much less frequent in men by an 8:1 ratio,[65] it appears in the same age distribution and with similar signs and symptoms as PTC in women.[66]

Children also may have PTC. While many retain or regain excellent visual function, permanent, profound visual loss occurs even in this age group.[67-69]

In its idiopathic form PTC may be a self-limiting disorder that resolves within months.[46] However, PTC may recur in up to 40% of patients,[70,64] and the disease may be prolonged over a period of several years. While PTC is usually a sporadic event, it has been reported in more than one family member.[71,72] The exact significance of this familial association is unknown.

*Pathogenesis.* The exact mechanism by which PTC is produced remains unknown. The theory most often advanced is that of increased arachnoid resistance to CSF drainage.[73,74] Other theories support an abnormality of the cerebral microvasculature causing increased cerebral blood volume. Proponents of this theory claim that intracranial hypertension is produced by brain tissue swelling due to increased water content.[75] This low level of edema was supported by increased white matter water signal seen on a heavily T2-weighted proton MRI scan using 1.5 T MRI.[45] These changes were not seen when 0.35 T MRI and different sequences were employed.[44] However, the role of MRI and CT is primarily to exclude other disorders that mimic PTC.

*Symptoms.* Headache is the most frequent symptom, being reported by 75% to 99% of patients. Diplopia, due to sixth nerve paresis, is a nonspecific sign of increased ICP. Visual disturbances include transient obscurations of vision, visual field defects, or decreased acuity.[76,47,64] Acuity is decreased in approximately 20% of patients with PTC.[77]

A review by Round and Keane[78] of 101 consecutive patients with PTC confirms that headache, nausea and vomiting, and visual disturbances are encountered most frequently. In their series, however, patients also experienced neck stiffness (31%), tinnitus (27%), paresthesias (22%), and arthralgias (13%).

The persistence of intracranial hypertension in PTC appears to have no consequences other than those resulting from the visual morbidity of chronic atrophic papilledema. Corbett et al.[36] found severe visual impairment in 14 of 57 patients with PTC observed for up to 41 years. Duration of papilledema does not appear to be a critical factor in the development of visual field loss. Progressive visual field defects may appear in weeks or may not occur even after years of chronic papilledema.[36,64] The only risk factor for visual loss in the series by Corbett et al.[36] was systemic hypertension. Orcutt et al.[38] described loss of visual function in 49% of eyes in 68 patients with PTC. Visual loss was more frequent in patients with high-grade or atrophic papilledema, peripapillary subretinal hemorrhages, anemia, older age, high myopia, optociliary shunt vessels, and transient visual obscurations.

The characteristic visual field defect in PTC is an enlarged blind spot, which may be a refractive scotoma due to induced peripapillary hyperopia.[79] The next most frequent defect is generalized constriction or loss of the inferonasal visual field. Visual field defects may be found with automated perimetry in up to 75% of eyes in pseudotumor patients.[77] The appearance or progression of a field defect on sequential perimetry necessitates the institution or intensification of treatment.

**Diagnosis.** Imaging and lumbar puncture are essential to the diagnosis of PTC. We prefer MRI to CT, since venous sinus thrombosis is more easily detected on MRI.

**Treatment.** The presence of papilledema in PTC is not in itself an indication for treatment. Some patients may tolerate years of papilledema with no visual consequences. Patients who develop signs of visual loss from chronic papilledema or those with intractable headache should be treated. Treatment varies, depending on the identification of a cause of the increased ICP.

*PTC induced by increased venous pressure.* Since thrombosed venous sinuses producing PTC will usually recanalize, the papilledema routinely subsides and as a rule does not produce permanent visual disability. If progressive visual loss occurs in the setting of prolonged papilledema, systemic corticosteroids should be given. Continued deterioration of vision despite this treatment is an indication for lumboperitoneal shunt or optic nerve sheath decompression (see Idiopathic PTC). Dehydrating agents should be avoided in this syndrome because they will aggravate the thrombosis. The use of heparin is advocated by some[80] but does not enjoy wide support.

*PTC induced by exogenous agents.* The withdrawal of any ingested agent that has produced PTC will result in resolution of the papilledema.

*PTC associated with systemic diseases.* In those rare instances of PTC associated with systemic disease (lupus, anemia), treatment of the associated disorder should be undertaken simultaneously with the treatment of PTC.

*Idiopathic PTC.* The treatment of idiopathic PTC is controversial, and many medical and surgical regimens have been advocated:

1. Repeated lumbar puncture: Because the CSF volume removed by lumbar puncture is re-formed within hours, we cannot advocate this form of therapy for the treatment of a chronic disorder. Lumbar puncture is also un-

comfortable for patients, who often fail to return for follow-up treatment.

2. Dehydrating agents: The pressure-lowering effect of oral dehydrating agents (glycerol and isosorbine) lasts only 4 hours. Oral glycerol is nauseatingly sweet and often results in poor patient compliance. It is also metabolized and is difficult to recommend in morbidly obese patients, who are often diabetics.

3. Carbonic anhydrase inhibitors: Acetazolamide (4 g daily) has been shown to decrease ICP in two patients with PTC who underwent continuous ICP recording.[81] This dose is better tolerated with the sustained-release form of the drug (Diamox Sequels), but numbness and tingling of the hands and feet, anorexia, malaise, a tinlike taste, and fatigue often limit the usefulness of therapy. If side effects result, methazolamide (Neptazane) may be substituted. Although no data are available, we have used this drug successfully to treat PTC. Diuretics such as furosemide and hydrochlorothiazide also have been used, but we do not find enough evidence to support their use.

4. Corticosteroids: The administration of oral corticosteroids will decrease ICP and promote the resolution of papilledema. However, PTC tends to be a chronic disorder, and chronic corticosteroid administration to already obese patients may aggravate this aspect of their problem. Steroid withdrawal is also implicated as a cause of PTC. Therefore we discourage the use of corticosteroids in this disorder.

5. Weight reduction: Loss of weight alone or in combination with other medical therapy may be beneficial in the treatment of PTC.[82] We urge weight reduction in all our obese patients with PTC, although enough weight loss to lower ICP is often difficult to achieve.

6. Surgical treatment: A variety of surgical procedures will relieve the chronic intracranial hypertension of PTC. Since the ventricles are not enlarged, shunting procedures are more easily performed via the lumboperitoneal route. These shunts may cease to function, and reoperation for shunt revision is often necessary.[83] Subtemporal decompression is rarely performed today since the advent of lumboperitoneal shunting operations.

Relief of papilledema also may be attained by incision of the sheath surrounding the intraorbital portion of the optic nerve.[29] While this approach effectively provides local relief to the optic nerve, it does not lower the increased ICP.[30] Sergott et al.[84] reported that optic nerve sheath fenestration via a nasal approach resulted in improved visual function postoperatively without the need for reoperation, oral corticosteroids, or diuretic agents in 21 of 23 patients with PTC. Optic nerve surgery even improved the visual function in six patients who had failed to recover vision after one or more lumbar peritoneal shunts.[84] This and other series[85] establish the efficacy of optic nerve sheath decompressive surgery in the treatment of the papilledema of PTC. Corbett et al.[86] performed a lateral orbitotomy for optic nerve sheath fenestration on 40 eyes in 28 PTC patients, with similar successful return of vision or halting of visual loss.[86] However, 16

## Management of Idiopathic Pseudotumor Cerebri

1. The patient who has papilledema with no symptoms and an otherwise normal ophthalmologic examination requires no treatment to lower the increased ICP. This patient must be reexamined monthly at onset to detect signs of early optic nerve compromise. If visual function remains normal for 3 months, the interval of reexamination may be extended (2 to 3 months). We urge weight loss and place all obese patients on a weight reduction regimen.

2. The patient with papilledema who has headache, transient visual obscurations, or signs of optic nerve dysfunction is begun on a regimen of acetazolamide (Diamox). The dose is 1 g daily initially but is increased to higher doses (2 to 4 g daily) depending on the patient's tolerance of the drug. In our experience, patients appear to tolerate acetazolamide sustained-release capsules (Diamox Sequels) better than acetazolamide tablets. The patient is reexamined every 2 to 3 weeks for signs of progressive optic nerve compromise.

3. The patient with papilledema who develops a progressive optic neuropathy while taking therapeutic doses of acetazolamide (or methazolamide) requires more aggressive treatment. These patients should have optic nerve sheath decompression, preferably via the nasal approach. Lumboperitoneal shunting should be performed as the primary procedure only if headache is a predominant part of the clinical picture.

permanent tonic pupils, 8 instances of visual loss postoperatively, and "trivial" facial scarring were reported with this approach to the optic nerve. The nasal approach appears to provide effective exposure with similarly successful visual results, but with fewer postoperative complications.

Our recommendations for the treatment of idiopathic PTC or progressive disc edema that requires treatment are illustrated in the chart on pp. 190-191.

**Further management.** Baseline evaluation of the patient with PTC ideally consists of determining visual acuity, color vision, contrast sensitivity (if available), visual fields, and optic disc photographs. At each subsequent visit optic nerve function is determined to detect any sign of progressing optic neuropathy. Visual field examination with particular attention to the arcuate nerve fiber bundle areas is performed every 3 to 4 months as long as disc edema persists.

Other ancillary tests are of questionable value in the evaluation of PTC. Bulens et al.[87] found spatial contrast sensitivity abnormalities in 16 (43%) of 37 nonamblyopic eyes in 20 patients with PTC, whereas impairment of visual acuity by Snellen testing was detected in only 6 eyes (16%). Verplanck et al.[88] reported that contrast sensitivity also was the most frequently abnormal test (18 [60%] of 30 eyes tested); in 9 eyes it was the only abnormal test. Goldmann visual fields were abnormal in only 13 (43%) of 30 eyes, whereas visual evoked potentials were abnormal in a mere 5 (17%) eyes. Contrast sensitivity testing may have a role in the diagnosis and evaluation of patients with PTC, but evoked potentials appear useless.

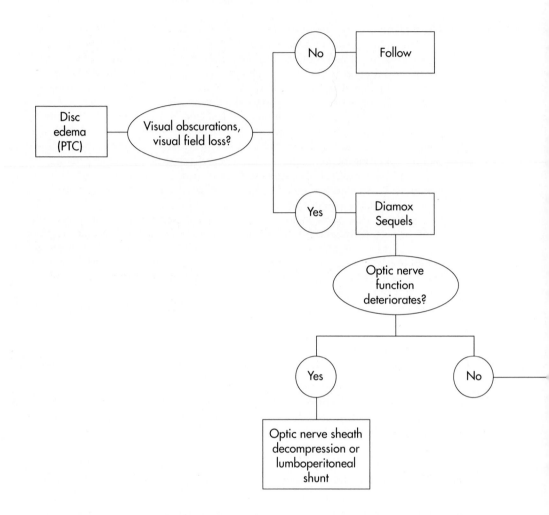

*Management of idiopathic pseudotumor cerebri*

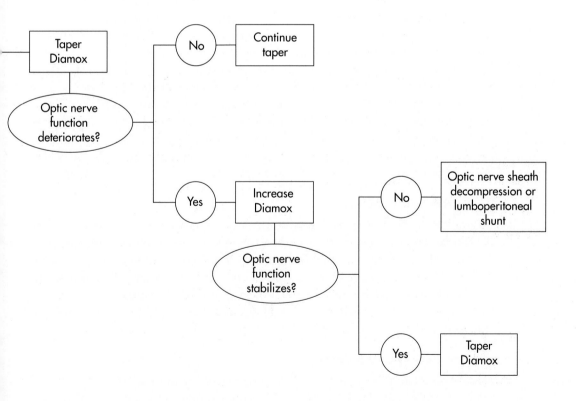

### ☐ Compressive optic neuropathy

Optic disc elevation and decreased acuity may be associated with optic nerve **tumors** (meningiomas or gliomas) (see Chapter 3) or **cysts,** or with a variety of orbital or canalicular tumors causing **optic nerve compression. Orbital inflammation** (orbital pseudotumor or Graves' ophthalmopathy) may cause compression of the optic nerve with resultant decreased acuity and disc edema. Inflammatory orbital disease usually is associated with proptosis or diplopia, so that the optic disc elevation is only one part of an overall constellation of signs and is rarely, if ever, an isolated finding (see Chapter 15). Optic nerve tumors are usually slow growing, and because they are intradural, they strangle the optic nerve, causing chronic optic disc elevation. Optociliary shunt vessels are another sign of chronic, progressive compression or infiltration of the optic nerve (Plate 8, *A*). However, these shunt vessels may be seen with chronic disc elevation from many causes.

### ☐ Hypertensive retinopathy with disc elevation

**Systemic hypertension** may produce optic disc elevation by causing ischemia to the optic nerve head or elevated ICP. Histopathologic changes in 23 eyes of 12 monkeys with accelerated renovascular hypertension showed the optic disc changes to be characteristic of local ischemia.[89] It is postulated that this optic neuropathy of hypertension is a form of anterior ischemic optic neuropathy.

Hypertensive patients also may have optic disc elevation due to papilledema and increased ICP. These patients with so-called **malignant hypertension** usually show other signs of a diffuse encephalopathy.

Treatment of this condition obviously entails bringing the systemic blood pressure into a more normal range. A rapid lowering of the blood pressure to normal or hypotensive levels may produce infarction of the swollen optic disc with permanent visual loss. While this is an unusual circumstance, it has even been reported to occur in children.[90] We therefore suggest a slowly graduated lowering of systemic blood pressure, especially if the optic discs are markedly elevated or show other signs of chronic elevation.

### ☐ Infiltrative optic neuropathy

Infiltration of the optic nerve may result in disc elevation in a variety of disorders. Inflammatory disorders, such as **sarcoidosis,** may produce disc elevation with or without abnormal cells being found in the spinal fluid. Malignant infiltration of the optic nerve may be seen in chronic[91] and acute[92] **leukemias** and **non-Hodgkin's lymphoma.**[93] In this group of disorders malignant cells in the spinal fluid, orbital involvement, or associated neurologic findings provide a clue to the etiology.

### ☐ Inflammatory optic neuropathy

Disc elevation and decreased acuity may be caused by **optic neuritis** (Plate 8, *B*). Optic neuritis may rarely produce bilateral simultaneous swollen discs (see Chapter 2). The correct diagnosis is made by the typical visual field abnormalities (see Chapters 1 and 2).

### ▣ Toxic and hereditary optic neuropathy

The presence of symmetric bilateral cecocentral scotomas with disc swelling usually implies a toxic or hereditary cause. However, most toxic or hereditary optic neuropathies do not have disc elevation, with the notable exception of acute methanol intoxication. An agent that produces a toxic optic neuropathy with disc edema is chloramphenicol.[94] Since this drug is often used in children with cystic fibrosis, the presence of a papillitis-like syndrome in this instance should suggest **chloramphenicol toxicity.** Vision recovers on drug withdrawal. Patients with **Leber's optic neuropathy** have nerve fiber layer edema and telangiectasia of the peripapillary region (see Chapter 2).

### ▣ Diabetic papillopathy

Another rare cause of acquired disc swelling is the disc elevation that occurs in type I (insulin-dependent) diabetics (Plate 8, *C*). This entity may present with few symptoms or with a host of visual findings, including central scotomas, arcuate visual field defects, and afferent pupillary defects. Disc edema is usually bilateral but may be unilateral. Acuity routinely improves within 3 months, although the disc edema itself may take a year to resolve.

The visual prognosis is generally but not uniformly favorable, with all patients (eight) experiencing visual recovery in one study[95] but four patients being left with permanent visual field defects and optic atrophy in another.[96]

The exact mechanism producing the disc swelling remains obscure. Fluorescein angiography does not show ischemia at the optic disc.[95] Barr et al.[96] speculate that optic nerve damage may result from anoxia secondary to failure of glucose utilization.

### ▣ Ischemic optic neuropathy

Acquired optic disc elevation with an altitudinal or arcuate visual field defect suggests infarction of the optic disc (Plate 8, *D*). Visual acuity may be normal or severely depressed (see Chapter 2).

### ▣ Central retinal vein occlusion and venous stasis retinopathy

Optic disc elevation, in one or both eyes, may be caused by central retinal vein occlusion (CRVO) or venous stasis retinopathy (Plate 8, *E*). Two major clinical forms of CRVO are seen: ischemic (hemorrhagic) and nonischemic. Both forms present with an elevated optic disc and intraretinal hemorrhages. The distinction between the two is the presence of numerous nerve fiber layer infarcts on ophthalmoscopy and capillary nonperfusion on fluorescein angiography, which identifies the ischemic form. The ischemic type is more likely than the nonischemic form to lead to neovascular glaucoma. Magargal et al.[97] indicate that panretinal photocoagulation (PRP) performed on 100 consecutive eyes with ischemic CRVO did prevent the development of neovascular glaucoma in all eyes. Although no double-masked study exists, we suggest immediate PRP in ischemic CRVO.

Kearns and Hollenhorst[98] described a form of optic disc edema associated with peripheral retinal hemorrhages and dilated retinal veins in patients with carotid occlusive disease. They named this condition *venous stasis retinopathy* (VSR), a term unfortunately used later by Hayreh[99] to describe the nonischemic form of retinal vein occlusion. One of the important factors distinguishing between the two conditions is that the retinal artery pressure in the retinopathy of carotid disease (VSR) is always decreased, whereas it is normal in retinal vein occlusions.[100] In addition, the retinal hemorrhages in CRVO extend further into the retinal periphery than do those of VSR.

CRVO and VSR may signify the presence of a variety of disorders. The most frequently associated diseases are **arterial hypertension, diabetes mellitus,** and **arteriosclerotic cardiovascular disease.**[101,102] Kohner et al.[103] reviewed 191 consecutive patients with CRVO and found the following percentages of intercurrent disease: hypertension, 44%; elevated blood urea, 25%; diabetes mellitus, 15%; elevated triglycerides, 40%; and elevated cholesterol, 30%. They also recommended an erythrocyte sedimentation rate and studies to detect hyperviscosity syndromes. The visual outcome was independent of the associated medical condition or its treatment. Chronic open-angle glaucoma is the ocular condition most frequently associated with CRVO, as it is found in approximately one third of all patients with CRVO.[104]

We recommend that patients with CRVO and VSR have a medical evaluation that includes the following tests:

Blood pressure determination
Two-hour postprandial blood glucose
Electrocardiogram
Complete blood count
Lipid profile
Serum protein electrophoresis
Prothrombin time/partial thromboplastin time (PT/PTT)

### ▣ Optic disc vasculitis

Some patients may present a fundus picture similar to that of CRVO or VSR, but pathologic examination reveals inflammation of the retinal veins.[105,106] This **phlebitis** may be identical to that form of disc swelling called **papillophlebitis** (Plate 8, *F*), which is encountered in young patients[107] and usually resolves without permanent visual sequelae. Cells may be detected in the vitreous overlying the optic disc.

A similar or possibly identical form of self-limiting, benign disc elevation seen in young, otherwise healthy individuals has been termed the **big blind spot syndrome.**[108] The only positive clinical findings are an elevated optic disc with venous overfilling, occasional retinal hemorrhages, and enlargement of the blind spot on visual field examinations. The etiology remains obscure, but this syndrome may represent optic neuritis without involvement of central acuity, or a mild form of venous occlusive disease.[109]

An enlarged blind spot without optic disc edema has been described.[110] This syndrome may be identical to the multiple evanescent white dot syndrome (see Chapter 1), a presumed viral retinopathy manifested by white lesions, primarily of the retinal pigment epithelium, throughout the fundus. Slight optic disc edema may be present acutely, but most nerve heads appear normal ophthalmoscopically.[111] The acute changes fade rapidly, leaving a fundus that appears normal but has a persistently enlarged blind spot on perimetry.[112,113]

## ☐ Uveitis or ocular hypotony

Optic disc elevation may occur in uveitis or ocular hypotony. Optic disc edema often accompanies diffuse posterior uveitis, pars planitis, or scleritis.

Bilateral posterior uveitis is becoming a frequently recognized manifestation of syphilis in human immunodeficiency virus (HIV)–infected patients[114] and may require more intensive antibiotic therapy than does syphilitic uveitis alone.[115] Becerra et al.[116] detected spinal fluid abnormalities of lues in 12 patients with uveitis and syphilis who were HIV positive. It is recommended that these patients be treated with 14 days of intravenous penicillin.

## REFERENCES

1. Radius RL, Maumenee AE. Optic atrophy and glaucomatous cupping. Am J Ophthalmol 1978;85:145-53.
2. Trobe JD, Glaser JS, Cassady J, et al. Nonglaucomatous excavation of the optic disc. Arch Ophthalmol 1980; 98:1046-50.
3. Romano PE. Simple photogrammetric diagnosis of optic nerve hypoplasia. Arch Ophthalmol 1989;107:824-6.
4. Mosier MA, Lieberman MF, Green WR, et al. Hypoplasia of the optic nerve. Arch Ophthalmol 1978;96:1437-42.
5. Frisén L, Holmegaard L. Spectrum of optic nerve hypoplasia. Br J Ophthalmol 1978;62:7-15.
6. Lambert SR, Hoyt CS, Narahara MH. Optic nerve hypoplasia. Surv Ophthalmol 1987;32:1-9.
7. Hoyt CS, Billson FA. Maternal anticonvulsants and optic nerve hypoplasia. Br J Ophthalmol 1978;62:3-6.
8. Van Dyk HJL, Morgan KS. Optic nerve hypoplasia and young maternal age [Letter]. Am J Ophthalmol 1980; 89:879.
9. Nelson M, Lessell S, Sadun AA. Optic nerve hypoplasia and maternal diabetes mellitus. Arch Neurol 1986;43:20-5.
10. Kim RY, Hoyt WF, Lessell S, et al. Superior segmental optic hypoplasia: a sign of maternal diabetes. Arch Ophthalmol 1989;107:1312-5.
11. Novakovic P, Taylor DSI, Hoyt WF. Localising patterns of optic nerve hypoplasia—retina to occipital lobe. Br J Ophthalmol 1988;72:176-82.
12. Bjork A, Laurell CG, Laurell U. Bilateral optic nerve hypoplasia with normal visual acuity. Am J Ophthalmol 1978;86:524-9.
13. Frisén L. Visual field defects due to hypoplasia of the optic nerve. In: Greve EL, ed. Third International Visual Field Symposium. The Hague: Dr W Junk, 1979:81-6. (Doc Ophthalmol Proc Ser;19.)
14. Skarf B, Hoyt CS. Optic nerve hypoplasia in children: association with anomalies of the endocrine and CNS. Arch Ophthalmol 1984;102:62-7.
15. Kaufman LM, Miller MT, Mafee MF. Magnetic resonance imagining of pituitary stalk hypoplasia: a discrete midline anomaly associated with endocrine abnormalities in septo-optic dysplasia. Arch Ophthalmol 1989; 107:1485-9.
16. Roessman U, Velasco ME, Small EJ, et al. Neuropathology of "septo-optic dysplasia" (de Morsier syndrome) with immunohistochemical studies of the hypothalmus and pituitary gland. J Neuropathol Exp Neurol 1987; 46:597-608.
17. Margalith D, Tze WJ, Jan JE. Congenital optic nerve hypoplasia with hypothalamic-pituitary dysplasia: a review of 16 cases. Am J Dis Child 1985; 139:361-6.
18. Brown GC, Shields JA, Patty BE, et al. Congenital pits of the optic nerve head. I. Experimental studies in collie dogs. Arch Ophthalmol 1979; 97:1341-4.

19. Goldhammer Y, Smith JL. Optic nerve anomalies in basal encephalocele. Arch Ophthalmol 1975;93:115-8.

20. Haik BG, Greenstein SH, Smith ME, et al. Retinal detachment in the morning glory anomaly. Ophthalmology 1984; 91:1638-47.

21. Young SE, Walsh FB, Knox DL. The tilted disk syndrome. Am J Ophthalmol 1976;82:16-23.

22. Rosenberg MA, Savino PJ, Glaser JS. A clinical analysis of pseudopapilledema. I. Population, laterality, acuity, refractive error, ophthalmoscopic characteristics, and coincident disease. Arch Ophthalmol 1979;97:65-70.

23. Wise GN, Henkind P, Alterman M. Optic disc drusen and subretinal hemorrhage. Trans Am Acad Ophthalmol Otolaryngol 1974;78:OP212-9.

24. Sanders TE, Gay AJ, Newman M. Hemorrhagic complications of drusen of the optic disk. Am J Ophthalmol 1971;71:204-17.

25. Levin BE. The clinical significance of spontaneous pulsations of the retinal vein. Arch Neurol 1978;35:37-40.

26. Gass JD, Braunstein R. Sessile and exophytic capillary angiomas of the juxtapapillary retina and optic nerve head. Arch Ophthalmol 1980;98:1790-7.

27. Schindler RF, Sarin LK, MacDonald PR. Hemangiomas of the optic disc. Can J Ophthalmol 1975;10:305-18.

28. Tso MOM, Hayreh SS. Optic disc edema in raised intracranial pressure. III. A pathologic study of experimental papilledema. Arch Ophthalmol 1977;95:1448-57.

29. Galbraith JEK, Sullivan JH. Decompression of the perioptic meninges for relief of papilledema. Am J Ophthalmol 1973;76:687-92.

30. Kaye AH, Galbraith JEK, King J. Intracranial pressure following optic nerve decompression for benign intracranial hypertension: case report. J Neurosurg 1981;55:453-6.

31. Kennedy F. Retrobulbar neuritis as an exact diagnostic sign of certain tumors and abscesses in the frontal lobes. Am J Med Sci 1911;142:355-68.

32. Kirkham TH, Sanders MD, Sapp GA. Unilateral papilloedema in benign intracranial hypertension. Can J Ophthalmol 1973;8:533-8.

33. Hoyt WF, Beeston D. The ocular fundus in neurologic disease: a diagnostic manual and stereo atlas. St Louis: Mosby–Year Book, 1966:2.

34. Okun E. Chronic papilledema simulating hyaline bodies of the optic disc. Am J Ophthalmol 1962;53:922-7.

35. Cogan DG. Blackouts not obviously due to carotid occlusion. Arch Ophthalmol 1961;66:180-7.

36. Corbett JJ, Savino PJ, Thompson HS, et al. Visual loss in pseudotumor cerebri: follow-up of 57 patients from five to 41 years and a profile of 14 patients with permanent severe visual loss. Arch Neurol 1982;39:461-74.

37. Green GJ, Lessell S, Loewenstein JI. Ischemic optic neuropathy in chronic papilledema. Arch Ophthalmol 1980; 98:502-4.

38. Orcutt JC, Page NGR, Sanders MD. Factors affecting visual loss in benign intracranial hypertension. Ophthalmology 1984;91:1303-12.

39. Morris AT, Sanders MD. Macular changes resulting from papilloedema. Br J Ophthalmol 1980;64:211-6.

40. Gittinger JW Jr, Asdourian GK. Macular abnormalities in papilledema from pseudotumor cerebri. Ophthalmology 1989;96:192-4.

41. Grehn F, Knorr-Held S, Kommerell G. Glaucomatous-like visual field defects in chronic papilledema. Albrecht Von Graefes Arch Klin Exp Ophthalmol 1981;217:99-109.

42. Spence JD, Amacher AL, Willis NR. Cerebrospinal fluid (CSF) pressure monitoring in the management of benign intracranial hypertension without papilledema [Abstract]. Neurology 1979;29:551.

43. Wolfe DR, Bird AC. The fundus. In: Lessell S, van Dalen JTW, eds. Neuro-ophthalmology: a series of critical surveys of the international literature, vol 2. Amsterdam: Excerpta Medica, 1980:9.

44. Silbergleit R, Junck L, Gebarski SS, et al. Idiopathic intracranial hypertension (pseudotumor cerebri): MR imaging. Radiology 1989;170:207-9.

45. Moser FG, Hilal SK, Abrams G, et al. MR imaging of pseudotumor cerebri. AJR Am J Roentgenol 1988;150:903-9.

46. Johnston I, Paterson A. Benign intracranial hypertension. I. Diagnosis and prognosis. Brain 1974;97:289-300.

47. Johnston I, Paterson A. Benign intracranial hypertension. II. CSF pressure and circulation. Brain 1974;97:301-12.

48. Hulcelle PJ, Dooms GC, Mathurin P, et al. MRI assessment of unsuspected dural sinus thrombosis. Neuroradiology 1989;31:217-21.

49. Chimowitz MI, Little JR, Awad IA, et al. Intracranial hypertension associated with unruptured cerebral arteriovenous malformations. Ann Neurol 1990;27:474-9.

50. Giles CL, Soble AR. Intracranial hypertension and tetracycline therapy. Am J Ophthalmol 1971;72:981-2.

51. Lubetzki C, Sanson M, Cohen D, et al. Hypertension intracrânienne bénigne et minocycline. Rev Neurol 1988; 144:218-20.

52. Cohen DN. Intracranial hypertension and papilledema associated with nalidixic acid therapy. Am J Ophthalmol 1973;76:680-2.

53. Mushet GR. Pseudotumor and nitrofurantoin therapy [Letter]. Arch Neurol 1977;34:257.

54. Hamed LM, Glaser JS, Schatz NJ, et al. Pseudotumor cerebri induced by danazol. Am J Ophthalmol 1989; 107:105-10.

55. Walker AE, Adamkiewicz JJ. Pseudotumor cerebri associated with prolonged corticosteroid therapy. JAMA 1964;188:779-84.

56. Lombaert A, Carton H. Benign intracranial hypertension due to A-hypervitaminosis in adults and adolescents. Eur Neurol 1976;14:340-50.

57. Selhorst JB, Waybright EA, Jennings S, et al. Liver lover's headache: pseudotumor cerebri and vitamin A intoxication [Letter]. JAMA 1984;252:3365.

58. Barber SG, Garvan N. Is "benign intracranial hypertension" really benign? J Neurol Neurosurg Psychiatry 1980;43:136-8.

59. Donaldson JO, Binstock ML. Pseudotumor cerebri in an obese woman with Turner syndrome. Neurology 1981; 31:758-60.

60. Britton C, Boxhill C, Brust JCM, et al. Pseudotumor cerebri, empty sella syndrome, and adrenal adenoma. Neurology 1980;30:292-6.

61. Carlow TJ, Glaser JS. Pseudotumor cerebri syndrome in systemic lupus erythematosus. JAMA 1974;228:197-200.

62. Guy J, Johnston PK, Corbett JJ, et al. Treatment of visual loss in pseudotumor cerebri asociated with uremia. Neurology 1990;40:28-32.

63. Jacobson DM, Frens DB. Pseudotumor cerebri syndrome associated with Lyme disease. Am J Ophthalmol 1989;107:81-2.

64. Rush JA. Pseudotumor cerebri: clinical profile and visual outcome in 63 patients. Mayo Clin Proc 1980;55:541-6.

65. Durcan FJ, Corbett JJ, Wall M. The incidence of pseudotumor cerebri: population studies in Iowa and Louisiana. Arch Neurol 1988;45:875-7.

66. Digre KB, Corbett JJ. Pseudotumor cerebri in men. Arch Neurol 1988; 45:866-72.

67. Lessell S, Rosman NP. Permanent visual impairment in childhood pseudotumor cerebri. Arch Neurol 1986; 43:801-4.

68. Baker RS, Carter D, Hendrick EB, et al. Visual loss in pseudotumor cerebri of childhood: a follow-up study. Arch Ophthalmol 1985;103:1681-86.

69. Couch R, Camfield PR, Tibbles JAR. The changing picture of pseudotumor cerebri in children. Can J Neurol Sci 1985;12:48-50.

70. Hamed LM, Winward KE, Glaser JS, et al. Optic neuropathy in uremia. Am J Ophthalmol 1989;108:30-5.

71. Traviesa DC, Schwartzman RF, Glaser JS, et al. Familial benign intracranial hypertension. J Neurol Neurosurg Psychiatry 1976;39:420-3.

72. Torlai F, Galassi G, Debbia A, et al. Familial pseudotumor cerebri in male heterozygous twins. Eur Neurol 1989; 29:106-8.

73. Aisenberg RM, Rottenberg DA. The pathogenesis of pseudotumor cerebri—a mathematical analysis. J Neurol Sci 1980;48:51-60.

74. Mann JD, Johnson RN, Butler AB, et al. Impairment of cerebrospinal fluid circulatory dynamics in pseudotumor cerebri and response to steroid treatment [Abstract]. Neurology 1979;29:550.

75. Raichle ME, Grubb RL Jr, Phelps ME, et al. Cerebral hemodynamics and metabolism in pseudotumor cerebri. Ann Neurol 1978;4:104-11.

76. Bulens C, De Vries WA, Van Crevel H. Benign intracranial hypertension: a retrospective and follow-up study. J Neurol Sci 1979;40:147-57.

77. Wall M, George D. Visual loss in pseudotumor cerebri: incidence and defects related to visual field strategy. Arch Neurol 1987;44:170-5.

78. Round R, Keane JR. The minor symptoms of increased intracranial pressure: 101 patients with benign intracranial hypertension. Neurology 1988;38:1461-4.

79. Corbett JJ, Jacobson DM, Mauer RC, et al. Enlargement of the blind spot caused by papilledema. Am J Ophthalmol 1988;105:261-5.

80. Bousser MG, Chiras J, Bories J, et al. Cerebral venous thrombosis—a review of 38 cases. Stroke 1985;16:199-213.

81. Gucer G, Viernstein L. Long-term intracranial pressure recording in the management of pseudotumor cerebri. J Neurosurg 1978;49:256-63.

82. Newborg B. Pseudotumor cerebri treated by rice reduction diet. Arch Intern Med 1974;133:802-7.

83. Rosenberg M, Smith C, Beck R, et al. The efficacy of shunting procedures in pseudotumor cerebri [Abstract]. Neurology 1989;39(suppl 1):209.

84. Sergott RC, Savino PJ, Bosley TM. Modified optic nerve sheath decompression provides long-term visual improvement for pseudotumor cerebri. Arch Ophthalmol 1988;106:1384-90.

85. Brourman ND, Spoor TC, Ramocki JM. Optic nerve sheath decompression for pseudotumor cerebri. Arch Ophthalmol 1988;106:1378-83.

86. Corbett JJ, Nerad JA, Tse DT, et al. Results of optic nerve sheath fenestration for pseudotumor cerebri: the lateral orbitotomy approach. Arch Ophthalmol 1988;106:1391-7.

87. Bulens C, Meerwaldt JD, Koudstaal PJ, et al. Spatial contrast sensitivity in benign intracranial hypertension. J Neurol Neurosurg Psychiatry 1988;51:1323-9.

88. Verplanck M, Kaufman DI, Parsons T, et al. Electrophysiology versus psychophysics in the detection of visual loss in pseudotumor cerebri. Neurology 1988;38:1789-92.

89. Kishi S, Tso MOM, Hayreh SS. Fundus lesions in malignant hypertension. II. A pathologic study of experimental hypertensive optic neuropathy. Arch Ophthalmol 1985;103:1198-206.

90. Taylor D, Ramsay J, Day S, et al. Infarction of the optic nerve head in children with accelerated hypertension. Br J Ophthalmol 1981;65:153-60.

91. Currie JN, Lessell S, Lessell IM, et al. Optic neuropathy in chronic lymphocytic leukemia. Arch Ophthalmol 1988;106:654-60.

92. Nikaido H, Mishima H, Ono H, et al. Leukemic involvement of the optic nerve. Am J Ophthalmol 1988;105:294-8.

93. Kay MC. Optic neuropathy secondary to lymphoma. J Clin Neuro Ophthalmol 1986;6:31-4.

94. Godel V, Nemet P, Lazar M. Chloramphenicol optic neuropathy. Arch Ophthalmol 1980;98:1417-21.

95. Pavan PR, Aiello LM, Wafai MZ, et al. Optic disc edema in juvenile-onset diabetes. Arch Ophthalmol 1980;98:2193-5.

96. Barr CC, Glaser JS, Blankenship G. Acute disc swelling in juvenile diabetes: clinical profile and natural history of 12 cases. Arch Ophthalmol 1980;98:2185-92.

97. Magargal LE, Brown GC, Augsburger JJ, et al. Neovascular glaucoma following central retinal vein obstruction. Ophthalmology 1981;88:1095-101.

98. Kearns TP, Hollenhorst RW. Venous-stasis retinopathy of occlusive disease of the carotid artery. Mayo Clin Proc 1963;38:304-12.

99. Hayreh SS. Central retinal vein occlusion: differential diagnosis and management. Trans Am Acad Ophthalmol Otolaryngol 1977;83:OP379-91.

100. Kearns TP. Differential diagnosis of central retinal vein obstruction. Ophthalmology 1983;90:475-80.

101. McGrath MA, Wechsler F, Hunyor ABL, et al. Systemic factors contributory to retinal vein occlusion. Arch Intern Med 1978;138:216-20.

102. Rubinstein K, Jones EB. Retinal vein occlusion: long-term prospects: 10 years' follow-up of 143 patients. Br J Ophthalmol 1976;60:148-50.

103. Kohner EM, Laatikainen L, Oughton J. The management of central retinal vein occlusion. Ophthalmology 1983; 90:484-7.

104. Green WR, Chan CC, Hutchins GM, et al. Central retinal vein occlusion: a prospective histopathologic study of 29 eyes in 28 cases. Retina 1981;1:27-55.

105. Appen RE, de Venecia G, Ferwerda J. Optic disk vasculitis. Am J Ophthalmol 1980;90:352-9.

106. Cogan DG. Retinal and papillary vasculitis. In: Cant JS, ed. The William Mackenzie Centenary Symposium on the Ocular Circulation in Health and Disease. St Louis: Mosby–Year Book, 1969:249-70.

107. Lonn LI, Hoyt WF. Papillophlebitis: a cause of protracted yet benign optic disc edema. Eye Ear Nose Throat Mon 1966;45:62 passim.

108. Miller NR. The big blind spot syndrome: unilateral optic disc edema without visual loss or increased intracranial pressure. In: Smith JL, ed. Neuro-ophthalmology update. New York: Masson, 1977:163-9.

109. Miller NR, ed. Walsh and Hoyt's clinical neuro-ophthalmology. 4th ed. Baltimore: Williams & Wilkins, 1982:223.

110. Fletcher WA, Imes RK, Goodman D, et al. Acute idiopathic blind spot enlargement: a big blind spot syndrome without disc edema. Arch Ophthalmol 1988;106:44-9.

111. Dodwell DG, Jampol LM, Rosenberg M, et al. Optic nerve involvement associated with the multiple evanescent white-dot syndrome. Ophthalmology 1990;97:862-8.

112. Hamed LM, Glaser JS, Gass JDM, et al. Protracted enlargement of the blind spot in multiple evanescent white dot syndrome. Arch Ophthalmol 1989;107:194-8.

113. Kimmel AS, Folk JC, Thompson HS, et al. The multiple evanescent white-dot syndrome with acute blind spot enlargement. Am J Ophthalmol 1989; 107:425-6.

114. Passo MS, Rosenbaum JT. Ocular syphilis in patients with human immunodeficiency virus infection. Am J Ophthalmol 1988;106:1-6.

115. Berry CD, Hooton TM, Collier AC, et al. Neurologic relapse after benzathine penicillin therapy for secondary syphilis in a patient with HIV infection. N Engl J Med 1987;316:1587-9.

116. Becerra LI, Ksiazek SM, Savino PJ, et al. Syphilitic uveitis in human immunodeficiency virus–infected and noninfected patients. Ophthalmology 1989;96:1727-30.

CHAPTER 8

# Gaze Disturbances

•   •   •   •   •   •   •   •   •   •   •   •   •   •   •   •

## The Ocular Motor System

The ocular motor system in humans has but one purpose: to place and maintain the image of regard on the foveas until the individual decides to look at something else. This physiologic state is accomplished through the coordinated output of a number of supranuclear control centers. With the exception of the vestibular apparatus and the superior colliculus, the initiation of various types of ocular movements is presumed to originate in cerebral hemispheric centers. Conceptually, these centers deal with capturing a target (saccadic center), maintaining acquired fixation (fixation center), pursuing a target (pursuit center), and keeping the eyes stabilized in space (vestibular apparatus). To presume that any center acts in total isolation would be simplistic. The following material represents a broad overview of experimental and clinical data that we believe is helpful in understanding gaze and vergence dysfunction.

The supranuclear centers produce the coordinated action of muscle groups and not of individual muscles. The output of these centers produces two types of eye movements[1]: (1) *conjugate movements,* in which both eyes move in the same direction, and (2) *vergence movements,* in which both eyes either turn in (convergence) or turn out (divergence).

Conjugate eye movements are of at least two types: fast and slow. *Fast eye movements* (Fig. 8-1) have a velocity that varies from 300 to 700 degrees/sec among individuals. If they are used to bring images of regard onto the fovea, they are called *saccades.* If they are part of a reflex such as a response to optokinetic or vestibular stimuli, they are generally termed *quick phases* that are corrective in nature (i.e., return the eye to the point of fixation).[2]* Three types of *slow (smooth) eye movements* exist: (1) foveal pursuit, which does not exceed 40 degrees/sec (if a faster movement is required, a "catch-up" saccade is programmed (Fig. 8-2); (2) the smooth movement of the vestibulo-ocular reflex, which may exceed 100 degrees/sec (Fig. 8-3); and (3) the slow movement induced by full-field optokinetic stimuli.

---

*In the clinical literature the term *saccade* is most often used to refer to all fast movements, and we will in certain instances take such a liberty.

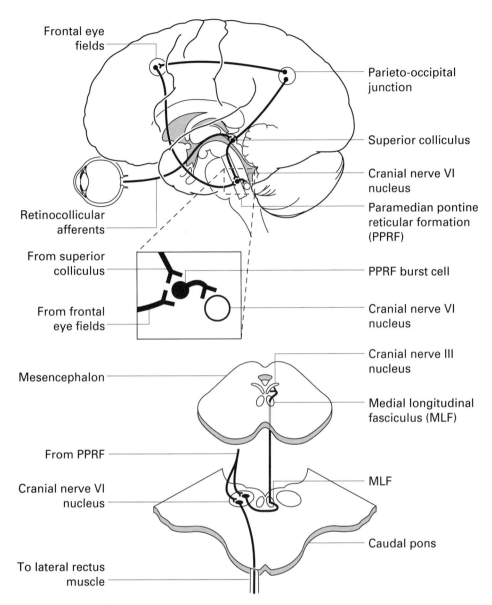

*Fig. 8-1.* Control of horizontal eye movements: saccadic pathway. Most saccades are primarily initiated in one or both cortical centers, the frontal eye fields and parieto-occipital junction, and in one subcortical center, the superior colliculus. (Quick phases of nystagmus are probably initiated in brainstem.) Messages are sent to caudal paramedian pontine reticular formation (PPRF). From there, commands for horizontal gaze are sent to sixth cranial nerve (abducens) nucleus, where they connect to two sets of neurons—those whose axons are destined to innervate lateral rectus muscle and those whose axons travel through medial longitudinal fasciculus (MLF) to activate medial rectus subnuclei of third cranial nerve. (Commands for vertical gaze are mediated through rostral PPRF and travel to rostral interstitial nucleus of MLF; see Fig. 8-4.)

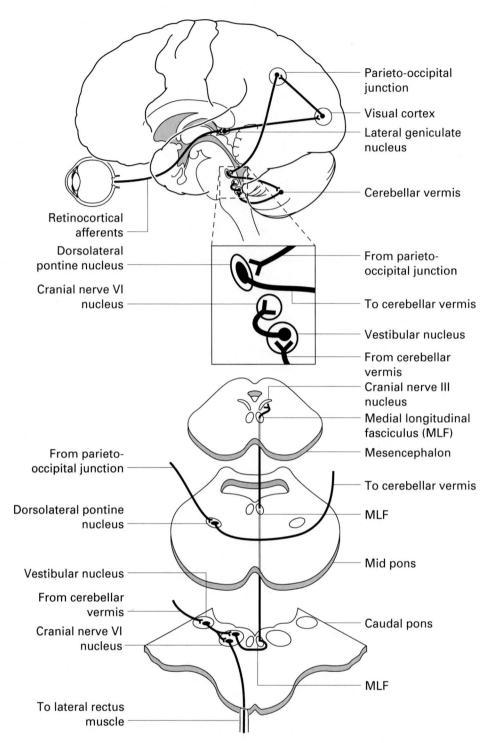

*Fig. 8-2.* Control of horizontal eye movements: pursuit pathway. Pursuit eye movements are activated by a slowly moving visual target that generates impulses in retinocortical pathway. Message then travels to parieto-occipital junction. From there, pathway in humans is uncertain but is believed to connect through dorsolateral pontine nuclei, cerebellar vermis, and vestibular nuclei. Efferents then carry signal to sixth nerve (abducens) nucleus. Rest of pathway is identical to that for saccades (see Fig. 8-1). Unlike saccadic pathway, pursuit pathway does not pass through PPRF.

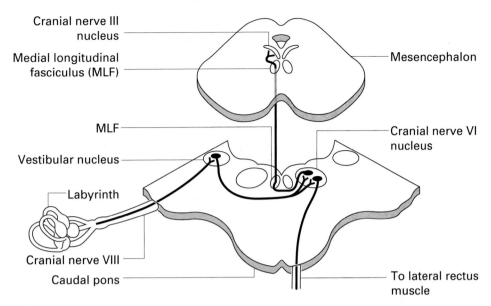

*Fig. 8-3.* Control of horizontal eye movements: vestibulo-ocular pathway. Acceleratory head movements activate this pathway via labyrinthine hair cells, which send signals to vestibular nuclei. Efferents carry excitatory message for all horizontal eye movements to contralateral sixth nerve (abducens) nucleus. Vertical eye movements are mediated by pathways carrying signals directly to midbrain.

Patients with damage or destruction of those areas of the brain producing conjugate gaze functions are usually unaware of their visual system disability, although they may complain of nondescript blurring of vision. On the other hand, patients with damage to mechanisms subserving vergence movements usually experience diplopia or blurring of vision, or both. Damage to the vestibular apparatus produces a type of oscillopsia, which is discussed in Chapter 12.

Gaze and vergence abnormalities almost never exist in neurologic isolation. The recognition of their presence can help localize a lesion anatomically and identify a specific nosologic entity. It is important to remember that extraocular muscle disease and disorders of the myoneural junction can mimic gaze and vergence disorders.

## CONJUGATE SYSTEMS

**FAST EYE MOVEMENT SYSTEMS.** As stated above, fast eye movements used to bring objects of interest onto the fovea are termed saccades and consist of intentional and reflexive types. These movements are generated when changing fixation and during pursuit of an object exceeding 40 degrees/sec. They can be generated volitionally. Fast eye movements can also occur during periods of noninterest (random eye movements) and during so-called rapid eye movement (REM) sleep. Fast movements that make up the corrective phase in all forms of nystagmus (vestibular and optokinetic) are termed quick phases.

Neurophysiologic evidence confirms specific activation of neurons within the frontal eye fields prior to the onset of contralateral visually guided saccades[3] (see Fig. 8-1). Studies using $^{15}OH_2$ with positron emission tomography (PET) demonstrate activity in the contralateral frontal eye fields (Brodmann's areas 8 α and γ) in the supplementary motor cortex and in the cerebellum during all fast eye movements.[4] The frontal eye fields send projections directly to the brainstem centers for horizontal and vertical gaze (paramedian pontine reticular formation).

Evidence indicates that the superior colliculus plays an important role in foveation (i.e., visually elicited saccades). The superior colliculus projects directly to the paramedian pontine reticular formation and to the rostral interstitial nucleus of the medial longitudinal fasciculus (MLF), mediating horizontal and vertical gaze. The superior colliculus receives input from the parieto-occipital junction and the frontal eye fields, as well as direct afferents from the retina. Experimental and clinical evidence[5,6] suggests that the ipsilateral frontal cortex can initiate ipsilateral saccades when the contralateral hemisphere has been damaged. Thus two (or more) parallel pathways capable of initiating saccades may exist. In addition, clinical and neuroanatomic evidence indicates that the posterior parietal cortex, specifically the inferior parietal lobule,[7] is involved with the control of visually guided saccades.[8]

The frontal eye fields and the superior colliculus send axons to the contralateral paramedian pontine reticular formation (PPRF)[9] (see Fig. 8-1). The projection from the frontal eye fields courses caudally and medially to pass through the anterior limb of the internal capsule near its knee adjacent to the globus pallidus. Here the fibers separate into two bundles:

1. The major pathway courses caudally and medially along the ventrolateral surface of the thalamus through the zona incerta and the fields of Forel. In the rostral midbrain these fibers are situated in the dorsomedial aspect of the corticospinal tract as part of the corticobulbar projection. Decussation occurs in the lower midbrain and upper pons at the level of the caudal end of the third nerve nucleus (just prior to the decussation of the central facial projections) to synapse in the PPRF just rostral to the abducens nuclei.
2. The minor pathway continues ipsilaterally rather than decussating before turning dorsally to enter the pontine tegmentum and the PPRF.

The exact pathways connecting all other supranuclear centers subserving saccadic function remain unknown. The dorsomedial aspect of the PPRF just rostral[9,10] to the sixth nerve nucleus acts as a brainstem center subserving conjugate ipsilateral horizontal saccadic movements. Pursuit movements have other brainstem generators (see Fig. 8-2). The PPRF sends axons to the ipsilateral sixth nerve nucleus, which serves as the final supranuclear center for all horizontal gaze movements, saccades, quick phases, and pursuit movements. The abducens nucleus consists of large motor cells whose axons form the ipsilateral sixth cranial nerve and small so-called interneurons whose axons cross immediately and ascend in the MLF, to end in one or more of the medial rectus subnuclei of the third cranial nerve[11,12] (see Fig. 8-1, *inset*).

Experiments in monkeys[13,14] indicate that the rostral end of the PPRF acts as a vertical gaze center from which arise projection pathways to the rostral interstitial nucleus of the medial longitudinal fasciculus (riMLF),[15,16] the final common pathway for conjugate vertical saccades. Pathologic studies in humans suggest that this area of the PPRF is rostral to the sixth nerve nucleus.[10] The riMLF lies dorsomedial to the anterior end of the red nucleus, rostral to the interstitial nucleus of Cajal (IC), and lateral to the nucleus of Darkschewitsch (Fig. 8-4). Evidence is good that the pathways for upgaze project dorsolaterally and that the tracts subserving downgaze project ventromedially.[16-18] Direct elevation and depression movements from the primary position require bilateral cortical input. The IC may contain interneurons sending axons to the contralateral superior rectus muscle.

**SLOW EYE MOVEMENT SYSTEMS.** The supranuclear system used for tracking continuously moving targets is called the foveal pursuit system. This system can maintain foveal fixation on targets with a maximum speed of 40 degrees/sec. The vestibular system can generate a smooth eye movement of higher speed to stabilize the object of regard on the fovea during head or background movements.

The cortical center for generating foveal smooth pursuit is generally agreed to be located within the broad region of the so-called parieto-occipital junction. Experimentally, the MST region in monkeys appears to be responsible for generating pursuit. It has as its homologue in humans parts of Brodmann's areas 37, 39, and the front of 19, which is compatible with the clinical findings implicating the inferior parietal lobule.[8] Experiments have shown that approximately two thirds of the neurons in the region of the superior temporal sulcus fire with ipsilateral pursuit and one third with contralateral pursuit.[19] The projection pathways of the pursuit system are unknown. In fact, the regions of the brainstem subserving smooth pursuit are not as well delineated as those subserving saccades. Experimental evidence suggests that the dorsolateral pontine nuclei (DLPN)[20] serve as the brainstem centers for ipsilateral foveal pursuit movements. Whether the DLPN project directly onto the sixth nerve nuclei or indirectly through the cerebellum (vermal lobules VI to X[21]) on the vestibular nuclei is not clear. In humans foveal pursuit is subserved by an anatomic pathway in the pons[10] separate from that producing the vestibulo-ocular reflex. In addition, the cerebellum and some of its pathways must be functioning normally to generate normal pursuit movements.

Hoyt and Daroff[22] postulated that a double decussation of the descending pursuit pathways takes place (probably in the brainstem), since control of pursuit is ipsilateral. That such a decussation exists has received support from the clinical finding of a lesion in the mesencephalon producing a contralateral saccadic and ipsilateral pursuit paresis.[23]

# VERGENCE SYSTEMS

Disjunctive eye movements enable the subject to fixate bifoveally at all points in space from infinity to the near point of convergence. This flexibility calls for active convergence and divergence. Vergence movements have a maximum veloc-

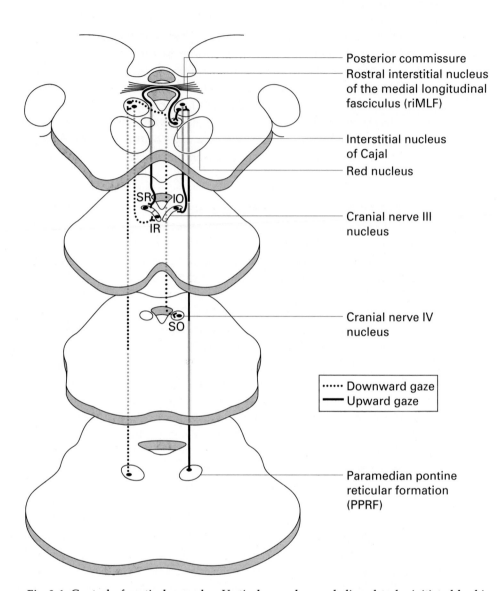

Posterior commissure

Rostral interstitial nucleus of the medial longitudinal fasciculus (riMLF)

Interstitial nucleus of Cajal

Red nucleus

Cranial nerve III nucleus

Cranial nerve IV nucleus

······ Downward gaze
—— Upward gaze

Paramedian pontine reticular formation (PPRF)

SR IO
IR
SO

*Fig. 8-4.* Control of vertical saccades. Vertical saccades are believed to be initiated by bi-hemispheric cortical signals that travel to rostral pontine paramedian reticular formation (PPRF). From there, signals travel along separate pathways—dorsally if eyes are to be moved up and ventrally if they are to be moved down. Both pathways end in rostral interstitial nucleus of medial longitudinal fasciculus (riMLF). Fibers mediating upgaze pass through posterior commissure before turning caudally to synapse on ipsilateral inferior oblique subnucleus and contralateral superior rectus subnucleus. Fibers to superior rectus synapse in interstitial nucleus of Cajal. Fibers mediating downgaze turn caudally to synapse on ipsilateral inferior rectus subnucleus and contralateral superior oblique nucleus. The fact that upgaze (but not downgaze) pathway passes through posterior commissure explains preferential paresis of upgaze by dorsal midbrain lesions.

ity of approximately 20 degrees/sec. Under normal conditions convergence is associated with pupillary miosis and accommodation, making up the triad of the near reflex.

Although the supranuclear substrates are unknown, electrical stimulation of regions in monkeys equivalent to Brodmann's areas 19 and 22 in humans activates different components of the near triad. Convergence and divergence cell groups have been identified in the mesencephalic reticular formation just dorsal and lateral to the oculomotor nucleus.[24] A convergence cell group has been identified more dorsally in the pretectal region rostral to the superior colliculus. Cells controlling divergence are much fewer than those controlling convergence.[24]

# Disorders Involving Supranuclear Control Pathways

As mentioned earlier, dysfunction of the supranuclear centers for saccadic and pursuit movements and their pathways produces conjugate gaze abnormalities. Most patients are not aware of any visual difficulty. Those who are symptomatic do not complain of conjugate deficits but attribute their symptoms (such as the inability to see food on their plates) to inappropriate glasses rather than inability to conjugately move their eyes downward. Patients with vergence problems usually complain of blurring of vision or frank diplopia, whereas patients with disorders of the vestibular system and its connections complain of oscillopsia.

Dysfunction of supranuclear gaze centers are discussed first in terms of isolated involvement of specific centers and then in terms of more diffuse central nervous system (CNS) disease. This is followed by a discussion of nuclear and infranuclear structures that mimic supranuclear disorders and diseases that involve the extraocular muscles.

## DISORDERS OF THE FAST EYE MOVEMENT SYSTEMS

Disorders of the fast eye movement systems can be caused by lesions that involve the frontal eye fields and their projections to the PPRF, and in turn the PPRF and its projections to the sixth nerve nuclei and the riMLF[10,25,26] (Figs. 8-1 and 8-2).

**UNILATERAL SACCADIC PARESIS** . Unilateral saccadic palsy can be produced by unilateral cerebral hemispheric damage involving the frontal eye fields and their projections. In the acute phase (following an ischemic, hemorrhagic, or traumatic event), these patients' eyes are deviated toward the side of the lesion. At this time the "doll's eye" (oculocephalic) maneuver (i.e., passive head turning) may or may not produce a full range of ocular movements. A caloric stimulus (cold or warm water instilled in the external auditory canal) will induce a full range of ocular movements (slow movement). The saccadic corrective quick phase is absent in the direction contralateral to the lesion.[14] As these patients become alert, their eyes assume the straight-ahead position, but the patients are unable to generate any fast movements to the side contralateral to the lesion. At this stage caloric stimuli still produce a tonic deviation of the eyes ipsilateral to the lesion, since the patient is unable to generate a contralateral corrective quick phase.

If the contralateral hemisphere is intact, the saccadic deficit will slowly improve. Initially the eyes will move a minimal distance eccentric to the midline contralaterally, but the eccentric gaze position will not be held and a coarse gaze-paretic nystagmus will develop with a drift toward the midline, followed by a corrective fast movement. Over weeks or months these contralateral fast eye movements become more normal with a concomitant disappearance of the gaze-paretic nystagmus. The saccades to the contralateral field always remain hypometric and slightly slow.[6]

**BILATERAL SACCADIC PARESIS.** Bilateral dysfunction of the frontobulbar system produces a loss of fast movements in both horizontal directions of gaze, termed *global saccadic palsy*. Pursuit, oculocephalic movements, and the slow movements in response to caloric stimuli remain unaffected. For unexplained reasons, vertical saccades are only variably affected.

**CONGENITAL OCULAR MOTOR APRAXIA.** Cogan and Adams[27] and Cogan[28] characterized congenital ocular motor apraxia (OMA) as the inability to make horizontal saccades when the head is immobilized. Some patients can generate random saccadic eye movements. Patients with OMA use head thrusts to induce compensatory eye movements by activating the vestibulo-ocular reflex system. The following is a typical sequence used to produce a movement to the right:

1. The lids are closed.
2. A rapid head thrust to the right drives the eyes tonically to the left; the head thrust overshoots the target and places the image of regard on the fovea of each eye in left gaze.
3. The object is held fixated by each eye, and the head is slowly rotated to the left until the eyes are in midposition (vestibulo-ocular reflex).

Head thrusts become less apparent with age as these patients develop some degree of saccadic function.

Most of these patients have normal vertical saccades and pursuit movements in all directions. On the other hand, they may have severe defects of the quick phases of induced optokinetic and caloric nystagmus.[29] The preservation of vertical saccades suggests a problem in the PPRF just rostral to the sixth nerve nuclei but caudal to that portion of the PPRF that mediates vertical gaze. Others maintain that this entity represents bihemispheric disease. Cogan[28] was the first to note that OMA may be asymmetric. Catalano et al.[30] observed an asymmetry of the apraxia in up to one third of the children they saw with congenital OMA.

Zee et al.[31] immobilized the heads of three patients with a form fruste of the complete syndrome and reported delayed initiation and hypometria of voluntary saccades. The fast phase of both optokinetic and vestibular nystagmus was almost normal. These patients used head thrusts to boost or trigger saccadic movements.

Our impression is that ocular motor apraxia in isolation is often seen in the context of developmental delay. If no other manifestations of neurologic or systemic disease are present, further workup is not indicated.

**ACQUIRED OCULAR MOTOR APRAXIA.** A variety of forms of volitional saccadic palsy exist. These patients may demonstrate a spectrum of dysfunction ranging from a complete loss of all saccades to delayed initiation and hypometria of voluntary saccades only.[27,32] Some of these patients maintain random saccadic eye movements; others have pursuit deficits as well.[33] Many of these patients use head thrusts to initiate slow movements. Pierrot-Deseilligny et al.[33] reported one such patient with bilateral watershed infarcts affecting the frontal lobes, as well as the posterior paramedian region of both hemispheres, nearly reaching the parieto-occipital junction. As Cogan[34] pointed out, in patients with acquired ocular motor apraxia, "The paradoxical maintenance of random eye movements with loss of purposeful eye movements often gives rise to the erroneous impression of hysterical blindness." Many of these patients have associated difficulty with initiating head movements and sometimes movements of the arms and legs. Considering the proximity of the cortical motor strip to the cortical eye movement center, this is not surprising.

**HUNTINGTON'S DISEASE.** Huntington's disease is inherited as an autosomally dominant trait. It has an insidious onset, usually beginning in the late thirties, with choreic movements and cognitive disturbances as its hallmark. The ocular motor abnormalities include random intrusions of saccadic movements during fixation, impaired initiation of saccades manifested by increased reaction time, and the inability to produce saccadic movement without head movement or blink. All fast movements become progressively slowed[35,36] and ultimately are lost. Interestingly, smooth pursuit is abnormal in the majority of patients, and vergences are abnormal in about a third of patients. The vestibulo-ocular reflex and the ability to hold eccentric fixation are preserved even late in the disease.

Mental deterioration begins a few years after the onset of the involuntary movements. Other findings include intermittent, nonstereotypical spasm of the facial muscles accompanied by periods of eyelid closure and periods during which the lids remain wide open. Leigh et al.[37] demonstrated a decrease in the number of large neurons in the riMLF pathologically in one of four patients with Huntington's disease who had difficulty in generating vertical saccades. They postulate that this deficiency in generating vertical saccades is due to a loss of supranuclear input, not to cell loss.

**MISCELLANEOUS.** Saccadic paralysis is reported in multiple sclerosis (MS), ataxia telangiectasia, Pelizaeus-Merzbacher disease, Wilson's disease, Whipple's disease, and spinocerebellar degeneration.[29,32] In addition, some patients with Wilson's disease develop a striking inability to maintain fixation for more than a few seconds, at which time they appear to be distracted and make a saccadic movement to a peripheral target.[38]

## DISORDERS OF THE SLOW EYE MOVEMENT SYSTEMS

Disorders of smooth pursuit may be caused by lesions involving the parieto-occipital junction, the projection pathway(s) to the brainstem, brainstem substrates, and the cerebellum.

**UNILATERAL PURSUIT PARESIS.** Unilateral loss of smooth pursuit is most often caused by lesions in the region of the parieto-occipital junction[39] or in a hemisphere of the cerebellum. In cerebral hemispheric disease involving the inferior parietal lobule, the loss of ipsilateral pursuit is often associated with a contralateral homonymous visual field defect and an attenuation of the optokinetic response when the stimulus is rotated toward the side of the lesion. Little, if any, recovery is noted in these patients over time.[39] Lesions of the cerebellar flocculus similarly produce ipsilateral pursuit deficits.

**BILATERAL PURSUIT PARESIS.** Bilateral saccadic pursuit can be produced by diffuse posterior hemispheric, cerebellar, or brainstem disease. In upper brainstem disease the saccadic pursuit movements are seen in the setting of more global deficits, such as those associated with Parkinson's disease. Many sedative drugs lower the maximum velocity at which smooth pursuit movements can be generated. In this group of patients intermittent "catch up" saccades will be noted even when they are tracking slow targets. Similar findings can be seen during the first 5 minutes following smoking a cigarette.[40]

## DISORDERS OF THE VERGENCE SYSTEM

**DIVERGENCE AND CONVERGENCE PARALYSIS.** Patients with either of these disorders usually have initial complaints of diplopia and therefore are discussed in Chapter 9.

**SPASM OF THE NEAR REFLEX.** A major complaint of patients with spasm of the near reflex is a general blurring of vision. A small number note diplopia, and an even smaller number note crossing of their eyes. Diagnosis is based on the findings of a variable esotropia associated with varying pupillary size. Spasm of the near reflex is often precipitated by acute stress. It has been associated with a variety of organic diseases, including encephalitis (usually accompanied by nystagmus), neurosyphilis, labyrinthine fistula, and trauma, but is more commonly a psychogenic illness. Some patients can voluntarily cross their eyes, and a small percentage use this ability to feign illness.

Spasm of the near reflex has been seen in patients with congenital horizontal gaze paralysis[41] as they attempt to fixate eccentrically. They may complain of diplopia and appear esotropic. Similar convergence movements can be seen in patients with MS as a substitute for conjugate gaze movements.

In patients with psychogenic spasm of the near reflex, supportive reassurance may be the best approach. For those in whom the spasm occurs during prolonged use of the eyes (e.g., studying for exams), taking a 5-minute "break" usually suffices to allow them to continue their work. At times using "tricks" to alleviate the spasm by inducing voluntary or reflex saccades may be necessary.

Some of these patients have recurrent prolonged bouts of spasm of the near reflex. In some patients various topical cycloplegic agents break the spasm and alleviate symptoms. A majority can slowly be withdrawn from the use of these cycloplegic agents. Paradoxically, Cogan and Freese[42] reported success using an artificially induced hyperopia (overminusing the spectacle correction by 1.50 to 2.50 diopters) in a large series of such patients. We have had no experience with this treatment modality.

**ACUTE THALAMIC ESOTROPIA.** In cases of infarction in the territory of penetrating branches of the mesencephalic artery, an acute monocular convergence spasm can be seen, termed *acute thalamic esotropia* by Gomez et al.[43] In these patients the pupils are uninvolved for the most part. These patients develop an acute esotropia with the involved eye turned in (sometimes slightly down) and immobile to all stimuli, whereas the fellow eye responds normally. Gomez et al.[43] suggest that this esotropia may be the "maximal expression of the phenomenon of 'pseudosixth' or 'pseudoabducens' palsy."[44] This misalignment is associated with stupor, impaired gaze, and long tract signs, which in many cases disappear rapidly, leaving a residua of impaired upgaze and convergence retraction nystagmus. All of these patients have lesions involving the thalamic-mesencephalic interface, demonstrated both neuropathologically[45] and by magnetic resonance imaging (MRI).[43]

## DISORDERS OF BOTH THE FAST AND SLOW EYE MOVEMENT SYSTEMS

Gaze palsies are defined[46] as an inability to move the eyes in a given direction by saccades (saccadic gaze palsy), smooth pursuit (pursuit gaze palsy), or both (global gaze palsy). Combined gaze palsies can be caused by lesions anywhere from the cerebral hemispheres (where diffuse damage involves both the frontal and parieto-occipital centers or pathways) to the primary and secondary gaze centers in the brainstem. Topographic localization depends on the extent of the deficit and accompanying neurologic signs.

**CONGENITAL ISOLATED HORIZONTAL GAZE DEFICITS.** A group of patients have either a sporadic or familial congenital paralysis of horizontal gaze.[47,48] In these individuals horizontal conjugate movements are absent, whereas vertical movements and convergence are variably affected. These patients may have a developmental anomaly affecting motor neurons and interneurons in the abducens nuclei.

*Möbius syndrome*[49] is a rubric for a heterogeneous group of patients who have in common facial diplegia and horizontal gaze paralysis. These patients may use the mechanism of accommodative convergence to increase their ability to look eccentrically by producing an esotropia and cross-fixating. Other congenital defects, including deafness and webbed or supernumerary digits, are variably found. A great many pathologic findings are reported in these patients, but one unifying feature is the involvement of the brainstem nuclei.[50]

Congenital horizontal gaze paresis is also reported in association with the

Klippel-Feil anomaly. Additional findings include hemifacial atrophy, ear dysplasia, and scoliosis.[41]

**ACQUIRED BILATERAL HORIZONTAL GAZE DEFICITS.** Abad and Wolintz[51] reported a patient who had bilateral paralysis of all horizontal eye movements with preservation of vertical eye movements. The patient had clinically definite MS, and pontine pathology was surmised. DeCarvalho et al.[52] described a patient with bilateral gaze paresis and difficulty with tandem gait and dysmetria of the right leg. The patient had metastatic lesions in the pontine tegmentum, as demonstrated by computed tomography (CT) imaging. Baloh et al.[53] reported two patients with pontine gliomas who had absent voluntary horizontal gaze in both directions but relatively normal horizontal reflex saccades and vertical gaze movements. Similar findings can been seen in patients with brainstem strokes.

**VARIOUS PONTINE GAZE DISORDERS.** Clinical findings associated with various pontine lesions allow the deduction of a number of physiologic concepts that reflect on ocular motor control. Lesions involving the abducens nucleus produce a combined ipsilateral saccadic and pursuit palsy. Involvement of the ipsilateral MLF produces a type of one-and-one-half syndrome.[54] This syndrome is characterized by a paralysis of horizontal gaze toward the side of the lesion due to involvement of the ipsilateral abducens nucleus, as well as failure of the ipsilateral eye to move contralaterally due to involvement of the ipsilateral MLF. Thus the eye on the side of the lesion is immobile during all conjugate gaze movements in either direction, whereas the contralateral eye abducts appropriately but floats back toward the midline in response to a conjugate gaze command ipsilateral to the lesion. A variant of the one-and-one-half syndrome, which includes an exotropia of the contralateral eye, is termed *paralytic pontine exotropia*.[55,56]

Lesions involving the PPRF just rostral to the sixth nerve nuclei produce saccadic conjugate gaze paresis with sparing of pursuit and vestibulo-ocular responses. The presumption is that pursuit is mediated through the sixth nerve nucleus but not the horizontal gaze center of the PPRF. Vestibular input feeds directly into the sixth nerve nucleus, which functions as the final common pathway for all horizontal conjugate gaze movements.[57,58] If in addition the ipsilateral MLF is involved, a saccadic one-and-one-half syndrome will be evident. Involvement of the dorsolateral pontine nuclei rostral to the sixth nerve nuclei can cause an ipsilateral smooth pursuit paresis.[10] As long as the abducens nucleus is intact, vestibular stimuli can produce full slow-phase movements with or without appropriate corrective quick phases,[25,26,59] depending on the extent of brainstem involvement.

One can differentiate between the sites of brainstem involvement (i.e., the PPRF versus the abducens nucleus) by the presence or absence of smooth pursuit movements and the response to vestibular stimuli. In lesions of the PPRF, smooth pursuit and vestibulo-ocular reflexes drive the eyes, whereas these movements are absent in lesions destroying the sixth nerve nucleus.[9,25,26]

**INTERNUCLEAR OPHTHALMOPLEGIA.** The hallmark of internuclear ophthalmoplegia (INO) is a lag of the ipsilateral medial rectus muscle in a conjugate gaze movement (*adduction* lag). INO is a sign of intrinsic brainstem disease involving the MLF between the abducens and the oculomotor nuclei. The adduction lag in a patient with an INO can be made more obvious by inducing repetitive saccadic movements into the field of action of the involved medial rectus muscle. For example, if a patient has a lesion of the right MLF with a right internuclear ophthalmoplegia, the lesion can be made clinically more apparent by rotating an optokinetic stimulus toward the right, inducing a fast corrective movement to the left, and thus stressing the right medial rectus muscle. Although often the most striking clinical finding to the casual observer, the presence of abducting nystagmus is not mandatory to make the diagnosis of INO.

A patient with minimal disruption of the MLF may complain of transient diplopia during the induced saccadic movement or nondescript visual blurring in the presence of the abducting nystagmus. With greater involvement of the MLF, the lag of the adducting eye increases, and it may be noted during smooth pursuit movements, as well with saccades. At this time diplopia may become a prominent complaint.

Bilateral INO is most likely due to MS, but over the age of 50 vertebrobasilar disease must be considered. A unilateral INO in a young adult is almost always due to MS, whereas similar findings in a patient over the age of 50 are most likely due to brainstem infarction. INO is often accompanied by vertical upbeat nystagmus in upgaze and a skew deviation.[60]

Although most often caused by pontine lesions, INO may be produced by a mesencephalic lesion. So-called anterior INO is usually bilateral, the eyes are aligned in primary position, and convergence is maintained. Thus the third nerve subnuclei are presumably spared, and only the MLF is involved bilaterally. In contrast, Lubow identified patients with a constellation of signs given the acronym WEBINO (wall-eyed bilateral internuclear ophthalmoplegia).[22] These patients are exotropic and have no convergence but have abducting nystagmus in right and left gaze. These signs are most likely due to bilateral involvement of the medial rectus subnuclei of the oculomotor nerve and the MLF. More caudal disease has been implicated in one case.[61]

**VERTICAL GAZE PALSIES.** Although somewhat inexact, an analogy can be drawn between the horizontal and the vertical gaze systems. The sixth nerve nucleus in horizontal gaze movements and the riMLF in vertical gaze movements act as the final generators of volitional movements receiving input from secondary gaze centers in the PPRF. Whereas involvement of the abducens nucleus produces a global horizontal gaze deficit, involvement of the riMLF produces a vertical gaze paresis, except that in such patients vertical movements can usually be induced by oculocephalic, optokinetic, or caloric stimuli.[26,57] Involvement of the third and fourth cranial nerve nuclei, or their fascicles, is necessary for loss of response to vestibular stimuli. Vertical gaze deficits also can be produced by pontine lesions involving the rostral PPRF.

**Downgaze deficits.** Isolated paralysis of downgaze is reported in a number of patients with pretectal disease.[8,15,16] These patients often have an accompanying apparent ptosis in downgaze: the lids move down, but the eye movements are limited. Histopathology has revealed bilateral lesions (stroke or metastases) of the medial ventral part of the riMLF just rostral to the third nerve nucleus and dorsomedial to the red nuclei in the pretectum.[15-17,62] One patient with bilateral downgaze deficits had bilateral ptosis[63] in primary position.

**Upgaze deficits.** Isolated upgaze paralysis is associated with infarction, infiltration, or compression involving the dorsolateral region of one riMLF and the contiguous posterior commissure. The control for ipsilateral monocular elevation requires projection to the contralateral superior rectus subnucleus of the oculomotor nucleus (which may involve a synapse in the IC [interneuron]), as well as to the ipsilateral inferior oblique subnucleus. This decussation takes place in the posterior commissure. Thus a unilateral destructive lesion causes a bilateral upgaze paresis and offers an explanation as to why the finding of upgaze paresis is more common than downgaze paresis.[64,65] Thames et al.[66] described a man with upgaze paralysis who had a single lesion of the brainstem confined to the periaqueductal gray matter between the levels of the superior and inferior colliculi. They suggested that the upgaze paresis was due to interruption of the fiber pathways going to or away from the riMLF.

*Parinaud's syndrome.* Generally, patients with Parinaud's syndrome (Koerber-Salus-Elschnig syndrome, sylvian aqueduct syndrome, dorsal midbrain syndrome) initially have a paresis of saccadic upgaze. Early in the evolution of the

---

### Ocular Signs and Symptoms of Parinaud's Syndrome

**Common**

1. Loss of saccadic upgaze
2. Pupillary mydriasis (4 to 5 mm in diameter)
3. Light-near dissociation
4. Convergence-retraction nystagmus (best elicited by rotating an optokinetic tape downward)
5. Papilledema

**Less common**

1. Skew deviation
2. Fourth cranial nerve palsy
3. Lid retraction
4. Loss of upgaze pursuit
5. Spontaneous convergence-retraction movements elicited by upgaze movements
6. Loss of downward saccades

**Infrequent**

1. Peduncular hallucinosis
2. Precocious puberty

syndrome, during attempts to look up, saccades are replaced by upward movements of the eyes that are serpentine in motion and require great effort. As the condition progresses, when the patient attempts to make an upward saccade, both eyes make a convergence movement while simultaneously being retracted into the orbit. This movement is produced by co-contraction of muscles supplied by the third nerve nucleus.[67] Convergence retraction nystagmus can be exaggerated by using an optokinetic stimulus rotating downward.[68] Late in the evolution of the syndrome, diplopia may be present as a result of a fourth nerve palsy or skew deviation.

Papilledema is a common finding secondary to obstructive hydrocephalus. Patients with papilledema may experience transient obscurations of vision. Other common findings include mid-dilated (4 to 5 mm in diameter) pupils that demonstrate light-near dissociation, convergence paresis, neurogenic lid retraction (Collier's sign[69]), convergence spasm, downgaze paresis, and anisocoria.

Precocious puberty and peduncular hallucinosis have been reported as part of the syndrome but must be rare. Peduncular hallucinosis is characterized by vivid-colored imagery that the patient does not perceive as being threatening[70-72] (see Chapter 6). Parinaud's syndrome is frequently caused by tumors of the pineal gland or aqueductal stenosis, but it is also reported to occur with infiltrating tumors in the region of the aqueduct and superior colliculus, as well as with neurosyphilis, MS, trauma, and stroke.

*Monocular elevation paresis.* Monocular elevation paresis is a rare acquired disorder in which supranuclear input is interrupted from the vertical gaze center in the pretectum to the oculomotor complex.[73,74] The characteristic findings are monocular loss of upgaze with diplopia in upward gaze only. The range of upgaze movements in response to oculocephalic maneuvers is fuller. No accompanying abnormalities of lid position or movement are present. Jampel and Fells[73] postulate a discrete ischemic lesion in the pretectum as being causative in their patients. Lessell[74] adds credence to their postulate by reporting a patient with bronchogenic carcinoma metastatic to the right pretectum who lost the ability to elevate his right eye.

**Combined upgaze and downgaze deficits.** Progressive supranuclear palsy and Parkinson's disease are two entities in which vertical gaze paresis is a prominent sign (Table 8-1). Strokes producing the so-called top of the basilar artery syndrome can also produce, among other findings, vertical gaze palsies. The underlying pathophysiology is supranuclear. Certain myopathies and mitochondrial encephalomyopathies may mimic both progressive supranuclear palsy and Parkinson's disease. Thus the mitochondrial encephalomyopathies must be included in the differential diagnosis in patients with what appear to be supranuclear ocular movement disorders.

The key to differentiating between the myopathies and supranuclear palsies is the presence of full ocular movements following vestibular stimuli early in the course of the disease in patients with supranuclear palsies. Late in the course of the disease when nuclear involvement is present, patients with supranuclear palsies also do not respond to vestibular stimuli.

| TABLE 8-1 | *Comparison of Selective Eye Signs in Progressive Supranuclear Palsy and Parkinson's Disease* |
|---|---|

| Progressive supranuclear palsy | Parkinson's disease |
|---|---|
| **LID DYSFUNCTION** | |
| 1. Apraxia of opening | 1. Apraxia of opening |
| 2. Decreased blinking | 2. Decreased blinking |
| 3. Loss of facial expression | 3. Loss of facial expression |
| | 4. Seborrheic dermatitis and blepharitis |
| **CONJUGATE GAZE ABNORMALITIES** | |
| 1. Early loss of saccadic downgaze followed by upgaze and horizontal gaze | 1. Hypometric saccades in all gaze directions, but upgaze is usually affected initially ("cogwheel") |
| 2. Pursuit eye movements preserved better than saccades | 2. Saccadic pursuit early in course of disease |
| 3. Normal oculocephalic movements | 3. Normal oculocephalic movements |
| | 4. Oculogyric crisis |
| **OTHER** | |
| 1. Axial dystonia greater than appendicular dystonia | 1. Appendicular dystonia greater than axial dystonia |

*Progressive supranuclear palsy.* Steele-Richardson-Olszewski syndrome[75] is a degenerative disease of the CNS characterized by progressive supranuclear palsy initially affecting voluntary downgaze, accompanied by axial rigidity. The inability of these patients to move their eyes downward is compounded by their difficulty in bending their necks. These patients often seek help for complaints such as "inability to read," "can't see the food on my plate," or "can't walk downstairs." The loss of vertical gaze function is associated with a delay in the vertical orientation of the eyes.[76] The ophthalmoplegia progresses to loss of voluntary upgaze, loss of horizontal gaze, and finally to loss of pursuit. During this time full ocular movements can be demonstrated by oculocephalic reflexes, but because of the nuchal rigidity this maneuver is often difficult to perform.

When the neck rigidity has progressed such that the head is almost immobile, caloric stimulation can demonstrate the integrity of nuclear and infranuclear pathways. Caloric stimulation produces a tonic deviation of the eyes. Other ophthalmologic findings may include the development of an inability to voluntarily open the lids (apraxia of eyelid opening; see Chapter 14).

As the disease progresses, patients may develop ocular misalignment and diplopia as a result of involvement of the ocular motor nuclei. Over time, facial expression is lost (masked facies) with the development of dystonia of the trunk muscles and progressive dementia. The progressive dementia is associated with increasing insomnia.[77] Very late in the evolution of the disease, the nuclear involvement becomes so severe that the eyes no longer move in response to caloric stimuli.

The disease has an equal sex distribution and for the most part is found in patients in the sixth and seventh decades. These patients usually have an inexorably progressive downhill course, with death ensuing in 8 to 10 years.

*Parkinson's disease.* Early in the course of Parkinson's disease, conjugate saccadic movements become hypometric. In addition, smooth pursuit movements become saccadic ("cogwheeling"). Masked facies, involuntary laughing, drooling, and difficulty swallowing mark disease progression. The patients may also demonstrate an apraxia of lid opening (see Chapter 14). In its most common form, Parkinson's disease is a degenerative condition of the extrapyramidal system in which a biochemical imbalance occurs between the dopaminergic and cholinergic systems within the basal ganglia. It can be seen in a postinfectious form, posttraumatic form, and after the use of methyl-4-phenyl-1,2,3,6-tetrahydropyridine (MPTP).[78] The complaint of diplopia in these patients is most often due to convergence weakness associated with near tasks.

**VERTICAL UPGAZE SPASMS.** Oculogyric crisis consists of a spasmodic involuntary upward deviation of the eyes and lids associated with neck hyperextension that lasts for several minutes to a few hours. Today it is most commonly seen as an acute side effect of phenothiazine therapy; in the past it was often seen in patients with postinfectious Parkinson's disease. Oculogyric crisis rarely occurs after trauma or in the setting of neurosyphilis.

Leigh et al.[79] have reported on three patients with oculogyric crisis accompanied by a variety of transient mood and thought disturbances, including slowing of thinking and ruminative obsessional thoughts. During the period of the crisis, all normal types of eye movements were present within the upper field of gaze, suggesting an imbalance of vertical gaze–holding mechanisms. All of these patients responded to treatment with anticholinergic agents.

# Myopathic Gaze Disorders

The following entities reflect ocular motor disorders associated with muscle disease in isolation or with CNS dysfunction. As such, they make up a group of disorders that clinically represent or mimic supranuclear eye movement disorders.

## MITOCHONDRIAL MYOPATHIES AND ENCEPHALOMYOPATHIES

Mitochondrial diseases[80,81] are defined by biochemical abnormalities of mitochondrial function or by the finding of "ragged red fibers" in muscle biopsy specimens. Mitochondrial diseases might be classified as those in which the disorder is limited to muscle (i.e., myopathies) and those in which diffuse involvement of many organ systems occurs (multisystem disorders). Progressive external ophthalmoplegia may be a prominent finding in either class of disease. It may also exist as an isolated finding, such as an ocular myopathy.

Molecular genetic research has demonstrated that chronic progressive external ophthalmoplegia, in itself or as part of multisystem disease, is sometimes associated with a deletion of mitochondrial DNA. Mitochondrial DNA is strictly maternal in origin. Thus the disease is passed through the so-called maternal line. Patients with myopathies or encephalomyopathies without progressive external ophthalmoplegia do not have deletions of mitochondrial DNA.[82] Certain cases of isolated ocular myopathies are associated with deletions of mitochondrial DNA.

## CHRONIC PROGRESSIVE EXTERNAL OPHTHALMOPLEGIA

The term *chronic progressive external ophthalmoplegia* (CPEO), as generally used, includes a number of different entities that have in common the development of a slowly progressive, generally symmetric, external ophthalmoplegia. The presence of CPEO suggests a mitochondrial related disease, but not all patients demonstrate such defects. The symmetry of the ophthalmoplegia makes these patients appear to have multidirectional gaze palsies similar to those seen in progressive supranuclear palsy. Progressive supranuclear palsy is differentiated from CPEO by the maintenance of full ocular rotations on oculocephalic maneuvers in the former.

Berenberg et al.[82] emphasize that the Kearns-Sayre syndrome[80,83-85] can be separated as an entity distinct from CPEO. Kearns-Sayre syndrome is characterized by the clinical triad of progressive external ophthalmoplegia, pigmentary degeneration of the retina, and heart block. The cerebrospinal fluid (CSF) protein is usually elevated, exceeding 100 mg/dl. The onset of disease is usually before age 20 years. The sequence of manifestations may vary, and the development of cardiomyopathy may be delayed for many years. The cardiomyopathy produces conduction defects, including intraventricular conduction deficits, bundle branch blocks, bifascicular disease, and complete heart block. These patients should be under the care of a cardiologist and be followed at least annually with electrocardiography. The patient and family should be aware of the possible need for a cardiac pacemaker.

Often other evidence indicates widespread neurologic disease affecting the cerebellum and auditory and vestibular pathways, as well as skeletal muscle. Less often intellectual dysfunction is present. The patients tend to be short and have delayed sexual maturation. The syndrome usually appears sporadically with no family history extractable. Skeletal or ocular muscle biopsy specimens in these patients, as well as in those with other forms of progressive external ophthalmoplegia, often reveal ragged red fibers (i.e., giant mitochondria) or other morphologic mitochondrial changes.[86] Postmortem brain specimens can demonstrate spongiform degeneration.[82,87]

A form of CPEO may exist in isolation, limited to the extraocular muscles and lids. Isolated CPEO appears to be hereditary with variable transmission. The isolated form tends to have its onset earlier in each succeeding generation.[88]

Lid crutches offer at best a temporary solution to the problem of ptosis, but one must be wary of performing ptosis surgery. The only successful surgery in these patients is a levator sling or brow suspension procedure. Because of the loss of upgaze and Bell's phenomenon, a great danger exists for these patients to develop exposure keratitis from inadequate lid closure, with subsequent corneal ulceration and visual loss.

# MUSCULAR DYSTROPHY

Oculopharyngeal muscular dystrophy is a slowly progressive disorder with onset around age 40 years, heralded by swallowing difficulties. Patients usually develop ptosis within 2 years of onset. Many patients have chronic progressive external ophthalmoplegia. Death is due to inanition. This condition is more common in French-Canadians and appears to be transmitted as an autosomal dominant disorder.[89] Muscle biopsy demonstrates a marked reduction in muscle fibers with advanced degenerative changes, including the absence of Z bands in remaining fibers.[90]

# CENTRONUCLEAR (MYOTUBULAR) MYOPATHY

Only patients with an early-onset form of centronuclear (myotubular myopathy) develop progressive external ophthalmoplegia. These patients have severe hypotonia at birth, delay in other developmental milestones, and diffuse muscle weakness that includes facial and masticatory muscles. The inheritance pattern is not clear.

# MYOTONIC DYSTROPHY

Myotonic dystrophy may be difficult to differentiate from mild forms of chronic progressive external ophthalmoplegia, at least initially. This rare disorder classically produces a mild symmetric external ophthalmoplegia, mimicking gaze paresis. In addition, these patients may have ptosis, lack of smooth ocular pursuit, orbicularis weakness, and myotonia on lid closure and in holding eccentric gaze. Occasionally diplopia may be a complaint.[91] Thompson et al.[92] have noted that these patients have sluggishly reactive pupils (see Chapter 13). These patients also have polychromatic cataracts and pigmentary changes of the retina, including the macula. Testicular atrophy, cardiac abnormalities, and frontal balding have also been noted.

# MYASTHENIA GRAVIS

Myasthenia gravis must be included in the differential diagnosis of any patient with either an apparent gaze paresis or diplopia. This disease process is discussed in detail elsewhere (see Chapter 10).

## REFERENCES

1. Dell'Osso LF, Daroff RB. Eye movement characteristics and recording techniques. In: Glaser JS, ed. Neuro-ophthalmology. Hagerstown, MD: Harper & Row, 1978:185-99.
2. Leigh RF, Zee DS. The neurology of eye movements. Philadelphia: FA Davis, 1983:1-11.
3. Goldberg ME, Bushnell MC. Behavioral enhancement of visual responses in monkey cerebral cortex. II. Modulation in frontal eye fields specifically related to saccades. J Neurophysiol 1981;46:773-87.
4. Fox PT, Fox JM, Raichle ME, et al. The role of cerebral cortex in the generation of voluntary saccades: a positron emission tomographic study. J Neurophysiol 1985;54:348-69.
5. Robinson DA, Fuchs AF. Eye movements evoked by stimulation of frontal eye fields. J Neurophysiol 1969;32:637-48.
6. Troost BT, Weber RB, Daroff RB. Hemispheric control of eye movements. I. Quantitative analysis of refixation saccades in a hemispherectomy patient. Arch Neurol 1972;27:441-8.

7. Lynch JC, Graybiel AM, Lobeck LJ. The differential projection of two cytoarchitectonic subregions of the inferior parietal lobule of macaque upon the deep layers of the superior colliculus. J Comp Neurol 1985;235:241-54.
8. Pierrot-Deseilligny CH, Gray F, Brunet P. Infarcts of both inferior parietal lobules with impairment of visually guided eye movements, peripheral visual inattention and optic ataxia. Brain 1986;109:81-97.
9. Henn V, Cohen B. Coding of information about rapid eye movements in the pontine reticular formation of alert monkeys. Brain Res 1976;108:307-25.
10. Pierrot-Deseilligny C, Goasguen J, Chain F, et al. Pontine metastasis with dissociated bilateral horizontal gaze paralysis. J Neurol Neurosurg Psychiatry 1986;49:159-64.
11. Baker R, Highstein SM. Vestibular projections to medial rectus subdivision of oculmotor nucleus. J Neurophysiol 1978;41:1629-46.
12. Highstein SM, Baker R. Excitatory termination of abducens internuclear neurons on medial rectus motoneurons: relationship to syndrome of internuclear ophthalmoplegia. J Neurophysiol 1978;41:1647-61.
13. Bender MB, Shanzer S. Oculomotor pathways defined by electric stimulation and lesions in the brain-stem of monkey. In: Bender MB, ed. The oculomotor system. New York: Harper & Row, 1964:81-140.
14. Kompf D, Gmeiner HJ. Gaze palsy and visual hemineglect in acute hemisphere lesions. Neuro-ophthalmology 1989;9:49-53.
15. Büttner-Ennever JA, Büttner U, Cohen B, et al. Vertical gaze paralysis and the rostral interstitial nucleus of the medial longitudinal fasciculus. Brain 1982;105:125-49.
16. Pierrot-Deseilligny CH, Chain F, Gray F, et al. Parinaud's syndrome: electrooculographic and anatomical analyses of six vascular cases with deductions about vertical gaze organization in the premotor structures. Brain 1982;105:667-96.
17. Goldman S, Cordonnier MJB, Sztencel J. Brainstem ischaemia presenting as naloxone-versible coma followed by downward gaze paralysis. J Neurol Neurosurg Psychiatry 1984;47:77-8.
18. Pierrot-Deseilligny C, Gaymard B. Eye movement disorders and ocular motor organization. Curr Opin Neurol Neurosurg 1990;3:796-801.
19. Desimone R, Ungerleider LG. Multiple visual areas in the caudal superior temporal sulcus of the macaque. J Comp Neurol 1986;248:164-89.
20. Glickstein M, Cohen JL, Dixon B, et al. Corticopontine visual projections in macaque monkeys. J Comp Neurol 1980;190:209-29.
21. Pierrot-Deseilligny C, Amarenco P, Roullet E, et al. Vermal infarct with pursuit eye movement disorders. J Neurol Neurosurg Psychiatry 1990;53:519-21.
22. Hoyt WF, Daroff RB. Supranuclear disorders of ocular control systems in man: clinical, anatomical, and physiological correlations—1969. In: Bach-y-Rita P, Collins CC, Hyde JE, eds. The control of eye movements. New York: Academic Press, 1971:175-235.
23. Zackon DH, Sharpe JA. Midbrain paresis of horizontal gaze. Ann Neurol 1984;16:495-504.
24. Mays LE, Porter JD, Gamlin PDR, et al. Neural control of vergence eye movements: neurons encoding vergence velocity. J Neurophysiol 1986;56:1007-21.
25. Bogousslavsky J, Miklossy J, Regli F, et al. One-and-a-half syndrome in ischaemic locked-in state: a clinico-pathological study. J Neurol Neurosurg Psychiatry 1984;47:927-35.
26. Bogousslavsky J, Meienberg O. Eye-movement disorders in brain-stem and cerebellar stroke. Arch Neurol 1987;44:141-8.
27. Cogan DG, Adams RD. A type of paralysis of conjugate gaze (ocular motor apraxia). Arch Ophthalmol 1953;50:434-42.
28. Cogan DG. Congenital ocular motor apraxia. Can J Ophthalmol 1966;1:253-60.
29. Cogan DG, Chu FC, Reingold D. Notes on congenital ocular motor apraxia: associated abnormalities. In: Glaser JS,

ed. Neuro-ophthalmology: symposium of the University of Miami and the Bascom Palmer Eye Institute, vol 10. St Louis: Mosby–Year Book, 1980:171-9.

30. Catalano RA, Calhoun JH, Reinecke RD, et al. Asymmetry in congenital ocular motor apraxia. Can J Ophthalmol 1988;23:318-21.

31. Zee DS, Yee RD, Singer HS. Congenital ocular motor apraxia. Brain 1977; 100:581-99.

32. Aicardi J, Barbosa C, Andermann E, et al. Ataxia—ocular motor apraxia: a syndrome mimicking ataxia-telangiectasia. Ann Neurol 1988;24:497-502.

33. Pierrot-Deseilligny C, Gautier J-C, Loron P. Acquired ocular motor apraxia due to bilateral frontoparietal infarcts. Ann Neurol 1988;23:199-202.

34. Cogan DG. Neurology of the ocular muscles. Springfield, IL: Charles C Thomas, 1956:106.

35. Leigh RJ, Newman SA, Folstein SE, et al. Abnormal ocular motor control in Huntington's disease. Neurology 1983; 33:1268-75.

36. Starr A. A disorder of rapid eye movements in Huntington's chorea. Brain 1967;90:545-64.

37. Leigh RJ, Parhad IM, Clark AW, et al. Brainstem findings in Huntington's disease: possible mechanisms for slow vertical saccades. J Neurol Sci 1985; 71:247-56.

38. Lennox G, Jones R. Gaze distractibility in Wilson's disease. Ann Neurol 1989;25:415-7.

39. Leigh RJ, Thurston SE. Recovery of ocular motor function in humans with cerebral lesions. In: Keller EL, Zee DS, eds. Adaptive processes in visual and oculomotor systems. Asilomar, CA 6/16-20/85 conference proceedings. Oxford: Pergamon Press, 1986:231-8.

40. Sibony PA, Evinger C, Manning KA. The effects of tobacco smoking on smooth pursuit eye movements. Ann Neurol 1988;23:238-41.

41. Safran AB, Roth A, Haenggeli CA. Congenital horizontal gaze paralysis and ear dysplasia—a syndrome. Ophthalmologica 1983;187:157-60.

42. Cogan DG, Freese CG Jr. Spasm of the near reflex. Arch Ophthalmol 1955; 54:752-9.

43. Gomez CR, Gomez SM, Selhorst JB. Acute thalamic esotropia. Neurology 1988;38:1759-62.

44. Caplan LR. "Top of the basilar" syndrome. Neurology 1980;30:72-9.

45. Castaigne P, Lhermitte F, Buge A, et al. Paramedian thalamic and midbrain infarcts: clinical and neuropathological study. Ann Neurol 1981;10:127-48.

46. Daroff RB, Troost BT, Leigh RJ. Supranuclear disorders of eye movements. In: Glaser JS, ed. Neuro-ophthalmology. 2nd ed. New York: JP Lippincott, 1990:299-323.

47. Safran AB, Roth A, Gauthier G. Le syndrome des spasmes de convergence: ou spasmes de convergence symptomatiques. Klin Monatsbl Augenheilkd 1982;180:471-3.

48. Yee RD, Duffin RM, Baloh RW, et al. Familial, congenital paralysis of horizontal gaze. Arch Ophthalmol 1982; 100:1449-52.

49. Möbius PJ. Ueber angeborene doppelseitige Abducens-Facialis-Lähmung. Münch Med Wschr 1888;35:91-4.

50. Towfighi J, Marks K, Palmer E, et al. Möbius syndrome: neuropathologic observations. Acta Neuropathol 1979; 48:11-7.

51. Abad VC, Wolintz A. Bilateral horizontal gaze palsy. Ann Ophthalmol 1982; 14:1046-8.

52. DeCarvalho C, Shuttleworth E, Knox D, et al. Bilateral gaze paralysis with positive computerized tomography findings: a clincoanatomic correlation. Arch Neurol 1980;37:184-6.

53. Baloh RW, Furman J, Yee RD. Eye movements in patients with absent voluntary horizontal gaze. Ann Neurol 1985;17:283-6.

54. Fisher CM. Some neuro-ophthalmological observations. J Neurol Neurosurg Psychiatry 1967;30:383-92.

55. Bronstein AM, Morris J, DuBoulay G, et al. Abnormalities of horizontal gaze: clinical, oculographic and magnetic resonance imaging findings. I. Abducens palsy. J Neurol Neurosurg Psychiatry 1990;53:194-9.

56. Sharpe JA, Rosenberg MA, Hoyt WF, et al. Paralytic pontine exotropia: a sign of acute unilateral pontine gaze palsy

and internuclear ophthalmoplegia. Neurology 1974;24:1076-81.

57. Hanson MR, Hamid MA, Tomsak RL, et al. Selective saccadic palsy caused by pontine lesions: clinical, physiological, and pathological correlations. Ann Neurol 1986;20:209-17.

58. Lang W, Henn V, Hepp K. Gaze palsies after selective pontine lesions in monkeys. In: Roucoux A, Crommelinck M, eds: Physiological and pathological aspects of eye movements. The Hague: Dr W Junk, 1982:209-18.

59. Bogousslavsky J, Fox AJ, Carey LS, et al. Correlates of brain-stem oculomotor disorders in multiple sclerosis: magnetic resonance imaging. Arch Neurol 1986;43:460-3.

60. Gonyea EF. Bilateral internuclear ophthalmoplegia: association with occlusive cerebrovascular disease. Arch Neurol 1974;31:168-73.

61. McGettrick P, Eustace P. The w.e.b.i.n.o. syndrome. Neuro-ophthalmology 1985; 5:109-15.

62. Ross RT. Paralysis of downward gaze. Neurology 1986;36:1540-1.

63. Büttner-Ennever JA, Acheson JF, Büttner U, et al. Ptosis and supranuclear downgaze paralysis. Neurology 1989; 39:385-9.

64. Bogousslavsky J, Miklossy J, DeRuaz JP, et al. Unilateral left paramedian infraction of thalamus and midbrain: a clinico-pathological study. J Neurol Neurosurg Psychiatry 1986;49:686-94.

65. Smith MS, Laguna JF. Upward gaze paralysis following unilateral pretectal infarction: computerized tomography correlation. Arch Neurol 1981;38:127-9.

66. Thames PB, Trobe JD, Ballinger WE. Upgaze paralysis caused by lesion of the periaqueductal gray matter. Arch Neurol 1984;41:437-40.

67. Gay AJ, Brodkey J, Miller JE. Convergence retraction nystagmus: an electromyographic study. Arch Ophthalmol 1963;70:456-61.

68. Smith JL, Zieper I, Gay AJ, et al. Nystagmus retractorius. Arch Ophthalmol 1959;62:864-7.

69. Collier J. Nuclear ophthalmoplegia, with especial reference to retraction of the lids and ptosis and to lesions of the posterior commissure. Brain 1927; 50:488-98.

70. Dunn DW, Weisberg LA, Nadell J. Peduncular hallucinations caused by brainstem compression. Neurology 1983;33:1360-1.

71. Geller TJ, Bellur SN. Peduncular hallucinosis: magnetic resonance imaging confirmation of mesencephalic infarction during life. Ann Neurol 1987; 21:602-4.

72. Lhermitte J, Lévy G, Trelles J. L'hallucinose pédonculaire (étude anatomique d'un cas). Rev Neurol 1932;1:382-8.

73. Jampel RS, Fells P. Monocular elevation paresis caused by a central nervous system lesion. Arch Ophthalmol 1968;80:45-57.

74. Lessell S. Supranuclear paralysis of monocular elevation. Neurology 1975; 25:1134-6.

75. Steele JC, Richardson JC, Olszewski J. Progressive supranuclear palsy: a heterogeneous degeneration involving the brain stem, basal ganglia and cerebellum with vertical gaze and pseudobulbar palsy, nuchal dystonia and dementia. Arch Neurol 1964;10:333-59.

76. Rafal RD, Posner MI, Friedman JH, et al. Orienting of visual attention in progressive supranuclear palsy. Brain 1988;111:267-80.

77. Aldrich MS, Foster NL, White RF, et al. Sleep abnormalities in progressive supranuclear palsy. Ann Neurol 1989; 25:577-81.

78. Burns RS, LeWitt PA, Ebert MH, et al. The clinical syndrome of striatal dopamine deficiency: parkinsonism induced by 1-methyl-4-phenyl-1,2,3,6-tetrahydropyridine (MPTP). N Engl J Med 1985;312:1418-21.

79. Leigh RF, Foley JM, Remler BF, et al. Oculogyric crisis: a syndrome of thought disorder and ocular deviation. Ann Neurol 1987;22:13-7.

80. Moraes CT, DiMauro S, Zeviani M, et al. Mitochondrial DNA deletions in progressive external ophthalmoplegia and Kearns-Sayre Syndrome. N Engl J Med 1989;320:1293-9.

81. Zeviani M, Bonilla E, DeVivo DC, et al.

Mitochondrial diseases. In: John WG, guest ed. Neurologic clinics. Vol 7. Neurogenetic diseases. Philadelphia, WB Saunders, 1989:123-56

82. Berenberg RA. Pellock JM, DiMauro S, et al. Lumping or splitting? "Ophthalmoplegia-plus" or Kearns-Sayre syndrome? Ann Neurol 1977;1:37-54.

83. Daroff RB. Chronic progressive external ophthalmoplegia: a critical review. Arch Ophthalmol 1969;82:845-50.

84. Kearns TP. External ophthalmoplegia, pigmentary degeneration of the retina, and cardiomyopathy: a newly recognized syndrome. Trans Am Ophthalmol Soc 1965;63:559-625.

85. Kearns TP, Sayre GP. Retinitis pigmentosa, external ophthalmoplegia, and complete heart bloc: unusual syndrome with histologic study in one of two cases. Arch Ophthalmol 1958; 60:280-9.

86. Adachi M, Torii J, Volk BW, et al. Electron microscopic and enzyme histochemical studies of cerebellum, ocular and skeletal muscles in chronic progressive ophthalmoplegia with cerebellar ataxia. Acta Neuropathol 1973; 23:300-12.

87. Daroff RB, Solitare GB, Pincus JH, et al. Spongiform encephalopathy with chronic progressive external ophthalmoplegia: central ophthalmoplegia mimicking ocular myopathy. Neurology 1966;16:161-9.

88. Cogan DG. Neurology of the ocular muscles. Springfield, IL: Charles C Thomas, 1956:123.

89. Murphy SF, Drachman DB. The oculopharyngeal syndrome. JAMA 1968; 203:1003-8.

90. Little BW, Perl DP. Oculopharyngeal muscular dystrophy: an autopsied case from the French-Canadian kindred. J Neurol Sci 1982;53:145-58.

91. Lessell S, Coppeto J, Samet S. Ophthalmoplegia in myotonic dystrophy. Am J Ophthalmol 1971;71:1231-5.

92. Thompson HS, Van Allen MW, von Noorden GK. The pupil in myotonic dystrophy. Invest Ophthalmol 1964; 3:325-38.

# CHAPTER 9

# Diplopia and Similar Sensory Experiences

• • • • • • • • • • • • • •

## Diagnosis

True diplopia is the awareness of seeing the same object located in two different places in visual space. This sensory experience is produced when the object of regard (the object at which the individual is looking) stimulates the fovea in one eye while simultaneously stimulating extrafoveal retinal elements in the other eye. When this situation occurs, foveal suppression occurs immediately in the nonfixing eye, presumably to avoid the totally unacceptable sensory experience of seeing two different images superimposed on one another ("visual confusion"). As we have defined it, *true diplopia* implies misalignment of the eyes. Many patients use the term "double vision" to describe another sensory experience that occurs with normal ocular alignment. This is a monocular sensory experience that is present when one or the other eye is occluded. For the most part, this experience is produced by a lack of uniformity of the various refractive surfaces and media within one or both eyes, which produces multiple images on the retina(s). This experience is best described as an overlapping of imagery similar to "ghosting" on a television set.

Some patients will not report diplopia, even when the eyes are misaligned, because vision is poor in one eye or both, suppression of the nonfixing eye has occurred, or they fail to appreciate or they misinterpret the sensory experience. For example, patients with a subtle internuclear ophthalmoplegia (INO) frequently fail to describe diplopia when the eyes are misaligned, although at that time they may complain of nondescript blurring of vision. Similarly, patients ordinarily do not verbalize the illusory to-and-fro movement of the environment that must occur during the period of nystagmus of the abducting eye. Patients with an incomplete sixth cranial nerve palsy may not describe diplopia as such but will be acutely aware of visual difficulty when the eyes move into the direction of gaze in which the underacting muscle is activated. The causes of diplopia and similar sensory experiences are listed in the box.

### DIPLOPIA BY HISTORY BUT NOT PRESENT AT EXAMINATION

Some patients experience diplopia only intermittently. They are asymptomatic at examination and do not demonstrate misalignment. A series of questions should

## Causes of Diplopia and Similar Sensory Experiences

I. No misalignment of the eyes
  A. Monocular
    1. Refractive abnormalities
      a. Corneal abnormalities
        (1) Astigmatism
        (2) Keratoconus
        (3) Cornea plana
        (4) Irregular astigmatism
          (a) Intrinsic corneal disease
          (b) Extrinsic pressure (e.g., chalazion)
      b. Iris abnormalities
        (1) Polycoria
        (2) Large, relatively nonreactive pupils in association with astigmatic refractive error or nuclear sclerotic lens changes
      c. Lens abnormalities
        (1) Nuclear sclerosis
        (2) Subluxated lens
    2. Following strabismus surgery in a patient with abnormal retinal correspondence
    3. Palinopsia
    4. Cerebral polyopia
    5. Psychogenic
  B. Binocular
    1. Aniseikonia
    2. Metamorphopsia
    3. Foveal displacement syndrome
    4. Physiologic
    5. Psychogenic
II. Misalignment of the eyes
  A. Supranuclear
    1. Skew deviation
    2. Convergence paresis
    3. Divergence paresis
    4. Accommodative convergence spasm (spasm of the near reflex)
    5. Convergence-retraction nystagmus
    6. Divergence spasm
    7. Loss of central fusion
    8. Hemifield slip
  B. Internuclear
  C. Nuclear*
    1. Third cranial nerve
    2. Fourth cranial nerve
  D. Infranuclear
    1. Fascicle
    2. Nerve
    3. Myoneuronal junction
    4. Extraocular muscle
      a. Restrictive
      b. Degenerative
      c. Developmental
  E. Following strabismus surgery with normal or abnormal retinal correspondence

*The sixth nerve nucleus contains motor neurons to the lateral rectus muscle and neurons to the contralateral medial rectus subnucleus of the third cranial nerve. A lesion in the nucleus should produce a gaze palsy and not diplopia.

### Causes of Intermittent Diplopia

1. Multiple sclerosis
2. Graves' ophthalmopathy
3. Myasthenia gravis
4. Decompensating phoria/intermittent tropia
5. Spasm of the near reflex
6. Convergence-retraction nystagmus
7. Hemifield slip
8. Ocular neuromyotonia
9. Refractive aberrations

be asked to extract specific historical data. Elucidating the circumstances under which diplopia occurs will suggest an underlying diagnosis (see box).

**MULTIPLE SCLEROSIS.** Patients with multiple sclerosis may experience transient blurring of vision, diplopia, or nystagmus with a rise in core body temperature of as little as 0.1° C.[1] Hot baths, hot showers, or exercise can induce or exacerbate these symptoms *(Uhthoff's phenomenon).*[2] Depending on the degree of demyelination, even walking upstairs or across the street can make the patient symptomatic. Whether it is the rise in body temperature or a change in the electrolytic milieu (decrease in pH and rise in lactic acid)[3] that produces the reversible conduction block is unknown; the patient's susceptibility depends on the degree of demyelination of axons. Uhthoff's phenomenon may be seen (rarely) in patients following optic neuropathy[4] of collagen vascular disease and in Leber's hereditary optic neuropathy.[5]

If the patient relates the symptoms to exercise or getting "overheated," the examiner can attempt to reproduce the symptoms. Core temperature can be artificially raised by having the patient run up and down three or four flights of stairs or by wrapping the patient in an electric blanket. Conversely, an improvement in overt diplopia or afferent visual system dysfunction may be seen with lowering of the core body temperature in many such patients. Preliminary evidence indicates that this group of patients may benefit from the use of digitalis-like compounds.[6,7]

**GRAVES' OPHTHALMOPATHY.** Patients with early congestive endocrine ophthalmopathy tend to have greater difficulty maintaining single binocular vision in the morning. This problem can be somewhat ameliorated by having the patient sleep in an almost sitting position. It is important to note that patients with Graves' disease have a predilection to develop other autoimmune diseases, including myasthenia gravis (0.6%).[8]

**MYASTHENIA GRAVIS.** Patients with myasthenia gravis or decompensating phorias tend to have diplopia later in the day. Specific note should be made of ptosis, which is a characteristic finding in at least 90% of patients with myasthenia gravis. Ptosis may be a cardinal sign of a concomitant myasthenic state in a patient with Graves' ophthalmopathy. During the evaluation of such a patient, the examiner should attempt to fatigue the extraocular muscles, including the levator, in an effort to produce or exacerbate either ptosis or diplopia. Arrangements may need to be made to examine the patient later in the day.

**DECOMPENSATING PHORIA OR AN INTERMITTENT TROPIA.** A history of childhood strabismus, or of having worn glasses or a patch as a child, or of squinting one eye in bright sunlight[9] (intermittent exotropia) suggests decompensation of a long-standing heretophoria. Supportive evidence includes the presence of a consistent head tilt or head turn, especially if a series of photographs can show it to have been present for a long period. Patching one eye for an hour or having the patient fixate on a remote target may unmask an intermittent strabismus (especially an "exo"-misalignment). The finding of large vertical fusional amplitudes (6 to 20 prism diopters) is diagnostic of a latent deviation of some chronicity, such as is seen in patients with so-called congenital superior oblique palsies.

**SPASM OF THE NEAR REFLEX.** The association of intermittent bouts of double vision and concurrent visual blurring during periods of stress (e.g., studying for exams) suggests the possibility of spasm of the near reflex (see Chapter 8). In general, spasm of the near reflex is not associated with organic disease. Marked overaction of the components of the near synkinesis produces overconvergence (i.e., esotropia and diplopia), as well as a blur for all objects remote from the accommodative near point. This blurring of vision, rather than the recognition of diplopia, is generally the complaint that prompts the patient to seek help. Pupillary constriction is an obligate component of the near reflex; miosis helps differentiate this entity from bilateral or unilateral lateral rectus paresis. Some individuals have learned to use the near synkinesis to mimic a palsy of the lateral rectus muscle(s) (see Chapter 8).

**CONVERGENCE-RETRACTION NYSTAGMUS.** The occurrence of diplopia is associated with the induced convergence movements accompanying attempted upgaze (see Chapter 8).

**HEMIFIELD SLIP.** A rare cause of intermittent diplopia is hemifield slip,[10] which occurs only when complete or nearly complete bitemporal hemianopia is present. In such patients there are no corresponding retinal areas that under normal physiologic circumstances lock the eyes together to produce an appropriate cyclopean perception of space (Fig. 9-1). In such patients the eyes may intermittently converge, producing a blank space between the vertical meridians (Fig. 9-1, C3) as the eyes "slip" inward. Ocular divergence produced when the eyes slip apart causes an overlapping of the vertical meridians (Fig. 9-1, C1), and vertical slip produces a displacement along the midline (Fig. 9-1, D).[10] Such symptomatology is an indication for formal visual field testing and imaging, since such patients will most likely have a large mass lesion compressing the chiasm.

**OCULAR NEUROMYOTONIA.** The occurrence of intermittent diplopia in a patient who has a history of an intracranial mass lesion treated by radiation should

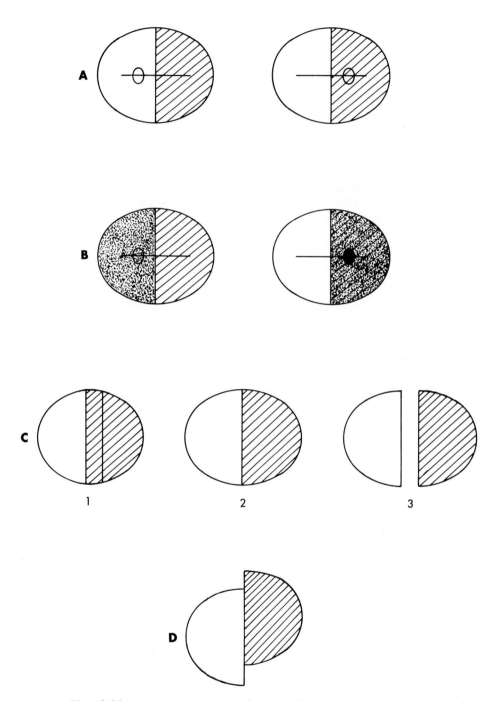

*Fig. 9-1.* Hemifields containing corresponding retinal areas. **A,** Full visual fields. Solid white areas and cross-hatched areas represent fields containing corresponding retinal areas. **B,** Bitemporal field loss *(dark areas)* superimposed on hemifields containing corresponding retinal areas. **C,** Hemifield slip cyclopean view: *1,* divergence; *2,* fusion; *3,* convergence. **D,** Hemifield vertical slip cyclopean view.

suggest the possibility of ocular neuromyotonia.[11-13] Patients with ocular neuro-myotonia experience paroxysmal binocular misalignment as a result of involuntary contraction of muscles innervated by the third, fourth, or sixth cranial nerves. The presumed cause is a radiation-induced cranial neuropathy manifesting a spontaneous discharge from axons with unstable cell membranes.[12] This produces a tonic contraction of one or more muscles. The paroxysms can occur 20 to 30 times daily.

Patients with third cranial nerve involvement may demonstrate lid retraction of the involved eye, as well as ocular misalignment with restriction of gaze in the direction opposite that of the induced myotonic movement. The neuromyotonia can be induced by sudden shifts of gaze into the field of action of the involved muscles. The paroxysms generally last several minutes and improve gradually. During the attacks the motility of the unaffected eye is normal, and between paroxysms the ocular motility of both eyes is normal. Treatment with carbamazepine is often effective in controlling the spasms.

**REFRACTIVE ABERRATIONS.** As discussed under Refractive Aberrations in the decision tree (see Chart 9-1), the wider the pupillary aperture, the greater the chance of paraxial rays being differentially refracted, producing a second defocused image. Myopic individuals and others with nuclear sclerotic lens changes may note monocular diplopia in one or both eyes under subdued lighting conditions. The symptoms may be reproduced by turning out all of the lights in the examining room. The sensory experience is alleviated by the use of a pinhole and the turning on of bright background lighting.

# A Decision Tree Approach to the Evaluation of Diplopia

The approach to a patient with the complaint of diplopia present at examination deviates from the classic format of the complete elucidation of a history followed by the performance of a physical examination. Each step is structured to provide information on which subsequent steps are based (Chart 9-1).

○ *Cover one eye, then the other.* The first procedure to do is to cover one of the patient's eyes, and then the other, to determine whether the diplopia remains or disappears.

☐ Diplopia present with either eye covered

▨ Monocular diplopia

If diplopia is present with one eye covered, the patient has monocular diplopia, a problem of different etiologic significance and, for the most part, less serious consequence than that of binocular diplopia. With few exceptions, monocular diplopia reflects optical aberrations within the refracting media of the eye. The next step is to acquire historical data.

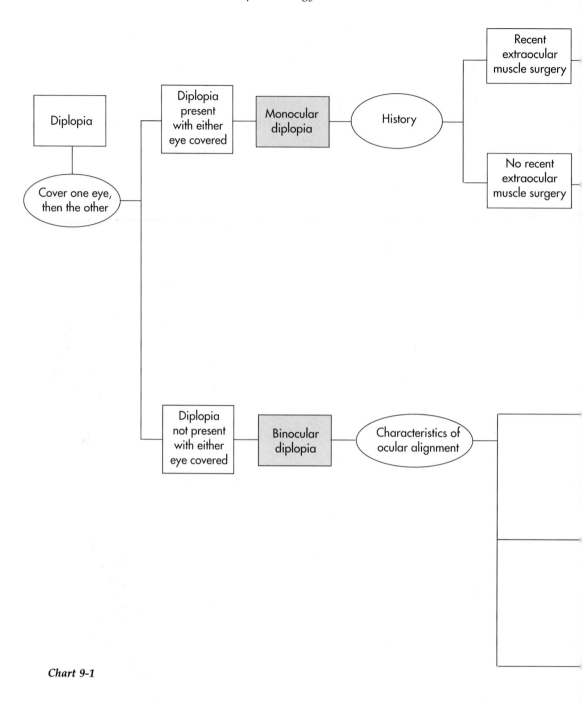

*Chart 9-1*

☐ Recent extraocular muscle surgery

▣ Abnormal retinal correspondence

The patient with a history of childhood strabismus and recent extraocular muscle surgery is likely to be experiencing diplopia due to a rare adaptive sensory phenomenon that may occur in patients with abnormal retinal correspondence (ARC). This sensory state, in which two retinal points in one eye function simul-

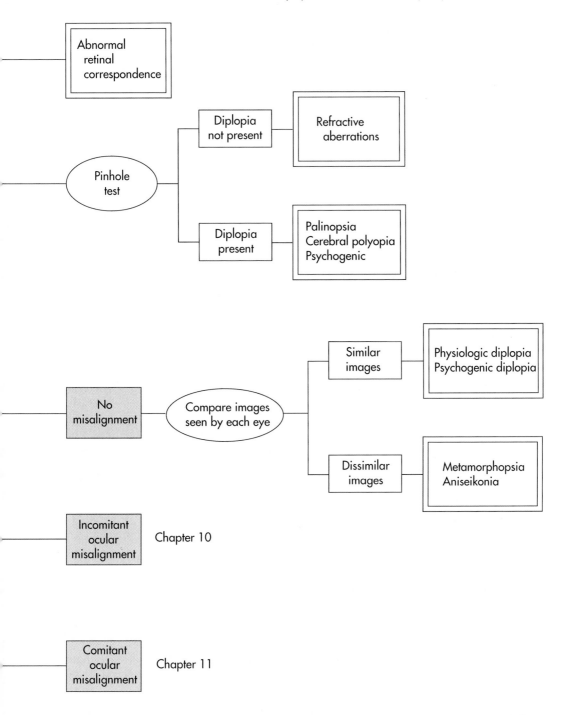

taneously, is transient (weeks to months) but has been known to persist.[14,15] It may represent a cortical failure of immediate sensory readaptation to motor re-alignment. Recent extraocular muscle surgery should suggest the presence of this peculiar phenomenon.

In patients with ARC the fovea of the misaligned eye gives up the primary visual direction to the extrafoveal area aligned with the fovea of the fixating eye. The fovea of the misaligned eye assumes the primary visual direction when it is forced to pick up fixation. The visual cortex can apparently adjust for changing sensory input, allowing the misaligned fovea to shift its visual direction depending on the testing situation. Following extraocular muscle surgery, a small group of patients with ARC experience monocular diplopia. This is due to the fact that with both eyes open, the previous pseudofovea maintains the primary visual direction, and the area of retina on which the image is projected following anatomic realignment fails to suppress. This produces monocular crossed or uncrossed diplopia, depending on the relationship of the stimulated retina to the pseudofovea (Fig. 9-2).

### ☐ No recent extraocular muscle surgery

○ *Pinhole test.* If the patient does not have a history of recent extraocular muscle surgery, a pinhole should be placed in front of the involved eye(s).

### ☐ Diplopia not present

If the diplopia disappears with the use of the pinhole, then one most likely is dealing with optical aberrations within the refracting media of the eye, although psychogenic disease cannot be fully excluded.

### ▣ Refractive aberrations

Although optical aberrations are usually associated with an overlapping of images similar to "ghosting," two separate images may be present. Almost all patients with myopic astigmatism can be made aware of ghosting in dim illumination but are unaware of its presence unless it is pointed out to them. Even with that proviso, **astigmatism** is probably the most frequent cause of monocular diplopia. Many astigmatic patients have lived with this experience all of their lives and rarely pay attention to it.

The most common cause of bothersome monocular diplopia is **lenticular nuclear sclerosis,** which produces a lamellar-like refractive effect. Such a lens can be likened to an onion cut in cross section, with a slightly different refractive effect occurring at each interface. The wider the pupillary aperture, the greater the chance of paraxial rays being differentially refracted, thus producing a secondary, superimposed but blurred image. As with the ghosting of myopic astigmatism, the ghosting of nuclear sclerosis is exaggerated in dim illumination and often is not present in bright light.

Other structural or pathologic changes in the cornea, iris, or lens can produce monocular diplopia by forming multiple retinal images. The changes in the ocular media may be so minimal that the only objective physical finding is a subtle alteration of the retinoscopic reflex.

Ghosting is so characteristic of alterations in the refractive media that if the patient sees two distinct images with one eye, rather than overlapping images, in the absence of gross ocular abnormalities (subluxation of the lens, polycoria), one is likely to be dealing with **psychogenic disease.**

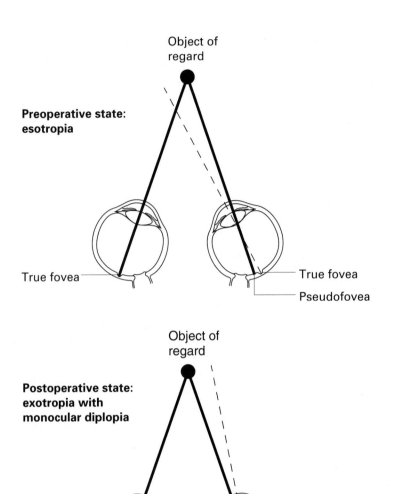

Object of
regard

**Preoperative state:
esotropia**

True fovea

True fovea

Pseudofovea

Object of
regard

**Postoperative state:
exotropia with
monocular diplopia**

Newly stimulated
retinal point

True fovea

Pseudofovea

*Fig. 9-2.* Diplopia after childhood strabismus surgery. *Top,* Before strabismus surgery, patient with abnormal retinal correspondence and strabismus surgery forms a single binocular image by fixating with fovea of left eye and an extrafoveal area (pseudofovea) of right eye. *Bottom,* After strabismus surgery that produces an exotropia, a new extrafoveal retinal area is stimulated. If previous pseudofovea is not suppressed, patient will experience binocular crossed diplopia (because newly stimulated retina is temporal to pseudofovea) and monocular diplopia with right eye.

☐ Diplopia present

▣ Palinopsia

If the patient lacks a history of recent strabismus surgery or diplopia is not relieved by use of the pinhole, then the examiner must ask explicit questions to determine whether the patient is seeing repetitive images or one image superimposed on another. If the patient's complaints are of repetitive or superimposed imagery, the likely diagnosis is palinopsia.

Critchley[16] defined palinopsia as "visual perseveration in time." The patient is unable to erase cortical images and sees one scene superimposed on another, not two images of the same scene. This sensory experience generally occurs episodically. It is a rare finding that occurs with occipitoparietal disease[17] (see Chapter 6).

▣ Cerebral polyopia

Some patients with signs and symptoms of posterior hemispheric dysfunction complain of seeing multiple images either monocularly or binocularly.[18] (For further discussion see Chapter 6.)

▣ Psychogenic

We use the broad generic term *psychogenic disease* to include both hysterical conversion reactions (unconscious dissembling) and malingering (conscious dissembling). If all of the possible causes of monocular diplopia have been clearly excluded, the only diagnosis left to the clinician is that of psychogenic diplopia. The answers obtained from certain patients with palinopsia may be so vague that separating these patients from the group of patients with psychogenic disease is impossible. In these litigious times, the feigning of diplopia is not a rare occurrence following a traumatic event.

☐ Diplopia not present with either eye covered

If covering one eye alleviates the diplopia, one is dealing with a binocular sensory experience (Chart 9-1, *A*).

◼ Binocular diplopia

○ *Characteristics of ocular alignment.* Binocular diplopia may occur either with or without ocular alignment. If the eyes are misaligned and the misalignment varies with gaze position, the misalignment is defined as *incomitant*. Incomitance is characteristic of cranial nerve palsies, restrictive disease, and myasthenia gravis (see Chapter 10). If the misalignment does not vary with gaze position, the misalignment is defined as *comitant*. Comitance is the hallmark of childhood strabismus (see Chapter 11).

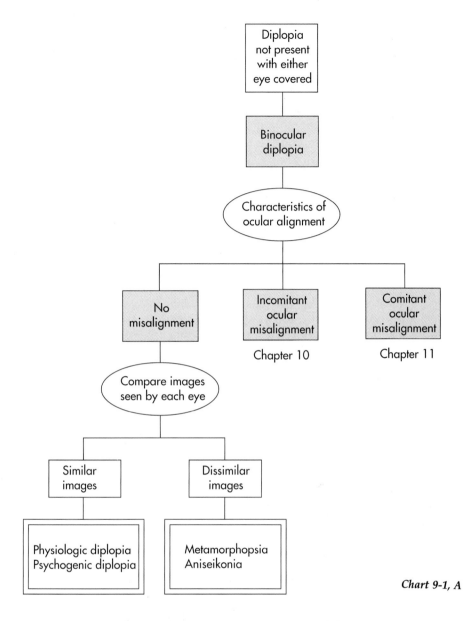

*Chart 9-1, A*

Ocular alignment can be determined subjectively by using the *red glass* test, or objectively by using prisms and the *cover-uncover test*. A comitant versus an incomitant misalignment may be determined by quantitating the amount of misalignment in the cardinal positions of gaze (Fig. 9-3) with the patient fixating at distance. Similar results can be obtained by making measurements using a near target for fixation, but they are more difficult to interpret).

**RED GLASS TEST.** When a red glass or filter is placed in front of one eye (by convention the right eye), a patient with binocular diplopia should become aware of two images: a red image (perceived by the right eye) and one without tint (perceived by the left eye). The untinted image is often not appreciated by the patient. The patient's awareness of this diplopic image can be facilitated by

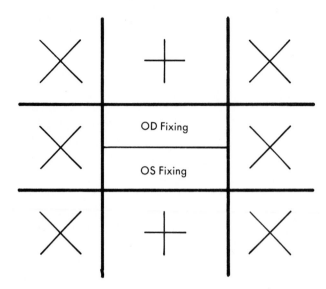

*Fig. 9-3.* The clinically important gaze positions in acquired strabismus are the primary position, right and left eye fixing in turn, and those marked by an X. Measurements in straight up and down position (+) are important in comitant strabismus (A and V patterns).

placing a green filter in front of the left eye or by alternately covering each eye and drawing the patient's attention to each image separately. The images of the right and left eyes are thus clearly identified. This improves the reliability of the subjective responses.

Ask the patient to look at a fixation light either at 20 feet (6 meters) or at about 20 inches (50 cm) in the straight-ahead (primary gaze) position. Ask the patient if he or she sees two lights separated in space, one red and one white (or green if a green filter has been used). The recognition of two separate images indicates ocular misalignment. Ask the patient to demonstrate with the fingers how far apart the images are in the various gaze positions. The amount of misalignment is determined in the cardinal positions of gaze.

**COVER-UNCOVER TEST.** The cover-uncover test is the objective counterpart of the red glass test. The patient should be wearing an appropriate refractive correction. Instruct the patient to hold the head straight and to fixate on an identifiable letter or object directly in front of him or her. First cover one eye and observe the other eye to see if it moves to pick up fixation. If the uncovered eye moves to pick up fixation, then a manifest misalignment, or *heterotropia* (tropia) is present. If the uncovered eye does not move, then that eye is fixing on the target appropriately. Then remove the occluder and observe the eye that was under the cover to see if it moves to pick up fixation, which would suggest the presence of a latent misalignment, or *heterophoria* (phoria). Repeat the sequence by covering the other eye, ultimately testing the patient in all cardinal positions of gaze with both distance and near fixation. By using the cover test with prisms, one can measure the amount of misalignment by neutralizing the induced ocular movement.

■ No misalignment

○ *Compare images seen by each eye.* If no misalignment is found, the patient is told to cover one eye at a time and is asked whether the images are similar.

☐ Similar images

If the patient observes similar images in both eyes, the patient has either physiologic or psychogenic diplopia. The patient's history may be helpful in this differentiation.

▣ Physiologic diplopia

If the diplopia is definitely present and the examination is normal, the examiner must determine if the patient has simply become aware of physiologic diplopia. In this case the patient will see one clear image with two blurred images. The examiner should demonstrate physiologic diplopia at near and distance. The patient is instructed to look at a pencil point held at 14 inches (35 cm) and to note if there is doubling of the background behind the examiner, and if this reproduces the symptoms. The patient is then instructed to fixate on a distant target and to place the two forefingers, one proximal and one distal, in his or her cyclopean line of sight. The patient is then asked if the doubling of images produced by fixation first on the proximal and then on the distal forefinger reproduces the sensory experience about which he or she is complaining.

▣ Psychogenic diplopia

Having excluded physiologic diplopia, the examiner must conclude that the patient's symptoms are not compatible with recognized pathologic states and represent psychogenic diplopia.

☐ Dissimilar images

If the images seen by the two eyes are dissimilar, then the patient has either metamorphopsia or aniseikonia.

▣ Metamorphopsia

If the patient has metamorphopsia from retinal disease, the image perceived by the involved eye is distorted (lines are curved, and segments are often indistinct). These findings can be confirmed subjectively by the use of an Amsler grid and indicate retinal disease. A type of metamorphopsia can be caused by cerebral disease. These patients complain of distorted imagery that is often bizarre in configuration. It is more often than not intermittent (see Chapter 6). These patients may complain of micropsia or teleopsia as well.

▣ Aniseikonia

The patient with aniseikonia will note a distinct difference in image size between the eyes, which may be meridional in nature. Both images will be distinct. This sensory phenomenon is produced by correcting refractive (usually large) differences between the two eyes with spectacles or contact lenses (e.g., aniseikonia is produced by correcting a refractive difference between the two eyes due to axial length with contact lenses or correcting an intrinsic refractive perturbation such as aphakia with spectacle lenses.

### ■ Incomitant ocular misalignment

Incomitant ocular misalignments are characterized by a variation of the angle of misalignment in different gaze directions (see Chapter 10).

### ■ Comitant ocular misalignment

Comitant ocular misalignments are characterized by a constant angle of misalignment in different gaze directions (see Chapter 11).

### REFERENCES

1. Persson HE, Sachs C. Visual evoked potentials elicited pattern reversal during provoked visual impairment in multiple sclerosis. Brain 1981;104:369-82.
2. Goldstein JE, Cogan DG. Exercise and the optic neuropathy of multiple sclerosis. Arch Ophthalmol 1964;72:168-70.
3. Selhorst J, Saul RF, Waybright EA. Optic nerve conduction: opposing effects of exercise and hyperventilation. Trans Am Neurol Assoc 1981;106:1-4.
4. Nelson D, Jeffreys WH, McDowell F. Effect of induced hyperthermia on some neurological diseases. Arch Neurol Psychiatry 1958;79:31-9.
5. Smith JL, Hoyt WF, Susac JO. Ocular fundus in Leber optic neuropathy. Arch Ophthalmol 1973;90:349-54.
6. Kaji R, Happel L, Sumner AJ. Effect of digitalis on clinical symptoms and conduction of variables in patients with multiple sclerosis. Ann Neurol 1990; 28:582-4.
7. Polman CH, van Diemen HA, van Dongen MMN, et al. 4-Aminopyridine in multiple sclerosis [Letter]. Ann Neurol 1990;28:589.
8. Puvanendran K, Cheah JS, Naganathan N, et al. Neuromuscular transmission in thyrotoxicosis. J Neurol Sci 1979; 43:47-57.
9. Wang FM, Chryssanthou G. Monocular eye closure in intermittent exotropia. Arch Ophthalmol 1988;106:941-2.
10. Nachtigäller H, Hoyt WF. Störungen des Seheindruckes bei bitemporaler Hemianopsie und Verschiebung Der Sehachsen. Klin Monatsbl Augenheilkd 1970;156:821-36.
11. Lessell S, Lessell IM, Rizzo JF III. Ocular neuromyotonia after radiation therapy. Am J Ophthalmol 1986;102:766-70.
12. Salmon JF, Steven P, Abrahamson MJ. Ocular neuromyotonia. Neuro-Ophthalmology 1988;8:181-5.
13. Shults WT, Hoyt WF, Behrens M, et al. Ocular neuromyotonia: a clinical description of six patients. Arch Ophthalmol 1986;104:1028-34.
14. Bielschowsky A. Uber monoculäre Diplopie ohne physikalische Grundlage nebts Bemerkungen über das Sehen Schielender. Graefes Arch Ophthalmol 1898;46:143-83.
15. Burian HM, von Noorden GK. Binocular vision and ocular motility: theory and management of strabismus. St Louis: Mosby–Year Book, 1974:260-1.
16. Critchley M. Types of visual perseveration: "palinopsia" and "illusory visual spread." Brain 1951;74:265-99.
17. Lessell S. Higher disorders of visual function: positive phenomenon. In: Glaser JS, Smith LJ, eds. Neuro-ophthalmology: symposium of the University of Miami and the Bascom Palmer Eye Institute, vol 8. St Louis: Mosby–Year Book, 1975:27-44.
18. Safran AB, Kline LB, Glaser JS, et al. Television-induced formed visual hallucinations and cerebral diplopia. Br J Ophthalmol 1981;65:707-11.

# CHAPTER 10

# *Incomitant Ocular Misalignment*

• • • • • • • • • • • • • • • • •

Incomitant ocular misalignments are differentiated from comitant ocular misalignments by the presence of a variation of the angle of misalignment in different gaze directions. A difference in the degree of misalignment depending on which eye is used for fixation (primary and secondary deviation)[1-3] is also characteristic.

Many patients with incomitant strabismus adopt a compensatory head posture to attempt to produce binocular single vision.[4] If this is not possible, patients may assume a head position in which the diplopia is made less bothersome. They do this by placing their eyes in such a position that either the nonfixating eye is occluded by the nose or the misalignment is maximized, making the diplopic image easier to ignore. In evaluating patients with adopted head posturing, old photographs are helpful in marking the chronicity of the problem. If such photographs are not available at the time of the initial examination, a series of sequential photographs dating back to childhood should be obtained. Adequate magnification for studying these pictures can be readily obtained with a +14-diopter magnifying lens or a slit lamp.[5]

## A Decision Tree Approach to the Evaluation of Incomitant Ocular Misalignment

As mentioned in Chapter 9, incomitance is characteristic of restrictive disease and myasthenia gravis, as well as of cranial nerve palsies. Thus before considering cranial nerve palsies as the cause of incomitant misalignments, one must exclude restrictive ophthalmopathy and myasthenia gravis (Chart 10-1). The modalities used to exclude these two processes are the forced duction and Tensilon tests.

○ *Forced duction test.* The presence of a mechanical restriction is most easily confirmed by the use of forced (passive) duction testing. Appropriate use of topical anesthetics makes forced duction testing comfortable for the patient, thus assuring the examiner of the best chance to detect minimal restrictions of movements.

Instill topical proparacaine solution in the inferior cul-de-sac of each eye.

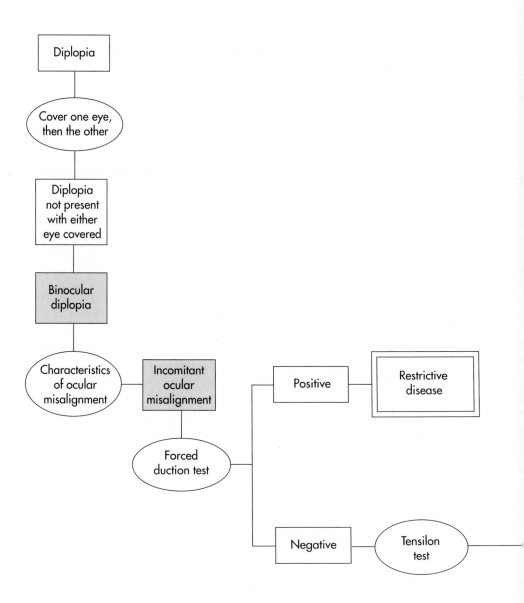

***Chart 10-1***

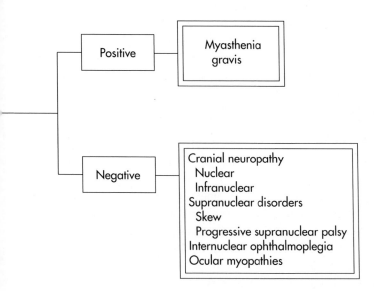

Then place a cotton-tipped applicator soaked in proparacaine (or cocaine) in the fornix over the insertion of the rectus muscles or region of the limbus to be manipulated for approximately 15 to 20 seconds. Ask the patient to look in the direction of the gaze limitation. Grasp either the conjunctiva and episcleral tissue at the limbus (180 degrees from the direction of restriction) or the insertion of the presumed restricted rectus muscle (antagonist to the muscle active in gaze movement) with a toothed forceps (0.1 to 0.5 mm). Then ask the patient to move the eyes in the direction of gaze restriction. Failure of movement or retraction of the globe into the orbit on passive movement signifies the presence of a restrictive process.

Repeat this same sequence with the other eye and compare the ease and range of passive movement of the globe. If the globe is pushed back into the orbit inadvertently as pressure is applied, an otherwise positive test may be made equivocal. Pushing the eye back into the orbit increases the relative length of the tethered muscle, allowing the eye to move more easily. The use of a forceps allows the examiner to make the diagnosis of even subtle restrictions. However, in some minimal ductional deficits due to restrictive processes, making an unequivocal judgment may be impossible.

Some patients may be unable to cooperate for these maneuvers. In this circumstance an alternative is to measure the intraocular pressure in the primary position and again with the eyes moved voluntarily into the direction of limited gaze. Although this measurement was originally described using Goldmann applanation tonometry, accurate results can be obtained more easily with a hand-held tonometer such as a pneumotonometer. A pressure rise of greater than 4 mm Hg in moving from one gaze position to another is diagnostic of a restrictive problem.[6,7] Patients with inferior rectus restriction often have apparently elevated intraocular pressures when such measurements are made in the primary position. If the physician is not aware of the underlying restrictive process or the associated pathophysiology, such patients may be identified mistakenly as glaucoma patients or "ocular hypertensives," because in the usual clinical setting patients are asked to elevate their eyes to reach the primary position in order to measure intraocular pressure. Unless evidence of progressive optic disc changes and visual field loss is present, no treatment is indicated.

☐ Positive forced duction test

▣ Restrictive disease

Although many disease processes cause mechanical limitation of extraocular movements, Graves' ophthalmopathy is the most common (see box).

The diagnosis of **Graves' ophthalmopathy** (see Chapter 15) is dependent on clinical features including lid retraction and lid lag, proptosis (unilateral or bilateral), conjunctival suffusion, engorgement of vessels over the horizontal recti, and restrictive muscle disease.[8] The restrictive muscle component can mimic supranuclear, nuclear, or peripheral ocular motor nerve paresis. Myasthenia gravis occurs in approximately 0.2% of cases of Graves' disease.[9] The finding of ptosis in the presence of Graves' ophthalmopathy should suggest the concur-

## Mechanical (Restrictive) Causes of Acquired Diplopia

Graves' ophthalmopathy
Brown's superior oblique tendon sheath syndrome
Orbital pseudotumor
Ocular myositis

Orbital mass lesions     Primary
                       Metastatic

Trauma       Orbital fracture
            Intrinsic muscle damage

rent diagnosis of myasthenia gravis and the need for a Tensilon test.[9]

Brown's **superior oblique tendon sheath syndrome,** which mimics an isolated inferior oblique palsy, is an often unrecognized entity. It can be either congenital or acquired. The acquired form often is associated with pain on attempted upgaze in the adducted position and tenderness in the region of the trochlea. The diagnosis is made by positive forced duction testing. Occasionally one can hear a "click" as the tendon slides through the trochlea, accompanied by a movement of the eye upward. Suggested treatment of the acquired form has included the use of systemic corticosteroids, as well as subtenon injections of corticosteroids in the region of the trochlea.[10,11] If the condition fails to resolve, a variety of surgical procedures have been suggested. Since spontaneous improvement often occurs over time without treatment, we believe that nothing more than observation is indicated.

☐ Negative forced duction test

◯ *Tensilon test.* If forced duction testing is negative, a Tensilon or neostigmine (Prostigmin) test should be performed to exclude myasthenia gravis. Tensilon (edrophonium hydrochloride) is supplied in single-dose, 10 mg/ml, break-neck vials (1 mg/0.1 ml).

For the Tensilon test, the examiner must choose a definite goal or end point. If ptosis is present, then a measured change in the amount of ptosis is satisfactory. (Polaroid pictures before and during the test are easily taken and are a good record. A copy given to the patient will save him or her from being "drowned in a veritable sea of Tensilon.") If no ptosis is present, a change in the deviation must be quantitated using a Hess or Lees screen or prism and cover test. Some clinicians choose to pretreat all patients with 0.4 mg of intravenous atropine, and others pretreat only when needed.

Two approaches are suggested for use with adults. In one approach, draw up Tensilon into a 1 cc tuberculin syringe. In another syringe containing 1 cc of tuberculin, draw up 0.4 mg of injectable atropine sulfate. Fill a third 10 cc syringe with injectable saline. Place a scalp-vein needle (21 or 23 gauge) into a dorsal hand vein. Use a multiswitch stopcock or change the syringes as necessary. Inject 1 ml of saline solution and observe for 1 minute. Then choose one of the following:

1. Inject 0.2 ml of Tensilon and flush tubing with 1 ml of saline; observe for 1 minute. If no response, inject a bolus of 0.8 ml of Tensilon and flush tubing with 1 ml of saline; connect atropine syringe to tubing; or
2. Inject 0.2 ml of Tensilon and flush with saline. Continue slow injection of Tensilon by slowly flushing with saline after priming tube with remaining 0.8 ml; or
3. Inject 0.2 ml of Tensilon and flush with saline; observe for 1 minute. Inject 0.4 ml of Tensilon and flush with saline; observe for 1 minute. Inject remaining 0.4 ml of Tensilon and observe for 1 minute.

Another approach in adults involves drawing Tensilon into a 1 cc tuberculin syringe with a ⅝-inch, 27-gauge needle. Inject directly with the tuberculin syringe and needle into a dorsal hand vein. Make sure the needle can be detached from the syringe before inserting it into the vein. The injections are the same as above.

A different approach is preferred in children, uncooperative adults, and patients in whom a long duration of action is desired. Administer intramuscular atropine, 0.4 mg, 15 minutes before an intramuscular injection of neostigmine. The dose of neostigmine is calculated as:

$$[\text{Weight (kg)} \div 70 \text{ kg}] \times 1.5 \text{ mg} = \text{Dose}$$

Reexamine the patient 30 to 45 minutes after injection.

### ☐ Positive Tensilon test

A positive Tensilon test, with improvement in extraocular muscle function, is generally diagnostic of myasthenia gravis.

### ☐ Myasthenia gravis

Myasthenia gravis may mimic any single or combined extraocular muscle palsy, or supranuclear or internuclear ophthalmoplegia (see box). Seventy-five percent of myasthenic patients[12] have ocular symptoms initially, and approximately 90% eventually develop ocular signs. If no systemic signs develop within 2 years, the disease is likely to remain localized to the extraocular muscles.[13] A feature of ocular myasthenia is muscle fatigue. In the presence of ptosis, sustained upgaze should produce a "window shade" effect of the involved lid(s) (i.e., the ptosis will get progressively worse). Measurements will vary during attempts to quantitate the ocular misalignment either subjectively or objectively. Testing the patient late in the afternoon rather than in the morning exaggerates this variability.

Moorthy et al.[14] point out that patients with compressive ocular motor palsies consequent to intracranial mass lesions may have positive Tensilon tests with clinical features mimicking those of myasthenia gravis. Of their eight patients, all of whom had intracranial mass lesions, four were believed to have myasthenia gravis, as well as compressive neuropathies, and four had compressive cranial neuropathies alone. Seven of these patients were Tensilon responsive, and four of five treated with anticholinesterase medications improved. Our impression, as well as that of others,[15,16] is that patients with cranial nerve paresis secondary to compressive lesions, as well as patients with recovering cranial nerve paresis, may in fact be somewhat responsive to Tensilon. The clinical

## Ophthalmic Signs of Myasthenia Gravis

Ptosis
Extraocular muscle palsies
Pseudogaze palsies
Pseudoconvergence paresis
Quiver movements

Pseudointernuclear ophthalmoplegia
Lid twitch
Orbicularis weakness
Nystagmus

course of such patients with cranial nerve palsies dictates the need for imaging.

In performing the Tensilon test, a measurable end point must be obtainable. One cannot rely on the subjective response of the patient or the qualitative judgment of the examiner. The only reliable indicator of a positive response is a quantitative change in the ptosis or measured ocular misalignment. If ptosis is present, a change in the amount is certainly the easiest parameter to quantitate; however, Eaton[17] has reported in his series of ocular myasthenics that 77% of patients who have diplopia have ptosis. This is not concordant with our clinical impression that ptosis is an almost universal finding in patients with ocular involvement in myasthenia gravis. Although these patients invariably demonstrate a characteristic "lid twitch" sign,[18] it is not specific for myasthenia gravis. In ocular myasthenia gravis ipsilateral orbicularis weakness is often present.[19] The Tensilon test may be negative initially in ocular myasthenia gravis and subsequently become positive.

Retzlaff et al.[20] have demonstrated the necessity of measuring the effect of Tensilon in more than one position of gaze using the Lancaster red-green test and have shown that the response varies according to gaze position. These changes must occur within 30 to 60 seconds of injection and return to the pretest measurements within 4 to 5 minutes. The changes must be repeatable on subsequent testing. Miller et al.[21] made similar observations using neostigmine.

Four responses to the Tensilon test are possible in patients with ocular involvement when measured in a single gaze position: one negative and three positive. A negative response (no change in the ocular alignment) generally means that the patient does not have myasthenia gravis but does not absolutely exclude the diagnosis. A few patients with myasthenia gravis have a negative response to intravenous injections of Tensilon. They may show a positive response to neostigmine or to more specialized tests (e.g., electromyography with repetitive nerve or single muscle fiber stimulation). Three types of positive responses may occur in any individual myasthenic patient, varying with the gaze position in which the misalignment is measured:

Type 1: An improvement in alignment
　　　　(Large tropia* → Small tropia → Fusion)
Type 2: A worsening of alignment
　　　　(Small tropia* → Large tropia)
Type 3: A reversal in alignment
　　　　(Right hypertropia → Left hypertropia)

*Vertical misalignment: minimum change $\geq 3^{\Delta}$. Horizontal misalignment: minimum change $\geq 5^{\Delta}$.

Paradoxical responses (types 2 and 3) to Tensilon include a worsening or a reversal of ocular misalignment (i.e., a right hypertropia would increase by more than $3^\Delta$, or a right hypertropia would become a left hypertropia). A similar reversal can be seen in a patient with ptosis wherein the lid develops retraction and the apparently normal lid becomes ptotic. Any of these responses may be seen in a small percentage (10%) of nonmyasthenic ophthalmoplegias.[14] Such responses may also be induced in patients with inadequately treated myasthenia gravis. Our impression is that using small increments (0.1 to 0.2 ml) of Tensilon often (but not always) produces a type 1 response in gaze positions that might otherwise demonstrate a type 2 or 3 response.

The side effects of Tensilon are those of cholinergic hyperactivity and include tearing, salivation, gastric distress, mild bradycardia, and lid fasciculations. The safety of the Tensilon test has been well documented.[22]

The treatment of patients with myasthenia gravis falls within the purview of a neurologist. The first line of treatment for ocular myasthenia gravis, as for generalized myasthenia gravis, is anticholinesterase agents such as pyridostigmine (Mestinon). Unfortunately, many patients do not respond to these agents. Alternatives include daily or alternate-day prednisone, 25 to 100 mg.[23,24] Although systemic corticosteroids may exacerbate systemic signs in patients with generalized myasthenia gravis, leading to extreme weakness and in some cases respiratory failure, this is unlikely to be a problem in patients with ocular myasthenia gravis.[23]

The elimination of diplopia in response to alternate-day steroids in patients with ocular myasthenia gravis is remarkable, approaching 90% to 100%. In our experience, patients with ocular myasthenia can be started on low doses of alternate-day or daily steroids (equivalent of 10 mg of prednisone). The dose is slowly increased until the desired effect is achieved. We estimate that about 80% of such patients become free of diplopia over a wide range of gaze positions. However, we believe that the side effects associated with the prolonged use of corticosteroids, even moderate doses of prednisone, preclude such intervention unless binocularity is an absolute necessity.

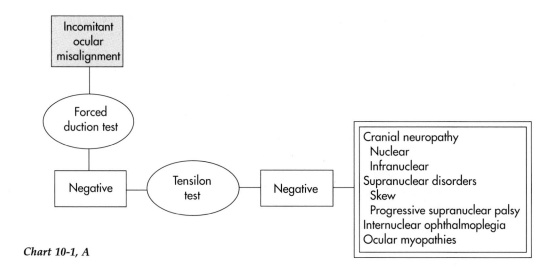

*Chart 10-1, A*

☐ Negative Tensilon test

Once both restrictive disease and myasthenia gravis have been excluded (Chart 10-1, *A*), the vast majority of patients with incomitant strabismus have processes affecting the **ocular motor nuclei,** their **fascicles,** or the **cranial nerves** themselves.

## OCULOMOTOR NERVE (THIRD CRANIAL NERVE)

**ANATOMY.** The third cranial nerve innervates five extraocular muscles: the levator palpebrae superioris; the superior, inferior, and medial rectus; and the inferior oblique. It also supplies the presynaptic parasympathethic outflow to the ciliary ganglion controlling pupillary sphincter function and accommodation. The anatomy of the oculomotor nuclear complex in primates as described by Warwick[25] has been modified in recent years by the work of Porter et al.,[26] among others,[27,28] using retrograde tracer substances (Fig. 10-1). The medial rectus subnucleus consists of three different cell masses.[29] The individual functions of these different subnuclei remain obscure. The medial and inferior rectus muscles, as well as the inferior oblique muscle, are ipsilaterally innervated.

As is classically held, the superior rectus subnucleus innervates the contralateral superior rectus muscle,[30] with the decussation occurring at the middle to caudal end of the nuclear complex. The central caudal nucleus innervates the levator palpebrae superioris bilaterally.[25] (It is assumed that these findings are applicable in humans, and clinically this appears to be true.)

The visceral nuclei extend from the rostral end of the somatic complex caudally.[27] The most rostral portion of the complex consists of paired central nuclei, the anterior median nuclei (one on each side of the midline). Dorsally and caudally at about the level where the somatic nuclei become recognizable, the Edinger-Westphal nucleus becomes evident. This part of the visceral complex consists of a central mass of cells that divide caudally into slender columns that

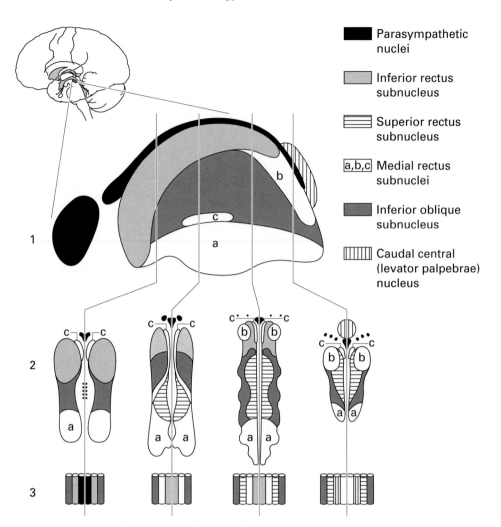

Parasympathetic
nuclei

Inferior rectus
subnucleus

Superior rectus
subnucleus

a,b,c Medial rectus
subnuclei

Inferior oblique
subnucleus

Caudal central
(levator palpebrae)
nucleus

*Fig. 10-1.* Third cranial nerve subnuclei. Schematic representation based on studies in nonhuman primates[25-30] and patients.[42-44] *1*, Parasagittal section of subnuclei; *2*, coronal sections of subnuclei; *3*, coronal sections of fascicles in midbrain.

subdivide again. Between the masses of the somatic motor nuclei is the nucleus of Perlia, which also makes up part of the visceral system. The visceral outflow is totally ipsilateral in projection.[27]

The oculomotor complex is cupped by the medial longitudinal fasciculi and lies ventral to the periaqueductal gray matter. Fascicles arise along its entire length and sweep ventrally to exit the midbrain as multiple rootlets in the interpeduncular fossa. A rostral caudal somatotopy exists among the fascicular fibers of the third nerve within the mesencephalon, with the visceral fibers being most cephalad,[27] followed by the inferior rectus and inferior oblique fibers, and, most caudally, the levator and superior rectus fibers.[30] Some evidence also indicates mediolateral somatotopy, with the superior rectus and inferior oblique being most lateral and the pupilloconstrictor fibers and the inferior rectus being most medial. Similarly, as the peripheral nerve itself is formed, a clear somato-

> ### Divisions of the Third Cranial (Oculomotor) Nerve
>
> 1. Superior division
>    a. Superior rectus muscle
>    b. Levator palpebrae superioris muscle
> 2. Inferior division
>    a. Medial rectus muscle
>    b. Inferior rectus muscle
>    c. Inferior oblique muscle
>    d. Parasympathetic innervation to sphincter pupillae muscle and ciliary muscles

topy of fibers is present, with the visceral fibers being superficial and dorsomedial, whereas the inferior and superior divisions are already segregated at this level. This segregation explains the occasional occurrence of divisional paresis with posterior lesions.[31,32]

The nerve then turns rostrally, traveling in the subarachnoid space and passing under the superior cerebellar and over the posterior cerebral arteries to enter the lateral wall of the cavernous sinus. The pupillary fibers travel in the dorsomedial portion of the nerve.[33,34] The nerve enters the orbit through the superior orbital fissure, dividing into a superior and inferior division in the anterior cavernous sinus or in the orbital fissure (see box). Because of the segregation of functional fiber bundles within the oculomotor pathway from the nucleus to the muscles, lesions at different sites tend to produce different signs.

• • •

The causes of cranial nerve palsies in adults[35-39] and children[40,41] are different. The information available in the published series is not derived from a similar population base, yet the results are remarkably comparable.

**THIRD NERVE PALSIES IN ADULTS.** The five major published series[35-39] of third nerve palsies consist of different population groups (Table 10-1). Some of these series include patients with neurologic deficits other than third nerve palsies but exclude involvement of the fourth and sixth cranial nerves,[37-39] whereas others deal with truly isolated nerve palsies.[36] An isolated cranial nerve palsy is one in which no other neurologic signs, not even headache, are present. The three major series from the Mayo Clinic[37-39] include a variety of patients with acquired impairment of ocular motility; some were ambulatory and had only diplopia, whereas others were hospitalized with serious illness. Although the patients with oculomotor nerve paresis had no other ocular motor (trochlear and abducens) palsies, many did have other accompanying neurologic signs. This is in contrast to the patients reported by Green et al.,[36] who had isolated oculomotor palsies.

The most common causes of third cranial nerve palsies in adults are aneurysms and presumed peripheral nerve infarction, although evidence is growing

| TABLE 10-1 | *Comparison of Causes of Third Cranial Nerve Palsy in Adults* | | | | | | | | | |
|---|---|---|---|---|---|---|---|---|---|---|
| | Rucker[37] (335 cases) | | Rucker[38] (274 cases) | | Green et al.[36] (130 cases) | | Goldstein and Cogan[35] (61 cases) | | Rush and Younge[39] (290 cases) | |
| | No. | % | No. | % | No. | % | No. | % | No. | % |
| Aneurysm | 64 | 19 | 50 | 18 | 38 | 30 | 11 | 18 | 40 | 14 |
| Vascular disease* | 63 | 19 | 47 | 17 | 25 | 19 | 28 | 47 | 60 | 21 |
| Trauma | 51 | 15 | 34 | 13 | 14 | 11 | 5 | 8 | 47 | 16 |
| Syphilis | 6 | 2 | 0 | 0 | 12 | 9 | 0 | 0 | 0 | 0 |
| Neoplasm | 35 | 11 | 50 | 18 | 5 | 4 | 6 | 10 | 34 | 12 |
| Undetermined | 95 | 28 | 55 | 20 | 33 | 23 | 7 | 11 | 67 | 23 |
| Miscellaneous | 21 | 6 | 38 | 12 | 5 | 4 | 4 | 6 | 42 | 14 |

*Including diabetes mellitus.

that fascicular damage in the brainstem may be a more frequent cause than previously thought.[32,42-44] These infarcts are more common in patients with hypertension, atherosclerosis, and diabetes mellitus. Aneurysms and infarcts each account for approximately 20% of the total number of oculomotor palsies. Trauma and tumors each account for 10% to 15% of cases. These tumors include pituitary tumors with lateral extension, parasellar mass lesions, and malignant lesions involving the brainstem and meninges.

A wide spectrum of miscellaneous neurologic and systemic diseases, including sinusitis, Hodgkin's disease, herpes zoster, temporal arteritis, meningitis, encephalitis, collagen vascular disease, Paget's disease, and acquired immunodeficiency syndrome (AIDS) with or without superimposed infections, as well as postoperative complications of neurosurgical procedures, have been implicated as causes of oculomotor paralysis. About 20% have been attributed to unknown cause, but since many of these patients have vascular risk factors and recover, it is assumed that many of these patients have had vascular infarction.

Diplopia has been reported to be the presenting sign in 12% of patients with giant cell arteritis.[45] Interestingly, in some of these patients no overt misalignment can be found, in spite of the presence of diplopia.[45] Others have a third or a sixth nerve palsy, and a few have presenting signs of total ophthalmoplegia due to severe orbital ischemia.[46] In our experience, the incidence of misalignment in giant cell arteritis is very low. However, because giant cell arteritis is a treatable disease, patients over the age of 55 years who have an ocular motor palsy(s) or intermittent diplopia, and who also have a history of polymyalgia rheumatica or headache, should have an erythrocyte sedimentation rate performed. Appropriate therapy should be instituted as necessary (see Chapter 2).

Recognition of differential involvement of components of the oculomotor nerve in an adult often helps to localize the offending lesion.

**Third nerve palsy involving all components** (Fig. 10-2). In an isolated total pa-

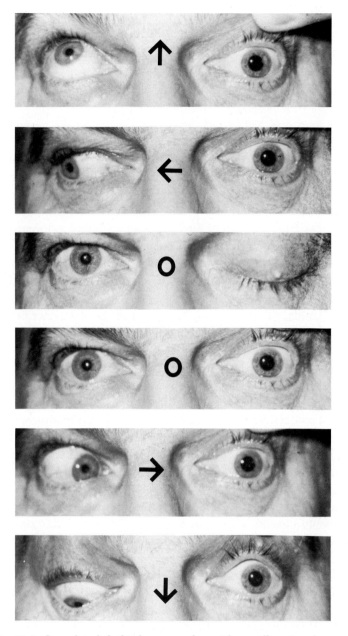

*Fig. 10-2.* Complete left third nerve palsy with pupillary involvement.

ralysis of the oculomotor nerve, the globe is turned out and slightly down. The pupil is dilated and unreactive to direct or consensual stimuli. The eye may float toward the midline with attempted gaze toward the contralateral side, and intorsion can be induced on attempted downgaze if the trochlear nerve is intact. Such findings usually indicate involvement between the base of the midbrain and the superior orbital fissure.

Patients with involvement of "all" the somatic components of the third nerve may demonstrate certain clinically apparent findings that are of diagnostic significance, such as pupillary sparing and aberrant regeneration.

*Pupillary sparing and its importance.* Most adult patients with retro-orbital or periorbital pain and the acute onset of an isolated third nerve palsy either have a posterior communicating aneurysm compressing the third nerve along its course or have suffered an infarction of the nerve substance itself (fasicles). The decision facing the clinician is to determine which patients are likely to have aneurysms and therefore are in need of arteriography with its associated morbidity and mortality. Rucker,[37] and subsequently Goldstein and Cogan,[35] pointed out that pupillary sparing (normal pupillary function) in the face of an almost total somatic palsy is the hallmark of a third nerve palsy, presumably due to vascular occlusion. Such pupillary sparing is found in 8% to 15% of patients with isolated third nerve palsies due to aneurysms.[47,48] Patients with aneurysmal third nerve palsies may have pupillary sparing on initial presentation, but if followed daily the pupil will be seen to become dilated and paretic within 3 to 5 days.[47]

Pupillary findings must be related to the remainder of third nerve function, since pupillary sparing is a relative concept. For example, if a patient has a total paresis of the extraocular muscles but the pupil on the involved side is only 1 to 2 mm larger than the other pupil and reacts fairly well to light stimuli (even though less briskly than its counterpart), we would consider this patient to have a *relative pupillary-sparing third nerve palsy*. However, if the extraocular muscles are not completely involved and the pupil is minimally, but definitely, involved, we would not consider the patient to have relative pupillary sparing (Fig. 10-3).

The explanation for pupillary sparing appears to lie in the anatomy of the third nerve and its blood supply. Pupillary fibers travel superficially and superonasally in the third nerve[33,34] and therefore are at risk for early involvement in compressive lesions (e.g., aneurysm or midline shift prior to herniation of the uncus through the tentorium cerebelli). Dreyfus et al.[49] and Asbury et al.[50] have demonstrated that patients with pupillary sparing have an ischemic infarct of the core of the nerve whereas the superficial fibers, including those destined for the pupil, remain unaffected. Hopf and Gutmann[42] reported 11 cases of isolated oculomotor palsies, 8 with pupillary sparing, in patients with diabetes mellitus. Three patients had magnetic resonance imaging (MRI) evidence of involvement of the ipsilateral oculomotor fascicles, and the others had electrophysiologic evidence of brainstem dysfunction. The authors concluded that an isolated diabetic third nerve palsy, with or without pupillary involvement, is much more likely to be caused by an infarct of the mesencephalon than by a peripheral nerve infarction. An appropriate explanation is the rostral medial segregation of pupillary fasicles in the midbrain.

Although discussion of pupillary-sparing third cranial nerve palsy has classically been limited to pointing out an association with diabetes mellitus, such palsies are most often found in patients who do not demonstrate abnormalities of glucose metabolism. The more general term *vasculopathic mononeuropathy* has been applied, implying small-vessel infarction associated with any number

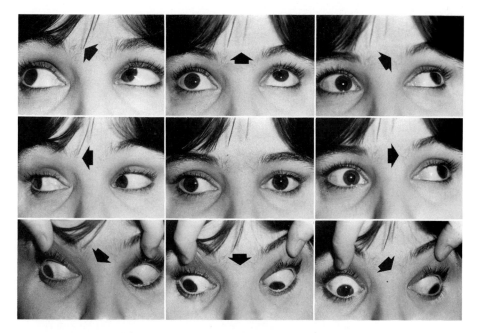

*Fig. 10-3.* Partial right third nerve palsy with minimal pupillary involvement.

of defined or undefined vascular diseases, such as diabetes mellitus, atherosclerosis, or hypertension. In general, vasculopathic mononeuropathy has implied a lesion in the peripheral nerve itself; however, it is now apparent that similar findings can be produced by brainstem infarction. A vasculopathic etiology has also been postulated as a frequent cause of isolated fourth and sixth cranial nerve palsies. Such palsies may be recurrent but almost always occur as a mononeuropathy. Total recovery within 3 to 4 months is the rule. These patients do not develop aberrant regeneration. If more than one ocular motor nerve is involved simultaneously, the diagnosis of a vasculopathic paresis should be held suspect.[51,52]

*Aberrant regeneration.* Aberrant regeneration of the oculomotor nerve (Fig. 10-4) consists of a constellation of findings, the most common of which is lid retraction in downgaze (pseudo-von Graefe's phenomenon[53]). Other abnormal findings include lid elevation or pupillary constriction on attempted adduction or unilateral globe retraction on upgaze or downgaze. Aberrant regeneration usually occurs following recovery from an acute third nerve palsy due to trauma or a compressive lesion, such as an aneurysm. Aberrant regeneration is presumed to be due to miswiring following a break in the axon cylinders within the third nerve with misdirection of sprouting axons.[28,54] One case of an acquired contralateral oculomotor synkinesis following trauma has been reported.[55] It is of interest that in two cases the patient's clinically evident "misdirection" was transient; one patient had ophthalmoplegic migraine,[56] and the other had pituitary apoplexy.[57] Ephaptic transmission has been postulated as a mechanism in these cases.

It was believed that aberrant regeneration almost always occurred follow-

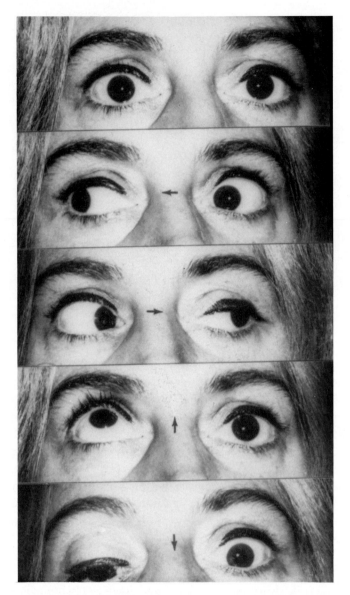

*Fig. 10-4.* Aberrant regeneration of left third cranial nerve. Left palpebral fissure widens on adduction, and left upper lid elevates on downgaze.

ing an acute oculomotor palsy, but Schatz et al.[58] noted aberrant regeneration without such a history. All of their patients had meningiomas of the cavernous sinus, and they believe that primary aberrant regeneration (i.e., aberrant regeneration without a previous history of a third nerve palsy) indicates an indolent mass lesion in the cavernous sinus. Cox et al.[59] have reported similar findings in a patient with an intracavernous aneurysm. Johnson et al.[60] reported three such patients with extracavernous lesions (neurilemoma, meningioma and unilaterally enlarged mamillary body).

**Divisional involvement.** As demonstrated by both experimental and clinical observation, divisional somatotopy is clearly evident within the ventral fascicles of the third nerve in the brainstem prior to formation of the rootlets. Although divisional paresis was previously believed to be the hallmark of an anterior cavernous sinus or superior orbital fissure lesion, we are now aware that divisional paresis can occur anywhere from the midbrain to the orbit.[31,32]

*Inferior divisional paresis.* Inferior divisional paresis is marked by internal ophthalmoplegia and paresis of the medial and inferior rectus muscles, as well as of the inferior oblique muscle. The lesions can be anywhere from the mesencephalon to the peripheral nerve in the orbit. Inferior divisional palsies have been reported with trauma, tumors, infarctions, and presumed viral insults. In presumed viral cases the paresis tends to recover spontaneously.[61]

*Superior divisional paresis.* Superior divisional paresis is marked by ptosis and superior rectus muscle paresis. Isolated superior divisional paresis is rare. Some cases, presumably of viral etiology, have been reported in which spontaneous recovery occurred.[62,63] Patients with intracavernous aneurysms have greater involvement of the superior division of the oculomotor nerve than they do of the inferior division.[64] Thus such a finding may suggest, in itself, a cavernous sinus lesion. Yet, Guy and Day[31] reported five patients with unilateral ptosis, limitation of supraduction, and normal pupillary reactivity who had basilar artery aneurysms. The most common location of the aneurysms was the interpeduncular fossa. Patients with cavernous sinus lesions, for the most part, have involvement of other cranial nerves (V and VI),[64] which helps in localization.

**Single muscle paresis.** Roper-Hall and Burde[43] reported a series of cases of isolated inferior rectus muscle palsies, presumed to be secondary to small-vessel occlusion in the brainstem. All of these patients recovered spontaneously. Warren et al.[44] reported a series of cases with partial third nerve palsies involving one or two muscles and the pupil. These deficits were accompanied by other signs of intrinsic midbrain disease, such as rubral tremor or cerebellar signs. Using Warwick's model of the component parts subserving individual muscle function within the third nerve nucleus, they postulated that lesions specifically located within the mesencephalon were the cause of the neurologic deficits.

Isolated paresis of the inferior oblique muscle of unknown etiology has also been reported.[65,66] In such cases a Brown superior oblique tendon sheath syndrome[67] must be excluded. The diagnosis is made by forced duction testing.

We do not consider the finding of a dilated unreactive pupil without other evidence of third nerve or neurologic dysfunction to be a sign of third nerve paresis. These patients should be evaluated for signs of possible ocular trauma, pharmacologic blockade, or Adie's syndrome (see Chapter 13). An isolated ptosis has been described as the presenting sign of a posterior communicating aneurysm,[68] but such a presentation is extraordinarily rare.

**THIRD NERVE PALSIES IN CHILDREN.** The causes of isolated third nerve palsies in children differ from those in adults[36,40,69] (Table 10-2). Between 43% and 47% of cases are congenital; 13% to 23% are traumatic; neoplasms account for approximately 10% and aneurysms for 7% of cases. Both Miller[69] and Harley[40]

| TABLE 10-2 | Comparison of Causes of Third Cranial Nerve Palsy in Children | | | | | |
|---|---|---|---|---|---|---|
| | Miller[69] (30 cases) | | Harley[40] (32 cases) | | Green et al.[36] (6 cases) | |
| | No. | % | No. | % | No. | % |
| Congenital | 13* | 43 | 15 | 47 | | |
| Aneurysm | 2 | 7 | | | | |
| Neoplasm | 3 | 10 | 3 | 9 | | |
| Vascular disease | | | 2† | 6 | | |
| Trauma | 6 | 20 | 4 | 13 | 4 | |
| Inflammation | 4 | 13 | 3 | 9 | 2 | |
| Miscellaneous | 2‡ | 7 | 5§ | 16 | | |

*Includes birth trauma.
†Ophthalmoplegic migraine.
‡Limited information.
§Three cases of ophthalmoplegic migraine.

have pointed out that a high percentage of their cases of congenital oculomotor palsy had aberrant regeneration (61% and 93%, respectively). Since most of these patients have nonprogressive defects and negative imaging studies, intrauterine or birth trauma is the most likely etiology.

Although aneurysm is responsible for 20% of isolated oculomotor palsies in adults, it is a much less common cause (3%) in children.[70] An angiogram may not be a necessary part of the workup in patients under age 10 with acquired third nerve palsies.[70]

A few cases of cryptogenic acute acquired complete oculomotor palsies have been reported in which good imaging techniques were used.[71] Abdul-Rahim et al.[72] reported five children between 3 and 17 years of age who developed slowly progressive oculomotor nerve palsies in whom no cause was found initially. Subsequent high-resolution computed tomography (CT) or 1.5 T MRI revealed a mass along the course of the involved nerve compatible with the diagnosis of schwannoma. They suggest, and we concur, that children with acquired oculomotor nerve palsies in whom no causative lesion can be found should undergo imaging studies every year.

**Cyclic oculomotor paresis.** Cyclic oculomotor paresis is a movement disorder usually present at birth, consisting of spasmodic movements of the muscles innervated by the third cranial nerve superimposed on an oculomotor paresis. These movements include lid elevation, adduction, pupillary miosis, and increased accommodation. The spasms occur at regular intervals, lasting 10 to 30 seconds.[41] Thus *cyclic oculomotor paresis* is a misnomer, since the paralysis is present most of the time. A better term would be *cyclic oculomotor spasm in association with oculomotor paresis.*

**Ophthalmoplegic migraine.** Ophthalmoplegic migraine is a rare syndrome that almost always has its onset in childhood. Patients with a migrainous ophthalmoplegia usually develop third cranial nerve palsy as the headache phase

## Management of Nontraumatic Isolated Third Cranial Nerve Palsies

1. In patients over the age of 10 who have pupillary-involving third nerve palsies, perform MRI. If the MRI scan shows either a mass compatible with an aneurysm or nothing, perform an angiogram.
2. Perform MRI in all children under age 10, regardless of the state of the pupil. If the MRI scan is negative, angiography is not necessary because of the low likelihood of aneurysm.
3. Perform MRI in patients between the ages of 10 and 40 who have pupillary-sparing third nerve palsies. If the results are normal, they should have a thorough medical evaluation and be observed sequentially. If the pupil becomes involved or signs and symptoms of subarachnoid hemorrhage develop, immediate angiography is required.
4. Observe patients daily for 5 to 7 days if they are in the vasculopathic age group (over age 40) and have pupillary-sparing (or relative pupillary-sparing) total somatic third nerve palsies. Then see these patients again at 6 weeks.

   An appropriate diagnostic workup includes measurement of the systemic blood pressure and at least a 2-hour postprandial blood glucose.

   Because 10% to 20% of patients with ischemic third nerve palsies have pupillary dysfunction,[35,37] even using these guidelines will result in a certain number of normal angiograms.
5. In patients over the age of 55 with third nerve palsies and symptoms of polymyalgia rheumatica, perform an immediate erythrocyte sedimentation rate, administer appropriate corticosteroid treatment, and perform temporal artery biopsy (see Chapter 2).
6. In patients with aberrant regeneration, except in cases of major head trauma, perform MRI with gadolinium to exclude the presence of a mass lesion.
7. Perform MRI in patients who develop a third cranial nerve palsy following minor head trauma. If the results are normal, follow them.
8. Do not subject patients with an isolated ptosis or dilated fixed pupil to invasive studies unless other signs or symptoms of greater somatic nerve or brainstem involvement become evident.

abates, although it may occur at any time in relation to the pain phase. In fact, the onset of the ptosis in many of these patients is the signal that the headache is about to disappear. The extraocular muscle weakness tends to last longer with each episode, and a few individuals develop a permanent oculomotor paresis[73] (see Chapter 16).

**Minimal trauma.** Parasellar mass lesions are reported to cause the acute onset of a third nerve palsy in association with a history of minimal trauma.[74]

## TROCHLEAR NERVE (FOURTH CRANIAL NERVE)

**ANATOMY.** The trochlear nerves arise from a pair of grouped motor neurons in the ventral mesencephalon under the inferior colliculi, contiguous to the caudal end of the third nerve complex. The fibers course dorsally to decussate completely in the anterior medullary velum, the roof of the fourth ventricle, where the fibers are vulnerable to traumatic injury. They emerge posterior to the inferior colliculi and travel rostrocaudally to enter the cavernous sinus just behind

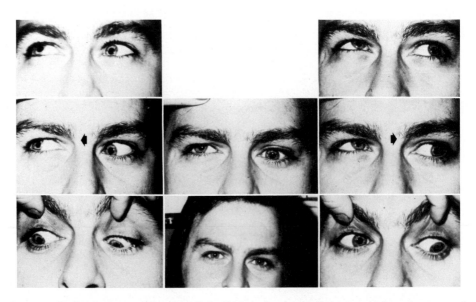

*Fig. 10-5.* Right superior oblique paresis. Patient has right hypertropia in primary position with head held relatively straight *(top middle)*. Patient keeps head tilted to the left to improve alignment and avoid diplopia *(bottom midle)*. Patient demonstrates greatest hypertropia in left gaze and left downgaze positions *(right middle and right bottom)*.

the posterior clinoid process. They lie inferior to the third nerves in the lateral walls of the cavernous sinuses and enter the orbits through the superior orbital fissures.

**FOURTH NERVE PALSIES IN ADULTS** (Fig. 10-5). Prior to 1970, reports of isolated trochlear nerve palsies were rare. Since then the literature has been replete with reports of varying entities causing isolated fourth cranial nerve palsies. This increase is most likely secondary to the improved diagnostic acumen of both ophthalmologists and neurologists. In the most recent series from the Mayo Clinic, Rush and Younge[39] report 172 cases of fourth nerve palsies recognized among 1000 patients with ocular motor palsies seen between 1966 and 1978. This is almost twice the number reported by Rucker in his previous series[37,38] surveying patients seen prior to 1966 in the same institution. The four largest series of fourth nerve palsies are listed in Table 10-3.[37-39,75] In spite of the availability of improved diagnostic techniques, the number of cases remaining without a specific diagnosis is still approximately 30%. The most common cause of fourth cranial nerve palsies is head trauma. Bilateral fourth nerve palsies are often seen following vertex blows to the head, such as occur in motorcycle accidents. The underlying mechanism is believed to be distention of the fourth ventricle, causing a physiologic disruption of the crossing fibers in the anterior medullary velum.

Vascular disease, including hypertension, atherosclerosis, and diabetes mellitus, accounts for approximately one fifth of the cases. Most isolated trochlear nerve palsies occurring in the fourth and fifth decades tend to improve

| TABLE 10-3 | *Comparison of Causes of Fourth Cranial Nerve Palsy* | | | | | | | |

| | Rucker[37] (67 cases) | | Rucker[38] (84 cases) | | Burger et al.[75] (33 cases) | | Rush and Younge[39] (172 cases) | |
|---|---|---|---|---|---|---|---|---|
| | No. | % | No. | % | No. | % | No. | % |
| Aneurysm | 0 | 0 | 0 | 0 | 1 | 3 | 3 | 2 |
| Vascular disease | 24 | 36 | 13 | 15 | 6 | 18 | 32 | 18 |
| Trauma | 24 | 36 | 22 | 27 | 13 | 39 | 55 | 32 |
| Neoplasm | 3 | 4 | 7 | 8 | 7 | 21 | 7 | 4 |
| Undetermined | 9 | 13 | 29 | 33 | 2 | 6 | 62 | 36 |
| Miscellaneous | 7 | 10 | 13 | 15 | 3 | 9 | 13 | 8 |

## Management of Isolated Nontraumatic Fourth Cranial Nerve Palsies

1. Patients of all ages with large vertical fusional amplitudes need no further evaluation. They have decompensating congenital fourth nerve palsies.
2. In patients who are in the nonvasculopathic age group without large vertical fusional amplitudes, and in whom the motility disorder is not quite classic or who demonstrate extraocular muscle fatigue, perform a Tensilon test to exclude myasthenia gravis. If the results are normal, perform MRI to rule out a posterior fossa tumor.
3. Evaluate patients without large fusional amplitudes in the vasculopathic age group for hypertension and diabetes mellitus. Imaging is not necessary, since nonischemic causes of neurologically isolated trochlear nerve palsies are rare.
4. Patients who demonstrate a progression of their fourth nerve palsy or who develop additional signs or symptoms of neurologic disease require thorough medical and imaging evaluation.

spontaneously over a period of 2 to 6 months, suggesting infarction of the peripheral nerve. Grimson and Glaser[76] described six patients with fourth nerve palsies following herpes zoster ophthalmicus. The onset of the fourth nerve palsy occurred from 2 days to 4 weeks following the onset of the cutaneous eruption. Three patients were left with permanent diplopia.

Rush and Younge[39] reported three cases of isolated trochlear nerve palsy due to aneurysm, one in the cavernous sinus. Miscellaneous causes include collagen vascular disease, neonatal hypoxia, hydrocephalus, encephalitis, complications of intracranial surgery, coronary angiography, and bypass surgery.

**FOURTH NERVE PALSIES IN CHILDREN.** In a review of 18 cases of trochlear nerve palsies, Harley[40] reported that the causes were quite different from those found in adults: 12 were considered to be congenital in origin (5 bilateral and 7 unilateral), 5 were secondary to head trauma, and 1 case followed encephalitis.

The sudden onset of an isolated superior oblique palsy in late childhood to the middle to late forties, in the absence of head trauma, should raise the possibility of decompensation of a "presumed" congenital trochlear nerve palsy.[77,78] These patients tend to have large fusional amplitudes, often being able to fuse $10^\Delta$ to $15^\Delta$ vertically from the neutral point. Old photographs demonstrating the presence of a head tilt, even in infancy, are extremely helpful. Vertical prisms often alleviate the patient's symptoms. If the vertical prisms are not successful, a torsional problem is usually present. Under these circumstances a variety of extraocular muscle surgical procedures should be considered.[79]

## ABDUCENS NERVE (SIXTH CRANIAL NERVE)

**ANATOMY.** The sixth cranial nerves arise from a paired group of motor cells whose location is marked as an elevation on the floor of the fourth ventricle (facial colliculi). This elevation is produced by the passage of the axons of the seventh cranial nerves over the sixth nerve nuclei on their way to exit laterally in the brainstem. Each nucleus consists of large motor cells that directly innervate the ipsilateral lateral rectus muscle and a group of smaller cells that innervate one of the medial rectus subnuclei of the contralateral third nerve nucleus.

The motor cells lie dorsal and medial to the vestibular nuclei and lateral to the medial longitudinal bundles. The fascicles course ventrally through the pontine tegmentum, without crossing, to exit ventromedially at the pontomedullary junction. After emerging, they take a sharp turn rostrally, being anchored to the tips of the petrous pyramids by the petrosphenoidal ligaments (Dorello's canals, Gruber's ligaments), to enter the substance of the cavernous sinuses and lie adjacent to the carotid arteries. They enter the orbits through the medial one third of the superior orbital fissures.

**SIXTH NERVE PALSIES IN ADULTS.** Sixth cranial nerve palsies are the most frequently reported ocular motor palsies (see Fig. 10-11). In the four largest series[37-39,80] (Table 10-4) approximately 25% of patients with sixth nerve involvement remained without a diagnosis. In three of these series[37-39] the sixth nerve palsies were not truly isolated. Other neurologic signs were often present. Slavin[81] found that many patients with isolated unilateral abducens palsies have unexplained hyperdeviations ranging from $4^\Delta$ to $18^\Delta$. If the abducens paresis was due to intrinsic brainstem disease, this hypertropia may be nothing more than a skew deviation.

Our clinical impression is that the most common cause of isolated sixth nerve palsy in patients over 40 years of age is infarction of the nerve trunk, as it is in isolated pupillary-sparing third nerve palsy and nontraumatic fourth nerve palsy. These patients often complain initially of periocular or retrobulbar pain for 5 to 7 days. The pain may precede the paresis. These vasculopathic palsies occur with greater frequency in patients with hypertension and diabetes mellitus. As in other mononeuropathies, nerve function typically returns completely within 3 to 6 months, which may be more in keeping with a peripheral rather than a brainstem lesion. On the other hand, as mentioned previously, evidence is accumulating to suggest fascicular infarction within the brainstem as causative. Other causes of sixth nerve palsy include trauma, multiple sclerosis, metastatic tumors, Wernicke's disease, sarcoidosis, mastoiditis, meningitis, migraine, and

| TABLE 10-4 | *Comparison of Causes of Sixth Cranial Nerve Palsy* | | | | | | | |
|---|---|---|---|---|---|---|---|---|
| | Rucker[37] (409 cases) | | Rucker[38] (515 cases) | | Shrader and Schlezinger[80] (104 cases) | | Rush and Younge[39] (419 cases) | |
| | No. | % | No. | % | No. | % | No. | % |
| Aneurysm | 16 | 4 | 15 | 3 | 0 | 0 | 15 | 3 |
| Vascular disease | 57 | 14 | 46 | 9 | 38 | 37 | 74 | 18 |
| Trauma | 57 | 14 | 55 | 11 | 3 | 3 | 70 | 17 |
| Neoplasm | 82 | 20 | 159 | 31 | 7 | 7 | 61 | 15 |
| Multiple sclerosis | 15 | 4 | 36 | 7 | 13 | 13 | 18 | 4 |
| Syphilis | 7 | 2 | 0 | 0 | 10 | 10 | 0 | 0 |
| Undetermined | 129 | 32 | 112 | 21 | 25 | 24 | 124 | 29 |
| Miscellaneous | 46 | 12 | 92 | 18 | 8 | 8 | 57 | 14 |

giant cell arteritis. Unilateral or bilateral abducens paresis may be seen following lumbar puncture or in association with raised intracranial pressure.

In patients with a past history of carcinoma, imaging studies are indicated. Metastatic carcinomas of the breast and prostate have been reported as causes of isolated sixth nerve palsy; these cases may be amenable to radiotherapy or chemotherapeutic intervention.[82,83] Interestingly, these metastatic lesions seem to be indolent, as most were discovered late in the course of the process.[82-84] With the exception of one patient, all of those reported to have such tumors had relatively stable neurologic deficits. Neurosurgical intervention was of little benefit.

Recent evidence indicates that the intramuscular injection of botulinum A toxin into the medial rectus muscle shortly after the onset of an abducens palsy not only allows the patient to maintain a small field of binocular vision, but also prevents the development of spastic contracture of the medial rectus muscle.[85,86] Spastic contracture will leave the patient with restrictive abduction deficit even in the face of full recovery of the sixth nerve paresis. Some believe that botulinum A toxin is of value in relieving contracture in patients with acute thyroid myopathy and in chronic sixth nerve palsies.[85-87]

**Bilateral sixth nerve palsies in adults.** Infarction should not be considered a cause of bilateral sixth nerve palsies at any age. In Keane's inpatient series of 125 cases,[88] 28 (25%) were caused by tumor, 17 (13%) by multiple sclerosis, 16 (14%) by subarachnoid hemorrhage, 12 (10%) by meningeal or parameningeal infection, and 11 (8%) by head trauma. Of the palsies caused by tumor, 56% were believed to be the result of local irritation or compression and 44% the result of increased intracranial pressure or a shift of brain substance related to a remotely situated mass.

Bilateral sixth nerve palsies have been reported following lumbar myelography and lumbar puncture.[89] Occasionally patients with Wernicke's encephalopathy may be seen with bilateral sixth nerve palsies. If such a patient is seen in the emergency room and appears dehydrated or stuporous, the use of intravenous glucose solutions is contraindicated without thiamine supplementation because of the danger of exacerbating Wernicke's encephalopathy.

## Management of Isolated Unilateral Nontraumatic Sixth Cranial Nerve Palsies

1. Patients under the age of 14 years do not require imaging because they are likely to have a benign sixth nerve palsy, unless they develop additional signs or symptoms of neurologic disease. Discuss with the parents the possibility that a compressive lesion may be present. If the parents are uncomfortable with not explicitly excluding the presence of a mass lesion, obtain an MRI scan.

   Initially we see these children every 2 weeks for 6 weeks to determine if the paresis is progressing or if additional neurologic problems are developing.

   If incomplete or no improvement occurs over a period of 6 months and the paresis remains isolated, obtain an MRI scan even though most such studies tend to be normal. These patients should undergo horizontal muscle surgery only after a period of 6 to 9 months has elapsed.

2. Patients between the ages of 15 and 40 years represent a controversial management problem. Although in many of these patients the problem is benign and remitting, we recommend MRI. If the MRI scan is negative, a thorough medical and neurologic examination, including a lumbar puncture, is indicated to exclude such entities as hypertension, collagen vascular disease, multiple sclerosis, Lyme disease,[98] and lues.

   If these investigations are negative, see the patient again in 6 weeks. If other systemic or neurologic abnormalities develop, if the paresis worsens, or if at 6 months after onset no improvement has occurred, completely reevaluate these patients, including imaging.[99]

3. Patients over age 40 should undergo a general medical evaluation, including a 2-hour postprandial blood glucose. If a patient over age 55 has symptoms of polymyalgia rheumatica, determine the erythrocyte sedimentation rate. Any patient with a sixth nerve paresis that has not remitted within 6 months should undergo imaging to exclude the presence of a basisphenoidal tumor.[82;83]

4. Suspect children and adults with bilateral sixth nerve palsies who do not have a history of severe head trauma of having raised intracranial pressure or meningeal-based disease. Obtain thorough imaging studies and if normal perform a lumbar puncture.

5. In any infant or child with an ocular motor paresis, always consider the diagnosis of battered child syndrome. Seek other stigmas of such maltreatment, such as bruises, basilar skull fracture, long bone fractures, and retinal hemorrhages.

**SIXTH NERVE PALSIES IN CHILDREN.** In children the abducens nerve is the most commonly affected of the ocular motor nerves, accounting for approximately 95% of the cases in Harley's series.[40] Trauma and neoplastic disease accounted for 40% and 33% of cases, respectively. Robertson et al.[90] reviewed 133 cases of acquired sixth nerve palsy in children and found that 52 cases (38%) were due to primary brainstem gliomas. In 15 (11%) of the 133 cases, an isolated abducens palsy was the first sign of disease. Packer et al.[91] emphasized the dismal course in children with brainstem gliomas. These tumors spread by infiltration, causing multiple cranial nerve deficits, pyramidal tract dysfunction, and cerebellar ataxia. One third of their patients (5 of 15) developed meningeal gliomatosis, and 3 of these patients had meningeal symptoms before other signs of posterior fossa involvement. Although cerebrospinal fluid (CSF) studies were universally abnormal, malignant cells were detected in the CSF in only one patient. Most of these patients die of local recurrence following a course of radiation therapy, with a median survival of 12 to 15 months.[92,93]

Of the 10 patients originally diagnosed as having Gradenigo's syndrome (a sixth nerve palsy with ipsilateral ear and facial pain) reported by Robertson et al.,[90] 3 subsequently proved to have mass lesions. With the exception of cases involving tumors, the prognosis for spontaneous improvement in their series was excellent. Robertson et al. found that any improvement in sixth nerve function was complete within 4 months of onset.

Knox et al.[94] and Robertson et al.[90] noted the occurrence of benign abducens nerve palsies in children. These pareses are always isolated and resolve within 10 to 16 weeks. A history of recent viral illness,[94] including varicella[95] or immunization,[96] is helpful but not necessary. Such postviral syndromes are benign; thus invasive procedures should be avoided unless progression occurs. These palsies may be recurrent and eventually may leave the patient with a persistent abduction deficit.[96,97]

**Bilateral sixth nerve palsies in children.** In an infant with symptoms of what appears to be bilateral abducens nerve palsies, the diagnosis of childhood strabismus should be considered. Lifting the child up, holding the child at arms' length, and spinning the child around with the examiner as the fulcrum will fail to induce full ocular rotations if the problem is one of abducens paresis. Robertson et al.[90] found that about 20% (29 of 133) of sixth nerve palsies in children were bilateral. Ten children had primary brainstem gliomas, five children had palsies associated with trauma, and seven children had inflammatory disease.

## NONISOLATED OCULAR MOTOR PALSIES

The topographic diagnosis of a lesion in a patient with nonisolated ocular motor palsy depends on the various combinations of associated neurologic deficits.

**INTRAAXIAL PALSIES.** The third nerve nucleus and fascicles are in close proximity to the medial longitudinal bundles, the red nucleus, the brachium conjunctivum, the substantia nigra, and pyramidal tracts. Involvement of the third nerve fascicles and the red nucleus produces an ipsilateral oculomotor paresis with an intention tremor of the contralateral foot, arm, and hand (Benedikt's syndrome).[44] Involvement of the pyramidal tract produces ipsilateral oculomotor paresis and contralateral hemiplegia (Weber's syndrome). Cerebellar ataxia with either unilateral or bilateral involvement of the oculomotor nerve due to midline lesions is called Nothnagel's syndrome. Various combinations of vertical gaze paresis, with or without convergence retraction nystagmus, may be associated with brainstem involvement of the oculomotor complex.

The fourth nerve nucleus is contiguous with the end of the oculomotor nucleus, and thus processes involving the third nerve nucleus may also involve the trochlear nucleus. Since the trochlear nerve exits the brainstem dorsally, it is less frequently associated with intraparenchymal pathology than either the third or sixth cranial nerves. Guy et al.[100] reported two patients with contralateral trochlear nerve paresis and ipsilateral Horner's syndrome due to intrinsic brainstem disease. This is due to a process involving the fourth cranial nerve nucleus

***Abduction Deficits***

1. Abducens paresis
   a. Simple abducens paresis
   b. Duane's syndrome
2. Pseudo–abducens paresis
   a. Restricted medial rectus muscle
      (1) Graves' ophthalmopathy
      (2) Inflammatory pseudotumor (myositis)
      (3) Orbital trauma (entrapment, muscle damage)
   b. Spasm of the near reflex
   c. Thalamic esotropia
   d. Myasthenia gravis

or the fascicles prior to decussation and the adjacent descending sympathetic fibers (first order neurons).

The abducens nucleus consists of both large and small motor cells and serves as the final center for all horizontal conjugate gaze movements. It is adjacent to a large number of structures associated with ocular movements, including medial longitudinal bundles, the paramedian pontine reticular formation, and the vestibular nuclei. In addition, the fibers of the seventh nerve loop around the sixth nerve nucleus, and the first order neurons subserving the sympathetic innervation to the iris travel laterally adjacent to the descending sensory root of the trigeminal nerve in the tegmentum. The fascicles of the abducens nerve pass through the corticospinal tracts as they exit the brain ventrally.

Pathologic processes involving the pons in the region of the sixth nerve nuclei can produce a variety of distinctive syndromes: (1) Foville's syndrome (anterior inferior cerebellar artery syndrome), which includes ipsilateral paralysis of gaze, facial palsy, loss of taste from the anterior two thirds of the tongue, Horner's syndrome, facial analgesia, and deafness; (2) Millard-Gubler syndrome, which includes ipsilateral sixth nerve paralysis with a contralateral hemiplegia; and (3) Duane's syndrome.

**Duane's syndrome.** The ophthalmologist or neurologist is often asked to evaluate a child or adult without diplopia who has "suddenly" been noted to have an abduction deficit and is presumed to have an abducens palsy. As mentioned previously, causes of apparent ocular motor palsies include both restrictive disease and myasthenia gravis (see box). On careful observation some such patients will demonstrate an adduction limitation as well, accompanied by retraction of the globe with narrowing of the palpebral fissure. Up or down shooting of the globe may be seen on attempted adduction as well. The patient may be orthophoric with or without a compensatory head turn to maintain single binocular vision or have a manifest misalignment. The condition may be bilateral, in which case retraction may be seen in vertical gaze as well.[101]

Such patients have Duane's syndrome,[102] which is due to agenesis of the abducens nerve and its nucleus. Aberrant innervation of the lateral rectus muscle from various branches of the third cranial nerve accounts for the variations seen both clinically and electromyographically.[103,104] A careful examination of old pictures, along with the absence of diplopia and the classical clinical findings, makes further evaluation unnecessary.

In addition, various combinations of sixth nerve paresis associated with horizontal gaze palsies and nystagmus should suggest pontine disease. Such findings have been reported following chiropractic manipulation.[105,106]

**EXTRAAXIAL PALSIES.** Sixth nerve paresis associated with fifth (corneal sensation), seventh, and eighth (vestibular and auditory) nerve dysfunction can occur with a cerebellopontine angle tumor. The acute onset of a sixth nerve palsy associated with ipsilateral facial or retroauricular pain, at any age, implies an inflammatory or neoplastic lesion involving the tip of the petrous pyramid. High-resolution CT scanning of this region including the mastoid bone is necessary. In an endemic area the onset of a cranial mononeuropathy should suggest the possibility of Lyme neuroborreliosis,[98] especially if the patient has a history of a rash (typically erythema chronicum migrans) or tick bite.

In children a sixth nerve paresis associated with ipsilateral facial pain and hearing loss indicates an osteitis of the tip of the petrous pyramid secondary to a chronic mastoiditis or middle ear infection (Gradenigo's syndrome). Involvement of the petrous pyramid by other processes such as cholesteatoma or metastatic carcinoma (usually in adults) produces a similar syndrome but without hearing loss and with less pain. The diagnosis in all of these cases is made most accurately with CT scanning.

## COMBINED THIRD, FOURTH, AND SIXTH NERVE PALSIES

Unilateral ophthalmoplegia involving the third, fourth, and sixth cranial nerves can be evaluated with the following scheme. Accompanying pain or altered sensation in the distribution of the first division of the trigeminal nerve with optic nerve involvement most likely implies orbital pathology. From the anterior cavernous sinus to the superior orbital fissure, the involved nerves can be the first division of the fifth nerve and the third, fourth, and sixth nerves. In lesions of the region of the posterior to midcavernous sinus, the involved nerves could include the first or second division of the fifth nerve and the third, fourth, and sixth nerves.

Inflammatory disease in this region can produce painful ophthalmoplegia, such as Tolosa-Hunt syndrome.[107,108] Cranial nerves II, III, IV, $V_1$, and VI are variably affected. The response to moderately high doses of oral corticosteroids (prednisone, 100 mg) is dramatic, with pain relief within 24 to 36 hours. Recovery of cranial nerve dysfunction lags behind the relief of pain.

In the retrocavernous space all three divisions of the trigeminal nerve can be involved, in addition to the optic chiasm or optic tract. The presence of other brainstem signs, of course, suggests posterior fossa disease.

Bilateral ophthalmoplegia is indicative of more widespread pathology. Lesions at the base of the brain or involving midline structures must be excluded. In all of these cases the particular distribution of neurologic deficits will mandate the appropriate diagnostic tests, including neuroradiologic, general medical, and CSF evaluation. The consecutive involvement of cranial nerves on both sides should suggest the possible diagnosis of a nasopharyngeal carcinoma. Focused imaging will identify most cases of nasopharyngeal lesions. In all cases in which multiple cranial nerve palsies are associated with polyradiculopathy, the diagnosis of AIDS or cytomegalic inclusion virus disease should be considered.

Two other entities should be included in the differential diagnosis of patients with ocular motor paresis: botulism and acute infectious polyradiculoneuropathy.

**BOTULISM.** Botulism may present in one of two forms: (1) floppy infant syndrome[109-111] in the first year of life secondary to colonization of the gut with *Clostridium botulinum* or (2) an acute form at any age following the ingestion of contaminated food.[112,113] The clinical syndrome this organism produces is due to the release of a species-specific exotoxin (A to E)[114] that interferes with cholinergic transmission. The exotoxins most often associated with ocular dysfunction are A and B.[114,115] The typical clinical picture of an alert patient with a dry mouth, swallowing difficulties, and flaccid paresis or weakness should alert the physician to the possibility of ingestion of botulinum toxin. The finding of dilated sluggish pupils with ptosis is an ominous sign, since these signs are present in almost all individuals who develop respiratory distress.[113] These patients are said to have accommodative paresis, but in most cases this is presumed on the basis of a complaint of blurred vision. The diagnosis is made by injecting graded dilutions of the sera from suspected cases into laboratory animals and determining the dilution that causes death by respiratory paresis. Treatment includes the use of polyvalent antitoxin and supportive care in cases of acute poisoning and decontamination of the gut with antibiotics in cases of floppy infant syndrome.

**ACUTE INFECTIOUS POLYRADICULONEUROPATHY.** Acute, infectious, demyelinating polyradiculoneuropathy can occur in an ascending Guillain-Barré-Strohl syndrome[116-118] or a bulbar variant described by Fisher[119] and others.[120] In the former state an ascending paresis with variable sensory loss progresses to involve the bulbar musculature, producing some degree of facial diplegia and unilateral or bilateral ocular motor palsies. If the oculomotor nerves are involved, usually both an internal and an external ophthalmoplegia is evident. The Fisher variant of the disease is characterized by areflexia, ataxia, and ocular motor palsies. In both syndromes involvement of the bulbar musculature may lead to respiratory and swallowing difficulties. These syndromes commonly follow a presumed "viral" illness.[116] Both variants are postulated to be due to a lymphocyte-mediated demyelination of the nerve roots, but this does not adequately explain the ataxia.

The diagnosis is confirmed by the finding of albuminocytologic dissociation on examination of the CSF (i.e, elevated protein in the absence of a pleocytosis). Systemic corticosteroids are indicated in cases of involvement of the bulbar musculature, but their efficacy remains open to question.[121] Plasmapheresis has been advocated early in patients with severe disease,[118,122] with a beneficial effect demonstrated with the use of continuous flow machines.[122] Therapy is supportive, including respiratory assistance in severe cases.

# Appendix

## ISOLATION OF PARETIC MUSCLE(S)

To isolate a single paretic muscle, if present, the examiner must determine the type of misalignment and its variability in various gaze positions, as well as the effect of head tilt maneuvers.

The first step is to establish whether the misalignment is horizontal, vertical, or diagonal. Place a red glass in front of the right eye and instruct the patient to show you how far apart the images are using fingers. By doing this, the patient will demonstrate whether the image separation is (1) horizontal (horizontal rectus muscles at fault) (Fig. 10-6) or (2) vertical or diagonal (vertical rectus or oblique muscles at fault) (Figs. 10-7 through 10-10).

**IDENTIFICATION OF PARETIC MUSCLE(S) IN HORIZONTAL MISALIGNMENT.** Having placed the red glass over the right eye, ask the patient if the red image is to the left or right of the white image. If the red image is to the left (crossed diplopia), the eyes are exotropic. Conversely, if the red image is to the right (uncrossed diplopia), the eyes are esotropic, as in Fig. 10-6. Thus the number of possible muscles involved is reduced to two. Place a dotted circle around the two medial rectus muscles or the two lateral recti.

In the case diagrammed (Fig. 10-6), the esotropia is greatest in right gaze, the gaze position in which the right lateral rectus muscle and the left medial rectus muscle are activated. Now place a circle around these two muscles. In the face of a horizontal misalignment, when two circles are placed around a muscle the paretic muscle has been identified, in this case the right lateral rectus muscle.

If a patient has a comitant (nonparalytic) strabismus, determine misalignment in the straight up and down position. Some of these patients demonstrate a quantitative change in the degree of misalignment between up, primary, and down positions. This variation is called vertical incomitance* and, according to the measurements, constitutes an **A** or **V** pattern.

**IDENTIFICATION OF PARETIC MUSCLE(S) IN VERTICAL MISALIGNMENT.** When examining a patient who complains of vertical or diagonal diplopia, ask if the red image is higher or lower, or have the patient point to the red light (Fig. 10-7). The hypertropic eye always produces the lower image. If the patient has a right hypertropia, the involved muscles are either the depressors of the right eye or the elevators of the left eye, and vice versa for a left hypertropia. The number of possibly affected muscles is thus reduced to four.

The number of possibly affected muscles can be further reduced to two by determining whether the misalignment is greater in right or left gaze (Fig. 10-8). These diagrams now reveal that of the two possible involved muscles, one has a

---

*Specifically, if a patient has an esotropia (i.e., is cross-eyed) and the horizontal misalignment is greater in upgaze than in downgaze, the patient has an **A** pattern esotropia. If the misalignment is greater in downgaze, the patient has a **V** pattern esotropia. The opposite is true for exotropia: if the misalignment is greater in upgaze, the pattern is a **V**; and if the misalignment is greater in downgaze, the pattern is an **A**.

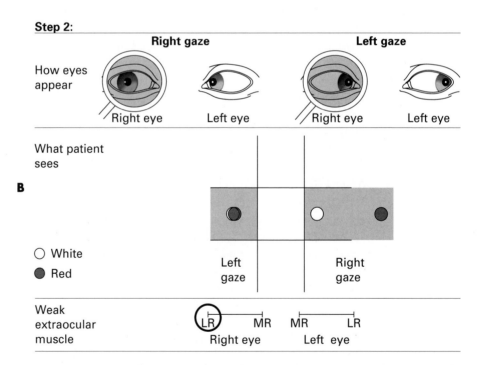

**Primary position**

How eyes
appear
(right lateral
rectus palsy)

Right eye     Left eye

**A**

What patient
sees

Left
gaze          Right
gaze

○ White
● Red

Possible weak
extraocular muscles

LR      MR    MR      LR

Right eye     Left eye

Step 2:

Right gaze                    Left gaze

How eyes
appear

Right eye    Left eye    Right eye    Left eye

What patient
sees

**B**

○ White
● Red

Left
gaze          Right
gaze

Weak
extraocular
muscle

LR      MR    MR      LR

Right eye     Left eye

*Fig. 10-6.* Isolating weak extraocular muscle in incomitant horizontal ocular misalignment. **A,** Step 1. Clinician notes relative location of red and white images as perceived by patient, whose eyes are in primary position (red glass in front of right eye). If there is a single paretic muscle, it may be either of the two lateral recti. **B,** Step 2. Clinician notes diplopia pattern in extremes of right and left gaze. Misalignment increases in right gaze. Right gaze is field of action of right lateral rectus muscle, and therefore the diagnosis of sixth nerve palsy is likely.

**Step 1:**

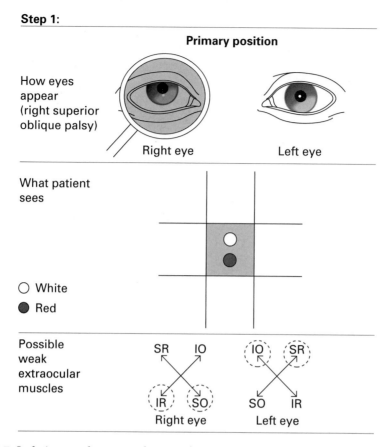

*Fig. 10-7.* Isolating weak extraocular muscle in incomitant vertical ocular misalignment: step 1. Solid circle represents red image as appreciated by patient, and open circle represents untinted image. In this example patient notes that diplopia is vertical and that red image (right eye) is lower, indicating that right eye is hypertropic (higher) eye, since image of hypertropic eye, by the laws of projection, is always the lower image. A right hypertropia can be produced by underaction of depressor muscles of right eye or elevator muscles of left eye. Thus at this point the number of involved extraocular muscles can be reduced to four.

field of action in upgaze and the other in downgaze (Fig. 10-9); thus it would appear that the final step is to determine if the misalignment is greater in right or left upgaze than in downgaze. If this is the case, the paretic muscle is identified by the field of action in which the patient demonstrates the greatest separation of images; however, patients who develop a vertical misalignment that becomes chronic often lose their vertical incomitance. (No measurable change occurs in misalignment in upgaze and downgaze.) This lack of a change in misalignment, or vertical comitance, is due to an adaptive phenomenon termed *inhibitional palsy of the contralateral antagonist.*[3] For example, if a patient has a right superior oblique paresis, with time an underaction of the left superior rectus muscle will develop. The yoke or agonist muscle of the right superior oblique muscle is the left inferior rectus muscle. The left superior rectus muscle

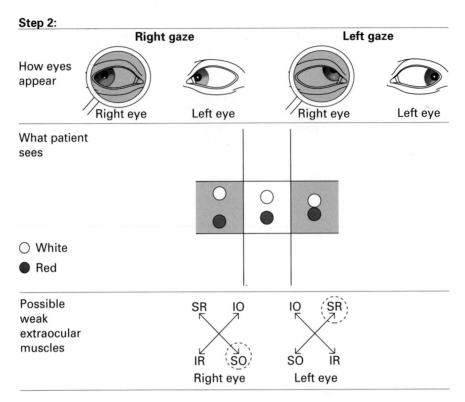

*Fig. 10-8.* Isolating weak extraocular muscle in incomitant ocular vertical misalignment: step 2. Patient is instructed to either judge or demonstrate change in image separation when object is placed first in right gaze and then in left gaze. In this example clinician notes that image separation is greatest on left gaze, reducing the possible weak extraocular muscles to two (i.e., muscles that act in left gaze being either right superior oblique muscle or left superior rectus muscle). Solid circle represents red image as perceived by patient's right eye, and open circle represents untinted image as perceived by patient's left eye.

*Fig. 10-9.* Isolating weak extraocular muscle in incomitant verticular ocular misalignment: step 3. **A,** In this example clinician notes that image separation in left gaze as reflected by patient is greatest in downgaze, or in field of action of right superior oblique muscle; thus it is the underacting extraocular muscle, suggesting a fourth cranial nerve palsy. **B,** Here clinician notes that image separation remains equal in all three positions of right gaze. A fourth step is now necessary to identify involved weak or underacting extraocular muscle (i.e., Bielschowsky head tilt test [see Fig. 10-10]).

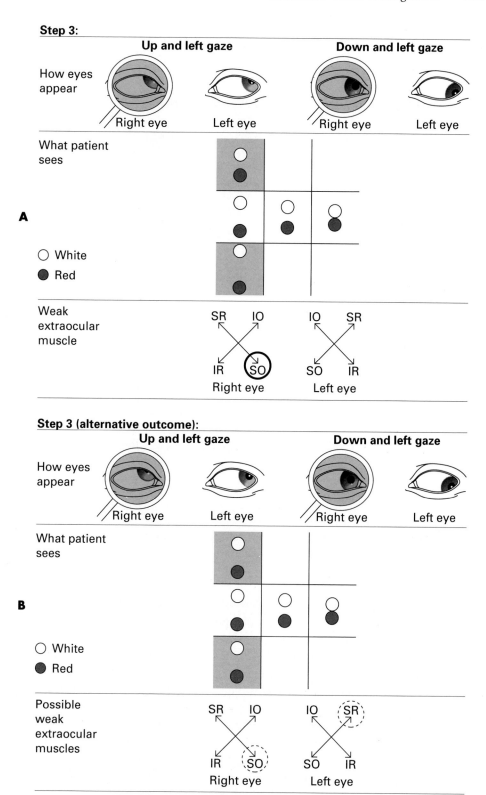

*Fig. 10-9.* For legend see opposite page.

**Step 4:**

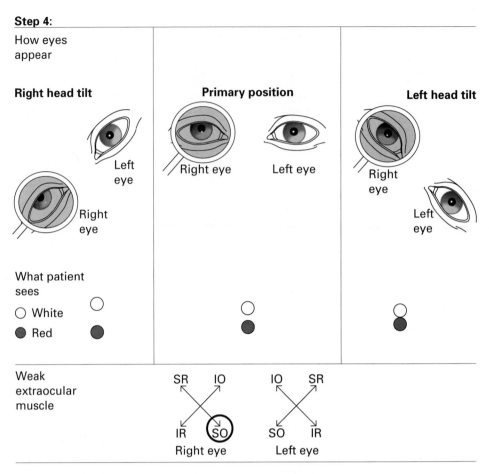

*Fig. 10-10.* Isolating weak extraocular muscle in incomitant vertical ocular misalignment: step 4. Bielschowsky head tilt test is performed by first having patient tilt head to the right and then to the left, quantifying image separation in each position. In this case image separation is greatest on right head tilt, a phenomenon virtually diagnostic of right superior oblique palsy.

is the direct antagonist of the left inferior rectus muscle or the contralateral antagonist of the right superior oblique muscle. Thus in a patient with a long-standing right superior oblique muscle paresis, a paresis of the left superior rectus muscle will be suggested. This adaptation, termed *spread of comitance,* is believed to be under cerebellar control.

In patients with vertical diplopia, additional information can be obtained by using the Bielschowsky head tilt test[1,4,123-126] (Fig. 10-10). The measured vertical misalignment increases when the head is tilted toward the side of the paretic muscle if the ipsilateral intorting muscles (the superior oblique and superior rectus muscles) are paretic, and to the opposite side if the extorting inferior muscles (inferior rectus and inferior oblique) are paretic. Misleading results can be obtained in the Bielschowsky test if the eyes are not maintained in the primary (straight-ahead) position.

**A**                    **B**

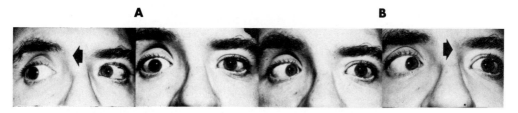

*Fig. 10-11.* Primary and secondary deviation. **A,** Esotropia with right (paretic) eye fixating (secondary deviation). **B,** Greater esotropia with left (nonparetic) eye fixating (primary deviation).

Since the head tilt test is dependent on gravitational changes on the utriculus of the vestibular apparatus, the patient must be sitting or standing for the test to work.

**PRIMARY AND SECONDARY DEVIATIONS.** In patients with the acute onset of an ocular motor palsy, the measured misalignment usually varies if the measurement is made with the patient first fixing with the involved eye and then with the uninvolved eye, or vice versa. The primary deviation is defined as the misalignment noted when the noninvolved eye (normal) is fixating (Fig. 10-11). The secondary deviation is that misalignment present when the eye with the affected muscle(s) is fixating. If the misalignment differs when fixating with one eye versus the other, nuclear or infranuclear pathology, either paretic or restrictive, is indicated. The larger deviation (greatest separation of images) occurs when the paretic eye is fixing (secondary deviation). The results of testing for such a change in misalignment are often equivocal late in the evolution of many cranial nerve palsies, especially those of great chronicity, such as "congenital" superior oblique palsies.

**TORSIONAL DIPLOPIA.** Many patients with paresis of oblique muscles (rarely with vertical rectus muscles) experience torsional diplopia with tilting of one or both images. This symptom may be accompanied by dizziness and nausea. Some patients experience a peculiar perception of the entire environment leaning in a particular direction. Torsional symptoms may occur with or without vertical misalignment.[79]

The demonstration of a torsional misalignment is helpful in isolating the paretic vertical muscle when spread of comitance has developed. The presence of a torsional misalignment is best demonstrated using double Maddox rods[127] (Fig. 10-12). Place the rods in the front cells of a trial frame with the bars parallel to the 0- to 180-degree axis. Place the appropriate spherical correction for distance in the back cell. Position the patient's head in the erect position and instruct the patient to look at a distance fixation light. Then tell the patient to turn the control knob until the two linear images are parallel and perpendicular to the horizon (straight up and down) (Fig. 10-13). Read the induced torsion secondary to the paresis in degrees from the 0- to 180-degree or the 90- to 270-degree axis on the trial frame. This test is invaluable for determining the presence

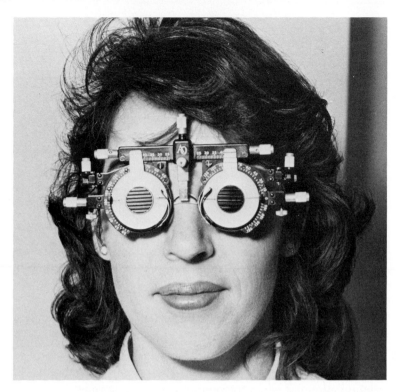

*Fig. 10-12.* Patient wearing double Maddox rod. The two Maddox rods are placed in trial frame in such a manner that both lines formed are perpendicular to horizon.

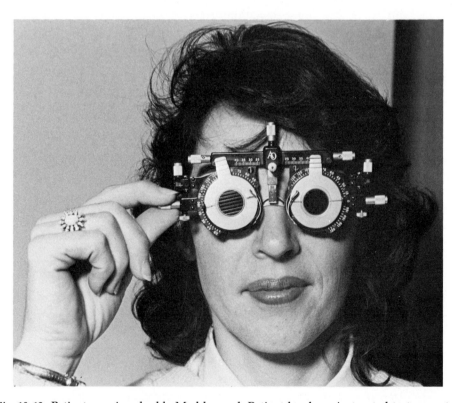

*Fig. 10-13.* Patient wearing double Maddox rod. Patient has been instructed to turn anterior cells to set linear images perpendicular to horizon and parallel to each other. Amount of induced cyclotorsion is then read in degrees of arc directly from trial frame.

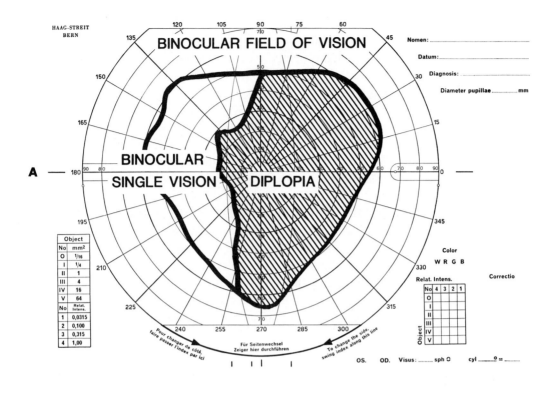

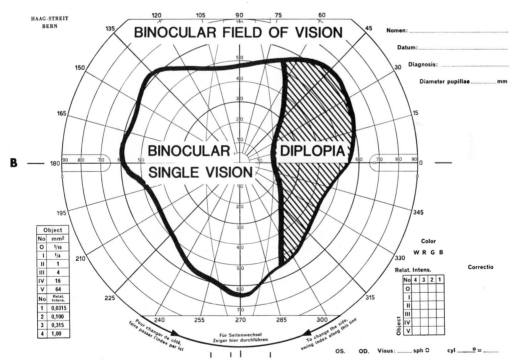

*Fig. 10-14.* **A,** Field of binocular single vision in patient with acute sixth nerve palsy secondary to trauma. **B,** Field of binocular single vision 3 months later.

of a torsional misalignment without vertical misalignment and for following the progression or regression of fourth cranial nerve palsies. The presence of any amount of torsion in a symptomatic patient is pathologic; a measured torsional misalignment that exceeds 10 degrees strongly suggests the diagnosis of bilateral superior oblique palsy.

**QUANTITATING CHANGES IN THE DEVIATION OVER TIME.** Repeatable quantitation of either the progression or regression of an extraocular muscle palsy is most easily achieved using the binocular single vision test adapted to the bowl perimeter.[128] In this test the patient is seated at a bowl perimeter (kinetic variety) with both eyes open, the head erect and centered, and the chin and head rest adjusted so that the fixation target is centered at eye level. Place the $III_4e$ test target within the patient's field of binocular single vision and instruct the patient to follow the light with the eyes. Move the light rapidly and outward in all directions, and ask the patient to report the onset of diplopia. The test quantitatively produces an outline of the area of binocular single vision (Fig. 10-14, *A*), can be performed in less than 10 minutes, and over time determines the stability of a given paresis (Fig. 10-14, *B*). Similar results can be obtained with the use of the Hess or Lees screen.

## REFERENCES

1. Feldon SE, Burde RM, Walonker CV. The extraocular muscles. In: Moses RA, Hart WM, eds. Adler's physiology of the eye. 8th ed. St Louis: Mosby–Year Book, 1987:89-182.
2. Hering E. Die Lehre vom binocullaren Sehen. Leipzig, Germany: Engelmann, 1868.
3. Hering E. Dr. Raumsin und die Bewegungen der Auges. In: Hermann L, ed. Handbuch der physiologie, vol 3, pt 1. 1879. English translation by CA Radde. Baltimore: American Academy of Optometry, 1942.
4. Roper-Hall G, Burde RM. The extraocular muscles. III. Clinical analysis of extraocular muscle paralysis. In: Moses RA, ed. Adler's physiology of the eye. 7th ed. St Louis: Mosby–Year Book, 1981:166-83.
5. Safran AB, Roth A. Using a slit lamp for the neuro-ophthalmologic evaluation of old photographs. Am J Ophthalmol 1983;95:558.
6. Gamblin GT, Harper DG, Galentine P, et al. Prevalence of increased intraocular pressure in Graves' disease—evidence of frequent subclinical ophthalmopathy. N Engl J Med 1983;308:420-4.
7. Zappia RJ, Winkelman JZ, Gay AJ. Intraocular pressure changes in normal subjects and the adhesive muscle syndrome. Am J Ophthalmol 1971;71:880-3.
8. Sergott RC, Glaser JS. Graves' ophthalmopathy: a clinical and immunologic review. Surv Ophthalmol 1981;26:1-21.
9. Burde RM. Graves' ophthalmopathy and the special problem of concomitant ocular myasthenia gravis. Am Orthoptic J 1990;40:37-50.
10. Hermann JS. Acquired Brown's syndrome of inflammatory origin: response to locally injected steroids. Arch Ophthalmol 1978;96:1228-32.
11. Wang FM, Wertenbaker C, Behrens MM, et al. Acquired Brown's syndrome in children with juvenile rheumatoid arthritis. Ophthalmology 1984;91:23-6.
12. Osserman KE. Ocular myasthenia gravis. Invest Ophthalmol 1967;6:277-87.
13. Grob D. Course and management of myasthenia gravis. JAMA 1953;153:529-32.
14. Moorthy G, Behrens MM, Drachman DB, et al. Ocular pseudomyasthenia

or ocular myasthenia "plus": a warning to clinicians. Neurology 1989; 39:1150-4.

15. Dirr LY, Donofrio PD, Patton JF, et al. A false-positive edrophonium test in a patient with brainstem glioma. Neurology 1989;39:865-7.

16. Schwab RS, Perlo VP. Syndromes simulating myasthenia gravis. Ann NY Acad Sci 1966;135:350-66.

17. Eaton L. As quoted in Retzlaff JA, Kearns TP, Howard FM Jr, et al. Lancaster red-green test in evaluation of edrophonium effect in myasthenia gravis. Am J Ophthalmol 1969;67:13-21.

18. Cogan DG. Myasthenia gravis: a review of the disease and a description of lid twitch as a characteristic sign. Arch Ophthalmol 1965;74:217-21.

19. Osher RH, Griggs RC. Orbicularis fatigue: the "peek" sign of myasthenia gravis. Arch Ophthalmol 1979;94:677-9.

20. Retzlaff JA, Kearns TP, Howard FM Jr, et al. Lancaster red-green test in evaluation of edrophonium effect in myasthenia gravis. Am J Ophthalmol 1969;67:13-21.

21. Miller NR, Morris JE, Maquire M. Combined use of neostigmine and ocular motility measurements in the diagnosis of myasthenia gravis. Arch Ophthalmol 1982;100:761-3.

22. Van Dyk HJL, Florence L. The Tensilon test: a safe office procedure. Ophthalmology 1980;87:210-2.

23. Fischer KC, Schwartzman RJ. Oral corticosteroids in the treatment of ocular myasthenia gravis. Neurology 1974;24:795-8.

24. Seybold ME, Drachman DB. Gradually increasing doses of prednisone in myasthenia gravis: reducing the hazards of treatment. N Engl J Med 1974;290:81-4.

25. Warwick R. Representation of the extra-ocular muscles in the oculomotor nuclei of the monkey. J Comp Neurol 1953;98:449-503.

26. Porter JD, Guthrie BL, Sparks DL. Innervation of monkey extraocular muscles: localization of sensory and motor neurons by retrograde transport of horseradish peroxidase. J Comp Neurol 1983;218:208-19.

27. Burde RM, Loewy AD. Central origin of oculomotor parasympathethic neurons in the monkey. Brain Res 1980;198:434-9.

28. Sibony PA, Evinger C, Lessell S. Retrograde horseradish peroxidase transport after oculomotor nerve injury. Invest Ophthalmol Vis Sci 1986;27:975-80.

29. Büttner-Ennever JA, Akert K. Medial rectus subgroups of the oculomotor nucleus and their abducens internuclear input in the monkey. J Comp Neurol 1981;197:17-24.

30. Bienfang DC. Crossing axons in the third nerve nucleus. Invest Ophthalmol 1975;14:927-31.

31. Guy JR, Day AL. Intracranial aneurysms with superior division paresis of the oculomotor nerve. Ophthalmology 1989;96:1071-6.

32. Ksiazek SM, Repka MX, Maguire A, et al. Divisional oculomotor nerve paresis caused by intrinsic brainstem disease. Ann Neurol 1989;26:714-8.

33. Kerr FWL, Hollowell OW. Location of pupillomotor and accommodation fibres in the oculomotor nerve: experimental observations on paralytic mydriasis. J Neurol Neurosurg Psychiatry 1964;27:473-81.

34. Sunderland S, Hughes ESR. The pupillo-constrictor pathway and the nerves to the ocular muscles in man. Brain 1946;69:301-9.

35. Goldstein JE, Cogan DG. Diabetic ophthalmoplegia with special reference to the pupil. Arch Ophthalmol 1960;64:592-600.

36. Green WR, Hackett ER, Schlezinger NS. Neuro-ophthalmologic evaluation of oculomotor nerve paralysis. Arch Ophthalmol 1964;72:154-67.

37. Rucker CW. Paralysis of the third, fourth and sixth cranial nerves. Am J Ophthalmol 1958;46:787-94.

38. Rucker CW. The causes of paralysis of the third, fourth and sixth cranial nerves. Am J Ophthalmol 1966;61:1293-8.

39. Rush JA, Younge BR. Paralysis of cranial nerves III, IV, and VI: cause and

prognosis in 1,000 cases. Arch Ophthalmol 1981;99:76-9.

40. Harley RD. Paralytic strabismus in children: etiologic incidence and management of the third, fourth, and sixth nerve palsies. Ophthalmology 1980; 87:24-43.

41. Loewenfeld IE, Thompson HS. Oculomotor paresis with cyclic spasms: a critical review of the literature and a new case. Surv Ophthalmol 1975; 20:81-124.

42. Hopf HC, Gutmann L. Diabetic 3rd nerve palsy: evidence for a mesencephalic lesion. Neurology 1990; 40:1041-5.

43. Roper-Hall G, Burde RM. Inferior rectus palsies as a manifestation of atypical IIIrd cranial nerve disease. Am Orthopt J 1975;25:122-30.

44. Warren W, Burde RM, Klingele TG, et al. Atypical oculomotor paresis. J Clin Neuro Ophthalmol 1982;2:13-8.

45. Hollenhorst RW, Brown JR, Wagener HP, et al. Neurologic aspects of temporal arteritis. Neurology 1960;10:490-8.

46. Barricks ME, Traviesa DB, Glaser JS, et al. Ophthalmoplegia in cranial arteritis. Brain 1977;100:209-21.

47. Kissel JT, Burde RM, Klingele TG, et al. Pupil-sparing oculomotor palsies with internal carotid-posterior communicating artery aneurysms. Ann Neurol 1983;13:149-54.

48. O'Connor PS, Tredici TJ, Green RP. Pupil-sparing third nerve palsies caused by aneurysm. Am J Ophthalmol 1983;95:395-7.

49. Dreyfus PM, Hakim S, Adams RD. Diabetic ophthalmoplegia: report of case, with postmortem study and comments on vascular supply of human oculomotor nerve. Arch Neurol Psychiatry 1957;77:337-49.

50. Asbury AK, Aldredge H, Hershberg R, et al. Oculomotor palsy in diabetes mellitus: a clinico-pathological study. Brain 1970;93:555-66.

51. Larson DL, Auchincloss JH. Multiple symmetric bilateral cranial nerve palsies in patients with unregulated diabetes mellitus: report of 3 cases. Arch Intern Med 1950;85:265-71.

52. Sergott RC, Glaser JS, Berger LJ. Simultaneous, bilateral diabetic ophthalmoplegia: report of two cases and discussion of differential diagnosis. Ophthalmology 1984;91:18-22.

53. Hepler RS, Cantu RC. Aneurysms and third nerve palsies: ocular status of survivors. Arch Ophthalmol 1967; 77:604-8.

54. Holland G. Elektromyographische Untersuchungen bei Fehlleitung regenerierender Nervenfasern nach Okulomotoriusparese. Klin Monatsbl Augenheilkd 1964;144:686-96.

55. Guy J, Engel HM, Lessner AM. Acquired contralateral oculomotor synkinesis. Arch Neurol 1989;46:1021-3.

56. Lepore FE, Glaser JS. Misdirection revisited: a critical appraisal of acquired oculomotor nerve synkinesis. Arch Ophthalmol 1980;98:2206-9.

57. Johnson LN, Pack WL. Transient oculomotor nerve misdirection in a case of pituitary tumor with hemorrhage. Arch Ophthalmol 1981;106:584-5.

58. Schatz NJ, Savino PJ, Corbett JJ. Primary aberrant oculomotor regeneration: a sign of intracavernous meningioma. Arch Neurol 1977;34:29-32.

59. Cox TA, Wurster JB, Godfrey WA. Primary aberrant oculomotor regeneration due to intracranial aneurysm. Arch Neurol 1979;36:570-1.

60. Johnson LN, Kamper CA, Hepler RS, et al. Primary aberrant regeneration of the oculomotor nerve from presumed extracavernous neurilemmoma, meningioma, and asymmetric mammillary body. Neuro-ophthalmology 1989; 9:227-32.

61. Susac JO, Hoyt WF. Inferior branch palsy of the oculomotor nerve. Ann Neurol 1977;2:336-9.

62. Derakhshan I. Superior branch palsy of the oculomotor nerve with spontaneous recovery. Ann Neurol 1978; 4:478-9.

63. Engelhardt A, Cedzich C, Kompf D. Isolated superior branch palsy of the oculomotor nerve in influenza-A. Neuro-ophthalmology 1989;9:233-5.

64. Trobe JD, Glaser JS, Post JD. Meningiomas and aneurysms of the cavernous sinus: neuro-ophthalmo-

logic features. Arch Ophthalmol 1978; 96:457-67.

65. Frey T. Isolated paresis of the inferior oblique. Ophthalmic Surg 1982;13: 936-8.

66. Scott WE, Nankin SJ. Isolated inferior oblique paresis. Arch Ophthalmol 1977;95:1586-93.

67. Brown HW. True and simulated superior oblique tendon sheath syndromes. Doc Ophthalmol 1973;34:123-36.

68. Good EF. Ptosis as the sole manifestation of compression of the oculomotor nerve by an aneurysm of the posterior communicating artery. J Clin Neuro Opthalmol 1990;10:59-61.

69. Miller NR. Solitary oculomotor nerve palsy in childhood. Am J Ophthalmol 1977;83:106-11.

70. Gabianelli EB, Klingele TG, Burde RM. Acute oculomotor nerve palsy in childhood: is arteriography necessary? J Clin Neuro Ophthalmol 1989;9:33-6.

71. Mizen TR, Burde RM, Klingele TG. Cryptogenic oculomotor nerve palsies in children. Am J Ophthalmol 1985;100:65-7.

72. Abdul-Rahim AS, Savino PJ, Zimmerman RA, et al. Cryptogenic oculomotor nerve palsy: the need for repeated neuroimaging studies. Arch Ophthalmol 1989;107:387-90.

73. Dalessio DJ, ed. Wolff's headache and other head pain. 4th ed. New York: Oxford University Press, 1980:111-3.

74. Eyster EF, Hoyt WF, Wilson CB. Oculomotor palsy from minor head trauma: an initial sign of basal intracranial tumor. JAMA 1972;220:1083-6.

75. Burger LJ, Kalvin NH, Smith JL. Acquired lesions of the fourth cranial nerve. Brain 1970;93:567-74.

76. Grimson BS, Glaser JS. Isolated trochlear nerve palsies in herpes zoster ophthalmicus. Arch Ophthalmol 1978; 96:1233-5.

77. Glaser JS. Infranuclear disorders of eye movement. In: Glaser JS, ed. Neuro-ophthalmology. Hagerstown, MD: Harper & Row, 1978:245-84.

78. Miller MT, Urist MJ, Folk ER, et al. Superior oblique palsy presenting in late childhood. Am J Ophthalmol 1970;70:212-4.

79. Metz HS, Lerner H. The adjustable Harada-Ito procedure. Arch Ophthalmol 1981;99:624-6.

80. Shrader EC, Schlezinger NS. Neuro-ophthalmologic evaluation of abducens nerve paralysis. Arch Ophthalmol 1960;63:84-91.

81. Slavin ML. Hyperdeviation associated with isolated unilateral abducens palsy. Ophthalmology 1989;96:512-6.

82. Currie J, Lubin JH, Lessell S. Chronic isolated abducens paresis from tumors at the base of the brain. Arch Neurol 1983;40:226-9.

83. Savino PJ, Hilliker JK, Casell GH, et al. Chronic sixth nerve palsies: are they really harbingers of serious intracranial disease? Arch Ophthalmol 1982;100:1442-4.

84. Sakalas R, Harbison JW, Vines FS, et al. Chronic sixth nerve palsy: an initial sign of basisphenoid tumors. Arch Ophthalmol 1975;93:186-90.

85. Elston JS, Lee JP. Paralytic strabismus: the role of botulinum toxin. Br J Ophthalmol 1985;69:891-6.

86. Scott AB, Kraft SP. Botulinum toxin injection in the management of lateral rectus paresis. Ophthalmology 1985; 92:676-83.

87. Wagner RS, Frohman LP. Long-term results: botulinum for sixth nerve palsy. J Pediatr Ophthalmol Strabismus 1989;26:106-8.

88. Keane JR. Bilateral sixth nerve palsy: analysis of 125 cases. Arch Neurol 1976;33:681-3.

89. Miller EA, Savino PJ, Schatz NJ. Bilateral sixth-nerve palsy: a rare complication of water-soluble contrast myelography. Arch Ophthalmol 1982;100: 603-4.

90. Robertson DM, Hines JD, Rucker CW. Acquired sixth-nerve paresis in children. Arch Ophthalmol 1970;83:574-9.

91. Packer RJ, Allen J, Nielsen S, et al. Brainstem glioma: clinical manifestations of meningeal gliomatosis. Ann Neurol 1983;14:177-82.

92. Epstein F, McCleary EL. Intrinsic brain-stem tumors of childhood: surgical indications. J Neurosurg 1986;64: 11-5.

93. Gjerris F. Clinical aspects and long-term prognosis of intracranial tumours in infancy and childhood. Dev Med Child Neurol 1976;18:145-59.

94. Knox DL, Clark DB, Schuster FF. Benign VI nerve palsies in children. Pediatrics 1967;40:560-4.

95. Nemet P, Ehrlich D, Lazar M. Benign abducens palsy in varicella. Am J Ophthalmol 1974;78:859.

96. Werner DB, Savino PJ, Schatz NJ. Benign recurrent sixth nerve palsies in childhood: secondary to immunization or viral illness. Arch Ophthalmol 1983;101:607-8.

97. Reinecke RD, Thompson WE. Childhood recurrent idiopathic paralysis of the lateral rectus. Ann Ophthalmol 1981;13:1037-9.

98. Halperin JJ, Luct BJ, Anand AK, et al. Lyme neuroborreliosis: central nervous system manifestations. Neurology 1989;39:753-9.

99. Moster ML, Savino PJ, Sergott RC, et al. Isolated sixth-nerve palsies in younger adults. Arch Ophthalmol 1984;102:1328-30.

100. Guy J, Day AL, Mickle JP, et al. Contralateral trochlear nerve paresis and ipsilateral Horner's syndrome. Am J Ophthalmol 1989;107:73-6.

101. Spielmann A. Bilateral vertical retraction syndrome in horizontal bilateral Duane's syndrome. Graefe's Arch Clin Exp Ophthalmol 1988;226:425-7.

102. Duane A. Congenital deficiency of abduction associated with impairment of adduction, retraction movements, contraction of the palpebral fissure and oblique movements of the eye. Arch Ophthalmol 1905;34:133-59.

103. Hotchkiss MG, Miller NR, Clark AW, et al. Bilateral Duane's retraction syndrome: a clinical-pathologic case report. Arch Ophthalmol 1980;98:870-4.

104. Miller NR, Kiel SM, Green WR, et al. Unilateral Duane's retraction syndrome (Type 1). Arch Ophthalmol 1982;100:1468-72.

105. Krueger BR, Okazaki H. Vertebral-basilar distribution infarction following chiropractic cervical manipulation. Mayo Clin Proc 1980;55:322-32.

106. Mueller S, Sahs AL. Brain stem dysfunction related to cervical manipulation. Neurology 1976;26:547-50.

107. Kline LB. The Tolosa-Hunt syndrome. Surv Ophthalmol 1982;27:79-95.

108. Schatz NJ, Farmer P. Tolosa-Hunt syndrome: the pathology of painful ophthalmoplegia. In: Smith JL, ed. Neuro-ophthalmology: symposium of the University of Miami and the Bascom Palmer Eye Institute, vol 6. St Louis: Mosby–Year Book, 1972:102-12.

109. Arnon SS, Midura TF, Damus K, et al. Honey and other environmental risk factors for infant botulism. J Pediatr 1979;94:331-6.

110. Midura TF, Arnon SS. Infant botulism: identification of *Clostridium botulinum* and its toxins in faeces. Lancet 1976;2:934-6.

111. Pickett J, Berg B, Chaplin E, et al. Syndrome of botulism in infancy: clinical and electrophysiologic study. N Engl J Med 1976;295:770-2.

112. Barker WH Jr, Weissman JB, Dowell VR Jr, et al. Type B botulism outbreak caused by a commercial food product: West Virginia and Pennsylvania, 1973. JAMA 1977;237:456-9.

113. Terranova W, Palumbo JN, Breman JG. Ocular findings in botulism type B. JAMA 1979;241:475-7.

114. Lewis GE Jr, Metzger JF. Botulism immune plasma (human). Lancet 1978;2:634-5.

115. Cherington M. Botulism: ten-year experience. Arch Neurol 1974;30:432-7.

116. Guillain G, Barré J-A, Strohl A. Sur un syndrome de radiculo-névrite avec hyperalbuminose du liquide céphalorachidien sans réaction cellulaire: remarques sur les caractères cliniques et graphiques des réflexes tendineux. Bull Mem Soc Méd Hop Paris 1916;40:1462-70.

117. Kennedy RH, Danielson MA, Mulder DW, et al. Guillain-Barré syndrome: a 42-year epidemiologic and clinical study. Mayo Clin Proc 1978;53:93-9.

118. Kleyweg RP, van der Meché FGA, Loonen MCB, et al. The natural history of Guillain-Barré syndrome in 18 children and 50 adults. J Neurol Neu-

rosurg Psychiatry 1989;52:853-6.

119. Fisher M. An unusual variant of acute idiopathic polyneuritis (syndrome of ophthalmoplegia, ataxia and areflexia). N Engl J Med 1956;255:57-65.

120. Blau I, Casson I, Lieberman A, et al. The not-so-benign Miller Fisher syndrome: a variant of the Guillain-Barré syndrome. Arch Neurol 1980;37:384-5.

121. Arnason BGW. Acute inflammatory demyelinating polyradiculoneuropathies. In: Dyck PJ, Thomas PK, Lambert EH, et al, eds. Peripheral neuropathy, vol. 2. Philadelphia: WB Saunders, 1984:2088-9.

122. McKhann GM, Griffin JW, Cornblath DR, et al. Plasmapheresis and Guillain-Barré syndrome: analysis of prognostic factors and the effect of plasmapheresis. Ann Neurol 1988;23:347-53.

123. Bielschowsky A. Lectures on motor anomalies. Hanover, NH: Dartmouth College Publications, 1943.

124. Hagedoorn A. A new diagnostic motility scheme. Am J Ophthalmol 1942;25:726-8.

125. Hardesty HH. Diagnosis of paretic vertical rotators. Am J Ophthalmol 1963;56:811-6.

126. Parks MM. Isolated cyclovertical muscle palsy. Arch Ophthalmol 1958;60:1027-35.

127. von Noorden GK, Maumenee AE. Atlas of strabismus. 2nd ed. St Louis: Mosby–Year Book, 1967:140.

128. Feibel RM, Roper-Hall G. Evaluation of the field of binocular single vision in incomitant strabismus. Am J Ophthalmol 1974;78:800-5.

# CHAPTER 11

# Comitant Ocular Misalignment

· · · · · · · · · · · · · · · · ·

If the examination of a patient with diplopia fails to reveal any change in the ocular misalignment in different gaze positions, then by definition the patient has a *comitant misalignment (strabismus)*.

The largest group of patients with comitant misalignment are those we categorize as having childhood strabismus. Childhood strabismus includes those cases of congenital and acquired misalignments dating from childhood that may be due to accommodative or nonaccommodative vergence abnormalities that remain to be defined. Helpful signs and symptoms in establishing the presence of early-onset ocular misalignment include amblyopia, absence of normal stereoacuity, dissociated vertical deviations, A and V patterns, latent nystagmus, a positive 4-diopter baseout prism test, or a recollection of patching and wearing glasses including bifocals. These patients do not complain of diplopia and therefore as a group are rarely seen in a neurologic context. Recognition of childhood strabismus is important in order to differentiate such patients from those with truly acquired misalignments, especially (1) in cases involving secondary gain and (2) in those patients who suddenly become aware of a previously unnoted ocular misalignment.

Orthophoria can be considered that condition of binocular vision in which there is no strain on fusional mechanisms. When a patient is fixating at distance or near, the cross-cover test will fail to demonstrate any shift of the eyes. Heterophoria is a misalignment kept latent by fusional mechanisms. An intermittent tropia is one in which fusional control is present part of the time, and a tropia is a manifest misalignment in which fusional control is not present.

## A Decision Tree Approach to the Evaluation of Comitant Ocular Misalignment (Chart 11-1)

☐ Decompensated phoria

Patients with a latent ocular misalignment may lose the ability to have single-binocular vision for reasons that remain oscure. In some patients decompensation has been associated with febrile illness, head trauma, and changing refractive needs. Prior to the development of either an intermittent tropia or a mani-

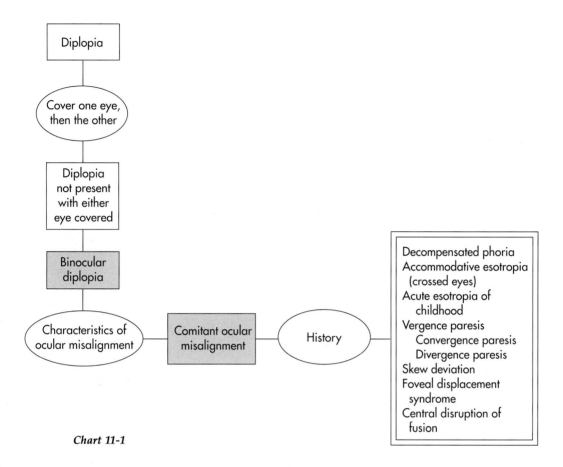

**Chart 11-1**

fest tropia, the patient may experience asthenopia (see Chapter 16) due to stresses placed on fusional mechanisms. With the loss of binocularity, a patient may reflexly squint one eye in the bright sunlight[1] to prevent the diplopia (intermittent exotropia) or may be aware of diplopia, either intermittently or constantly. Evidence helpful in making the diagnosis of a latent misalignment or decompensated phoria includes the presence of an adaptive head posture and large fusional amplitudes.

Fusional amplitudes can be measured using loose prisms, a prism bar, or a rotary prism. With the patient fixating on either a distant or near target, any manifest tropia should be neutralized. Then, a sequence of progressively stronger prisms is introduced in front of one eye to produce the desired fusional movement (e.g., baseout prism for convergence). The prism strength is increased until the patient reports insuperable diplopia. The amount of prism needed to produce diplopia over that needed to neutralize the tropia (if present) represents the fusional amplitude for that particular vergence movement (Table 11-1).

### Accommodative esotropia (crossed eyes)

Sudden development of esotropia between ages 1 and 7 years occasionally associated with trauma or a febrile illness should suggest a diagnosis of accommo-

| **TABLE 11-1** | *Normal Vergence Amplitudes in Prism Diopters* | | |
|---|---|---|---|
| | **Convergence** | **Divergence** | **Sursumvergence** |
| Distance | 16-20 | 6-8 | 2-4 |
| Near | 26-40 | 12-14 | 2-4 |

dative esotropia. This misalignment is usually intermittent in the beginning. Most of these children will not complain of diplopia and can easily become amblyopic if the condition is not recognized by the presence of the misalignment.

Depending on the classification, four or more types of accommodative esotropia have been recognized. The important point differentiating this entity from acute esotropia of childhood is the presence of binocularity with the appropriate use of corrective lenses and prisms if amblyopia has not developed.

### Acute esotropia of childhood

Acute-onset acquired esotropia in a child should not be confused with divergence paralysis. In acute acquired comitant esotropia the measured distance and near misalignment are approximately equal. This entity is considered for the most part to have a benign course and responds to surgery with the reestablishment of motor fusion.[2] The acute onset of comitant esotropia has been associated with a CNS malignancy.[3-6] Williams and Hoyt[6] described six such children ranging in age from 3 to 10 years who were found to have tumors of the brainstem or cerebellum. In three of their cases, the onset of this esotropia was associated with the presence of nystagmus, and they emphasize the importance of this combination of findings in suggesting the necessity of a neurologic evaluation in this group of patients. Three of their patients had no additional signs of neurologic disease. Any child who fits into this category and who does not develop motor fusion following the use of optical devices or extraocular muscle surgery should have a neurologic evaluation. The mechanism underlying the onset of acute comitant esotropia in patients with brain tumors is unknown, and obviously some of these patients have no tell-tale signs to indicate the need for further evaluation.

Although we have very little collective experience, we suggest that all patients with the acute onset of comitant esotropia who do not demonstrate motor fusion with appropriate hyperopic spectacles (accommodative esotropia) or with prisms have a neurologic evaluation including imaging.

### Vergence paresis

**CONVERGENCE PARESIS.** Convergence paresis is a condition in which the patients are orthotropic at a distance but complain of diplopia when looking at near objects. They can fully adduct their eyes during conjugate gaze movements. The deviation is comitant across the field of gaze for a given distance. This diagnosis must be made with caution, since the amplitude of convergence depends,

among other things, on patient effort. Because of the need for patient cooperation, this condition can be feigned easily. Pupillary miosis is a good objective
sign of attempted convergence, being an obligate part of the near synkinesis.
Unfortunately, in many patients with convergence paralysis, pupillary and accommodative functions are disturbed as well; thus the absence of miosis does
not necessarily imply psychogenic disease. The diagnosis of convergence paresis
depends on consistency of objective findings during successive examinations.
An appropriate accommodative target should be used consistently in an attempt
to activate the near reflex (convergence).

Although convergence paresis occurs with structural disease, such as infarction or demyelination within the brainstem, it also occurs in isolation as a
sequela of "flu" syndromes and following head trauma. In the latter case it may
be transient or permanent. When convergence paresis exists in isolation (i.e.,
without accommodative or pupillary involvement or evidence of central nervous system [CNS] disease), differentiating it from *convergence insufficiency* may
be difficult, although convergence paresis usually has an acute onset. A patient
with a history that implies chronicity of complaints (asthenopic symptoms of
long duration) associated with near fixation is more likely to have a diagnosis of
convergence insufficiency than convergence paresis.

The diagnosis of convergence insufficiency depends on the finding of decreased amplitudes of convergence at near (Table 11-1) associated with a remote
near point. These amplitudes can be measured with free prisms, a prism bar, or
a haploscope. Although the accompanying asthenopia is usually of long and un-
determined duration (i.e., insidious in onset), the symptoms may be of recent
and acute onset associated with a new prescription for spectacles to correct a relatively high hypermetropic or myopic refractive error of 5 to 6 diopters[7] or as an
accompaniment of an initial presbyopic correction. These patients always demonstrate miosis on attempted near fixation.

**DIVERGENCE PARESIS.** Divergence paresis is a supranuclear paralysis heralded
by the sudden onset of esotropia accompanied by diplopia.[8] The misalignment
is horizontally comitant for all gaze positions. In spite of esotropia, horizontal
versions are normal. At near, there is a small range in which the patients are able
to fuse. More proximal to this fusional space, patients may have convergence insufficiency and may become exotropic.

Some debate exists over whether divergence paresis really exists as a nosologic entity or whether the findings represent a mild symmetric binocular lateral
rectus paresis.[9] Our opinion is that divergence paresis differs from bilateral sixth
cranial nerve palsies, convergence spasm, and decompensating latent esotropia
of the divergence insufficiency type.[7] In our experience, most often divergence
paresis is benign and self-limited. We have seen it following head trauma, lumbar puncture, epidural anesthetic blocks, and presumed viral illnesses, as well as
in an idiopathic form. Occasional reports associate divergence paralysis with encephalitis, demyelinating disease, neurosyphilis, trauma, and tumors in and
around the cerebellum.[10] We believe all such patients should have magnetic resonance imaging (MRI).

Stern and Tomsak[11] reported a case of divergence paralysis in which other signs suggested the site of the pathology to be in the area of the pontomedullary junction. MRI demonstrated what was interpreted as a demyelinating plaque in the lower pons along the floor of the ventricle.

## Skew deviation

The occurrence of vertical diplopia that cannot be isolated to a single extraocular muscle or muscles is defined as a skew deviation once restrictive and myoneural junction disease are excluded. The hypertropic eye may vary with gaze position and in such cases is associated with downbeat nystagmus.[12] Skew deviation may appear as a comitant or incomitant misalignment but is not associated with the presence of a primary or secondary deviation. Skew deviation may be intermittent[13,14] and can periodically alternate.[15,16] No torsional misalignment will be present.[17]

The presence of a skew deviation implies posterior fossa disease, and the search for other signs and symptoms involving this broad region should be instituted. In our experience, skew deviation rarely occurs in isolation. However, the associated findings may be subtle and may involve only disorders of ocular movement (i.e., saccadic pursuit or nystagmus). The only time that a skew deviation has localizing significance with respect to the side of a brainstem lesion is when it is accompanied by an internuclear ophthalmoplegia. In this circumstance the adduction lag points to the side of the lesion.[18]

## Foveal displacement syndrome

Some patients with subretinal neovascular membranes before or after photocoagulation therapy may develop binocular diplopia due to displacement of the foveomacular receptor elements.[19] Misalignment of foveal elements between the two eyes produces a rivalry between central and peripheral fusional mechanisms, since peripheral corresponding areas will not be aligned. A similar picture may be seen in patients with proliferative diabetic retinopathy.[20] Thus if the eyes are aligned (the usual circumstance, since peripheral fusional mechanisms are stronger than central mechanisms), the fovea of the involved eye is displaced (dragged) relative to the fovea of the normal eye, and the patient experiences diplopia. If the diplopia is neutralized by prisms, a small comitant deviation will be induced; however, in spite of prescribing the neutralizing prism, diplopia recurs within minutes as the stronger peripheral mechanisms realign the eyes. Little can be done to make these patients binocularly comfortable, but a few can tolerate a small central occluder in the visual axis of their spectacle correction in front of the involved eye.[19]

## Central disruption of fusion

In 1973 Wade[21] described a patient with a loss of fusion following head trauma. Patients acquiring this fusional dysfunction can only momentarily superimpose targets even if the targets are presented bifoveally by a synoptophore. These patients are almost always exotropic and may in addition have an associated hypotropia and excyclotorsion. Quantifying the misalignment is difficult, since most of these patients develop a bobbing movement of the nondominant eye in the vertical plane. Reports document such a loss of fusion following head trauma,[21-23] the development of a dense unilateral cataract not treated by relatively prompt cataract extraction,[24,25] and cataract surgery without correcting the aphakic state for a period of time.[25] Patients with unilateral congenital cataract in spite of surgery during the first few months of life have, as a rule, an inability to fuse foveally. The underlying mechanism in these children is presumed to be different.

Interestingly, these patients are aware of movement of the environment observed by the bobbing of the nonfixing eye. Attempts at surgical realignment of the eyes makes these patients more symptomatic because they can no longer as easily ignore the diplopic image as it is moved closer to the real fixated image. These patients must occlude one eye to function.

## REFERENCES

1. Wang FM, Chryssanthou G. Monocular eye closure in intermittent exotropia. Arch Ophthalmol 1988;106:941-2.
2. Burian HM, Miller JE. Comitant convergent strabismus with acute onset. Am J Ophthalmol 1958;45:55-64.
3. Anderson WD, Lubow M. Astrocytoma of the corpus callosum presenting with acute comitant esotropia. Am J Ophthalmol 1970;69:594-8.
4. Zweifach PH. Childhood esotropia with delayed appearance of cerebellar tumor. Neuro-Ophthalmology 1981;1:291-3.
5. Mickatavage RC. Neuro-ophthalmological disease presenting as orthoptic problems. Am Orthoptic J 1972;22:44-6.
6. Williams AS, Hoyt CS. Acute comitant esotropia in children with brain tumors. Arch Ophthalmol 1989;107:376-8.
7. von Noorden GK. Binocular vision and ocular motility: theory and management of strabismus. 4th ed. St Louis: Mosby–Year Book, 1990:395.
8. Roper-Hall G, Burde RM. Diagnosis and management of divergence paresis. Am Orthoptic J 1987;37:113-21.
9. Kirkham TH, Bird AC, Sanders MD. Divergence paralysis and raised intracranial pressure: an electro-oculographic study. Br J Ophthalmol 1972;56:776-82.
10. Cogan DG. Neurology of the ocular muscles. 2nd ed. Springfield, IL: Charles C Thomas, 1956:133-4.
11. Stern RM, Tomsak RL. Magnetic resonance images in a case of "divergence paralysis." Surv Ophthalmol 1986;30:397-401.
12. Moster ML, Schatz NJ, Savino PJ, et al. Alternating skew on lateral gaze (bilateral abducting hypertropia). Ann Neurol 1988;23:190-2.
13. Allerand CD. Paroxysmal skew deviation in association with brain stem glioma: report of an unusual case. Neurology 1962;12:520-3.
14. Hedges TR III, Hoyt WF. Ocular tilt reaction due to an upper brainstem lesion: paroxysmal skew deviation, torsion, and oscillation of the eyes with head tilt. Ann Neurol 1982;11:537-40.
15. Corbett JJ, Schatz NJ, Shults WT, et al. Slowly alternating skew deviation: description of a pretectal syndrome in three patients. Ann Neurol 1981;10:540-6.
16. Mitchell JM, Smith JL, Quencer RM. Periodic alternating skew deviation. J Clin Neuro Ophthalmol 1981;1:5-8.
17. Trobe JD. Cyclodeviation in acquired vertical strabismus. Arch Ophthalmol 1984;102:717-20.
18. Keane JR. Ocular skew deviation: analysis of 100 cases. Arch Neurol 1975;32:185-90.
19. Burgess D, Roper-Hall G, Burde RM. Binocular diplopia associated with subretinal neovascular membranes. Arch Ophthalmol 1980;98:311-7.
20. Bresnick GH, Smith V, Pokorny J. Visual function abnormalities or macular heterotopia caused by proliferative diabetic retinopathy. Am J Ophthalmol 1981;92:85-102.

21. Wade SL. Loss of fusion following brain damage. Br Orthoptic J 1965;22:81-3.
22. Pratt-Johnson JA. Central disruption of fusional amplitude. Br J Ophthalmol 1973;57:347-50.
23. Pratt-Johnson JA, Tillson G. Acquired central disruption of fusional amplitude. Ophthalmology 1979;86:2140-2.
24. Hamed LM, Helveston EM, Ellis FD. Persistent binocular diplopia after cataract surgery. Am J Ophthalmol 1987;103:741-4.
25. Pratt-Johnson JA, Tillson G. Intractable diplopia after vision restoration in unilateral cataract. Am J Ophthalmol 1989;107:23-6.

# CHAPTER 12

# Nystagmus and Other Ocular Oscillations

• • • • • • • • • • • • • • • •

The term *nystagmus* is used to describe oscillatory ocular movements that are "to a certain extent rhythmic."[1] Ocular movements that are oscillatory, but not rhythmic, are called nystagmoid movements. In recent years elegant recording techniques have been used to study the waveforms, amplitudes, velocities, and other characteristics of ocular oscillatory movement disorders. From these data rather structured and complex classification systems have been established. Mathematical modeling based on inferred neurophysiologic control centers and integrators has also provided insight into the underlying pathology. Despite this rapid proliferation of knowledge, little has been gained that is clinically applicable to improving treatment at this time.

Classically nystagmus has been divided into two broad categories depending on the clinical appearance of the movements. Pendular nystagmus is characterized by ocular oscillations that are approximately equal in velocity in both directions.[2] These oscillations may vary in speed and amplitude and are almost always horizontal. They often have a jerk component in eccentric gaze, with the fast phase in the direction of gaze. Jerk nystagmus is characterized by rhythmic oscillations in which the movement in one direction is recognizably faster than the movement in the other direction. The slow movement is the pathologic movement, and the fast movement is corrective. Even so, jerk nystagmus is named (defined) according to the direction of the fast-phase or corrective movement. Both pendular and jerk nystagmus may have a gaze position in which the intensity (amplitude and frequency) of the ocular oscillation is at a minimum (position of relative stability); this point or area of gaze is termed the *null point*.

The clinician should develop a method, usually diagrammatic (Figs. 12-1 and 12-2), to record the patterns of nystagmus or nystagmoid movements and how they are affected by movement into the various gaze positions. In addition, the clinician should observe the patient for a few minutes to determine if the observed movements change with time. Examples of such time-dependent changes include the reversal of direction of nystagmus in periodic alternating nystagmus or intermittent breaks in fixation of ocular flutter or square wave jerks. Stimulating the ocular motor system may be necessary to induce or unmask certain disorders, such as ocular dysmetria, superior oblique myokymia, or positional nystagmus. The discipline of diagramming is important for several

**289**

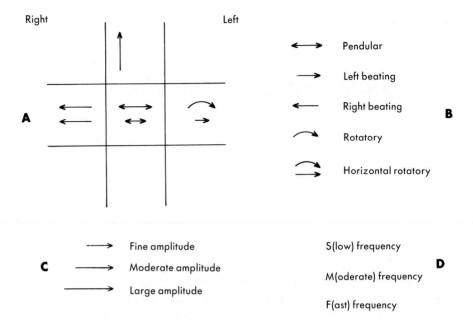

Fig. 12-1. Method of depicting nystagmus. **A,** Depict movements in nine positions of gaze, right eye over left. **B,** Arrows point in direction of fast phase of nystagmus. **C,** Length of arrow reflects amplitude. **D,** *S, M,* and *F* designate frequency.

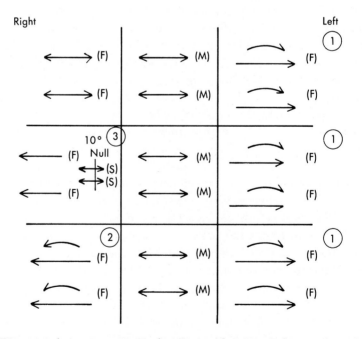

Fig. 12-2. Diagram of eye movements of patient with congenital nystagmus. *1,* Rotatory component in left gaze; *2,* rotatory component in right downgaze; *3,* null point 10 degrees to right of primary position with small-amplitude, slow-frequency movement.

reasons. First, the mechanical diagramming assists the clinician in extracting all of the available information from the observed movement. Furthermore, diagramming serves as a permanent record of the stability of the oscillation over prolonged periods. Finally, the examiner should observe the patient's responses to optokinetic stimuli and note abnormal head posture and head movements. Eye movement recordings may be of value when a diagnostic conundrum remains in spite of careful clinical observation, and when such information could affect future management.

# A Decision Tree Approach to the Evaluation of Nystagmus

Nystagmus and nystagmoid movements have been classified in various ways. The decision tree approach we use (Chart 12-1) does not attempt to formally classify ocular oscillations, but rather suggests a series of pragmatic steps intended to help the physician recognize a particular movement disorder.

○ *History.* Certain historical data are helpful in attuning the clinician to the presence and type of oscillatory disturbance. The acute onset of complaints (vestibular or visual) is usually predictive of an acquired disorder. The symptoms of acute vestibular dysfunction are vertigo, tinnitus, and nausea. The visual symptom associated with acquired nystagmus is most often oscillopsia; the symptom associated with congenital nystagmus is blurring of vision (degradation of visual function), particularly when the eyes move away from the null point.

Oscillopsia is best described as an illusory perception of environmental movement and may be gaze induced, position dependent, or affected by activity. Oscillopsia may assume four forms:

1. Associated with acquired jerk nystagmus. The patient reports that the environment is moving in one direction, opposite to the slow phase of the nystagmus (i.e., in the direction of the fast phase). No movement is perceived during the fast phase, since the visual threshold is elevated during fast eye movements.
2. Associated with pendular nystagmus. The patient perceives a to-and-fro movement of the environment.
3. Associated with superior oblique myokymia. The patient experiences a peculiar jellylike quivering of the environment during the rapid firing of the superior oblique muscle.
4. Associated with bilateral labyrinthine dysfunction. The patient complains of a continuous "jiggling" of the environment, which at rest may be in rhythm with the heartbeat. With magnification, even when the patient is symptomatic, no ocular movement is apparent.

Patients with acquired oscillations should be asked about drug use and abuse (current and past), including medications such as tranquilizers, antiepileptics, antibiotics, and alcohol. Many drugs can induce ocular oscillations at therapeutic as well as toxic levels. A history of significant head trauma, neuro-

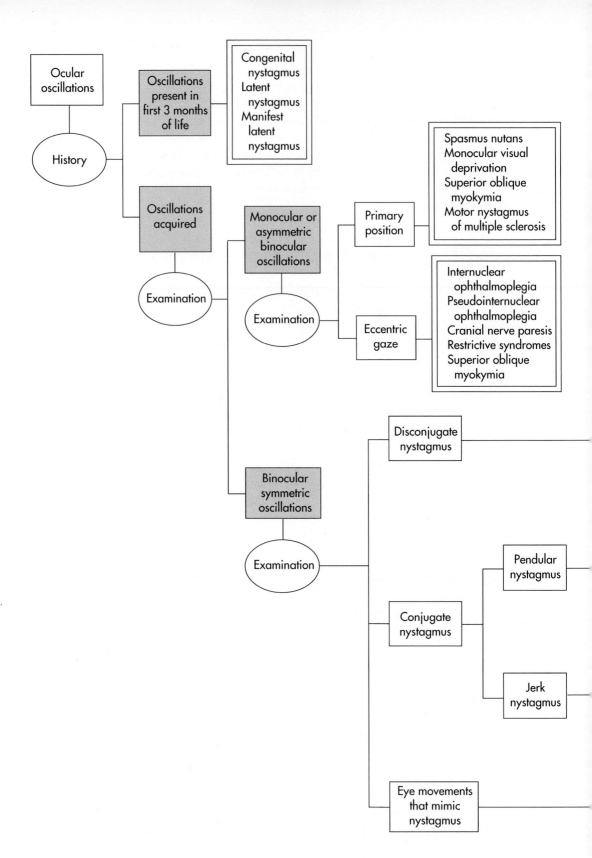

*Chart 12-1*

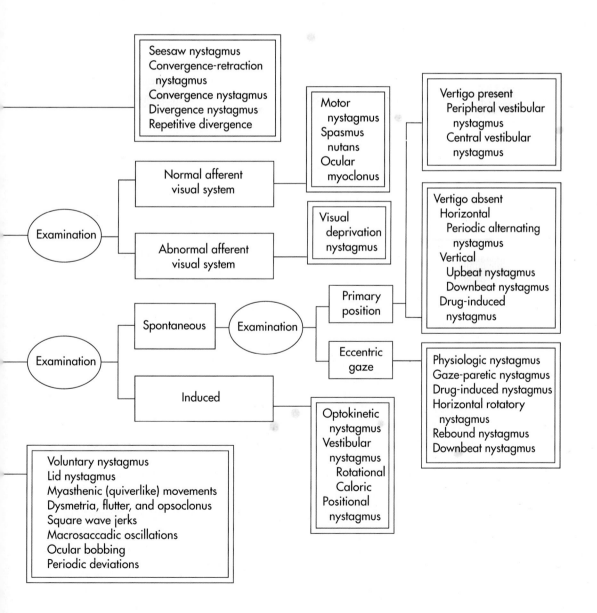

surgical intervention, or seizures suggests the possibility of an underlying structural abnormality.

If a parent brings in a child with so-called dancing eyes, the examiner must inquire whether the oscillations were present in the first 3 months of life.

## ▨ Oscillations present in first 3 months of life

### ▧ Congenital nystagmus

Congenital nystagmus is an ocular oscillatory movement disorder caused by a motor instability that can exist with or without afferent visual system dysfunction. This entity is defined both clinically and by waveform. Congenital nystagmus associated with afferent visual system dysfunction is more common than that without afferent visual system dysfunction (10:1).[3]

Congenital nystagmus unassociated with poor visual acuity is usually present in the perinatal period. Some patients with poor visual potential at the time they might be expected to begin to develop central fixation will unmask an underlying gain/delay problem (inherited [?] or familial [?]), allowing a latent nystagmus to become manifest.[4] Thus some patients with poor visual potential develop congenital nystagmus whereas others do not. An example would be the development of congenital nystagmus with congenitally poor vision at age 3 to 4 months, or earlier in patients with Leber's congenital amaurosis. Deafferentation of patients with such a propensity even later in life can produce an ocular oscillatory movement indistinguishable from congenital nystagmus. Patients deafferented at any age who do not have the underlying propensity to develop congenital nystagmus develop pendular-like, nonrhythmic, wandering eye movements.

Clinically, congenital nystagmus may vary from an overt jerk nystagmus to what appears to be a purely pendular movement disorder. The terms *jerk* and *pendular* do not really reflect the complexity of the underlying foveational strategies.[5] At least 12 waveforms of congenital nystagmus consisting of combinations of jerk and pendular movements have been noted in sophisticated eye movement recordings.[6] The nystagmus may be irregular but is almost always conjugate and horizontal, and rarely purely vertical.

The underlying defect in congenital nystagmus remains elusive. Some[5] consider it to be a failure of the slow eye movement control subsystem; others[3] suggest a defect in the subcortical optokinetic system. In any case, the result is fixation instability that can be aggravated by poor visual acuity.[4] The primary eye movement is a drift away from fixation, whereas the corrective movement is aimed at recovering fixation, which may or may not be achieved.[7] Attempted fixation tends to exaggerate the oscillations. Patients who have decreased vision for other reasons will also have a more severe nystagmus with attempted fixation.

Even in the absence of a history of neonatal onset, the diagnosis of congenital motor nystagmus is relatively straightforward, since this movement disorder has certain characteristic findings. The nystagmus is bilateral and grossly symmetric in amplitude and frequency. The nystagmus remains horizontal in all gaze directions (even vertical), although a rotary component may be superimposed in lateral gaze (Fig. 12-2). In spite of almost continuous eye movements, patients with congenital nystagmus do not complain of oscillopsia. The nystagmus disappears during sleep.

Patients who have congenital nystagmus almost always have a relative null point or area where the oscillatory movements are minimized. This null area may differ slightly for each eye (Fig. 12-2). These patients often assume a head turn to place the null point in the straight-ahead position, thereby maximizing their distance acuity. The development of a face turn to improve vision is unusual in acquired nystagmus. Patients with congenital nystagmus and no afferent visual system disease always have much better reading vision than distance vision (e.g., 20/40 versus 20/80 to 20/200), since convergence damps the nystagmus. Two types of head movements are associated with congenital nystagmus: (1) an involuntary head movement that does not affect visual acuity and (2) a synchronous compensatory head movement opposite in direction to the beating of the nystagmus fast phase, which does improve visual acuity.[1,6,8] These patients may demonstrate a reverse response to optokinetic stimuli, as well as a superimposed latent nystagmus (see below).

Various treatments have been tried to maximize vision in the straight-ahead position in these patients. Dell'Osso[7] has recommended the use of prism glasses with two goals: (1) to optically place the null point in the straight-ahead position, obviating the need for a head turn, and (2) to induce convergence in order to improve distance acuity. This method of treatment has not been widely accepted for the following possible reasons: (1) the prisms are heavy and unsightly; (2) the prismatic shift, especially that associated with chronic convergence, produces asthenopia; and (3) in patients who are fixating bifoveally, neither an appropriate horizontal shift nor convergence can be induced.

On the other hand, the Kestenbaum procedure, which attempts to move the null point from an extremely eccentric position to the primary position by surgically recessing one pair of horizontal yoke muscles while simultaneously resecting the other, is extremely effective. This procedure not only allows the patient to assume a more nearly normal head position, but damps the nystagmus as well.[9-11]

Differentiating congenital from acquired nystagmus other than by history or by accompanying signs of neurologic dysfunction suggesting an acquired lesion may be virtually impossible.

Gelbart and Hoyt[3] reported 132 patients with infantile nystagmus, 104 of whom had sensory defects. Associated abnormalities included 41 patients with optic nerve hypoplasia, 33 patients with Leber's congenital amaurosis, 16 patients with oculocutaneous albinism, 7 patients with cone dystrophies, and the remainder with varied underlying etiologies. Many patients had paradoxical pupillary responses.[3]*

---

*Paradoxical pupillary responses may be demonstrated by decreasing the ambient illumination and finding pupillary constriction or by starting in subdued illumination, switching the lights on, and noting pupillary dilatation.[12-14]

### ☐ Latent nystagmus

Latent nystagmus is a congenital jerk nystagmus induced by monocular occlusion; it is characterized by a slow-phase drift toward the covered eye, followed by a fast-phase corrective movement toward the uncovered eye. The movements are bilateral and symmetric, similar in amplitude and frequency. Latent nystagmus usually occurs if either eye is covered but may be induced by covering one eye only. Latent nystagmus may also be induced with neutral density filters or high plus lenses placed in front of one eye. Although a congenital condition, latent nystagmus is not generally recognized until later in life, when an attempt is made to determine monocular visual acuity during vision screening at school. Children with latent nystagmus have poor acuity if each eye is tested individually with occlusion of the other. Patients with latent nystagmus who develop visual loss in one eye immediately develop a constant nystagmus indistinguishable from congenital nystagmus[15] (i.e., manifest latent nystagmus).

Latent nystagmus is a marker of a congenital ocular motor disturbance. Thus in a patient with nystagmus, the presence of a superimposed latent component labels the oscillation as congenital. It has been reported to occur in association with congenital esotropia and dissociated vertical deviations as well.

Accurate determination of visual acuity in patients with latent nystagmus is accomplished most easily by placing a central dot of tape on a plano lens in front of one eye and blocking central fixation but allowing the eye to remain open while refracting the other eye. Similar results may be obtained by using a polarized acuity chart with polarizing lenses.

### ☐ Manifest latent nystagmus

Manifest latent nystagmus is an oscillation that occurs in patients with strabismus who have a jerk nystagmus in the direction of the fixing eye (i.e., a right-beating nystagmus when fixing with the right eye and a left-beating nystagmus when fixing with the left eye).[16-18] This change in direction differentiates manifest latent nystagmus from other forms of nystagmus. This nystagmus may be converted from a manifest to a latent oscillation if the eyes are surgically aligned.[19]

### ■ Oscillations acquired

If the nystagmus is not present within the first 3 months of life, we consider it to be acquired.

○ *Examination.* Observation of the patient will reveal almost immediately whether the acquired oscillation primarily involves one or both eyes.

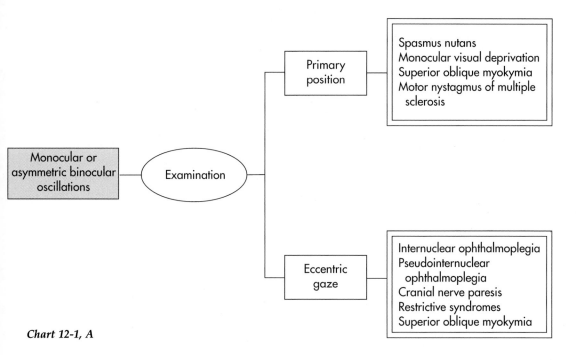

*Chart 12-1, A*

### ▓ Monocular or asymmetric binocular oscillations

If the oscillation is confined to one eye (monocular) or involves mainly one eye (i.e., markedly asymmetric [dissociated]), the movement disorder may then be further subdivided (Chart 12-1, A) by determining if oscillation is present in the primary position or whether it is evoked by assuming an eccentric gaze position (gaze evoked).

### ▢ Primary position

### ▣ Spasmus nutans

Spasmus nutans is a rare, most often benign triad of nystagmus, torticollis, and head nodding, which may appear monocular by gross inspection.[20,21] It usually has its onset between the ages of 4 and 14 months but has been reported as late as 3½ years.[22] Cogan[23] states, "Indeed it is the most common if not the only cause of unilateral horizontal nystagmus in infancy." Only two of the three characteristic findings of the triad need to be present to make the diagnosis.

Spasmus nutans often lasts less than 1 month but may last several months or years (average 12 to 24 months) and usually disappears by age 5. The head nodding usually appears first, is rhythmic, and disappears with sleep and changes of head position. The pendular eye movement appears monocular. Closer inspection with a slit lamp or with a +15 diopter lens dialed into a direct ophthalmoscope, however, reveals the condition to be binocular with a fine conjugate shimmering movement in the apparently uninvolved eye. In our experience, spasmus nutans may be horizontal, vertical, or rotary, and its amplitude and frequency tend to vary with gaze position.

Spasmus nutans occurs occasionally in association with developmental central nervous system (CNS) disorders,[24] but no cause-effect relationship has been established. It has been reported as a complication of the fetal alcohol syndrome.[25] Acquired monocular nystagmus with head oscillations and tilt mimicking spasmus nutans can be the initial signs of chiasmal gliomas[26-28] and third ventricular tumors.[29,30] In all of these cases associated with structural pathology, the spasmus nutans tends not to disappear with time.[22,25]

All children with an acquired monocular or primarily monocular oscillation(s) should have magnetic resonance imaging (MRI) to exclude afferent visual system tumors.[4] Since adequate sedation is a necessity for this procedure (general anaesthesia may be required), a concomitant fundus examination should be performed to look for optic disc abnormalities (e.g., nerve fiber bundle dropout).

### ☐ Monocular visual deprivation

Adults or children who sustain monocular visual loss may develop an ipsilateral vertical ocular oscillation (Heimann-Bielschowsky phenomenon) that can range in amplitude from barely perceptible to coarse.[31,32] This oscillation may only be noted with the magnification of the slit lamp or during ophthalmoscopy. Monocular adults (i.e., who sustain visual loss in their only seeing eye) may develop a similar oscillation.[32] This oscillation can develop years after the unilateral visual loss and can disappear immediately on surgical reestablishment of useful vision.[31]

### ☐ Superior oblique myokymia

Superior oblique myokymia is a monocular tremor caused by spontaneous firing of superior oblique muscle fibers.[33] The patient complains of episodes of tilting of the image seen by one eye (episodic intorsion), oscillopsia, or shimmering, or of the awareness of ocular movement. The episodes are brief (seconds) but occur repeatedly, and patients are acutely aware of their onset and cessation. These episodes may be induced by looking into the field of gaze of the involved superior oblique muscle or by moving the eye from that field back to the primary position.

Rosenberg and Glaser[34] emphasize that superior oblique myokymia can also manifest as a slower, large-amplitude, intorsional movement causing vertical and torsional diplopia. This oscillation may exist independently or be superimposed on the monocular microtremor. Other associated ocular motor findings include intermittent overaction of the superior oblique muscle, ipsilateral underaction of the superior oblique, and intermittent inability to elevate the eye in adduction.

Hoyt and Keane[33] report rapid phasic activity by electromyography in the involved superior oblique muscle and the absence of reciprocal phasic inhibition of the inferior oblique muscle. They postulate that this movement disorder is best explained by dysfunction involving the fascicles of the fourth cranial nerve in the brainstem. Electromyographic findings typical of denervation with subsequent reinnervation have been recorded.[35,36]

Two patients with superior oblique myokymia, one of whom had a large astrocytoma involving the midbrain, have been reported.[37] Both patients had similar oculographic findings demonstrating bursts of tonic and phasic intorsion, depression, and miniature oscillations. If, as it appears from this case, superior oblique myokymia can be the only presenting sign of an intracranial mass lesion, we must recommend that neuroimaging be obtained in all such patients.

The natural course of superior oblique myokymia includes spontaneous remissions and relapses. In those who are sufficiently symptomatic, a trial of carbamazepine is indicated.[38] Unfortunately, in our experience, as well as that of others,[34] carbamazepine has not been uniformly successful in treating these patients. Intrasheath tenotomy of the superior oblique muscle alone or in combination with an inferior oblique weakening procedure has been suggested to be effective in recalcitrant cases.[33,38,39] Unfortunately, many of these patients will be left with symptomatic diplopia or continue to experience bouts of oscillopsia.

## ▣ Motor nystagmus of multiple sclerosis

Motor or efferent nystagmus is an acquired pendular nystagmus of low frequency and amplitude found in patients with multiple sclerosis (MS). It may be monocular or binocular, conjugate or disconjugate, and have a nystagmus waveform that does not vary with gaze position.[40,41] This nystagmus is usually multivectorial rather than predominantly horizontal. Patterns of movement can include circular, elliptical,* and oblique ("windmill") oscillations.[40,42,43] The nystagmus may be synchronous with other involuntary movements or be associated with head tremor. Other evidence of MS is always present. These patients complain bitterly of oscillopsia. This nystagmus is believed to be due to a lesion either in the brainstem or in the cerebellum.[41]

In these patients systemic scopolamine may damp the nystagmus and relieve the oscillopsia.[41] Carbamazepine, baclofen, and the benzodiazepines have also been recommended. We have not found these drugs to be consistently effective. Isoniazide in conjunction with baseout prisms appears to have promise.[44] Some of these patients may obtain short-term ability to read with the use of extremely high minus contact lenses,[45,46] which stabilize the image.

## ☐ Eccentric gaze

In another group of primarily monocular oscillatory movement disorders, the nystagmus is not present in primary position but only in eccentric gaze position.

## ▣ Internuclear ophthalmoplegia

Internuclear ophthalmoplegia (INO) is discussed in detail elsewhere (see Chapter 8). INO is seen as a lack or lag of movement of the adducting eye, with nystagmus of the abducting eye occurring at the completion of a horizontal conjugate gaze movement. The impaired movement of the adducting eye is caused by an interruption of the fibers to the agonist medial rectus muscle traveling in the medial longitudinal fasciculus (MLF). These fibers arise in the contralateral abducens nucleus and cross at the level of the sixth nerve nucleus to course ros-

---

*Paradoxically, in both circular and elliptical oscillations the apparent movement of the environment in these patients will be in the same direction as the oscillation.

trally in the MLF (see Fig. 8-1). The presence of an INO is indicative of intrinsic brainstem pathology. Numerous hypotheses have been offered to explain the presence of the nystagmus of the abducting eye, none of which has received universal acceptance.[47-49] The report by Zee et al.[49] adds credence to the hypothesis that the abduction nystagmus is a manifestation of a normal adaptive response. They suggest that cerebellar output is adjusted to compensate for the slow movement of the involved medial rectus muscle, at which time by Hering's law an increase in innervational energy is sent to the yoke contralateral lateral rectus muscle. This action produces an overshoot of the abducting eye with a subsequent oscillation around the eccentric fixation point.

When the dissociation during the conjugate movement is subtle, it may be made clinically more apparent by the use of an optokinetic stimulus.[50] The weakness is exaggerated when the optokinetic target is moved toward the side of the lesion, thus activating the involved medial rectus muscle during each corrective saccade.

Whether it is unilateral or bilateral, INO in a younger age group (under 40 to 50 years) is most often due to MS; in an older age group (over 40 to 50 years) stroke from atherosclerotic vertebrobasilar disease must be considered causative.

### ☐ Pseudointernuclear ophthalmoplegia

In any case of innervational or restrictive impairment of adduction, an abducting nystagmus may be seen. This combination of findings will mimic INO. Glaser reported three patients with myasthenia gravis in whom these findings disappeared after the injection of Tensilon.[51] We have also observed these findings in partial third nerve palsies and restrictive lateral rectus disease. Similar types of monocular nystagmoid movements may be seen in the involved yoke

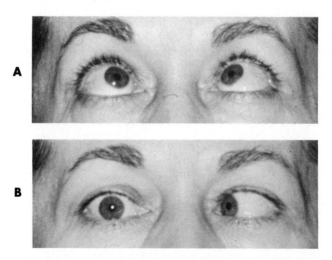

*Fig. 12-3.* Graves' disease with convergence-retraction nystagmus. **A,** Marked bilateral medial deviation of eyes on attempted upgaze. **B,** Left esotropia in primary position with right eye fixing. Bilateral lid retraction may be a sign of either Graves' disease or midbrain dysfunction.

muscle of any affected agonist; for example, if the right superior rectus muscle is weak, the left eye may demonstrate a nystagmoid movement in upgaze.

### Cranial nerve paresis

In a patient who has a partial paresis of one of the extraocular muscles, a monocular oscillation may occur in the involved eye or its yoke during an ocular movement into the field of action of the involved muscle. Once the eye has been moved as far as possible into the field of action of the paretic muscle, it will begin to drift back toward the primary position. This drift will be halted clinically by a fast corrective movement toward the eccentric gaze position.

### Restrictive syndromes

Monocular oscillations may also be seen in restrictive syndromes in the field of action in which the tethering is occurring. For example, in a patient with a blowout fracture of the orbit who has a trapped inferior rectus muscle, the involved eye would not move upward well and a unilateral jerk nystagmus would appear on attempted upgaze. In certain cases of severe restrictive disease (e.g., Graves' ophthalmopathy), convergence-retraction movements can be produced (Fig. 12-3).

### Superior oblique myokymia

Superior oblique myokymia may be induced by moving the eyes into or away from the field of action of the involved superior oblique muscle (see earlier heading, Superior Oblique Myokomia).

## Binocular symmetric oscillations

If the ocular oscillations involve both eyes to a relatively equal degree (Chart 12-1, *B*), the first decision to be made is whether the movement is disconjugate (the eyes moving in opposite directions) or conjugate (both eyes moving in the same direction), or falls into a category best termed *peculiar or distinctive eye movements* (i.e., eye movements that mimic nystagmus).

### Disconjugate nystagmus

If the nystagmus is disconjugate, the examiner should note whether the oscillations are vertical or horizontal.

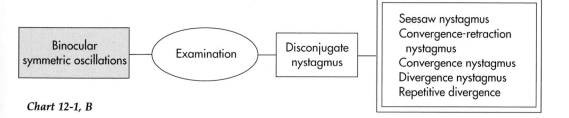

*Chart 12-1, B*

### ☐ Seesaw nystagmus

Seesaw nystagmus is the only vertical disconjugate movement disorder. It is a rare oscillatory movement characterized by an alternate elevation and depression of one eye accompanied by a similar movement, but in the opposite direction, in the other eye (seesaw motion). It can occur in both a congenital and an acquired form. In the more common acquired form the rising eye intorts and the descending eye extorts, whereas in the congenital form either the torsional component is absent or the pattern is opposite (i.e., extorsion on elevation and intorsion on depression).[52,53] The torsional movements are present in all fields of gaze, whereas in general the seesaw effect is limited to the primary position.[54]

For the most part, these patients have large parasellar tumors producing chiasmal and optic nerve compression. Thus vision may be decreased in one or both eyes with bitemporal visual field loss. Patching of the eye with poorer vision may damp the seesaw movement, improve visual acuity, and reduce the accompanying motion sickness feeling induced by the oscillopsia.[55] Brainstem infarct, septo-optic dysplasia, and head trauma have also been implicated as causes of this peculiar movement disorder.[54-58]

### ☐ Convergence-retraction nystagmus

Convergence-retraction nystagmus (a horizontal oscillatory disorder) occurs as part of the dorsal midbrain syndrome (Parinaud's syndrome) (see Chapter 8). These lesions are most often extrinsic masses, but similar signs are seen with intrinsic lesions (usually infiltrative), as well as in patients with hydrocephalus. Initially most of these patients have a selective loss of the ability to voluntarily elevate their eyes; that is, upward saccades are replaced by a slow, undulating upward movement (side-to-side movement superimposed on the vertical movement). With time the patient loses the ability to make upward smooth pursuit movements, and eventually any attempt to produce upward saccades induces a bilateral convergence movement with the eyes retracting into the orbits. This peculiar movement is demonstrated most easily by using an optokinetic stimulus moving downward to induce sequential corrective upward saccades.

### ☐ Convergence nystagmus

Convergence nystagmus is a pendular nystagmus induced by convergence. The oscillation may be convergent, horizontal, or vertical and may be accompanied by lid nystagmus. This rare condition may be congenital or acquired.[59,60] A unique pendular convergence oscillation with the characteristics of normal vergence movements, accompanied by contraction of the muscles of mastication or in synchrony with palatal and mandibular muscular activity, has been termed *oculomasticatory myorhythmia*.[61-63] This finding is considered to be pathognomonic of Whipple's disease. It is usually accompanied by supranuclear ophthalmoparesis, especially of vertical gaze, progressive somnolence, and intellectual deterioration. Recognition of this peculiar complex of findings is important, since early treatment with trimethoprim/sulfamethoxazole may be beneficial.

### ◙ Divergence nystagmus

Divergence nystagmus is a rare form of jerk nystagmus characterized by fast-phase movements away from the nose. It is postulated to be due to cerebellar dysfunction.[59]

### ◙ Repetitive divergence

Repetitive divergence is quite different, consisting of a slow divergent movement followed by a rapid return to the primary position at regular intervals. It has been seen in patients with hepatic encephalopathy.[64]

### ☐ Conjugate nystagmus

The acquired binocular conjugate oscillations can be divided into two major categories by clinical waveform: pendular nystagmus and jerk nystagmus.

### ☐ Pendular nystagmus

If the oscillations are conjugate and pendular, the examiner must determine if they are associated with a normal afferent visual system or with blindness (Chart 12-1, C).

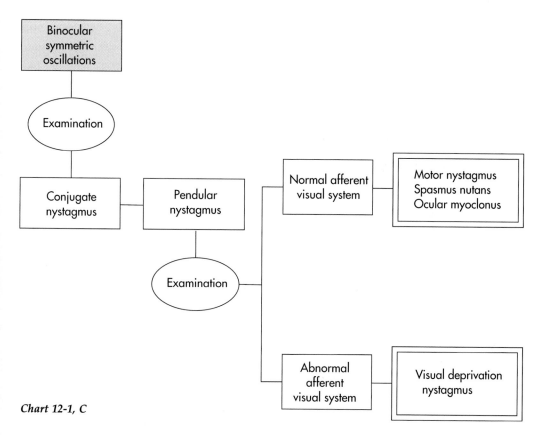

*Chart 12-1, C*

☐ Normal afferent visual system

▣ Motor nystagmus

Motor nystagmus due to MS or brainstem ischemia may be conjugate and binocular, as well as asymmetric. Oblique (diagonal) nystagmus and an oblique nystagmus in which the directional vectors continuously change, producing so-called windmill nystagmus, have been reported.[43] Vertical pendular nystagmus following brainstem hemorrhage has been reported to markedly improve with chronic trihexyphenidyl treatment[65] (see earlier under Monocular or Asymmetric Binocular Oscillations).

▣ Spasmus nutans

Spasmus nutans is discussed in detail earlier in this chapter (see earlier heading, Spasmus Nutans).

▣ Ocular myoclonus

Ocular myoclonus[66] is a continuous, rhythmic, to-and-fro pendular oscillation, usually vertical and often occurring with similar synchronous movements of the face and palate. The ocular movement is a nonspecific form of acquired pendular nystagmus that becomes specific because of the accompanying simultaneous muscle movements.[41] These combined simultaneous movements, termed *oculo-palatal myoclonus,* indicate damage in the "myoclonic triangle" formed by the ipsilateral red nucleus and inferior olivary nucleus and the contralateral dentate nucleus of the cerebellum and their interconnecting fiber tracts. Histopathologic examination reveals hypertrophy of the inferior olivary nucleus. A latency period of weeks to months following the acute lesion (usually infarction) passes before pendular eye movements develop. These movements are present during sleep[67] and usually persist forever.

☐ Abnormal afferent visual system

▣ Visual deprivation nystagmus

Patients who become blind at any age may develop pendular nystagmus. A jerk component may be seen in lateral gaze.

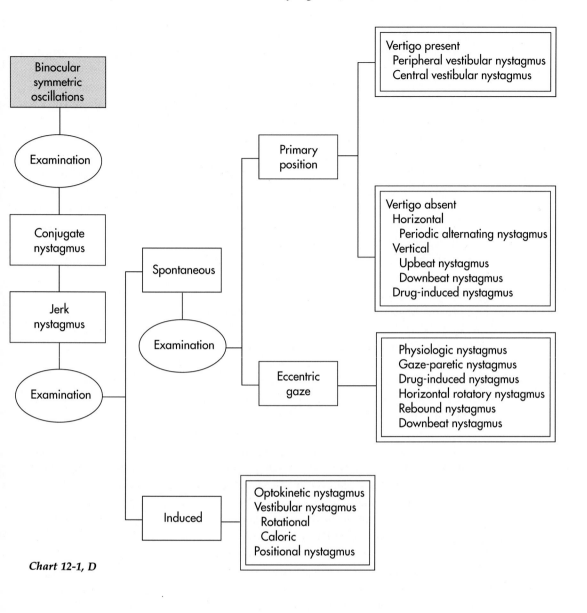

*Chart 12-1, D*

☐ Jerk nystagmus

Jerk nystagmus may be divided into that which is present spontaneously and that which is induced (Chart 12-1, *D*).

☐ Spontaneous jerk nystagmus

Spontaneous jerk nystagmus may in turn be divided into forms present in the primary position and that which is present on eccentric gaze.

☐ Primary position

Jerk nystagmus present in the primary position can be subdivided according to the presence or absence of vertigo.

□ Vertigo present

The presence of vertigo indicates a lesion involving the membranous labyrinth, the eighth cranial nerve, or the vestibular nuclear complex and its connections. Labyrinthine or **peripheral vestibular nystagmus** is a rotary (torsional), horizontal-rotary, or purely horizontal jerk nystagmus present in the primary position that increases in intensity when the eyes are moved in the direction of the fast phase (Alexander's law[68,69]).

Lesions of the vestibular apparatus act as destructive lesions and can be mimicked by ipsilateral irrigation of the ear with cold water. Thus a patient with a disease affecting the right vestibular apparatus will have a left-beating nystagmus, and the environment will appear to move toward the left. A normal individual who undergoes cold water irrigation of the right ear will develop a similar left-beating nystagmus. The patient may experience the sensation of spinning to the right, will pastpoint to the right, and on standing (especially with eyes closed) will tend to fall to the right.

Jerk nystagmus also may be produced by central vestibular dysfunction (i.e., **central vestibular nystagmus**). Peripheral and central vestibular dysfunction may be differentiated by the features listed in Table 12-1. Patients with nystagmus due to peripheral vestibular lesions have a fast phase that beats in the same direction independent of gaze position. Patients with central lesions have nystagmus that may reverse direction as the gaze position changes. Patients with mixed signs (direction of the nystagmus and vertigo, pastpointing, and falling) most likely have a central lesion.

A common form of central vestibular nystagmus is Wallenberg's lateral medullary syndrome.[71] This consists of a distinct constellation of signs and symptoms including ipsilateral loss of pain and temperature sensation in the face and contralateral loss in the trunk and limbs, ipsilateral Horner's syndrome, dysarthria and dysphagia, ataxia of the ipsilateral limbs, vertigo, and a distinctive type of nystagmus. With the eyes open, a horizontal rotary jerk nystagmus beats away from the side of the lesion. With a disruption of fixation (e.g., closing the eyes), the nystagmus either stops or reverses.[72] This syndrome is caused by an infarct in the territory of the posterior inferior cerebellar artery. Depending on the amount of underlying cerebellar and brainstem damage, the physical findings vary considerably.[72] Often these patients experience an illusionary tilting of the environment by 90 or 180 degrees. These patients may demonstrate ocular lateropulsion[73,74] (i.e., a tendency for the eyes to deviate toward the side of the lesion during vertical saccades). In addition, many of these patients complain that their eyes are being pulled toward the side of the lesion. (A veering of the eyes toward the side of the lesion is noted on vertical gaze movements.) Saccades are hypometric and pursuit is impaired away from the lesion, whereas saccades are hypermetric and pursuit is normal toward the side of the lesion. Patients with an infarction in the territory of the superior cerebellar artery may experience contrapulsion (i.e., the eyes are pushed away from the side of the lesion).[75]

| TABLE 12-1 | *Peripheral Versus Central Vestibular Disease* | |
|---|---|---|
| | **Peripheral** | **Central** |
| Severity of vertigo | Marked | Mild to moderate |
| Duration of symptoms | Finite | May be chronic |
| Tinnitus/deafness | Common | Rare |
| Type of nystagmus | Usually mixed horizontal-rotary | May be purely horizontal, rotary, or vertical* |
| Visual fixation | Inhibits nystagmus | Has no effect on nystagmus |
| Common causes | Infectious | Acoustic neuroma |
| | Inflammatory | Ischemia |
| | Toxic | Demyelinating disease |
| | Trauma | Trauma |

*Three cases of primary position upbeating nystagmus due to middle ear disease have been reported.[70]

□ Vertigo absent

Those patients having primary position jerk nystagmus without vertigo may be subdivided according to the plane of ocular oscillation.

**Horizontal jerk nystagmus** is limited to the entity of periodic alternating nystagmus, which is a jerk nystagmus with a cyclically moving or wandering null point.[76] Thus if the eyes are observed in one position of gaze, they pass through a repetitive sequence consisting of a 10-second null period in which the eyes do not move or may beat downward, followed by a period of ascending and descending intensity (amplitude and frequency) of unidirectional jerk nystagmus lasting approximately 90 seconds, followed by a null period and then a repeat of crescendo nystagmus but with the fast phase in the opposite direction. Pathologic[77] and experimental[78] data suggest that the lesion is in the vestibular nucleus. *Periodic alternating nystagmus* may be accompanied by other neurologic findings implicating posterior fossa disease, specifically of the cervicomedullary junction.[76,79] At this time the evaluation of these patients consists of MRI of the posterior fossa. On the basis of a single report[80] that baclofen causes the disappearance of periodic alternating nystagmus, we advocate a trial of this agent in all patients. Reis et al.[81] reported patients with encephalitis who had a type of short-period alternating nystagmus in which the nystagmic bursts changed direction every 3 to 4 seconds. This nystagmus was superimposed on an underlying slow oscillation of the eyes. These patients had encephalitis due to infectious mononucleosis (Epstein-Barr virus).

**Vertical jerk nystagmus** present in the primary position may be subdivided according to the direction of the fast phase into upbeat (fast phase up) and downbeat (fast phase down) varieties. Both upbeat and downbeat nystagmus may represent defects in the smooth pursuit mechanism in the direction of the fast phase.[4,82] *Upbeat nystagmus*[83,84] always represents an intrinsic lesion of the cerebellar vermis or the pontomedullary region of the brainstem; therefore these patients require imaging. Sibony et al.[85] have demonstrated that tobacco smoking in normal subjects induces a transient primary upbeat nystagmus. *Downbeat nystagmus* can occur in any position of gaze and usually indicates cervicomedullary structural disease.[86] Downbeat nystagmus can be present in the primary position but more often occurs in downgaze or in lateral or lateral and down gaze. In the latter instance nystagmus may be present only in left or right gaze and can assume a diagonal vector. Causes of downbeat nystagmus include stroke, MS, Chiari malformation, platybasia, and spinocerebellar degeneration.[87-89] It has also been noted in the setting of a paraneoplastic degeneration,[90] communicating hydrocephalus,[91] or magnesium deficiency,[92] and in phenytoin,[93] lithium,[94] and carbamazepine[95] intoxication. We recommend that all patients with downbeat nystagmus have MRI of the posterior fossa and cervical cord.

**Drug-induced nystagmus** has also been reported. Eight epileptic patients, six of whom were taking both phenytoin and carbamazepine, developed intermittent recurrent visual disturbances (diplopia with ocular misalignment and oscillopsia with horizontal and vertical nystagmus).[96] Discontinuation and reintroduction of these drugs led to cessation and recurrence of the visual disturbances.

### ☐ Eccentric gaze

Jerk nystagmus can also be induced by assuming an eccentric gaze position.

### ☐ Physiologic nystagmus

Physiologic or endpoint nystagmus is a low-amplitude jerk nystagmus of irregular frequency with the fast phase toward the field of gaze. It is poorly sustained. It usually does not occur until the eyes have been held eccentrically for a few seconds. This form may be minimally asymmetric.

### ☐ Gaze-paretic nystagmus

Gaze-paretic nystagmus represents a failure to maintain an eccentric gaze position. Patients with gaze paresis or who are recovering from a gaze palsy pass through a stage where they are able to make a conjugate gaze movement but are unable to maintain the eccentric position. Following an adequate saccadic movement the eyes drift back toward the primary position, at which time a corrective saccade is initiated. A similar movement can be seen in patients with cerebellar disease. Normal subjects in the dark have similar ocular oscillations on eccentric gaze.[97] These movements have been reproduced in cerebellectomized animals[78,98] and thus are considered to represent some deficit of cerebellar modulation of brainstem function.[99]

### ☐ Drug-induced nystagmus

The most common causes of pathologic gaze-evoked nystagmus are tranquilizers or anticonvulsant medications. The nystagmus is usually horizontal but may have a rotary component. Upbeat nystagmus is more frequent than downbeat nystagmus. Drug-induced upbeat nystagmus is the most common form of vertical nystagmus noted clinically. Drug-induced downbeat nystagmus is rare.

### Horizontal rotary nystagmus

Acquired horizontal rotary nystagmus is a common nonspecific finding associated with brainstem dysfunction due to intrinsic or extrinsic causes.

**Bruns' nystagmus** is a combination of gaze-paretic and horizontal rotary nystagmus. Patients with lesions in the cerebellopontine angle often have a distinctive gaze-evoked pattern of nystagmus. Patients with right-sided lesions have slow, large-amplitude, right-beating nystagmus on gaze to the right; left-beating nystagmus of medium amplitude and frequency in primary position; and fine horizontal rotary left-beating nystagmus in left gaze.[100,101] Most of these lesions are acoustic neuromas, which grow so slowly that the patients do not develop vertigo because of the adaptive ability of the vestibular system.

### Rebound nystagmus

Rebound nystagmus, a horizontal jerk nystagmus, is divided into two types. Type 1 occurs when a patient with cerebellar hemispheric degeneration due to alcohol abuse is made to sustain an eccentric gaze position. At first a gaze-evoked nystagmus will be seen that slowly habituates and is followed by the development of a jerk nystagmus in the opposite direction (i.e., fast phase toward the primary position).[102] Rebound nystagmus type 2 is a transient primary position nystagmus that occurs when the eyes are returned to the primary position following sustained eccentric gaze. The nystagmus has its fast phase in the direction opposite to the sustained deviation and represents cerebellar parenchymal disease[103] not limited to the effects of alcohol.

### Downbeat nystagmus

Downbeat nystagmus is frequently seen in eccentric gaze only (see previous discussion).

### Induced jerk nystagmus

Jerk nystagmus can be produced in all normal individuals by either optokinetic or vestibular stimulation. Some people develop a transient jerk nystagmus when they place their heads into particular positions (positional nystagmus). Positional nystagmus always indicates an abnormality of the vestibular system.

### Optokinetic nystagmus

Optokinetic nystagmus (OKN) is a type of induced nystagmus easily elicited in all alert persons whose vision permits them to count fingers. It represents activation of pursuit (slow-movement) mechanisms followed by a fast-phase movement either foveating or at least corrective in the opposite direction. It is usually induced clinically by the use of a striped tape or rotating drum. The eyes involuntarily follow a moving stripe until it passes beyond the range of fixation, at which time a fast movement is made in the opposite direction. A sustained optokinetic response is more consistently evoked with targets moving in the horizontal plane than in the vertical plane. Although the underlying physiologic mechanisms are not known, the response is involuntary and cannot be suppressed if the optokinetic stimulus fills the entire visual field.

An OKN abnormality is seen in patients with deep lesions of the occipito-parietal lobes but not in patients with lesions limited to the occipital lobes. This response consists of a reduced amplitude of movement when the tape is rotated toward the side of the lesion. The optokinetic response can be reduced or absent in brainstem disease involving the ocular motor mechanisms. Optokinetic stimuli are also useful in exaggerating the dissociated movements of subtle INO and in inducing convergence-retraction nystagmus in midbrain syndromes. Since the optokinetic response cannot be suppressed, its presence can be used to infer visual function in patients suspected of malingering.

### Vestibular nystagmus

The vestibular apparatus plays a major role in controlling and coordinating the tone of the body musculature, including the extraocular muscles. Response to linear acceleration is controlled by the otoliths in the utricle and saccule, whereas responses to angular acceleration are controlled by the hair cells in the semicircular canals. Varying degrees of nystagmus and vertigo can be produced in a normal person by stimulating the peripheral vestibular apparatus by either rotational or caloric testing. Such tests are useful clinically to determine the integrity of the membranous labyrinth and its central connections.

**ROTATIONAL NYSTAGMUS.** The interpretation of both rotational and caloric testing assumes that horizontal canal function reflects the functional capability of the vertical canals as well. Rotational testing is, for the most part, relegated to the laboratory because of the need for sophisticated equipment. A gross but effective type of rotational testing is often done in infants. The examiner lifts and spins the child around with the head appropriately supported and the examiner acting as the fulcrum. The infant's head is tilted 30 degrees forward. Under normal conditions, when the examiner spins to the left the infant's eyes will be conjugately driven to the infant's left, with the development of an after-nystagmus to the right. The infant's vertical eye movements can be checked by use of vertical oculocephalic movements.

**CALORIC NYSTAGMUS.** Caloric testing depends on producing convection currents in the endolymph of the membranous labyrinth by the use of a caloric stimulus introduced into the external auditory canal. To isolate and maximize this effect on the horizontal canal, the patient's head must be positioned so that the horizontal canal lies in the vertical plane. This is accomplished in the seated patient by tilting the patient's head backward 60 degrees, or in the supine patient by tilting the patient's head forward 30 degrees. Thermal stimulation produces a directional jerk nystagmus most easily remembered by the mnemonic COWS—Cold, Opposite; Warm, Same—with *cold* and *warm* referring to the type of stimulus and *opposite* and *same* referring to the direction of the fast-phase response with respect to the side being stimulated. The advantage of the caloric test is that the vestibular apparatus on each side can be tested separately, and no sophisticated equipment is required.

In comatose individuals or those with loss of voluntary supranuclear control mechanisms (e.g., progressive supranuclear palsy), the integrity of the brainstem mechanisms may be determined by calorics or by moving the patient's head in a horizontal and then a vertical plane. The latter manipulation produces contraversive eye movements, the so-called oculocephalic or doll's eye maneuver.

The aminoglycosides (including streptomycin and gentamicin) can produce sudden, irreversible failure of vestibular function.[4,104] In some cases a return of vestibular function over a period of weeks has been noted after discontinuing the use of the drugs. Deafness occurs in some patients, although it is rarely complete. The major complaint of individuals so affected is the almost continuous presence of oscillopsia in the absence of any apparent concomitant eye movements. When at rest, some individuals note a synchrony with the pulse. The oscillopsia is made worse on ambulation or riding over a bumpy road.

### ▣ Positional nystagmus

Positional nystagmus is a jerk nystagmus induced by altering the position of the body or the head. The patient complains about the acute onset of vertigo with changes in body orientation. Two types of positional nystagmus exist: (1) central, involving the vestibular nerve, nuclei, or their connections, and (2) peripheral, involving the membranous labyrinth.[105]

In *central positional nystagmus* the nystagmus begins immediately on changing to the inducing head position, does not fatigue or habituate if the test is repeated, and is associated with mild vertigo. The central type has been associated with a variety of disorders, including neoplasm, infarct, demyelination, and degeneration of the cerebellum and brainstem.[106] Evaluation will depend on accompanying neurologic markers.

*Peripheral positional nystagmus* has a measurable latency before onset after moving the head into the appropriate position, fatigues within a short period of time, habituates with repeat testing, and is associated with severe but transient vertigo. This variety of positional nystagmus, although bothersome to the patient, is almost always a benign disorder and thus has been termed *benign paroxysmal positional nystagmus*. It is indicative of labyrinthine disease. It has been reported following trauma, but in most cases the etiology remains obscure. In the absence of other neurologic signs, no investigation is warranted.

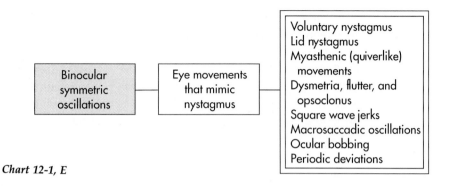

| Binocular symmetric oscillations | → | Eye movements that mimic nystagmus | → | Voluntary nystagmus<br>Lid nystagmus<br>Myasthenic (quiverlike)<br>   movements<br>Dysmetria, flutter, and<br>   opsoclonus<br>Square wave jerks<br>Macrosaccadic oscillations<br>Ocular bobbing<br>Periodic deviations |

*Chart 12-1, E*

☐ Eye movements that mimic nystagmus

The remaining entities are part of a collection of distinctive movement disorders in which no unifying feature is apparent (Chart 12-1, *E*).

▣ Voluntary nystagmus

To the observer, voluntary nystagmus appears to be a low-amplitude, high-frequency pendular oscillation that occurs in bursts and cannot be maintained for more than a few seconds. Eye movement recordings have established voluntary nystagmus to be a series of sequential saccades.[107] The ability to produce this nystagmus is frequently a familial trait[108] and is often used as a parlor trick. The importance of recognizing this syndrome is the identification of patients feigning illness with the complaint of sudden onset of oscillatory movements following an alleged injury. This movement will completely disappear if patients are forced to keep their eyes open, since it requires tremendous volitional effort and cannot be sustained for prolonged periods.

▣ Lid nystagmus

Lid nystagmus is a rhythmic upward jerking of the upper eyelids that usually accompanies vertical ocular nystagmus. Three types of lid nystagmus exist. The first is the exaggeration of the normal lid movement that accompanies vertical nystagmus; only the amplitude of the lid movement exceeds that of the ocular movement. The second type is evoked on lateral gaze, and the fast movements of the lids and horizontal nystagmus are synchronous.[109] The third type has been associated with convergence effort[110] and is seen in the lateral medullary syndrome, as well as in the sylvian aqueduct syndrome.

▣ Myasthenic (quiverlike) movements

In patients with myasthenia gravis with marked involvement of all their muscles, a jellylike bilateral quiver movement may be clinically recognized after the initiation of a saccadic movement.[111] This quiver movement is considered to be specific for myasthenia gravis. In addition, myasthenic patients with ocular involvement may appear to have a gaze paresis, including the development of a gaze-paretic type of nystagmus that may be vertical.[112] This nystagmus fatigues rapidly with the eyes assuming a position short of the target. Similarly, a pseudointernuclear ophthalmoplegia may be seen. All of these movement disorders are markedly improved by the injection of Tensilon.

### ☐ Dysmetria, flutter, and opsoclonus[113]

Inappropriate saccades or saccadic intrusions consist of a group of disorders that interfere with foveal fixation. They include ocular dysmetria, ocular flutter, and opsoclonus, as well as square wave jerks, macrosquare wave jerks, and macro-saccadic oscillations. Dysmetria, flutter, and opsoclonus[113] constitute a group of ocular oscillations that, in listed order, occur with increasing degrees of cerebellar dysfunction.[114]

*Ocular dysmetria*[113] occurs at the end of refixation saccades. It is often more apparent when the eyes move from the lateral gaze position to the primary position than in the opposite direction. Ocular dysmetria manifests either as a binocular conjugate undershooting or overshooting followed by a to-and-fro saccadic oscillation around the fixation point before foveation is accomplished, or as a conjugate overshoot followed by a single corrective saccade in large-amplitude refixation movements.

*Ocular flutter*[113] is a spontaneous binocular break in fixation followed by horizontal oscillations around fixation consisting of back-to-back saccades without an intersaccadic interval. It is almost never present in the absence of dysmetria, and its presence probably represents a further deterioration of cerebellar function.

*Opsoclonus*, or *saccadomania* (rapid, involuntary, continuous, repetitive, conjugate saccadic eye movements in all directions), occurs when cerebellar input to the paramedian pontine reticular formation is entirely disrupted. Hattori et al.[115] have demonstrated this disorder in two patients with purely pontine lesions. These movements persist during sleep. Patients who recover go through a reverse sequence in which brief periods of opsoclonus interrupt stable periods of fixation, followed by a period in which flutter and dysmetria are present. The flutter then disappears, and finally with total recovery the dysmetria also disappears.

Opsoclonus in both children and adults can occur as part of a paraneoplastic syndrome and is associated with ataxia, myoclonus, and irritability. Opsoclonus in children should be considered to be due to occult neuroblastoma[116] until imaging studies of the abdomen and thorax exclude the diagnosis. Such remote effects may be seen in adult patients with carcinoma[117] (usually oat cell of the lung) and may be thiamine responsive.[118]

Opsoclonus can occur as part of a postinfectious syndrome with ataxia, extremity myoclonus, and tremulousness. This postinfectious syndrome is somewhat responsive to corticosteroid therapy. Opsoclonus has been associated with hyperosmotic nonketotic coma,[119,120] drug toxicity,[121,122] mesencephalic glioma, ischemic and hemorrhagic stroke, hydrocephalus, and trauma.[117]

### ☐ Square wave jerks

Square wave jerks and macrosquare wave jerks[123] are ocular movement disorders in which an observable break in fixation occurs because of an intrusion of an unwanted saccade, followed by a rapid single movement of refoveation after a nearly normal intersaccadic interval. On inspection, both square wave and macrosquare wave jerks may look like primary position horizontal nystagmus but are identified by their characteristic electronystagmographic pattern. Square wave jerks are subtle and may be easily missed clinically (amplitude, 0.5 to 3 degrees; latency to refixation, 200 ms), whereas macrosquare wave jerks are quite easily seen (amplitude, 4 to 30 degrees; latency to refixation, 50 to 150 ms). Both types of disorder are in general associated with neurodegenerative states, especially progressive supranuclear palsy and Parkinson's disease.

### Macrosaccadic oscillations

Macrosaccadic oscillations consist of a saccadic intrusion followed by a series of hypermetric saccades bypassing the object of regard with an appropriate intersaccadic interval. These oscillations reflect the patient's inability to program a small enough saccade to produce fixation and are related to cerebellar dysfunction.

### Ocular bobbing

Ocular bobbing indicates severe brainstem dysfunction and is not precisely localizable.[124] In ocular bobbing the eyes repeatedly move briskly downward from the primary position, remain eccentric for a few seconds, and then slowly drift back to the primary position.[125] The movement may be more apparent in one eye than in the other.[126] Usually, horizontal eye movements are completely absent. Ocular bobbing has been classically associated with intrinsic brainstem lesions, including strokes,[127] pontine glioma,[128] toxic[129] and metabolic[127,130] encephalopathies, MS,[131] and encephalitis.[132] It has been reported with extraaxial lesions compressing the brainstem as well.[127,133]

*Reverse bobbing*[127,134,135] consists of a rapid deviation of the eyes upward and a slow return to the horizontal.

*Ocular dipping,* or *inverse bobbing,* is an arrhythmic, slow downward movement followed by a fast upward component. This disorder has been reported with intracerebral hematomas and metabolic encephalopathy.[125] In patients with reverse or inverse bobbing, horizontal eye movements are usually absent. The vertical movements are postulated to represent the function of the only intact eye motor system.

### Periodic deviations

Periodic deviations are of two types: periodic alternating gaze deviation and periodic alternating "Ping-Pong" gaze.

*Periodic alternating gaze deviation*[136] is an involuntary, continuous cyclic disorder of eye movements that disappears during sleep. A cycle consists of a binocular horizontal slow deviation of the eyes to one eccentric gaze position; the eyes remain in lateral gaze for about 2 minutes, and then a slow conjugate movement of the eyes occurs to the opposite lateral gaze position, where the eccentric position is maintained for 2 minutes, and then the cycle begins again.

*Periodic alternating Ping-Pong gaze* is a cyclic disorder of eye movements in which the eyes deviate briefly far to the right and then rapidly reverse direction to the left with a periodicity of a few seconds.[137-139]

Both of these movements are seen in comatose patients with extensive bihemispheric infarction or posterior fossa hemorrhage. The underlying pathology remains speculative. Most patients die, although Ping-Pong gaze has been seen in a patient with reversible coma due to an overdose of monoamine oxidase inhibitors.[140]

The *ocular tilt reaction* is an extremely rare intermittent movement disorder consisting of paroxysmal tonic skew deviation and torsion of the eyes, coupled with a pendular nystagmus and head tilt due to a lesion in the region of the zona incerta of the diencephalon.[141] It can be produced experimentally in the monkey by stimulation near the interstitial nucleus of Cajal.[142]

Defects in normal ocular counterrolling mechanisms, especially the lack of sustained compensatory torsion, have been found in patients with spasmodic torticollis.[143] This finding, along with spontaneous vertical nystagmus in the dark and directional preponderance with caloric stimulation, implies that the cause of the ocular tilt reaction and spasmodic torticollis is a disruption of central vestibular pathways.

## REFERENCES

1. Cogan DG. Neurology of the ocular muscles. 2nd ed. Springfield, IL: Charles C Thomas, 1956:184.
2. Cogan DG. Neurology of the ocular muscles. 2nd ed. Springfield, IL: Charles C Thomas, 1956:189.
3. Gelbart SS, Hoyt CS. Congenital nystagmus: a clinical perspective in infancy. Graefe's Arch Clin Exp Ophthalmol 1988;226:178-80.
4. Dell'Osso LF, Daroff RB, Troost BT. Nystagmus and saccadic intrusions and oscillations. In: Glaser JS, ed. Neuro-Ophthalmology. Philadelphia: JB Lippincott, 1990:325-56.
5. Dell'Osso LF, Daroff RB. Congenital nystagmus waveforms and foveation strategy. Doc Ophthalmol 1975;39:155-82.
6. Gresty M, Page N, Barratt H. The differential diagnosis of congenital nystagmus. J Neurol Neurosurg Psychiatry 1984;47:936-42.
7. Dell'Osso LF. Improving visual acuity in congenital nystagmus. In: Smith JL, Glaser JS, eds. Neuro-ophthalmology: symposium of the University of Miami and the Bascom Palmer Eye Institute, vol 7. St Louis: Mosby–Year Book, 1973:98-106.
8. Gresty MA, Halmagyi GM. Abnormal head movements. J Neurol Neurosurg Psychiatry 11979;42:705-14.
9. D'Esposito M, Reccia R, Roberti G, et al. Amount of surgery in congenital nystagmus. Ophthalmologica 1989;198:145-51.
10. Helveston EM. The value of strabismus surgery. Ophthalmic Surg 1990;21:311-7.
11. Sigal MB, Diamond GR. Survey of management strategies for nystagmus patients with vertical or torsional head posture. Ann Ophthalmol 1990;22:134-8.
12. Barricks ME, Flynn JT, Kushner BJ. Paradoxical pupillary responses in congenital stationary night blindness. In: Smith JL, ed. Neuro-ophthalmology update. New York: Masson Publishing, 1977:31-8.
13. Freeman MI, Burde RM, Gay AJ. A case of true paradoxical pupillary reaction. Arch Ophthalmol 1966;75:740-1.
14. Goldhammer Y. Paradoxical pupillary reaction. In: Smith JL, ed. Neuro-ophthalmology update. New York: Masson Publishing, 1977:39-42.
15. Ohm J. Der latente Nystagmus nach Verlust eines Auges. Albrecht von Graefes Arch Ophthalmol 1942;144:617-22.

16. Dell'Osso LF, Schmidt D, Daroff RB. Latent, manifest latent, and congenital nystagmus. Arch Ophthalmol 1979; 97:1877-85.

17. Dell'Osso LF, Abel LA, Daroff RB. Latent/manifest latent nystagmus reversal using an ocular prosthesis: implications for vision and ocular dominance. Invest Ophthalmol Vis Sci 1987;28:1873-6.

18. Kestenbaum A. Clinical methods of neuro-ophthalmological examination. 2nd ed. New York: Grune & Stratton, 1961:344.

19. Zubcov AA, Reinecke RD, Gottlob I, et al. Treatment of manifest latent nystagmus. Am J Ophthalmol 1990; 110:160-7.

20. Spicer WTH. The nystagmus of spasmus nutans in infants. Br Med J 1901;1:1120.

21. Weissman BM, Dell'Osso LF, Abel LA, et al. Spasmus nutans: a quantitative prospective study. Arch Ophthalmol 1987;105:525-8.

22. Norton EWD, Cogan DG. Spasmus nutans: a clinical study of twenty cases followed two years or more since onset. Arch Ophthalmol 1954; 52:442-6.

23. Cogan DG. Neurology of the ocular muscles. 2nd ed. Springfield, IL: Charles C Thomas, 1956:192.

24. Jayalakshmi P, Scott TFM, Tucker SH, et al. Infantile nystagmus: a prospective study of spasmus nutans, congenital nystagmus, and unclassified nystagmus of infancy. J Pediatr 1970;77:177-87.

25. Bray PF. Can maternal alcoholism cause spasmus nutans in offspring? N Engl J Med 1990;322:554.

26. Donin JF. Acquired monocular nystagmus in children. Can J Ophthalmol 1967;2:212-5.

27. Kelly TW. Optic glioma presenting as spasmus nutans. Pediatrics 1970; 45:295-6.

28. Schulman JA, Shults WT, Jones JM Jr. Monocular vertical nystagmus as an initial sign of chiasmal glioma. Am J Ophthalmol 1979;87:87-90.

29. Antony JH, Ouvrier RA, Wise G. Spasmus nutans: a mistaken identity. Arch Neurol 1980;37:373-5.

30. Halpern J. Spasmus nutans. Arch Neurol 1980;37:737-8.

31. Smith JL, Flynn JT, Spiro HJ. Monocular vertical oscillations of amblyopia: the Heimann-Bielschowsky phenomenon. J Clin Neuro Ophthalmol 1982; 2:85-91.

32. Yee RD, Jelks GW, Baloh RW, et al. Uniocular nystagmus in monocular visual loss. Ophthalmology 1979; 86:511-8.

33. Hoyt WF, Keane JR. Superior oblique myokymia: report and discussion on five cases of benign intermittent uniocular microtremor. Arch Ophthalmol 1970;84:461-7.

34. Rosenberg ML, Glaser JS. Superior oblique myokymia. Ann Neurol 1983; 13:667-9.

35. Herzau V, Körner F, Kommerell G, et al. Obliquus superior-myokymie: Eine klinische und elektromyographische studie. In: Kommerell G, ed. Disorders of ocular motility: neuro-physiological and clinical aspects. Munich: Bergmann, 1978:81-90.

36. Kommerell G, Schaubele G. Superior oblique myokymia: an electromyographical analysis. Trans Ophthalmol Soc UK 1980;100:504-6.

37. Morrow MJ, Sharpe JA, Ranalli PJ. Superior oblique myokymia associated with a posterior fossa tumor: oculographic correlation with an idiopathic case. Neurology 1990;40:367-70.

38. Susac JO, Smith JL, Schatz NJ. Superior oblique myokymia. Arch Neurol 1973;29:432-4.

39. Palmer EH, Shults WT. Superior oblique myokymia: preliminary results of surgical treatment. J Pediatr Ophthalmol Strabismus 1984;21:96-101.

40. Aschoff JC, Conrad B, Kornhuber HH. Acquired pendular nystagmus with oscillopsia in multiple sclerosis: a sign of cerebellar nuclei disease. J Neurol Neurosurg Psychiatry 1974; 37:570-7.

41. Gresty MA, Ell JJ, Findley LJ. Acquired pendular nystagmus: its characteristics, localising value and pathophysiology. J Neurol Neurosurg Psychiatry 1982;45:431-3.

42. Leigh RJ, Zee DS. The neurology of

eye movements. Philadelphia: FA Davis, 1983:204.

43. Sanders MD. Alternating windmill nystagmus. In: Smith JL, Glaser JS, eds. Neuro-ophthalmology: symposium of the University of Miami and the Bascom Palmer Eye Institute, vol 7. St Louis: Mosby–Year Book, 1973:133-6.

44. Traccis S, Rosati G, Monaco MF, et al. Successful treatment of acquired pendular elliptical nystagmus in multiple sclerosis with isoniazid and base-out prisms. Neurology 1990;40:492-4.

45. Leigh RJ, Rushton DN, Thurston SE, et al. Effects of retinal image stabilization in acquired nystagmus due to neurologic disease. Neurology 1988;38:122-7.

46. Rushton DN. Geometrical optics of the retinal image stabilisation device. J Neurol Neurosurg Psychiatry 1989;52:137-8.

47. Burde RM, Lehman RAW, Roper-Hall G, et al. Experimental internuclear ophthalmoplegia. Br J Ophthalmol 1977;61:233-9.

48. Kommerell G. Unilateral internuclear ophthalmoplegia: the lack of inhibitory involvement in medial rectus muscle activity. Invest Ophthalmol Vis Sci 1981;21:592-9.

49. Zee DS, Hain TC, Carl JR. Abduction nystagmus in internuclear ophthalmoplegia. Ann Neurol 1987;21:383-8.

50. Smith JL, David NJ. Internuclear ophthalmoplegia: two new clinical signs. Neurology 1964;14:307-9.

51. Glaser JS. Myasthenic pseudo-internuclear ophthalmoplegia. Arch Ophthalmol 1966;75:363-6.

52. Slatt B, Nykiel F. See-saw nystagmus. Am J Ophthalmol 1964;58:1016-21.

53. Williams IM, Dickinson P, Ramsay RJ, et al. See-saw nystagmus. Aust J Ophthalmol 1982;10:19-25.

54. Daroff RB. See-saw nystagmus. Neurology 1965;15:874-7.

55. Lourie H. Seesaw nystagmus: case report elucidating the mechanism. Arch Neurol 1963;9:531-3.

56. Davis GV, Shock JP. Septo-optic dysplasia associated with see-saw nystagmus. Arch Ophthalmol 1975;93:137-9.

57. Kanter DS, Ruff RL, Leigh RJ, et al. See-saw nystagmus and brainstem infarction. Neuro-ophthalmology 1987;7:279-83.

58. Schmidt D, Kommerell G. Schaukel-Nystagmus (seesaw nystagmus) mit bitemporaler Hemaniopie als Folge von Schädelhirntraumen. Albrecht von Graefes Arch Klin Exp Ophthalmol 1969;178:349-66.

59. Cogan DG. Convergence nystagmus: with notes on a single case of divergence nystagmus. Arch Ophthalmol 1959;62:295-9.

60. Sharpe JA, Hoyt WF, Rosenberg MA. Convergence-evoked nystagmus: congenital and acquired forms. Arch Neurol 1975;32:191-4.

61. Grotta JC, Pettingrew LC, Schmidt WA, et al. Oculomasticatory myorhythmia. Ann Neurol 1987;22:395-6.

62. Miller NR, ed. Walsh and Hoyt's clinical neuro-ophthalmology, vol 2. 4th ed. Baltimore: Williams & Wilkins, 1985:892-931.

63. Schwartz MA, Selhorst JB, Ochs AL, et al. Oculomasticatory myorhythmia: a unique movement disorder occurring in Whipple's disease. Ann Neurol 1986;20:677-83.

64. Noda S, Ide K, Umezaki H, et al. Repetitive divergence. Ann Neurol 1987; 21:109-10.

65. Herishanu Y, Louzoun Z. Trihexyphenidyl treatment of vertical pendular nystagmus. Neurology 1986; 36:82-4.

66. Chokroverty S, Barron KD. Palatal myoclonus and rhythmic ocular movements: a polygraphic study. Neurology 1969;19:975-82.

67. Tahmoush AJ, Brooks JE, Keltner JL. Palatal myoclonus associated with abnormal ocular and extremity movements. Arch Neurol 1972;27:431-40.

68. Alexander G. Die Ohrenkrankheiten im Kindesalter. In: Pfaundler M, Schlossmann A, eds. Handbuch der Kinderheilkunde. Leipzig: Vogel, 1912: 84-96.

69. Doslak MJ, Dell'Osso LF, Daroff RB. Alexander's law: a model and resulting study. Ann Otol Rhinol Laryngol 1982;91:316-22.

70. Gresty MA, Bronstein AM, Brookes GB, et al. Primary position upbeating

nystagmus associated with middle-ear disease. Neuro-ophthalmology 1988;8:321-8.

71. Wallenberg A. Acute Bulbäraffection (Embolie der Art. cerebellar. post. inf. sinistr.). Arch Psychiatr Nervenkr 1895;27:504-40.

72. Duncan GW, Parker SW, Fisher CM. Acute cerebellar infarction in the PICA territory. Arch Neurol 1975; 32:364-8.

73. Kommerell G, Hoyt WF. Lateropulsion of saccadic eye movements: electro-oculographic studies in a patient with Wallenberg's syndrome. Arch Neurol 1973;28:313-8.

74. Meyer KT, Baloh RW, Krohel GB, et al. Ocular lateropulsion: a sign of lateral medullary disease. Arch Ophthalmol 1980;98:1614-6.

75. Ranalli PJ, Sharpe JA. Contrapulsion of saccades and ipsilateral ataxia: a unilateral disorder of rostral cerebellum. Ann Neurol 1986;20:311-6.

76. Daroff RB, Dell'Osso LF. Periodic alternating nystagmus and the shifting null. Can J Otolaryngol 1974;3:367-71.

77. Karp JS, Rorke LB. Periodic alternating nystagmus. Arch Neurol 1975; 32:422-3.

78. Burde RM, Stroud MH, Roper-Hall G, et al. Ocular motor dysfunction in total and hemicerebellectomized monkeys. Br J Ophthalmol 1975;59:560-5.

79. Keane JR. Periodic alternating nystagmus with downward beating nystagmus: a clinicoanatomical case study of multiple sclerosis. Arch Neurol 1974; 30:399-402.

80. Halmagyi GM, Rudge P, Gresty MA, et al. Treatment of periodic alternating nystagmus. Ann Neurol 1980;8:609-11.

81. Reis J, Eber AM, Warter JM, et al. Alternating nystagmus and infectious mononucleosis. Neuro-ophthalmology 1989;9:289-92.

82. Zee DS, Friendlich AR, Robinson DA. The mechanism of downbeat nystagmus. Arch Neurol 1974;30:227-37.

83. Daroff RB, Troost BT. Upbeat nystagmus. JAMA 1973;225:312.

84. Gilman N, Baloh RW, Tomiyasu U. Primary position up-beat nystagmus: a clinicopathologic study. Neurology 1977;27:294-8.

85. Sibony PA, Evinger C., Manning KA. The effects of tobacco smoking on smooth pursuit eye movements. Ann Neurol 1988;23:238-41.

86. Cogan DG. Down-beat nystagmus. Arch Ophthalmol 1968;80:757-68.

87. Farris BK, Smith JL, Ayyar R. Neuro-ophthalmologic findings in vestibulo-cerebellar ataxia. Arch Neurol 1986;43: 1050-3.

88. Halmagyi GM, Rudge P, Gresty MA, et al. Downbeating nystagmus: a review of 62 cases. Arch Neurol 1983;40:777-84.

89. Kapila A, Elble R, Ratcheson RA, et al. Radiologic demonstration of dorsal medullocervical spur in adult Chiari malformation. J Clin Neuro Ophthalmol 1982;2:235-40.

90. Posner JB. Paraneoplastic syndromes involving the nervous system. In: Aminoff MJ, ed. Neurology and general medicine: the neurological aspects of medical disorders. New York: Churchill Livingstone, 1989:341-64.

91. Phadke JG, Hern JEC, Blaiklock CT. Downbeat nystagmus—a false localising sign due to communicating hydrocephalus. J Neurol Neurosurg Psychiatry 1981;44:459.

92. Saul RF, Selhorst JB. Downbeat nystagmus with magnesium depletion. Arch Neurol 1981;38:650-2.

93. Alpert JN. Downbeat nystagmus due to anticonvulsant toxicity. Ann Neurol 1978;4:471-3.

94. Williams DP, Troost BT, Rogers J. Lithium-induced downbeat nystagmus. Arch Neurol 1988;45:1022-3.

95. Wheeler SD, Ramsay RE, Weiss J. Drug-induced downbeat nystagmus. Ann Neurol 1982;12:227-8.

96. Remler BF, Leigh RJ, Osoria I, et al. The characteristics and mechanisms of visual disturbance associated with anticonvulsant therapy. Neurology 1990;40:791-6.

97. Becker W, Klein HM. Accuracy of saccadic eye movements and maintenance of eccentric eye positions in the dark. Vision Res 1973;13:1021-34.

98. Westheimer G, Blair SM. Oculomotor defects in cerebellectomized monkeys. Invest Ophthalmol 1975;12:618-21.

99. Robinson DA. The effect of cerebellec-

tomy on the cat's vestibulo-ocular integrator. Brain Res 1974;71:195-207.

100. Baloh RW, Konrad HR, Dirks D, Honrubia V. Cerebellar-pontine angle tumors: results of quantitative vestibuloocular testing. Arch Neurol 1976;33: 507-12.

101. Schatz NJ, Savino PJ. Nystagmus. In: Symposium on neuro-ophthalmology: transactions of the New Orleans Academy of Ophthalmology. St Louis: Mosby–Year Book, 1976:84-9.

102. Hood JD, Kayan A, Leech J. Rebound nystagmus. Brain 1973;96:507-26.

103. Zee DS, Yee RD, Cogan DG, et al. Ocular motor abnormalities in hereditary cerebellar ataxia. Brain 1976;99: 207-34.

104. Marra TR, Reynolds NC Jr, Stoddard JJ. Subjective oscillopsia ("jiggling" vision) presumably due to aminoglycoside ototoxicity: a report of two cases. J Clin Neuro Ophthalmol 1988;8:35-8.

105. Harrison MS, Ozsahinoglu C. Positional vertigo: aetiology and clinical significance. Brain 1972;95:369-72.

106. Kattah JC, Kolsky MP, Luessenhop AJ. Positional vertigo and the cerebellar vermis. Neurology 1984;34:527-9.

107. Shults WT, Start L, Hoyt WF, et al. Normal saccadic structure of voluntary nystagmus. Arch Ophthalmol 1977;95:1399-404.

108. Aschoff JC, Becker W, Rettelbach R. Voluntary nystagmus in five generations. J Neurol Neurosurg Psychiatry 1976;39:300-4.

109. Daroff RB, Hoyt WF, Sanders MD, et al. Gaze-evoked eyelid and ocular nystagmus inhibited by the near reflex: unusual ocular motor phenomena in a lateral medullary syndrome. J Neurol Neurosurg Psychiatry 1968; 31:362-7.

110. Sanders MD, Hoyt WF, Daroff RB. Lid nystagmus evoked by ocular convergence: an ocular electromyographic study. J Neurol Neurosurg Psychiatry 1968;31:368-71.

111. Cogan DG, Yee RD, Gittinger J. Rapid eye movements in myasthenia gravis. Arch Ophthalmol 1976;94:1083-5.

112. Keane JR, Hoyt WF. Myasthenic (vertical) nystagmus: verification by edrophonium tonography. JAMA 1970; 212:1209-10.

113. Cogan DG. Ocular dysmetria: flutterlike oscillations of the eyes, and opsoclonus. Arch Ophthalmol 1954; 451:318-35.

114. Ellenberger C Jr, Keltner JL, Stroud MH. Ocular dyskinesia in cerebellar disease: evidence for the similarity of opsoclonus, ocular dysmetria and flutter-like oscillations. Brain 1972; 95:685-92.

115. Hattori T, Hirayama K, Imai T, et al. Pontine lesion in opsoclonus-myoclonus syndrome shown by MRI. J Neurol Neurosurg Psychiatry 1988; 51:1572-5.

116. Solomon GE, Chutorian AM. Opsoclonus and occult neuroblastoma. N Engl J Med 1968;279:475-7.

117. Wolpow ER. Discussion. In: Wolpow ER, Richardson EP Jr, eds. MGH case records (case 9-1988): a 57-year-old woman with worsening opsoclonus. In: Case records of the Massachusetts General Hospital. N Engl J Med 1988;318:563-70.

118. Nausieda PA, Tanner CM, Weiner WJ. Opsoclonic cerebellopathy: a paraneoplastic syndrome responsive to thiamine. Arch Neurol 1981;38:780-1.

119. Noda S, Takao A, Itoh H, et al. Opsoclonus in hyperosmolar nonketotic coma. J Neurol Neurosurg Psychiatry 1985;48:1186-7.

120. Weissman B, Devereaux M, Krishan C. Opsoclonus and hyperosmolar stupor. Neurology 1989;39:1401-2.

121. Pullicino P, Aquilina J. Opsoclonus in organophosphate poisoning. Arch Neurol 1989;46:704-5.

122. Scharf D. Opsoclonus-myoclonus following intranasal usage of cocaine. J Neurol Neurosurg Psychiatry 1989; 52:1447-8.

123. Leigh RJ, Zee DS. The neurology of eye movements. Philadelphia: FA Davis, 1983:61.

124. Bosch EP, Kennedy SS, Aschenbrener CA. Ocular bobbing: the myth of its localizing value. Neurology 1975; 25:949-53.

125. Fisher CM. Ocular bobbing. Arch Neurol 1964;11:543-6.

126. Newman N, Gay AJ, Heilbrun MP. Disconjugate ocular bobbing: its relation to midbrain, pontine, and medullary function in a surviving patient. Neurology 1971;21:633-7.

127. Susac JO, Hoyt WF, Daroff RB, et al. Clinical spectrum of ocular bobbing. J Neurol Neurosurg Psychiatry 1970; 33:771-5.

128. Daroff RB, Waldman AL. Ocular bobbing. J Neurol Neurosurg Psychiatry 1965;28:375-7.

129. Paty DW, Sherr H. Ocular bobbing in bromism: a case report. Neurology 1972;22:525-6.

130. Rai GS, Buxton-Thomas M, Scanlon M. Ocular bobbing in hepatic encephalopathy. Br J Clin Pract 1976;30:202, 205.

131. Ash PR, Keltner JL. Neuro-ophthalmic signs in pontine lesions. Medicine 1979;58:304-20.

132. Rudick R, Satran R, Eskin TA. Ocular bobbing in encephalitis. J Neurol Neurosurg Psychiatry 1981;44:441-3.

133. Finelli PF, McEntee WJ. Ocular bobbing with extra-axial haematoma of the posterior fossa. J Neurol Neurosurg Psychiatry 1977;40:386-8.

134. Knobler RL, Somasundaram M, Schutta HS. Inverse ocular bobbing. Ann Neurol 1981;9:194-7.

135. Ropper AH. Ocular dipping in anoxic coma. Arch Neurol 1981;38:297-9.

136. Goldberg RT, Gonzalez C, Breinin GM, et al. Periodic alternating gaze deviation with dissociation of head movement. Arch Ophthalmol 1965; 73:324-30.

137. Masucci EF, Fabara JA, Saini N, et al. Periodic alternating ping-pong gaze. Ann Ophthalmol 1981;13:1123-7.

138. Senelick RC. "Ping-pong" gaze: periodic alternating gaze deviation. Neurology 1976;26:532-5.

139. Stewart JD, Kirkham TH, Mathieson G. Periodic alternating gaze. Neurology 1979;29:222-4.

140. Watkins HC, Ellis CJK. Ping pong gaze in reversible coma due to overdose of monoamine oxidise inhibitor. J Neurol Neurosurg Psychiatry 1989; 52:539.

141. Hedges TR III, Hoyt WF. Ocular tilt reaction due to an upper brainstem lesion: paroxysmal skew deviation, torsion, and oscillation of the eyes with head tilt. Ann Neurol 1982;11:537-40.

142. Westheimer G, Blair SM. The ocular tilt reaction—a brainstem oculomotor routine. Invest Ophthalmol 1975;14: 833-9.

143. Diamond SG, Markham CH, Baloh RW. Ocular counterrolling abnormalities in spasmodic torticollis. Arch Neurol 1988;45:164-9.

# CHAPTER 13

# Anisocoria and Abnormal Pupillary Light Reactions

• • • • • • • • • • • • • • • • • •

The two major pupillary problems that concern the clinician are (1) anisocoria (a difference in pupillary size between the two eyes) and (2) reduced pupillary response to light stimulation. Analysis of pupillary abnormalities requires a basic understanding of the anatomic pathways and physiologic reactions underlying normal pupillary function.

## Anatomy and Physiology

Although pupillary size and reactivity and ciliary muscle tone are basically controlled by the opposing limbs of the autonomic nervous system, the major role is played by the parasympathetic system because of the mechanical superiority of the iris sphincter muscle.

### PARASYMPATHETIC CONTROL

Parasympathetic tone originates in a complex group of paired midline nuclei including the anterior median nucleus, the Edinger Westphal complex, and Perlia's nucleus lying contiguous to the somatic oculomotor nucleus in the midbrain. Projection pathways from the parasympathetic nuclei include the fascicles of the third cranial nerve and the nerve itself (Fig. 13-1). The exact function of each parasympathetic nucleus is unknown, but accommodation appears to be represented more rostrally than pupillary function.[1]

When an individual is asleep, the pupils are miotic, reflecting unopposed parasympathetic tone. On awakening, this parasympathetic tone is modified by psychogenic factors (fear, alertness, stress, and noise) that inhibit the parasympathetic nuclei directly. In addition, the response to the presence or absence of light is relayed through the pretectal nuclei to modify parasympathetic tone.

Afferent input to the pretectal nuclei (sublentiform and superior olivary nuclei in the primate) originates in the retinal ganglion cells subserving, for the most part, macular function with spectral sensitivity similar to that of visual afferents. Whether this afferent limb consists of a single system subserving both vision and pupillomotor functions with divergent axon collaterals arising proxi-

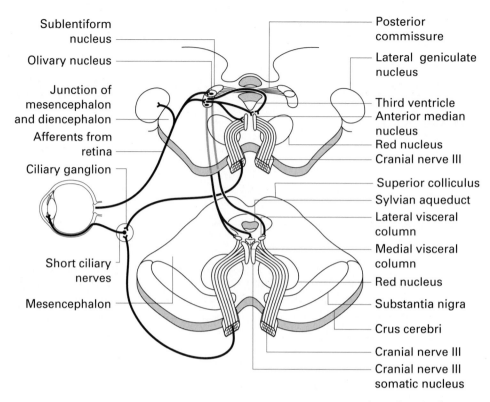

*Fig. 13-1.* Pupillary light reflex. Afferents arising in retina project to lateral geniculate nucleus and pretectal (sublentiform and olivary) nuclei. Fibers arising from pretectal nuclei project above and below third ventricle and Sylvian aqueduct to anterior median nucleus and to medial and lateral visceral columns of Edinger-Westphal complex. These nuclei send axons through fascicles of cranial nerve III to synapse in ciliary ganglion. Fibers arising from this ganglion project to eye via short ciliary nerves.

mal to the lateral geniculate body, or whether it consists of separate but parallel pathways is not clear.

Fiber projections from the pretectal nuclei decussate both dorsally and ventrally around the Sylvian aqueduct and synapse in the parasympathetic nuclei in the mesencephalon. Axons arising in these nuclei traverse the mesencephalon in the rostral fascicles of the third cranial nerve to enter the peripheral nerve in the interpeduncular fossa. Fibers arising caudally sweep rostrally before turning ventrally to form the rostral fascicles of the oculomotor nerve. Divisional somatotopy[2] exists within the fascicles and nerve rootlets of the oculomotor nerve in the midbrain (see Chapter 10). The parasympathetic fibers travel in the superior medial part of the peripheral nerve, enter the orbit as part of its inferior division, and arrive at the main ciliary ganglion or accessory ciliary ganglia by means of the motor nerve to the inferior oblique muscle. The vast majority of the pupillomotor fibers synapse in the main or accessory ganglia and reach the iris sphincter muscle via the short ciliary nerves. Interruption in this pathway from the mesencephalon to the sphincter muscle causes pupillary dilatation and decreased speed and amplitude of constriction.

Pupillary constriction (miosis) is also a component of a number of synki-

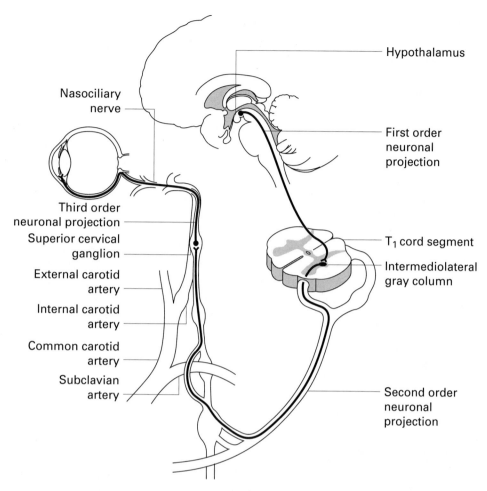

*Fig. 13-2.* Sympathetic innervation of dilator muscle of iris. Cell bodies of first order sympathetic neurons in hypothalamus project axons through brainstem to intermediolateral gray column of lower cervical and upper thoracic spinal cord. Second order neurons project via white rami communicantes through paravertebral sympathetic chain to superior cervical ganglion. On left side, chain in its course splits around subclavian artery. Third order neurons travel within pericarotid plexus to cavernous sinus, where they join sixth cranial nerve briefly before entering orbit on first division of trigeminal nerve. These axons enter globe to innervate iris dilator muscle.

netic reactions involving parasympathetic activity, including (1) near reflex (miosis, accommodation, and convergence); (2) Bell's phenomenon (levator inhibition, superior rectus muscle activation, and miosis); and (3) Westphal-Piltz reaction (orbicularis contraction and unilateral or bilateral pupillary miosis).

## SYMPATHETIC CONTROL

The oculosympathetic pathway is composed of a three-neuron arc (Fig. 13-2). *First order neurons* arise in the hypothalamus, and their axons descend through the reticular formation. At the level of the caudal end of the third nerve nucleus, they are located in a position contiguous to the fourth nerve nucleus or its fascicles, and at the pontomedullary junction they have moved laterally to pass near the vestibular nuclei. The axons of the first order neurons synapse in the intermediolateral gray substance of the lower cervical and upper thoracic spinal cord (ciliospinal center of Budge-Waller, C8-T1).

The axons of the *second order neurons* arise in the intermediolateral gray column, exit in the ventral spinal roots, and travel via the white rami communicantes to ascend without synapse through the sympathetic paraspinal chain to synapse in the superior cervical ganglion, which lies at about the level of the angle of the mandible. On the left side the sympathetic chain splits around the subclavian artery; the posterior branch (ansa subclavia) lies near the apex of the lung. Most of the fibers destined for the eye travel in the anterior branch. These two neuronal projections make up the preganglionic portion of the three-neuron sympathetic arc.

From the superior cervical ganglion, the postganglionic axons of the *third order neurons* travel on the surface of the common carotid artery. At the bifurcation of the common carotid artery, sympathetic fibers destined for the eye follow the course of the internal carotid artery, whereas those destined to control facial sweating follow the course of the external carotid artery. In some individuals an aberrant group of fibers that control sweating of a small patch of skin over the superior orbital notch travel on the surface of the internal carotid artery, along with the fibers destined for the eye and lid. In the cavernous sinus these eye and lid fibers join the sixth cranial nerve[3,4] before appending themselves to the first division of the fifth cranial nerve and entering the orbit via the superior orbital fissure. Fibers destined for the dilator muscle enter the eye via the long posterior ciliary nerves.

## PUPILLARY SIZE

The size of the pupil is in a continual state of flux, adjusting to changes in ambient illumination, fixation distance, and psychosensory stimuli. Pupillary diameter tends to be smaller in infants and older adults than in young adults, and smaller in brown eyes than in blue eyes. To accurately determine pupillary size and light reactivity, the patient must fixate on a distant target so that variances in pupillary size produced by components of the near reflex are controlled.

A subtle anisocoria is the rule rather than the exception.[5-8] A difference in pupillary size of 0.3 to 0.4 mm is easily recognized clinically and has been found in approximately 20% of the normal population under age 17. Roarty and Keltner[9] have noted a 21% prevalence of anisocoria in infants. The prevalence of anisocoria increases with age, with about 33% of the population over age 60 years having anisocoria.[10]

Lam et al.[6] photographically recorded pupillary size and measured the pupillary diameter twice a day for 5 consecutive days in 128 normal patients. Of these, 41% had an anisocoria of greater than 0.4 mm at some time; on inspection of photographs, anisocoria of greater than 0.2 mm could be measured in 80%. Anisocoria of any degree was more obvious when the pupils were small. The pupillary size inequality was the same under all lighting conditions, and the pupillary light reactions were equally brisk. This combination of physical findings is considered to be diagnostic of physiologic, essential or "central" anisocoria.[7]

**LIGHT REACTION.** As mentioned previously, the response of the pupil to light is determined with the patient fixating at distance to prevent activation of the near reflex. The direct and consensual responses should be equal in all aspects. The amplitude, latency, and speed of the pupillary contraction to a light stimulus should somewhat parallel the patient's visual acuity, with the exception of decreased vision due to circumscribed foveal and bilateral occipital lobe disease involving the macular projection areas. In patients with limited foveal disease, visual acuity may be severely affected, but the majority of pupillary afferents from the macular region will be functioning normally and the pupillary light reflex will be brisk and full. Patients with dysfunction of both tips of the occipital lobes also have decreased vision but normal pupillary reactions to light. This disparity is due to the anatomic fact that the retinal fibers that drive the pupillary light reaction diverge from visual fibers (which will synapse in the lateral geniculate nucleus) anterior to the lateral geniculate nucleus and thus are unaffected by posterior lesions.

In infants who are crying, it is impossible to determine the adequacy of the pupillary response accurately, because each time the baby squeezes his or her eye(s) closed, the pupil constricts (Westphal-Piltz phenomenon). Ordinarily if such a child is lifted and tilted toward the examiner, the child will immediately stop crying and reflexly open his or her eyes. At this time a light may be projected into each pupil by an assistant and the status of the light reflex determined.

Children, adolescents, anxious adults, and psychiatrically ill patients often have sluggish pupillary light reflexes that normalize during the course of examination. Such pupils are called Bumke's or "anxiety" pupils.[11] These pupils tend to be slightly larger than normal initially. This complex of findings is believed to be caused by excess sympathetic tone.

**NEAR REACTION.** The near reaction is a synkinesis consisting of convergence, accommodation, and pupillary miosis. The near reaction may be checked even in a blind person by having the patient fix on his or her own finger. Checking the pupillary reaction to a near stimulus is superfluous if the light reaction is normal and if the patient has no difficulty with close work.

If the patient complains of difficulty at the reading position, then each of the components of the near reaction—convergence, accommodation, and pupillary constriction—must be tested individually. Activation of the near reflex requires volitional effort. The only objective sign of the patient's cooperating during these tests is the presence of miosis on near fixation (see Chapters 8 and 11).

# A Decision Tree Approach to the Evaluation of Anisocoria

The decision tree (Chart 13-1) for the evaluation of anisocoria and abnormal pupillary light reactions is a modification of that proposed by Thompson and Pilley.[12]

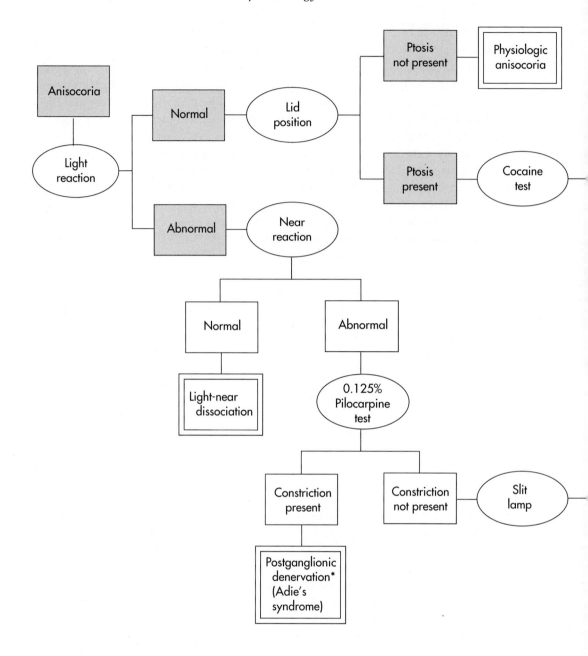

*Can occur as part of a third nerve palsy, but in isolation constriction
generally signifies postganglionic denervation.

**Chart 13-1**

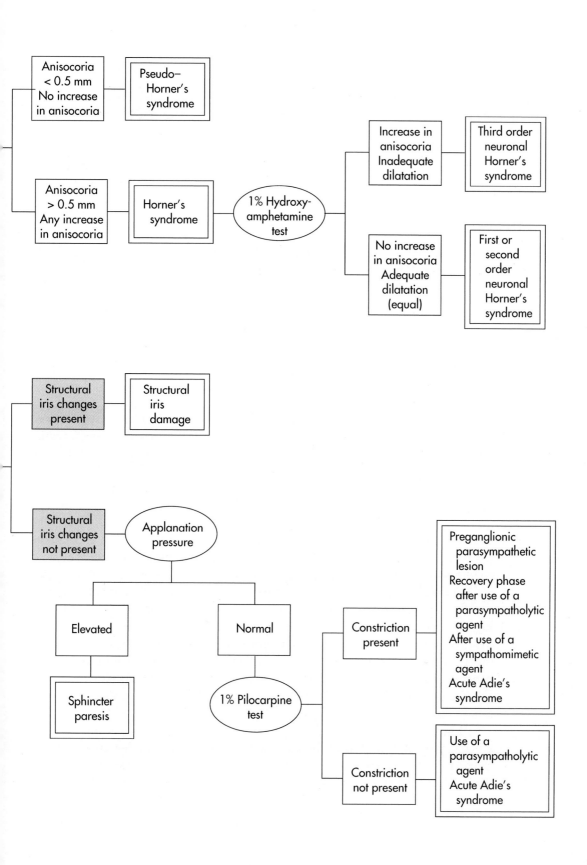

■ Anisocoria

○ *Light reaction.* If the size of the two pupils differs, the first step is to study the pupillary light reaction.

■ Normal light reaction

If the pupillary response is normal (i.e., brisk bilateral constriction occurs with the light projected into either eye), the anisocoria is either **physiologic** (essential, central) or the patient has **Horner's syndrome.**

○ *Lid position.* If the light reaction is normal in both eyes, the next step is to determine if an ipsilateral lid position abnormality is present, such as upper lid ptosis or lower lid elevation (inverse ptosis).

■ Ptosis not present

If no evidence of ptosis is found, the diagnosis is **physiologic anisocoria.** In such patients the anisocoria may vary during the examination.

■ Ptosis present

If ptosis is present or equivocal (Chart 13-1, *A*), the examiner must exclude oculosympathetic paresis (Horner's syndrome), which includes relative miosis, dilatation lag, ptosis, inverse ptosis, and sometimes increased accommodation with or without ipsilateral facial anhidrosis.[13] We recommend sequential pharmacologic testing using cocaine and hydroxyamphetamine to verify the diagnosis of Horner's syndrome.[14]

○ *Cocaine test.* Instill 4%, 5%, or 10% cocaine in both eyes (one drop each at 5-minute intervals). Measure the patient's pupillary diameter under the same lighting conditions before and approximately 30 minutes after cocaine instillation. Under normal conditions cocaine produces pupillary dilatation because it blocks the reuptake of norepinephrine released tonically by the postganglionic synaptic endings. If sympathetic tone is interrupted anywhere from the hypothalamus to the iris dilator muscle, the amount of norepinephrine released will decrease and the involved pupil will not dilate to the same extent as the uninvolved pupil. In patients with dark irides, the response to cocaine may be extremely slow. If mydriasis has not occurred in either eye after 1 hour, administer an additional instillation of cocaine and observe the patient for 1 to 2 hours.[15]

Kardon et al.[16] have demonstrated that measuring postcocaine anisocoria is a better predictor of Horner's syndrome than calculating the net change in anisocoria. If the postcocaine anisocoria exceeds 0.8 mm, the mean odds ratio of having Horner's syndrome is approximately 1054:1; at 0.5 mm the mean odds ratio is 77:1. At present we suggest that the examiner measure both the change

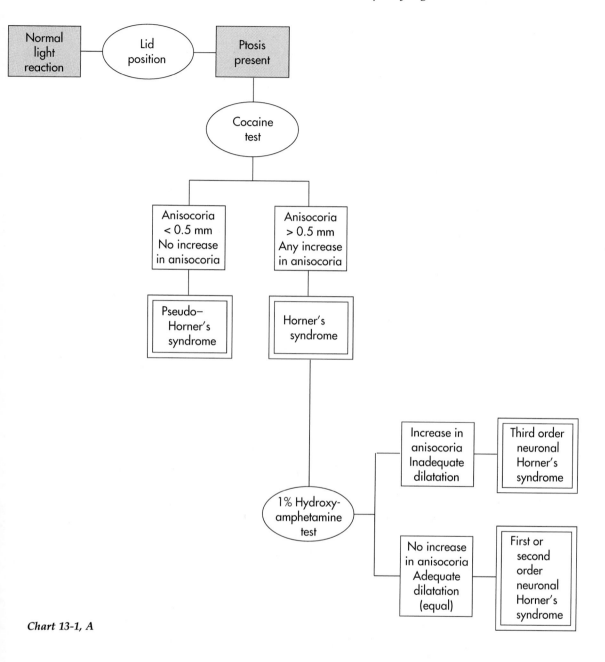

*Chart 13-1, A*

in anisocoria and the absolute difference in postcocaine pupil size.

Since random drug screening for drug abuse is becoming a common occupational occurrence, inform the patient that topical cocaine was used, since urine will test positive for cocaine derivatives for at least 36 hours (24 hours: 100%; 36 hours: 53%).[17]

☐ Anisocoria <0.5 mm or no increase in anisocoria

If anisocoria does not increase after the instillation of cocaine, or if the measured difference between the two pupils is less than 0.5 mm, the diagnosis is pseudo–Horner's syndrome.[18]

⬚ Pseudo–Horner's syndrome

Thompson et al.[18] have emphasized that the occurrence of ipsilateral ptosis and miosis does not make the diagnosis of Horner's syndrome. They reported 18 patients with ipsilateral ptosis and miosis referred for evaluation of Horner's syndrome who, on pharmacologic testing, were found not to have oculosympathetic paresis. They emphasize that miosis with a drooping lid can be produced by causes unrelated to oculosympathetic paresis. The majority of their patients had physiologic anisocoria with ipsilateral lid dysfunction due to such diverse entities as levator aponeurotic dehiscence, dermatochalasis, and myasthenia gravis.

☐ Anisocoria >0.5 mm or any increase in anisocoria

⬚ Horner's syndrome

If the pupillary inequality increases after the topical use of cocaine or the post-dilatation difference exceeds 0.5 mm, Horner's syndrome is confirmed. Minimal pupillary dilatation occurs frequently in patients with partial interruption of the sympathetic pathway.[19] Partial interruption is probably the explanation for the minimal pupillary dilatation seen in patients with first order neuron involvement.[19,20] The response to cocaine provides no information about the site of the causative lesion but merely confirms the existence of an oculosympathetic paresis. Once the diagnosis of Horner's syndrome has been established, hydroxyamphetamine testing provides a method of differentiating between postganglionic third order neuronal lesions and first and second order neuronal lesions.

○ *1% Hydroxyamphetamine test.* Use of 1% hydroxyamphetamine can differentiate between preganglionic and postganglionic lesions causing Horner's syndrome. Hydroxyamphetamine releases norepinephrine from the sympathetic vesicles at synaptic endings; thus its efficacy in dilating the pupils depends on the integrity of the third order neuron (superior cervical ganglion to the dilator pupillae muscle). If the suspect pupil fails to dilate 45 minutes after instillation of hydroxyamphetamine, or only partially dilates, then a **sympathetic postganglionic third order neuronal lesion** is present. However, if the involved pupil dilates to the same extent or more than the normal pupil, the lesion is **preganglionic,** involving either the **first or second order sympathetic neurons.**[21,22]

Thompson and Mensher[19] have shown that the results of hydroxyamphetamine testing are prejudiced by the immediate preceding use of cocaine and suggest waiting 24 to 48 hours between tests. This has led investigators[22,23] to attempt to bypass the use of cocaine and use a single-drop hydroxyamphetamine test. Maloney et al.[23] performed pharmacologic testing in 162 patients with Horner's syndrome in whom the location of the causative lesion within the three-neuron chain (central, intermediate, or peripheral) was known (Table 13-1). They found a lack of pupillary dilatation in 89 patients tested topically with hydroxyamphetamine. Of these, 75 patients (84%) had third order lesions. The other 14 patients whose miotic pupil did not dilate had first or second order neuronal sympathetic lesions that had been incorrectly localized. Thus for third order neuronal lesions, hydroxyamphetamine had a diagnostic specificity of 84%

| **TABLE 13-1** | *Pupillary Response to 1% Hydroxyamphetamine* | | | | |
|---|---|---|---|---|---|
| **Known location of lesion** | **Failed to dilate** | **Dilated** | **Equivocal** | **Total** | **Diagnostic sensitivity** |
| Third order neuron | 75 | 2 | 1 | 78 | 96% |
| First/second order neuron | 14 | 70 | 0 | 84 | 84% |
| TOTAL | 89 | 72 | | | |
| Diagnostic specifity | 84% | 97% | | | |

Data from Maloney WF, Younge BR, Mayer NJ. Am J Ophthalmol 1989;90:394-402.

(75/89). Of the 78 patients who had a third order neuronal lesion, the pupil failed to dilate in 75, yielding a sensitivity of 96%.

Maloney et al.[23] reported a diagnostic specificity for hydroxyamphetamine of 97% for more proximal lesions; of 72 patients who dilated to hydroxyamphetamine, 70 had preganglionic lesions. Of the 84 patients with known first or second order neuronal lesions, 70 dilated, for a sensitivity of 84% for proximal lesions. Van der Wiel and Van Gijn[24] challenged the value of the hydroxyamphetamine test, finding that an abnormal test reliably indicates a lesion of the third order neuron but with a sensitivity of only 40%.

Recently Cremer et al.[22] studied hydroxyamphetamine mydriasis in 54 patients with Horner's syndrome confirmed both by dilatation lag of the smaller pupil and cocaine testing. The location of the causative lesion was known with reasonable certainty; 24 were preganglionic lesions and 30 were postganglionic lesions. The authors compared the pupillary size before and after the instillation of hydroxyamphetamine (i.e., the difference in dilatation between the two eyes). Although the separation between preganglionic and postganglionic groups was not absolute, a zero difference in dilatation gave the best separation. The amount of anisocoria increased in 93% of postganglionic cases. No change or a decrease in the amount of anisocoria after hydroxyamphetamine occurred in 90% of patients with preganglionic lesions. We believe any measurable increase in anisocoria following instillation of hydroxyamphetamine should be considered diagnostic of a third order lesion.

In Horner's syndrome neither the relative miosis (range of 0.5 to 1 mm) nor the ptosis (range 1 to 2 mm) is marked. The upper lid ptosis is associated with ipsilateral loss of the lid crease. The lower lid elevation is subtle and due to relaxation of the lower lid retractors. A defect of the third order neuron proximal to the carotid bifurcation will produce ptosis, miosis, and ipsilateral facial anhidrosis with the exception of a small patch of skin above the supraorbital notch. A lesion distal to the bifurcation tends to produce ptosis and miosis without anhidrosis. Patients with Horner's syndrome often have a transient increase in their amplitude of accommodation.

Not only do patients who have a disruption of sympathetic innervation to the eye early in life demonstrate Horner's syndrome, but also they do not develop iris pigmentation on the involved side, because the formation of pigment granules by stromal melanocytes is under sympathetic control. Thus the color differs between the two irides (*heterochromia iridis*). Heterochromia accompanied

## Management of Horner's Syndrome

1. In all children with Horner's syndrome without evidence of birth trauma, perform imaging studies to exclude cervical or mediastinal tumors.
2. In adults confirm the diagnosis of Horner's syndrome by cocaine testing. Localize the lesion by using topical hydroxyamphetamine.
   a. If the first or second order neurons are involved, carefully question the patient to determine the presence of arm pain. Perform imaging studies of the midthorax to the angle of the jaw if warranted.
   b. If the third order neuron is involved in isolation, no further studies are indicated. If accompanying signs or symptoms are present, they dictate the evaluation.
3. Use other signs or symptoms that accompany Horner's syndrome to guide imaging.

by ipsilateral ptosis and miosis with or without anhidrosis is highly suggestive of *congenital Horner's syndrome*. An occasional patient with congenital Horner's syndrome will have straight hair on the involved side and curly hair on the uninvolved side.[25]

This disruption of oculosympathetic tone is generally produced by natal or perinatal trauma, which may also damage the brachial plexus.[26-28] A single case of acquired heterochromia has been reported in a sympathetically denervated adult.[29]

In all children the presence of Horner's syndrome without evidence of birth trauma necessitates appropriate imaging to exclude the presence of cervical or mediastinal neuroblastoma.[26,27,30-32] Since iris coloration is established only after several months of age, heterochromia is not a helpful feature during the perinatal period. Children who acquire Horner's syndrome most often have a lesion of the second order neuron.[25,27,31,32] Causative lesions include malignant tumors of neural crest origin,[27,31] benign tumors,[25] and trauma.[31]

In adults Maloney et al.[23] found that:

1. In contrast to the report of Giles and Henderson,[19] malignant neoplasm is not as frequent a cause of Horner's syndrome as was previously believed. (Maloney et al.[23] found malignant neoplasm in only 37 of 450 patients.)
2. Only 13 (3%) of 450 patients with Horner's syndrome had a previously undetected malignancy. Of these, 10 had involvement of the superior pulmonary sulcus. Nine of these patients had arm pain as their sole symptom or as one of their primary initial complaints, indicating lower brachial plexus involvement (C8, T1) (Pancoast's syndrome).[33] Thus 9 of 13 patients with undetected malignancy could have been identified by history alone.
3. Malignancies producing Horner's syndrome[14,19] involved the first or second order neurons in 31 of 37 (84%) cases, typically, the second order neurons.

The likelihood of a particular type of lesion causing Horner's syndrome is biased by the location of the interruption of the sympathetic outflow, which is reflected by accompanying signs and symptoms. Involvement of the first order neuron within the brainstem rarely if ever occurs in isolation. Horner's syndrome involving the first order neurons has been reported (1) with hypothalamic infarction producing hemianhidrosis, ptosis, miosis, contralateral hemiplegia, and homonymous field loss, as well as aphasia *(telodiencephalic syndrome)*[34,35]; (2) with a contralateral trochlear nerve palsy[36]; (3) with bilateral abducens palsy due to pontine infarction[37]; and (4) as part of Wallenberg's syndrome.

Horner's syndrome involving the second order neurons and their axonal projections is usually due to trauma,[38-40] neoplasm,[20,23,33] or internal carotid dissection.[41-42] Since first or second order neuronal lesions are often due to malignant neoplasm,[2,20,30] a patient should have a complete neurologic examination, palpation of the neck and thyroid gland, and a chest x-ray study with thoracic outlet views or imaging of the mediastinum and neck.

In a patient with *isolated* Horner's syndrome localized to the third order neuron, no investigation is necessary.[33,38,43] Third order neuronal lesions are almost always benign.

### Abnormal light reaction

In the presence of anisocoria and a normal afferent visual system, if one pupil does not react as well to a direct light stimulus (decreased speed and/or amplitude of response), there must be a disturbance of the parasympathetic pathways to the sphincter muscle or a structural defect of the iris sphincter muscle. In a patient with anisocoria associated with an abnormal light reaction, the involved pupil tends to be the larger of the two. The failure of the pupil to constrict may be limited to a sector, or it may involve the entire sphincter muscle.

If the light reaction is abnormal, the next step is to determine the pupillary response to a near target (Chart 13-1, *B*). The near reaction can be normal or abnormal (absent, sluggish, or tonic).

### Near reaction

#### Normal near reaction

If the difference in pupillary response to light versus that to near stimuli is substantial, the condition is termed **light-near dissociation.** The most likely cause of light-near dissociation is a lesion of the anterior afferent visual system. Other possible causes include diabetes mellitus and pretectal lesions (compressive and luetic).

#### Abnormal near reaction

If the near response is abnormal, the next step is to apply weak solutions of pilocarpine topically.

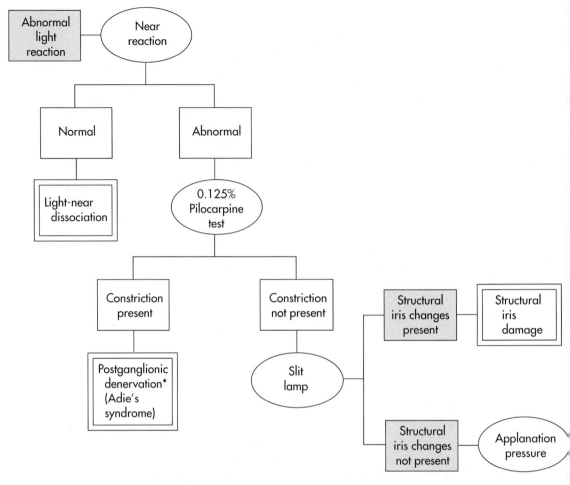

*Chart 13-1, B*

*Can occur as part of a third nerve palsy, but in isolation constriction generally signifies postganglionic denervation.

⬭ *0.125% Pilocarpine test.* Apply 0.125% pilocarpine to test for cholinergic supersensitivity. With rare exception, cholinergic supersensitivity is the hallmark of postganglionic denervation.[44,45]

☐ Constriction present

Pupillary constriction in response to the topical application of weak parasympathomimetic solutions is considered diagnostic of postganglionic denervation. Ponsford et al.[46] have called attention to some apparent exceptions to this rule. They studied the pupillary responses to 2.5% methacholine in 14 patients with solely unilateral partial or complete third nerve palsies, 14 patients with Adie's syndrome, normal control subjects, and patients with neurologic disease not accompanied by third nerve dysfunction with normal pupils. They found that the involved pupils in both preganglionic third nerve palsies and Adie's syndrome responded to 2.5% methacholine by becoming miotic.

Subsequently, similar findings using 0.125% pilocarpine have been reported in patients with intracranial lesions (preganglionic), including two with lateral extension of pituitary adenomas and one with a midbrain hemorrhage.[47] In such patients the pupillary abnormalities do not exist in isolation. At present no adequate explanation for preganglionic supersensitivity is available.[48] Jacobson[49] has postulated two possible mechanisms: transsynaptic degeneration or a mechanical basis. In the latter he suggests that a relatively larger pupil appears to constrict more to any miotic agent than does its mate.

### ☐ Postganglionic denervation (Adie's syndrome)

The most common cause of postganglionic denervation is Adie's syndrome.[50] This disorder of pupillary function usually consists of areas of sector paresis of the iris sphincter with interposed sections of actively constricting muscle (vermiform movements[51]). Sector paresis produces a shifting of the iris stroma toward area(s) of active contraction, a phenomenon called "iris streaming."[52]

Extraordinarily slow constriction of the pupil to either light and near stimuli with very slow pupillary redilatation is termed *tonic reaction*. Tonic reaction and hypersensitivity to weak cholinergic agents are characteristic of Adie's syndrome. In addition, patients with Adie's syndrome have regional corneal hypesthesia due to interruption of fibers of the ophthalmic division of the trigeminal nerve as they pass through the ciliary ganglion. These patients (90%) also have diminished or absent deep tendon reflexes.[53,54]

Adie's syndrome is seen most often in young women (second to fourth decade) (70%). When first seen, these patients may have a dilated and fixed pupil that does not demonstrate cholinergic supersensitivity. In fact, in acute Adie's syndrome, the pupil may not react to strong solutions of pilocarpine (1%), thus making it indistinguishable from pupils that are pharmacologically blockaded (by anticholinergic drugs) and from some cases of acute traumatic iridoplegia. Over time, effective contractions of parts of the pupillary sphincter become evident. This apparent reinnervation is assumed to be due to resprouting of axons from the damaged ciliary ganglion. Aberrant reinnervation of the pupillary sphincter is invoked as an explanation for pupillary and ciliary muscle tonicity.

Cholinergic supersensitivity develops in 80% of patients.[45,55] Although Adie's syndrome is initially a unilateral condition (90%), it may become bilateral.[50] The affected pupil will become more miotic with time and in unilateral cases may eventually become smaller than the unaffected pupil.[52]

The lack of pupillary response to light often causes problems with glare outdoors or difficulty with fluorescent lamps. The glare problem in some of these patients may be alleviated by weak solutions of pilocarpine, which produce miosis. The ciliary muscle also demonstrates varying amounts of cholinergic supersensitivity, and some of these patients develop ciliary spasm with the use of pilocarpine.

Accommodative difficulties due to ciliary muscle paresis often cause the patient to have problems with near tasks. If a sector paresis of the ciliary muscles exists, lenticular astigmatism may cause visual distortion while reading. Some individuals are acutely aware of their inability to relax accommodation following prolonged close work. Patients with difficulties in reading often are helped somewhat either by the use of bilateral and equal bifocal or reading corrections fixing the reading distance for both eyes, or by the use of unilateral or bilateral unequal bifocal corrections.

Other causes of postganglionic denervation of the pupillary sphincter occur relatively infrequently and include ciliary nerve damage produced by varicella,[56,57] orbital injury (including surgical), orbital or choroidal tumors, diffuse laser photocoagulation of the retina and choroid, extensive cryotherapy of the retina and choroid, and retrobulbar alcohol injections.

## ☐ Constriction not present

If the pupil does not constrict to 0.125% pilocarpine, a slit lamp examination should be performed to exclude structural changes in the iris.

## ◯ Slit lamp examination

## ▪ Structural iris changes present

Slit lamp examination can reveal structural changes in the iris such as sphincter rupture(s). Transillumination of the iris may demonstrate subtle breaks in the iris sphincter or stroma. Structural iris damage can be due to active or old inflammatory disease (keratitic precipitates, cells, flare, iris nodules, anterior or posterior synechiae, or ectropion uveae) or previous ocular surgery. Evidence of acquired heterochromia raises the possibility of a retained metallic intraocular foreign body or infiltrating iris melanoma.[58]

## ▪ Structural iris changes not present

If no miosis develops after application of a dilute solution of pilocarpine and slit lamp examination reveals no evidence of structural iris damage, the next step is to measure the intraocular pressure.

## ◯ Applanation pressure (Chart 13-1, C )

## ☐ Elevated intraocular pressure

At pressure levels of 40 to 45 mm Hg, a relative **sphincter muscle paresis** occurs, believed to be a result of hypoxia of the iris muscles.[59] An occasional patient with acute-angle glaucoma or asymmetric chronic angle-closure glaucoma may have no other symptoms.

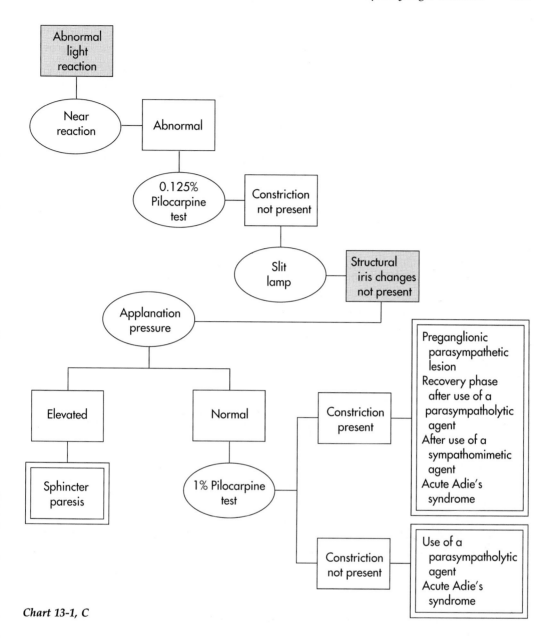

*Chart 13-1, C*

☐ Normal intraocular pressure

If the intraocular pressure is normal, the examiner must exclude the presence of cholinergic blockade by the use of 1% pilocarpine.[60]

◯ *1% Pilocarpine test.* In the absence of structural iris changes, the instillation of 1% pilocarpine should produce pupillary constriction except in some cases of acute Adie's syndrome, or after the use of strong cycloplegic agents.

☐ Constriction present

Constriction after the application of 1% pilocarpine implies either a **preganglionic parasympathetic lesion,** prior instillation of a **parasympatholytic agent that is "wearing off,"** the use of a **sympathomimetic agent,** or **acute Adie's syndrome.**

Patients with isolated anisocoria and subnormal or absent pupillary reactions who do not have evidence of iris damage or postganglionic denervation supersensitivity are often suspected of having an acquired third nerve palsy due to a posterior communicating or basilar artery aneurysm. We do not believe that an aneurysm causes an *isolated* dilated nonreactive pupil *without* disturbing extraocular muscle function. However, two cases of an isolated internal ophthalmoplegia as the presenting sign of an intracranial aneurysm have been reported.[61,62] Therefore patients with such an isolated pupillary finding should be screened with high-resolution magnetic resonance imaging (MRI) and, if the findings are normal, should be observed at regular intervals. This dictum holds regardless of the presence of headache.

An additional cause of a unilaterally dilated, sluggishly reactive pupil is the topical application of a strong sympathomimetic agent such as 2.5% or 10% phenylephrine. These pupils always constrict to a strong light stimulus such as an indirect ophthalmoscope and to 1% pilocarpine. The diagnosis is often clinically apparent, since they also have ipsilateral lid retraction.

Patients who are in the recovery phase from the effects of the application of parasympatholytic agents may also demonstrate pupillary constriction to the application of 1% pilocarpine (partial cholinergic blockade; see below).

☐ Constriction not present

In any patient with an isolated internal ophthalmoplegia, the physician should be alert to the possibility of exposure to atropine-like substances producing **pharamcologic blockade.** Patients, their families, and medical personnel often contaminate their eyes unintentionally. People who picnic or work in areas where jimson weed grows may inadvertently get the belladonna alkaloid from this plant in one or both eyes. In addition, individuals using retroauricular scopolamine patches (Transderm Scop) to combat motion sickness may also have unilaterally or bilaterally dilated pupils.[63,64] Others may place these substances in their eyes in an attempt to feign illness. Such individuals have accommodative, as well as pupillary, paresis. These patients are usually seen in a hospital emergency room because of the dilated, nonreactive pupil(s) and accommodative paresis, often with additional complaints of blurred vision. In mydriasis due to pharmacologic blockade, the pupillary response to 1% pilocarpine is decreased or absent. The amount of miosis produced by 1% pilocarpine varies in relation to the strength of the mydriatic used and the time elapsed since its instillation.

Patients with **Adie's syndrome** of recent onset may have a fixed dilated pupil that will fail to constrict to light or even strong solutions of pilocarpine (e.g., 1%).

# Intermittent Pupillary Syndromes

Some pupillary abnormalities are difficult to characterize because they are intermittent and their reactions to pharmacologic agents have not been well studied.

## BENIGN EPISODIC PUPILLARY DILATATION

Benign episodic pupillary dilatation (BEPD)[61,65,66] is often seen in young healthy people, some of whom have migraine headaches.[58,65,67] An attack is heralded by the patient's acute awareness that something is wrong with one eye, accompanied by mild blurring of vision. The patient generally looks in the mirror and notes that one pupil is widely dilated (springing pupil).[68] Some patients note difficulty with accommodation, which has led investigators to question the possibility of cholinergic blockade.[65,66,69] Some of these patients develop a nondescript headache following the episode. This is a benign condition.

## "TADPOLE" PUPILS

Thompson et al.[70] have reported 26 patients with sectoral pupillary dilatation. This is an intermittent pupillary abnormality in which the pupil can be seen to be distorted in one segment for a minute or more and then return to normal. The episodes recur multiple times throughout the day and usually continue for several days or a week and disappear spontaneously. Infrequently the patient may experience a recurrence of a cluster of these episodes. Almost all of the patients Thompson et al. reported experienced some unusual sensation in the affected eye, drawing attention to the pupil. Seventeen of the 26 patients complained of concomitant blurring of vision. Eight had definite or probable migraine. These authors postulate that the underlying pathophysiology is a segmental spasm of the iris dilator muscle, and they refer to this distortion as tadpole-shaped pupils.

## UNCAL HERNIATION

Patients with incipient uncal herniation with lateral brainstem compression due to a shift of midline structures[71] may pass through a phase of intermittent mydriasis with sluggish pupillary reactions to light.[72] Other neurologic findings, such as the patient's state of consciousness and motor function, contribute to the diagnosis.

## SEIZURE DISORDERS

Unilateral pupillary dilatation is an uncommon manifestation of seizure disorders. The anisocoria may occur during the seizure or in the postictal phase.[73-75] During these periods the dilated pupil has been reported to be sluggishly reactive to light.

## MIGRAINE

Many authors [58,65,67,76,77] have reported isolated unilateral pupillary mydriasis, decreased light reaction, and loss of accommodation in patients with migraine headaches. The internal ophthalmoplegia tends to be transient, although some suggest it remains for longer periods with each subsequent attack.

## CLAUDE BERNARD SYNDROME[78]

Vijayan[40] reported seven patients who sustained neck trauma with recurrent unilateral frontotemporal throbbing headaches associated with ipsilateral mydriasis, lid retraction, and facial hyperhidrosis (Claude Bernard syndrome—mydriasis, lid retraction, and excessive facial perspiration). After the headache had abated, four of these patients had transient ipsilateral Horner's syndrome (lasting 3 days). During the headache-free intervals, pharmacologic testing suggested the existence of partial sympathetic denervation. Vijayan postulated that the probable site of the causative (irritative) lesion was in the neck after the fibers had emerged from the T1 segment.

## ALTERNATING ANISOCORIA

Patients who have cervical cord lesions, such as from old trauma or syringomyelia, may have alternating anisocoria.[39,65,79] From one episode to the next, first one pupil, and then the other, is larger. To state categorically whether this anisocoria is due to an interruption of the sympathetic pathways, producing alternating Horner's syndrome, or is secondary to irritative phenomena, producing alternating Claude Bernard syndrome, is impossible.[39,40,80] The mechanism can be determined only by pharmacologic testing at the time of the anisocoria,[39,80] and the results of such testing are not, for the most part, adequately reported.

Saito and Nakazawa[81] reported a single such patient in whom the mydriatic pupil was sluggishly reactive to light and constricted to 0.5% pilocarpine. Results of pharmacologic testing during the nonmydriatic phase were contradictory, with failure to dilate to 1.25% epinephrine or 4% tyramine. These patients have identifiable accompanying neurologic deficits such as limb weakness, paresthesias, or radicular pain.

## BILATERALLY REDUCED PUPILLARY LIGHT REACTIONS

*Light-near dissociation* is that state in which a patient's visual function is normal or near normal, the pupillary light reflexes in both eyes are sluggish, and the near reaction is normal. Light-near dissociation can be seen in dorsal midbrain syndrome, diabetes mellitus, and in tabes dorsalis (Argyll Robertson pupils).

In patients with *dorsal midbrain syndrome,* the pupils are usually 4 to 5 mm in size, round, and regular. Any disease affecting the intercalated fibers between the pretectal nucleus and the parasympathetic nuclei can produce light-near dissociation. The best known cause is external pressure on the mesencephalon from a pineal mass lesion. Other causes include any type of intrinsic dorsal mesencephalic lesion and hydrocephalus.

Similarly, light-near dissociation with mid-dilated pupils can be seen in *diabetes mellitus.* These findings are presumed to be due to a peripheral autonomic neuropathy. Sigsbee et al.[82] have shown that 75% of patients with long-standing diabetes mellitus show cholinergic supersensitivity. A similar picture can be seen following panretinal photocoagulation or extensive peripheral retinal cryotherapy.

The initial interest in light-near dissociation was due to the report of Argyll Robertson, who noted this finding in patients with central nervous system (CNS) syphilis, most often *tabes dorsalis*.[83] The criteria Argyll Robertson used to describe these pupils included (1) miotic irregular pupils, (2) total absence of a light response in the face of a retina sensitive to light (good vision), (3) brisk pupillary constriction to near stimuli, (4) further pupillary constriction to physostigmine, and (5) poor dilatation to belladonna alkaloids.

Apter[84] demonstrated unilateral Argyll Robertson pupils in 12 of 46 patients with neurosyphilis. Hooshmand et al.[85] noted light-near dissociation in 86 (44%) of 241 patients with neurosyphilis. In our opinion, patients with unilateral or bilateral miotic irregular pupils, normal vision, and light-near dissociation should have a VDRL followed by an FTA-Abs (fluorescent treponemal antibody-absorption test) if the VDRL is positive. The location of the causative lesion has not been indisputably settled.

## BILATERALLY REDUCED PUPILLARY LIGHT AND NEAR REACTIONS

In some patients the pupils respond sluggishly to both light and near stimuli. They may be divided by pupillary size into those whose pupils are either relatively mydriatic or miotic.

**RELATIVELY MYDRIATIC PUPILS.** These patients should be tested with topical 0.125% pilocarpine. Bilateral constriction indicates bilateral postganglionic denervation, most likely as part of Adie's syndrome (see earlier under Postganglionic Denervation [Adie's Syndrome]). Other entities in which bilateral segmental palsies of the iris with cholinergic hypersensitivity may be seen include a form of acute infectious demyelinating polyradiculoneuropathy called Fisher's variant[86,87] of Guillain-Barré syndrome and peripheral neuropathies with autonomic components (diabetes mellitus, Riley-Day syndrome, and multiple-system atrophy). Some patients with multiple-system atrophy demonstrate sympathetic denervation as well, with failure to dilate to psychosensory stimuli, cocaine, or hydroxyamphetamine.

Patients with hereditary motor sensory neuropathy types 1 and 2 (Charcot-Marie-Tooth Disease) have bilateral pupillary abnormalities that resemble those of Adie's tonic pupil syndrome. Keltner et al.[88] reported a kindred of 15 patients with hereditary motor sensory neuropathy, 13 of whom had pupillary abnormalities. These patients go through a sequence of changes reflecting the presence of progressive parasympathetic denervation. They often receive symptomatic relief from glare and reading problems with the use of topical 0.025% pilocarpine four times daily.

**RELATIVELY MIOTIC PUPILS.** Patients with myotonic dystrophy tend to have pupils that are smaller in diameter than age-matched controls and are sluggishly reactive (amplitude and velocity) to light and near stimuli.[89,90] These pupils dilate well in response to psychosensory stimuli. No evidence of cholinergic supersensitivity exists, since these pupils do not become more miotic in response to the topical application of 2.5% methacholine.[90]

**PHARMACOLOGIC BLOCKADE.** Sluggish pupillary responses may be seen in patients taking systemic drugs with anticholinergic actions, such as those used to treat diarrhea, Parkinson's disease, or depression, or be secondary to the effect of various bacterial toxins (botulinum or diphtheria). Similarly, late in the course of parasympatholytic therapy or during sympathomimetic therapy, patients have sluggish light and near reactions. All of these patients demonstrate pupillary constriction to 1% pilocarpine.

## OTHER PUPILLARY CONDITIONS

**PREMATURE NEONATES.** Isenberg et al.[91] recently reported that the pupils of premature neonates are large (mean of 4.7 mm) at 26 weeks postconceptional age and are nonreactive. The pupils become progressively smaller, reaching 3.4 mm by 29 weeks, but do not react to light until 31 weeks. The authors emphasize that pupils unresponsive to light should not suggest blindness until 32 weeks postconception. Similarly, the examiner must remember that as an individual ages the pupils tend to become progressively more miotic.[10]

**EXTREME MIOSIS.** Bilateral extreme miosis may be caused by the binocular application of strong parasympathomimetic agents, pontine hemorrhage, or the use of narcotics. Unilateral extreme miosis suggests the use of a strong topical parasympathomimetic agent.[92] The differential diagnosis is of great importance, especially when the patient is comatose. If surgical intervention is required, as when the coma is secondary to trauma, the use of succinylcholine would be contraindicated in the face of prior use of cholinesterase inhibitors. The use of the narcotic antagonist naloxone topically produces pupillary dilatation in patients under the influence of narcotics, thus separating this cause from other causes of pinpoint pupils.[93]

**MIDBRAIN CORECTOPIA.** Selhorst et al.[94] noted intermittent corectopia (eccentric or oval pupils) in a patient with bilateral rostral midbrain infarction who subsequently died. This condition is believed to represent selective central inhibition of sphincter tone. The iris sphincter appears to consist of 70 to 80 separate motor units, which in a normal individual can be seen to fire somewhat asynchronously in low background illumination. In patients with midbrain pathology this asynchrony can be carried to an extreme.

Marshall et al.[95] suggest that midbrain corectopia represents a transitional stage in the development of third nerve compression during transtentorial herniation. They reported the finding of oval pupils in 15 patients on a neurosurgical service, 14 of whom had raised intracranial pressure. Eleven of these patients had suffered closed head injuries. In 9 of the 14 patients with intracranial hypertension, the oval pupil disappeared with relative normalization of the intracranial pressure. On the other hand, Fisher[71,96] believes that third nerve involvement in such patients is secondary to a shift of midline structures, and that the transtentorial herniation is a late and irreversible epiphenomenon. In our opinion, the finding of oval pupils in the setting of severe neurologic dysfunction can represent either intrinsic midbrain dysfunction or shift of midline supratentorial structures.

**PARADOXICAL PUPILLARY LIGHT REACTIONS.** Most perplexing is the finding of a bilateral paradoxical pupillary response to light stimuli (i.e., pupillary constriction to the lowering of ambient illumination and pupillary dilatation to the raising of ambient illumination). This phenomenon has been reported in patients with (1) congenital stationary night blindness, (2) congenital achromatopsia, (3) bilateral optic neuritis, (4) dominant optic atrophy, (5) Leber's congenital amaurosis, (6) anomalies of optic nerve development, (7) congenital nystagmus, and (8) strabismus and amblyopia. Although this paradoxical response was at one time considered to indicate retinal dysfunction, this generalization is no longer tenable. The underlying pathophysiology remains unknown.[97]

## REFERENCES

1. Jampel RS, Mindel J. The nucleus for accommodation in the midbrain of the macaque: the effect of accommodation, pupillary constriction, and extraocular muscle contraction produced by stimulation of the oculomotor nucleus on the intraocular pressure. Invest Ophthalmol 1967;6:40-58.

2. Ksiazek SM, Repka MX, Maguire A, et al. Divisional oculomotor nerve paresis caused by intrinsic brainstem disease. Ann Neurol 1989;26:714-8.

3. Parkinson D. Bernard, Mitchell, Horner syndrome and others? Surg Neurol 1979;11:221-3.

4. Johnston JA, Parkinson D. Intracranial sympathetic pathways associated with the sixth cranial nerve. J Neurosurg 1974;40:236-43.

5. Czarnecki JSC, Pilley SFJ, Thompson HS. The analysis of anisocoria: the use of photography in the clinical evaluation of unequal pupils. Can J Ophthalmol 1979;14:297-302.

6. Lam BL, Thompson HS, Corbett JJ. The prevalence of simple anisocoria. Am J Ophthalmol 1987;104:69-73.

7. Loewenfeld IE. "Simple central" anisocoria: a common condition, seldom recognized. Trans Am Acad Ophthalmol Otolaryngol 1977;83:832-9.

8. Meyer BC. Incidence of anisocoria and difference in size of palpebral fissures in five hundred normal subjects. Arch Neurol Psychiatry 1947;57:464-8.

9. Roarty JD, Keltner JL. Normal pupil size and anisocoria in newborn infants. Arch Ophthalmol 1990;108:94-5.

10. Loewenfeld IE. Pupillary changes related to age. In: Thompson HS, Daroff RB, Frisén L, et al, eds. Topics in neuro-ophthalmology. Baltimore: Williams & Wilkins, 1979:129.

11. Bumke [O]. Beiträge zur Kenntnis der Irisbewegungen. Centralbl Nervenh Psychiatr 1904;27:89-99.

12. Thompson HS, Pilley SFJ. Unequal pupils: a flow chart for sorting out the anisocorias. Surv Ophthalmol 1976;21:45-8.

13. Pilley SFJ, Thompson HS. Pupillary "dilation lag" in Horner's syndrome. Br J Ophthalmol 1975;59:731-5.

14. Grimson BS, Thompson HS. Drug testing in Horner's syndrome. In: Glaser JS, Smith JS, eds. Neuro-ophthalmology: symposium of the University of Miami and the Bascom Palmer Eye Institute, vol 8. St Louis: Mosby–Year Book, 1975:265-70.

15. Friedman JR, Whiting DW, Kosmorsky GS, et al. The cocaine test in normal patients [Letter]. Am J Ophthalmol 1984;98:808-10.

16. Kardon RH, Denison CE, Brown CK, et al. Critical evaluation of the cocaine test in the diagnosis of Horner's syndrome. Arch Ophthalmol 1990;108:384-7.

17. Bralliar BB, Skarf B, Owens JB. Ophthalmic use of cocaine and the urine test for benzoylecgonine [Letter]. N Engl J Med 1989;320:1757-8.

18. Thompson BM, Corbett JJ, Kline LB, et al. Pseudo-Horner's syndrome. Arch Neurol 1982;39:108-11.

19. Thompson HS, Mensher JH. Adrenergic mydriasis in Horner's syndrome: hydroxyamphetamine test for diagnosis of post-ganglionic defects. Am J Ophthalmol 1971;72:472-80.

20. Giles CL, Henderson JW. Horner's syndrome: an analysis of 216 cases. Am J Ophthalmol 1958;46:289-96.

21. Cremer SA, Thompson HS, Digre KB, et al. Hydroxyamphetamine mydriasis in normal subjects. Am J Ophthalmol 1990;110:66-70.

22. Cremer SA, Thompson HS, Digre KB, et al. Hydroxyamphetamine mydriasis in Horner's syndrome. Am J Ophthalmol 1990;110:71-6.

23. Maloney WF, Younge BR, Moyer NJ. Evaluation of the causes and accuracy of pharmacologic localization in Horner's syndrome. Am J Ophthalmol 1980;90:394-402.

24. Van der Weil HL, Van Gijn L. Localization of Horner's syndrome: use and limitations of the hydroxyamphetamine test. J Neurol Sci 1983;59:229-35.

25. Shewmon DA. Unilateral straight hair in congenital Horner syndrome due to stellate ganglion tumor. Ann Neurol 1983;13:345-6.

26. Jaffe N. Reply to: Spigelblatt L, Benoit P, Jacob JL, et al. Neuroblastoma with heterochromia and Horner syndrome [Letter]. J Pediatr 1976;88:1067-8.

27. Jaffe N, Cassady R, Petersen R, et al. Heterochromia and Horner syndrome associated with cervical and mediastinal neuroblastoma. J Pediatr 1975; 87:75-7.

28. Kestenbaum A. Clinical methods of neuro-ophthalmologic examination. 2nd ed. New York: Grune & Stratton, 1961:467.

29. Makley TA, Abbott K. Neurogenic heterochromia: report of an interesting case. Am J Ophthalmol 1965;59:927-8.

30. Musarella MA, Chan HS, DeBoer G, et al. Ocular involvement in neuroblastoma: prognostic implications. Ophthalmology 1984;91:936-40.

31. Sauer C, Levingohn MW. Horner's syndrome in childhood. Neurology 1976; 26:216-20.

32. Spigelblatt L, Benoit P, Jacob JL. Neuroblastoma with heterochromia and Horner syndrome [Letter]. J Pediatr 1976;88:1067-8.

33. Pancoast HK. Superior pulmonary sulcus tumor: tumor characterized by pain, Horner's syndrome, destruction of bone and atrophy of hand muscles. JAMA 1932;99:1391-6.

34. Schiffter R. Telodiencephalic ischemic syndrome [Letter]. Arch Neurol 1987; 44:1218-9.

35. Stone WM, de Toledo J, Romanul FC. Horner's syndrome due to hypothalamic infarction: clinical, radiologic, and pathologic correlation. Arch Neurol 1986;43:199-200.

36. Guy J, Day AL, Mickle JP, et al. Contralateral trochlear nerve paresis and ipsilateral Horner's syndrome. Am J Ophthalmol 1989;107:73-6.

37. Kellen RI, Burde RM, Hodges TF III, et al. Central bilateral sixth nerve palsy associated with a unilateral preganglionic Horner's syndrome. J Clin Neuro Ophthalmol 1988;8:179-84.

38. Goldhammer Y, Nathan H, Luchansky E. Compression of the superior cervical ganglion by the internal carotid artery demonstrated by anatomic studies: a possible etiology for Horner's syndrome in the elderly. Presented at the Fourth Annual Meeting of the International Neuro-Ophthalmologic Society, Hamilton, Bermuda, June 1982.

39. Ottomo M, Heimburger RF. Alternating Horner's syndrome and hyperhidrosis due to dural adhesions following cervical spinal cord injury: case report. J Neurosurg 1980;53:97-100.

40. Vijayan N. A new post-traumatic headache syndrome: clinical and therapeutic observations. Headache 1977;17: 19-22.

41. Bogousslavsky J, Despland PA, Regli F. Spontaneous carotid dissection with acute stroke. Arch Neurol 1987;44:137-40.

42. Goldberg HI, Grossman RI, Gomori JM, et al. Cervical internal carotid artery dissecting hemorrhage: diagnosis using MR. Radiology 1986;158:157-61.

43. Havelius U, Hindfelt B. Minor vessels leaving the extracranial internal carotid artery: possible clinical implications. Neuro-Ophthalmology 1985;5:51-6.

44. Adler FH, Scheie HG. The site of the disturbance in tonic pupils. Trans Am Ophthalmol Soc 1940;38:183-92.

45. Ramsay DA. Dilute solutions of phenylephrine and pilocarpine in the diag-

nosis of disordered autonomic innervation of the iris: observations in normal subjects and in the syndromes of Horner and Holmes-Adie. J Neurol Sci 1986;73:125-34.

46. Ponsford JR, Bannister R, Paul EA. Methacholine pupillary responses in third nerve palsy and Adie's syndrome. Brain 1982;105:583-97.

47. Slamovits TL, Miller NR, Burde RM. Intracranial oculomotor nerve paresis with anisocoria and parasympathetic hypersensitivity. Am J Ophthalmol 1987;104:401-6.

48. Burde RM. Direct parasympathetic pathway to the eye: revisited. Brain Res 1988;463:158-62.

49. Jacobson DM. Pupillary responses to dilute pilocarpine in preganglionic 3rd nerve disorders. Neurology 1990;40: 804-8.

50. Thompson HS. A classification of "tonic pupils." In: Thompson HS, Daroff R, Frisén L, et al, eds. Topics in neuro-ophthalmology. Baltimore: Williams & Wilkins, 1979:95-6.

51. Münch K. Zur Frage der wurmförmigen Zuckungen am Sphinkter pupillae. Klin Monatsbl Augenheilkd 1912;50: 745-9.

52. Thompson HS. Segmental palsy of the iris sphincter in Adie's syndrome. Arch Ophthalmol 1978;96:1615-20.

53. Holmes G. Partial iridoplegia associated with symptoms of other disease of the nervous system. Trans Ophthalmol Soc UK 1931;51:209-28.

54. Thompson HS, Bourgon P, Van Allen MW. The tendon reflexes in Adie's syndrome. In: Thompson HS, Daroff R, Frisén L, et al, eds. Topics in neuro-ophthalmology. Baltimore: Williams & Wilkins, 1979:104-13.

55. Bourgon P, Pilley FJ, Thompson HS. Cholinergic supersensitivity of the iris sphincter in Adie's tonic pupil. Am J Ophthalmol 1978;85:373-7.

56. Dubois HF, van Bijsterveld OP. Internal ophthalmoparesis: an uncommon complication of varicella, a common disease. Ophthalmologia 1977;175:263-8.

57. Noel LP, Watson AG. Internal ophthalmoplegia following chickenpox. Can J Ophthalmol 1976;11:267-9.

58. Miller NR, Keltner JL, Gittinger JW Jr, et al. Intermittent pupillary dilation in a young woman. Surv Ophthalmol 1986;31:65-8.

59. Thompson HS. The pupil. In: Moses RA, ed. Adler's physiology of the eye: clinical application. 7th ed. St Louis: Mosby–Year Book, 1981:343.

60. Thompson HS, Newsome DA, Loewenfeld IE. The fixed dilated pupil: sudden iridoplegia or mydriatic drops? A simple diagnostic test. Arch Ophthalmol 1971;86:21-7.

61. Walsh FG, Hoyt WFL. Clinical neuro-ophthalmology, vol 1. Baltimore: Williams & Wilkins, 1969:253.

62. Payne JW, Adamkiewicz J Jr. Unilateral internal ophthalmoplegia with intracranial aneurysm. Am J Ophthalmol 1969;68:349-52.

63. Carlston JA. Unilateral dilated pupil from scopolamine disk [Letter]. JAMA 1982;248:31.

64. McCrary JA III, Webb NR. Anisocoria from scopolamine patches. JAMA 1982; 248:353-4.

65. Edelson RN, Levy DE. Transient benign unilateral pupillary dilation in young adults. Arch Neurol 1974;31:12-4.

66. Hallett M, Cogan DG. Episodic unilateral mydriasis in otherwise normal patients. Arch Ophthalmol 1970;84:130-6.

67. Woods D, O'Connor PS, Fleming R. Episodic unilateral mydriasis and migraine. Am J Ophthalmol 1984; 98:229-34.

68. Bach L: Pupillenlehre. Berlin: S Karger, 1908:153-7.

69. Boghen D. Transient benign unilateral pupillary dilation [Letter]. Arch Neurol 1975;32:68-9.

70. Thompson HS, Zackon DH, Czarnecki JSC. Tadpole-shaped pupils caused by segmental spasms of the iris dilator muscle. Am J Ophthalmol 1983;96:467-77.

71. Fisher CM. Observations concerning brain herniation [Abstract]. Ann Neurol 1983;14:110.

72. Plum F, Posner JB. The diagnosis of stupor and coma. 2nd ed. Philadelphia: FA Davis, 1972:87.

73. Gadoth N, Margalith D, Bechar M.

Unilateral pupillary dilatation during focal seizures. J Neurol 1981;225:227-30.

74. Pant SS, Benton JW, Dodge PR. Unilateral pupillary dilatation during and immediately following seizures. Neurology 1966;16:837-40.

75. Zee DS, Griffin J, Price DL. Unilateral pupillary dilatation during adverse seizures. Arch Neurol 1974;30:403-5.

76. Dalessio DJ, ed. Wolff's headache and other head pain. 4th ed. New York: Oxford University Press, 1980:111.

77. Miller MR, ed. Walsh and Hoyt's clinical neuro-ophthalmology, vol 2. 4th ed. Baltimore: Williams & Wilkins, 1985: chap 31.

78. Bonnet P. L'historique du syndrome de Claude Bernard: le syndrome paralytique du sympathique cervical. Arch Opht 1957;17:121-38.

79. Furukawa T, Toyokura Y. Alternating Horner syndrome. Arch Neurol 1974; 30:311-3.

80. Burde RM. Alternating Horner's syndrome or Bernard's sympathetic irritation [Letter]. J Neurosurg 1980;53:866.

81. Saito H, Nakazawa S. Episodic unilateral mydriasis after neck trauma. Neuro-Ophthalmology 1990;10:209-16.

82. Sigsbee B, Torkelson R, Kadis G, et al. Parasympathetic denervation of the iris in diabetes mellitus: a clinical study. J Neurol Neurosurg Psychiatry 1974; 37:1031-5.

83. Argyll Robertson D. On an interesting series of eye symptoms in a case of spinal disease, with remarks on the action of belladonna on the iris. Edinburg Med J 1869a;14:696-708.

84. Apter JT. The significance of the unilateral Argyll Robertson pupil. I. A report of 13 cases. Am J Ophthalmol 1954; 38:34-43.

85. Hooshmand H, Escobar MR, Kopf SW. Neurosyphilis: a study of 241 patients. JAMA 1972;219:726-9.

86. Keane JR. Tonic pupils with acute ophthalmoplegic polyneuritis. Ann Neurol 1977;2:393-6.

87. Okajima T, Imamura S, Kawasaki S, et al. Fisher's syndrome: a pharmacological study of the pupils. Ann Neurol 1977;2:63-5.

88. Keltner JL, Swisher CN, Gay AJ, et al. Myotonic pupils in Charcot-Marie-Tooth disease: successful relief of symptoms with 0.025% pilocarpine. Arch Ophthalmol 1975;93:1141-8.

89. Morone G. Ricerche pupillografiche nella distrofia miotonica. Boll d'Ocul 1948;27:481-506.

90. Thompson HS, Van Allen MW, von Noordern GK. The pupil in myotonic dystrophy. Invest Ophthalmol 1964; 3:325-38.

91. Isenberg SJ, Molarte A, Vasquez M. The fixed and dilated pupils of premature neonates. Am J Ophthalmol 1990;110:168-71.

92. Fogelholm R, Laru-Sompa R. Brain death and pinpoint pupils [Letter]. J Neurol Neurosurg Psychiatry 1988; 51:1002.

93. Creighton FJ, Ghodse AH. Nalaxone applied to the conjunctiva as a test for physical opiate dependence. Lancet 1989;1:748-50.

94. Selhorst JB, Hoyt WF, Feinsod M, et al. Midbrain corectopia. Arch Neurol 1976;33:193-5.

95. Marshall LF, Barba D, Toole BM, et al. The oval pupil: clinical significance and relationship to intracranial hypertension. J Neurosurg 1983;58:566-8.

96. Fisher CM. Oval pupils. Arch Neurol 1980;37:502-3.

97. Frank JW, Kushner BJ, France TD. Paradoxic pupillary phenomena: a review of patients with pupillary constriction to darkness. Arch Ophthalmol 1988; 106:1564-6.

# CHAPTER 14

# Eyelid Disturbances

• • • • • • • • • • • • • • • •

## PART I: PTOSIS

Blepharoptosis (ptosis) is the downward displacement of the upper lid caused by a dysfunction of the lid elevators. True ptosis must be distinguished from pseudoptosis (Chart 14-1).

## A Decision Tree Approach to the Evaluation of Ptosis

### Pseudoptosis

Pseudoptosis is an apparent narrowing of the palpebral fissure that is not associated with a myopathy, neuropathy, or myoneural dysfunction involving the upper lid elevators.

### Blepharospasm

Blepharospasm is a voluntary or involuntary lowering of the upper lid caused by orbicularis contraction, which is always associated with elevation of the lower lid and lowering of the brow (see Part III). The inferior corneal limbus is covered by the lower lid; this does not occur in true ptosis except with Horner's syndrome. Blepharospasm is frequently accompanied by visible twitching movements of the orbicularis muscle (Fig. 14-1, A).

### Apraxia of lid opening

Apraxia of lid opening is the inability to initiate lid opening voluntarily in the presence of normal spontaneous lid elevation. Frontalis muscle contraction is normal, and no evidence of concurrent orbicularis oculi muscle contraction, no ocular motor nerve dysfunction, no ocular sympathetic dysfunction, and no ocular myopathy is present. Most patients have extrapyramidal disease, but unilateral and bilateral hemispheric disease has been implicated in causing lid opening apraxia.[1] Patients may manually lift these lids or at times use a head-thrusting movement.[2]

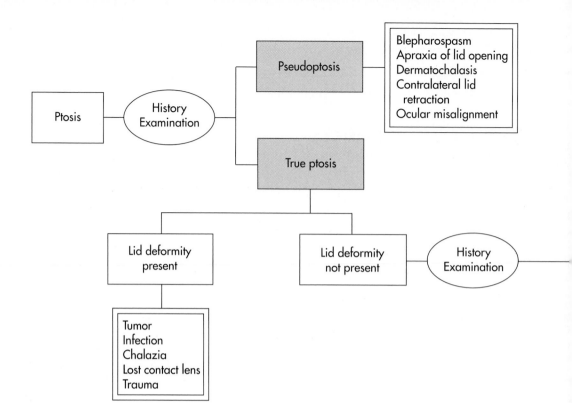

*Chart 14-1*

☐ Dermatochalasis

Dermatochalasis is the presence of redundant skin on the upper lid causing narrowing of the interpalpebral fissure. This condition is usually seen in older patients and is often accompanied by external signs of protrusion of orbital fat through an incompetent orbital septum (Fig. 14-1, *B*).

☐ Contralateral lid retraction

Subtle lid retraction of one upper lid may make the other lid appear ptotic even though it is in its normal position. Normally the upper lid covers the superior corneoscleral limbus when the eyes are in the primary position. Visibility of sclera above the superior limbus indicates upper lid traction and suggests that the suspected "ptotic" lid is in a normal position (Fig. 14-1, *C*).

☐ Ocular misalignment

The upper lid may appear ptotic when an eye is relatively hypotropic to its fellow. When the hypotropic eye fixates, the apparent ptosis disappears.

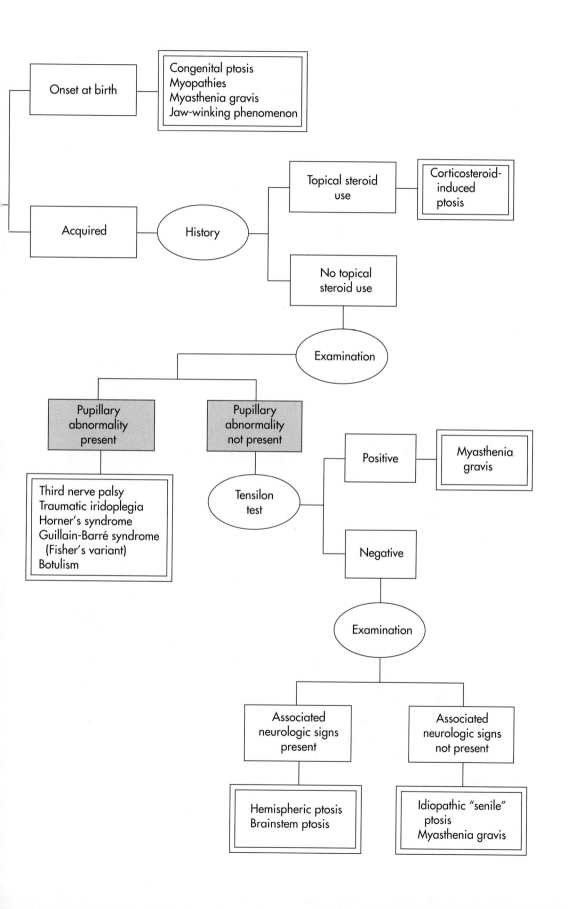

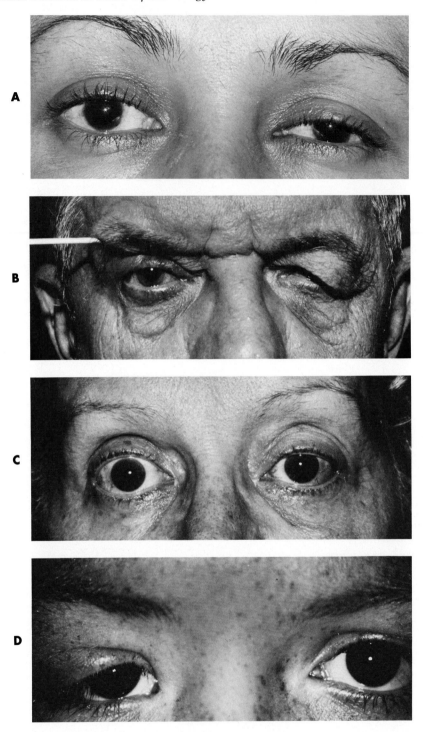

*Fig. 14-1.* Pseudoptosis. **A,** Blepharospasm: narrower lid fissure on left is due to lower upper lid but also to elevation of lower lid. Note flattening of left brow. **B,** Dermatochalasis: redundant folds of upper lid skin diminish apparent width of interpalpebral fissure. Elevation of right fold shows upper lid in its normal position. **C,** Contralateral lid retraction: right upper lid retracted, exposing sclera above superior corneoscleral limbus. Left upper lid is in normal position. **D,** Lid deformity: thickened, S-shaped right upper lid is due to a neurofibroma in this patient with neurofibromatosis.

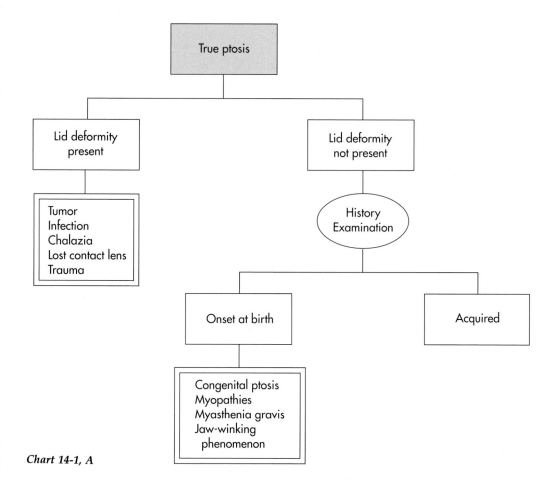

*Chart 14-1, A*

True ptosis

Once the examiner has determined that the patient has true ptosis and not pseudoptosis, local lid abnormalities that may weigh down the upper lid should be eliminated as causes (Chart 14-1, *A*).

☐ Lid deformity present

Any extra mass added to the upper lid will, by the force of gravity and thickening of the lid itself, result in its drooping. **Tumors** of the upper lid (Fig. 14-1, *D*) or **infectious processes,** which may be acute **(preseptal cellulitis)** or chronic **(chalazia),** may produce ptosis. Patients who are **contact lens** wearers should be asked about previously "lost" lenses. A contact lens may become trapped under the upper lid, and a granulomatous reaction around this retained foreign body can cause ptosis.[3] Double eversion of the upper lid will reveal the true nature of this ptosis. True lowering of the upper lid may occur after **trauma.** While lid deformity may be absent, it is usually detectable.

☐ Lid deformity not present

If no lid deformity or mass is apparent, the next critical distinction is to determine if the ptosis was present at birth or was acquired later in life.

☐ Onset at birth

⬜ Congenital ptosis

Congenital ptosis is present from birth. It may be isolated or associated with difficulty in elevation of the ipsilateral eye due to underaction of the levator palpebrae superioris and superior rectus muscles, both of which are derived from the same superior mesodermal complex.[4] At times ptosis may be part of a more complex syndrome of multiple congenital anomalies (Turner's syndrome, Smith Lemli-Opitz syndrome[5]). If doubt exists as to the presence of ptosis from birth, old photographs should be reviewed. Often a previously undetected congenital ptosis may be documented in this manner, thus avoiding the necessity for further evaluation.

⬜ Myopathies

Ptosis at birth may be part of a generalized myopathic disorder such as myotubular myopathy, congenital fiber-type disproportion, or congenital myotonia. In these conditions other signs of systemic involvement, incuding ophthalmoplegia, generalized extremity weakness, and hypotonia, accompany ptosis (see Chapter 8).

⬜ Myasthenia gravis

**NEONATAL MYASTHENIA.** Children born of myasthenic mothers may show evidence of ptosis or other signs of myasthenia beginning within 24 hours of birth. The syndrome of neonatal myasthenia may last for weeks and may require supportive treatment with anticholinesterase agents. This transient form of myasthenia is produced by the passage across the placenta of antibodies against acetylcholine receptors.[6]

**GENETIC FORMS OF MYASTHENIA.** These forms of myasthenia are due to a variety of pathophysiologic mechanisms, but symptoms typically appear in the neonatal period or early infancy. Unlike other forms of myasthenia, the genetic form is not antibody mediated.[7]

⬜ Jaw-winking phenomenon

Infants may manifest intermittent retraction of a ptotic lid during chewing, jaw movement, or sucking. This movement (Marcus Gunn, jaw-winking phenomenon) results from a presumed miswiring between the oculomotor and trigeminal motor pathways. Jaw winking may become less marked as the patient grows older. These patients do not require a neurologic evaluation.

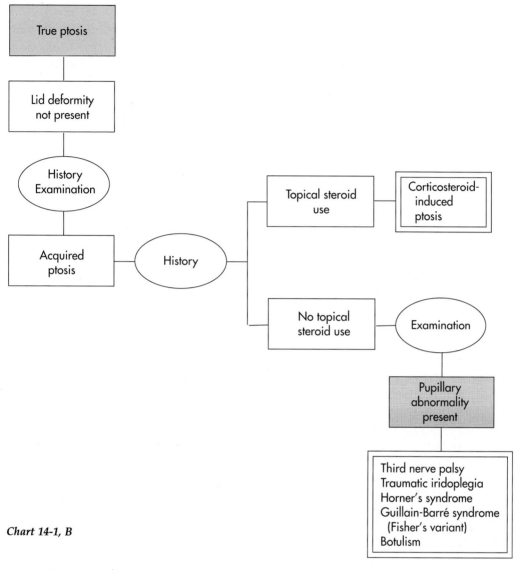

*Chart 14-1, B*

☐ Acquired ptosis

When it has been determined that the ptosis is acquired (Chart 14-1, *B*), the patient should be questioned about the use of topical corticosteroids, which have been implicated in the production of ptosis.[8] The true incidence of **corticosteroid-induced ptosis** must be small, given the amount of topical corticosteroid dispensed without apparent difficulty.

If no medication can be implicated as the cause of the ptosis, close inspection of pupillary size and reactivity should be performed.

☐ No topical steroid use

▨ Pupillary abnormality present

Several forms of pupillary abnormality may be associated with ptosis. The presence of a dilated, poorly reactive pupil ipsilateral to the ptotic lid suggests a

**third cranial nerve palsy** (see Chapter 10). **Trauma** may result in ptosis and a large pupil, but iris sphincter ruptures or tears will be detected on slit lamp examination. The association of ptosis and ipsilateral miosis suggests an oculo-sympathetic paresis **(Horner's syndrome)** (see Chapter 13). Rarely, **Fisher's variant of Guillain-Barré syndrome** and **botulism** may present with ptosis and mydriasis early in the course of their evolution.

■ Pupillary abnormality not present (Chart 14-1, C)

Acquired ptosis in the presence of normal pupils must be considered to be caused by myasthenia gravis until proved otherwise. Myasthenia is a disorder involving skeletal and not visceral musculature; therefore the pupils and accommodation are normal. The intravenous administration of edrophonium chloride (Tensilon test) should be carried out in all patients with acquired ptosis and normal pupils.

○ *Tensilon test.* When a variable or fatigable ptosis suggests myasthenia, the intravenous administration of edrophonium chloride (Tensilon) is warranted. An unequivocally positive Tensilon test strongly suggests, but does not prove, the diagnosis of myasthenia gravis (Fig. 14-2). False-positive tests are rare but may occur with other myopathies or neuropathies.[9-11] More frequently myasthenia may exist even in the face of a negative Tensilon test, and one negative test does not exclude myasthenia as the cause of ptosis.

☐ Positive tensilon test

▣ Myasthenia gravis

Myasthenia gravis is characterized by impaired transmission of impulses across the myoneural junction. The impaired transmission is due to the presence of antibodies to acetylcholine receptors in the motor end-plate of striated muscle. These antibodies block the receptor, and some also cause accelerated receptor degradation.[12] Ocular signs, particularly ptosis, may be the initial manifestation of myasthenia in up to 75% of patients.[13] If these ocular signs remain the only indications of myasthenia for longer than 2 years, systemic myasthenia is not likely to develop. The ocular form of myasthenia occurs in approximately 20% of myasthenic patients.[13,14]

Variability of clinical signs and fatigability of specific muscle groups on repeated function are the hallmarks of myasthenia. Ptosis is improved or absent on awakening but becomes pronounced as the day progresses. Marked ptosis may be produced by having the patient sustain upgaze (Fig 14-3). This curtain effect of the lids to sustained upward gaze is a useful office test in detecting my-

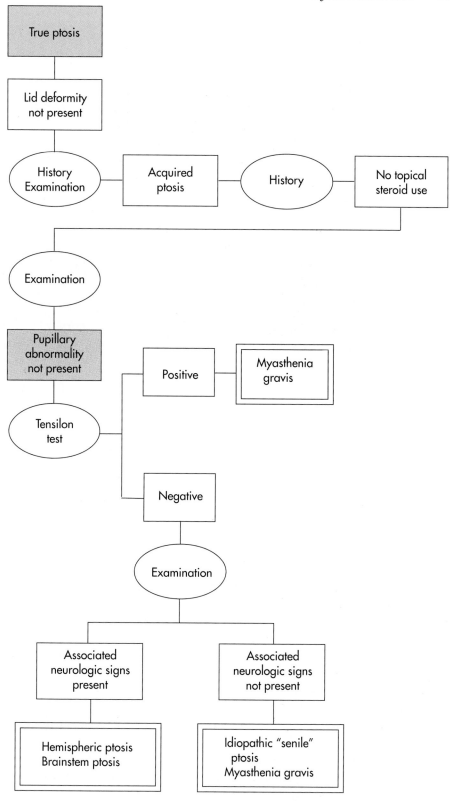

*Chart 14-1, C*

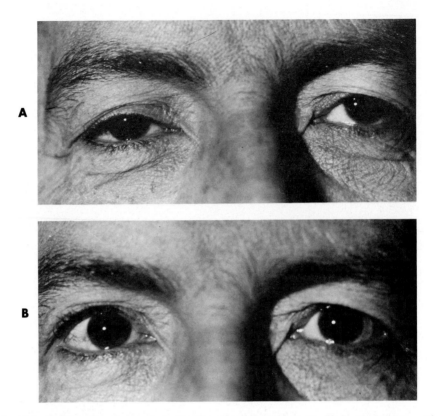

*Fig. 14-2.* Positive Tensilon test. **A,** Pre-Tensilon bilateral ptosis. **B,** Postinjection, widened interpalpebral fissures with resolution of bilateral ptosis.

asthenic ptosis. Because ptosis from any cause may worsen during the day, fatigability is suggestive of but not specific for myasthenia.

When the ptosis is asymmetric, the patient may use the frontalis muscle to elevate both lids, producing what appears to be lid retraction on one side. If the examiner manually elevates the more ptotic lid, the previously retracted lid will fall (Fig. 14-4). This fall of the apparently retracted upper lid has been termed *enhanced ptosis*[15] and probably is explained by invoking Hering's law of equal innervation as applied to the levator palpebrae superioris. Lid retraction of Graves' orbitopathy is not affected by manually elevating the contralateral lid.

Cogan[16] has described the lid-twitch sign as being characteristic of myasthenic ptosis. The patient looks down for 10 to 15 seconds and is then asked to make a rapid refixational eye movement to the primary position. A positive lid-twitch sign consists of an upward overshoot of the lid, which then will slowly drop to its previous ptotic position. We have seen this sign with nonmyasthenic ptosis, however.

Myasthenic ptosis is frequently associated with orbicularis weakness. For example, while the patient attempts forced lid closure, the examiner can manually separate the lids, often with little effort.

Ocular motility disturbances often accompany myasthenic ptosis. The ocu-

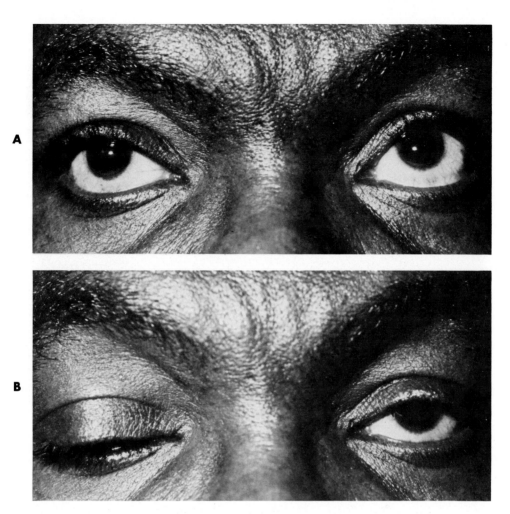

***Fig. 14-3.*** Lid fatigue: myasthenic patient is asked to look up continually. Initially lids are open, **A.** However, after sustaining upgaze, lids droop, producing an almost complete right ptosis and a marked left ptosis, **B.**

lar motility defects may resemble an isolated extraocular muscle weakness, cranial nerve palsy, or supranuclear motility disturbance (see Chapter 10).

Myasthenia gravis and Graves' disease, both immunologically mediated disorders, are often associated. Circulating antithyroid antibodies have been found in 30% to 40% of myasthenic patients.[17] When these disorders occur together, the ptosis of myasthenia may be masked by the lid retraction of Graves' disease (see Part II). Connective tissue diseases also are found more frequently in myasthenia than in the general population.

Electromyographic (EMG) demonstration of neuromuscular fatigue may be present when pharmacologic testing is equivocal or negative.[6] In patients with purely ocular myasthenia, the presence of an abnormal repetitive stimulation test in clinically uninvolved muscles does not predict that the disease will become clinically generalized.[18]

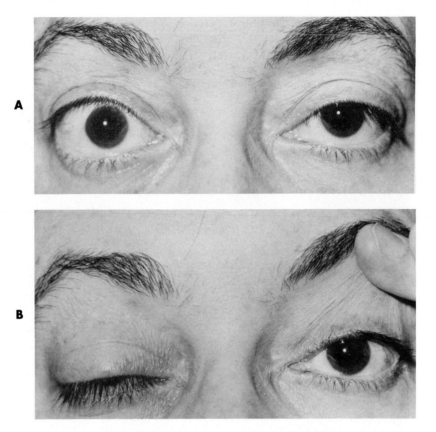

*Fig. 14-4.* Enhanced ptosis. **A,** Myasthenic patient has left ptosis and right upper lid retraction. **B,** Left lid is elevated manually, which produces a complete ptosis of previously retracted right upper lid.

Acetylcholine-receptor antibody levels, routinely elevated in generalized myasthenia, may be normal in the ocular form of the disorder. The sensitivity of antibody levels is estimated to approach 90% in generalized myasthenia but is only approximately 65% in the ocular form of the disease.[19] However, the clinical characteristics of the seronegative patients do not differ from those of patients in the same clinical group who have high antibody titers.[20] The exact reason for this phenomenon is unknown.[21]

An unequivocally positive Tensilon test is highly suggestive of myasthenia, but because false-positive responses occur, we recommend obtaining acetylcholine receptor antibody levels in all patients. We reserve EMG testing for patients in whom the Tensilon test and antibody levels produce equivocal results.

Once the diagnosis of myasthenia has been established, the patient should be referred to a neurologist to determine the extent of disease and for treatment. Even if ocular signs appear to be the only manifestation of myasthenia, treatment by a nonneurologist should be discouraged unless the treating physician is comfortable managing the bulbar aspects of myasthenia and the side effects of myasthenic treatment regimens.

Many treatment options are now available to the myasthenic patient. The time-honored initial treatment usually consists of oral pyridostigmine bromide (Mestinon). Systemic corticosteroids may be administered in conjunction with anticholinesterase medications if remission does not occur. Azathioprine[22] and plasmapheresis have also proved effective. Myasthenic patients should have imaging of the chest to detect the presence of an enlarged thymus gland due to hyperplasia or a thymoma. Surgical removal of thymic masses often results in the remission of myasthenia. Some have suggested that all young patients with generalized myasthenia, irrespective of the chest imaging findings, should undergo thymectomy.[6] We do not advise thymectomy in patients with purely ocular myasthenia unless a thymic mass is detected by imaging.

Certain medications that may further compromise nerve conduction should be avoided in myasthenic patients. The aminoglycosides (gentamicin, colistin, polymyxin, neomycin, kanamycin, tobramycin) have a curarelike effect on the neuromuscular junction and must be used cautiously in myasthenic patients and only when other antibacterial agents are not efficacious.[23]

A myasthenic-like syndrome may be produced by penicillamine, although the exact mechanism remains unknown. Since this drug is used frequently to treat rheumatoid arthritis, an arthritic patient who develops myasthenic symptoms should be asked about ingestion of penicillamine.[24] Myasthenic patients treated for cardiac arrhythmias with quinidine or procainamide may experience worsening of their myasthenia.[25]

### ☐ Negative tensilon test

When the Tensilon test is negative, the examiner must determine if other neurologic signs are present or if the ptosis is truly isolated. Ocular motility disturbances associated with acquired ptosis and normal pupils may indicate a pupillary-sparing third cranial nerve palsy, the syndrome of multiple–cranial nerve involvement, chronic progressive external ophthalmoplegia, myotonic dystrophy,[26] Fisher's variant of the Guillain-Barré syndrome, or botulism (see Chapter 8).

### ☐ Associated neurologic signs present

#### ☐ Hemispheric ptosis

Ptosis produced by cerebral hemispheric dysfunction is reported to be bilateral (symmetric or asymmetric) or unilateral.[27,28] A more thorough description of this entity is provided by Lepore,[29] who found bilateral ptosis in 13 patients with right hemisphere stroke. The complete syndrome includes right gaze deviation or preference, left facial weakness and hemiparesis, and left hemisensory loss. Lepore attributes the asymmetry of ptosis in his patients to the presence of a unilateral facial weakness.

#### ☐ Brainstem ptosis

Lesions of the brainstem may produce bilateral ptosis by involving the levator subnucleus of the third cranial nerve.[30] Bilateral ptosis occurring with bilateral downgaze paresis has been attributed to destruction of brainstem premotor input to the levator subnucleus.[31] An alternative explanation may be the intact normal inhibition mechanism of the levator muscles on attempted downgaze. Thus, while the eyes do not descend below the midline, the lids do depress as if the eyes were in downgaze. This "reverse Collier's sign" is thought to represent the disruption of the normal synkinesis between the levator muscles and the vertically acting extraocular muscles.[32]

☐ Associated neurologic signs not present

▣ Idiopathic ("senile") ptosis

An isolated ptosis in the nonmyasthenic older patient may be classified as "senile" ptosis. This noninherited form of ptosis is believed to be due to disinsertions or dehiscences of the levator aponeurosis.[33] The superior lid sulcus deepens, and the lid fold becomes lower because of levator dehiscence. When the ptosis becomes a functional or cosmetic disturbance, surgical correction may be considered.

▣ Myasthenia gravis

It should be recalled that ptosis with or without accompanying ocular motility disturbance may still be myasthenic despite repeatedly negative Tensilon tests.

### REFERENCES

1. Johnston JC, Rosenbaum DM, Picone CM, et al. Apraxia of eyelid opening secondary to right hemisphere infarction. Ann Neurol 1989;25:622-4.
2. Goldstein JE, Cogan DG: Apraxia of lid opening. Arch Ophthalmol 1965; 73:155-9.
3. Yassin JG, White RH, Shannon GM. Blepharoptosis as a complication of contact lens migration. Am J Ophthalmol 1971;72:536-7.
4. Sevel D. Ptosis and underaction of the superior rectus muscle. Ophthalmology 1984;91:1080-5.
5. Gellis SS, Feingold M. Atlas of mental retardation syndromes: visual diagnosis of facies and physical findings. US Rehabilitation Services Administration, Division of Mental Retardation. Washington, DC: US Department of Health, Education, and Welfare. US Government Printing Office, 1968.
6. Drachman DB. Myasthenia gravis [first of two parts]. N Engl J Med 1978; 298:136-42.
7. Misulis KE, Fenichel GM. Genetic forms of myasthenia gravis. Pediatr Neurol 1989;5:205-10.
8. Fraunfelder FT: Drug-induced ocular side effects and drug interactions. 3rd ed. Philadelphia: Lea & Febiger, 1989.
9. Dirr LY, Donofrio PD, Patton JF et al. A false-positive edrophonium test in a patient with a brainstem glioma, Neurology 1989;39:865-7.
10. Moorthy G, Behrens MM, Drachman DB, et al. Ocular pseudomyasthenia or ocular myasthenia "plus": a warning to clinicians. Neurology 1989;39:1150-4.
11. Oh SJ, Cho HK. Edrophonium responsiveness not necessarily diagnostic of myasthenia gravis. Muscle Nerve 1990; 13:187-91.
12. Drachman DB, Adams RN, Josifek LF, et al. Functional activities of autoantibodies to acetylcholine receptors and the clinical severity of myasthenia gravis. N Engl J Med 1982;307:769-75.
13. Osserman KE. Ocular myasthenia gravis. Invest Ophthalmol 1967;6:277-87.

14. Daroff RB. Ocular myasthenia: diagnosis and therapy. In: Glaser JS, ed. Neuro-ophthalmology, vol 10. St Louis: Mosby–Year Book, 1980:62-71.

15. Gorelick PB, Rosenberg M, Pagano RJ. Enhanced ptosis in myasthenia gravis. Arch Neurol 1981;38:531.

16. Cogan DG. Myasthenia gravis: a review of the disease and a description of lid twitch as a characteristic sign. Arch Ophthalmol 1965;74:217-21.

17. Kiessling WR, Pflughaupt KW, Ricker K, et al. Thyroid function and circulating antithyroid antibodies in myasthenia gravis. Neurology 1981;31:771-4.

18. Bever CT Jr, Aquino AV, Penn AS, et al. Prognosis of ocular myasthenia. Ann Neurol 1983;14:516-9.

19. Phillips LH II, Melnick PA. Diagnosis of myasthenia gravis in the 1990s. Semin Neurol 1990;10:62-9.

20. Soliven BC, Lange DJ, Penn AS, et al. Seronegative myasthenia gravis. Neurology 1988;38:514-7.

21. Mossman S, Vincent A, Newsom-Davis J. Myasthenia gravis without acetylcholine-receptor antibody: a distinct disease entity. Lancet 1986;1:116-9.

22. Witte AS, Cornblath DR, Parry GJ. Azathioprine in the treatment of myasthenia gravis [Abstract]. Ann Neurol 1983;14:112.

23. Howard JF Jr. Adverse drug effects on neuromuscular transmission. Semin Neurol 1990;10:89-102.

24. Bocanegra T, Espinoza LR, Vasey FB, et al. Myasthenia gravis and penicillamine therapy of rheumatoid arthritis. JAMA 1980;244:1822-3.

25. Lisak RP, Barchi RL. Myasthenia gravis. Vol 2. Major problems in neurology. Philadelphia: WB Saunders, 1982:6.

26. Lessell S, Coppeto J, Samet S. Ophthalmoplegia in myotonic dystrophy. Am J Ophthalmol 1971;71:1231-5.

27. Caplan LR. Ptosis. J Neurol Neurosurg Psychiatry 1975;37:1-7.

28. Nutt JG. Lid abnormalities secondary to cerebral hemisphere lesions. Ann Neurol 1977;1:149-51.

29. Lepore FE: Bilateral cerebral ptosis. Neurology 1987;37:1043-6.

30. Growdon JH, Winkler GF, Wray SH. Midbrain ptosis: a case with clinicopathologic correlation. Arch Neurol 1974;30:179-81.

31. Büttner-Ennever JA, Acheson JF, Büttner U, et al. Ptosis and supranuclear downgaze paralysis. Neurology 1989;39:385-9.

32. LoBue TD, Feldon SE. Reverse Collier's sign: pseudoblepharoptosis associated with downgaze paralysis [Letter]. Am J Ophthalmol 1983;95:120-1.

33. Dortzbach RK, Sutula FC. Involutional blepharoptosis: a histopathological study. Arch Ophthalmol 1980;98:2045-9.

# PART II: LID RETRACTION

In the absence of primary position ocular misalignment, the upper lid covers the superior limbus by 1 to 2 mm. If sclera is visible between the superior limbus and the upper lid, the upper lid is considered to be retracted. While marked proptosis due to an orbital mass lesion may produce a widened interpalpebral fissure, lid retraction is most often caused by either cicatricial or innervational contraction of the lid elevators.

## GRAVES' OPHTHALMOPATHY

Lid retraction is caused most frequently by Graves' disease. The patient may have a typical "stare" appearance, and the widened palpebral fissure may produce the appearance of proptosis even if none is present. The upper lid may be delayed in following the eyes as they move into downward gaze. This momentary "hang up" of the upper lid is termed *lid lag.*

The retracted upper lid remains elevated in downgaze in Graves' disease (Fig. 14-5) This differentiates Graves' lid retraction from midbrain lid retraction (Collier's sign), wherein the lids also are retracted in the primary position but are normal in downgaze. Lid lag without retraction in primary position has also been described in Guillain-Barré syndrome but is associated with peripheral facial paralysis.[1]

The cause of dysthyroid lid retraction remains unknown. It is believed that initially the retraction is innervational but in the chronic state becomes cicatricial. Lid retraction is not related to the state of thyroid function. Retraction may remit when the hyperthyroid state is treated successfully, but it may remain unchanged or even worsen. No particular form of thyroid therapy appears to predictably influence lid retraction. Corticosteroid administration concomitant with the initial treatment of the hyperthyroid state may decrease all signs of Graves' ophthalmopathy.[2]

Graves' lid retraction should be treated when it results in corneal exposure or a severe cosmetic blemish. Many surgical approaches are available, and the type of lid surgery required differs from patient to patient. Lateral tarsorrhaphy has been used as a temporizing procedure to protect the cornea. However, we caution against tarsorrhaphy because of the potential to increase intraorbital pressure. Definitive lid surgery should be delayed until the ophthalmopathy is quiescent and stable for at least 6 months and until other surgery (orbital or extraocular muscle) has been completed. Topically applied guanethidine and thymoxamine will alleviate the lid retraction of Graves' disease early in the course of the disease. However, these drugs cause a chemical keratitis, are poorly tolerated, and are not approved by the Food and Drug Administration for topical ocular use.[3]

## NON-GRAVES' CICATRICIAL LID RETRACTION

Upper lid retraction may result from alteration of the lid tissues themselves. Following trauma, scar formation may produce retraction of the upper lid. Scarring that follows lid inflammation may cause retraction, such as after an attack of herpes zoster. This form of lid retraction is almost invariably accompanied by

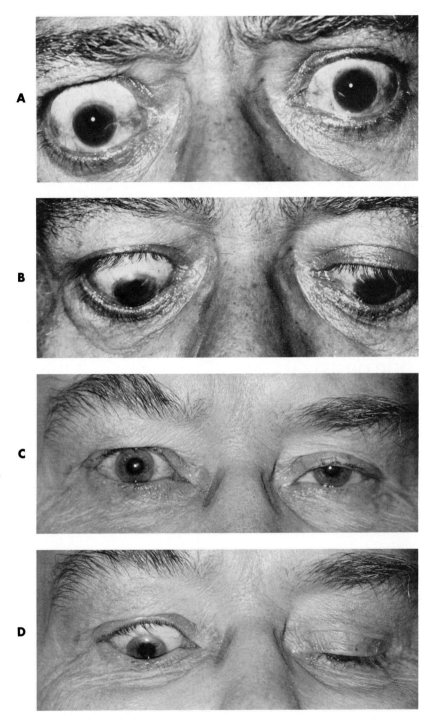

*Fig. 14-5.* Lid retraction Graves' ophthalmopathy. Lid retraction may be marked in primary position, **A,** and persist on downward gaze, **B.** The retraction also may be mild in primary position, **C,** but become evident by appearance of severe retraction in downward gaze, **D.**

visible deformities of the lid itself. Surgical recession of the superior rectus muscles also may result in upper eyelid retraction.

## MIDBRAIN LID RETRACTION (COLLIER'S SIGN)

A variety of lesions in the region of the dorsal midbrain may produce lid retraction. Masses in the periaqueductal gray region, especially pinealoma, are the most frequent causes in young adults, whereas hydrocephalus from any cause may produce this sign in young children. The combination of lid retraction and downward displacement of the eye gives infants the typical "setting-sun" sign.

Midbrain lid retraction is usually bilateral and symmetric but is occasionally unilateral.[4] It is frequently associated with upgaze paresis and light-near dissociation of the pupils (Parinaud's syndrome). No lid retraction in downward gaze occurs as in Graves' ophthalmopathy (Fig. 14-5). A patient with Collier's sign requires imaging of the third ventricular region.

## SYMPATHETIC IRRITATION (CLAUDE BERNARD SYNDROME)

Claude Bernard syndrome, a relatively rare phenomenon and the opposite of Horner's syndrome, consists of lid retraction and an enlarged ipsilateral pupil. It is said to be due to irritation of the sympathetic chain.[5] In our experience, this is a very uncommon finding (see Chapter 13).

## METABOLIC LID RETRACTION

Lid retraction without evidence of Graves' disease has been reported in 13 patients with hepatic cirrhosis.[6] Although thyroid studies were "normal," the more modern stimulation or suppression tests were not performed. Lid retraction due exclusively to cirrhosis must truly be a rare phenomenon.

## VOLITIONAL LID RETRACTION

The patient may produce lid retraction as a volitional act. This is usually seen in anxious or psychotic patients. This form of bilateral lid retraction is accompanied by furrowing of the brow, indicating contribution by the frontalis musculature.

### REFERENCES

1. Neetens A, Smet H. Lid lag in Guillain-Barré-Strohl syndrome. Arch Neurol 1988;45:1046-7.
2. Bartalena L, Marcocci C, Bogazzi F, et al. Use of corticosteroids to prevent progression of Graves' ophthalmopathy after radioiodine therapy for hyperthyroidism. N Engl J Med 1989;321:1349-52.
3. Dixon RS, Anderson RL, Hatt MU. The use of thymoxamine in eyelid retraction. Arch Ophthalmol 1979;97:2147-50.
4. Walsh FB, Hoyt WF. Clinical neuro-ophthalmology. 3rd ed. Baltimore: Williams & Wilkins, 1969:305.
5. Kestenbaum A. Clinical methods of neuro-ophthalmologic examination. 2nd ed. New York: Grune & Stratton, 1961: 449.
6. Summerskill WHJ, Molnar GD: Eye signs in hepatic cirrhosis. N Engl J Med 1962;266:1244-8.

# PART III: BLEPHAROSPASM

The term *blepharospasm* refers to intermittent or constant narrowing of the palpebral fissure caused by contraction of the orbicularis oculi. It may be confused with two other conditions that produce eyelid closure: (1) ptosis and (2) apraxia of eyelid opening or, more correctly, "involuntary inhibition of levator contraction."[1] In blepharospasm, unlike these latter conditions, the brow will be lower than normal (usually below the superior orbital rim) because of orbicularis oculi contraction. Another distinguishing feature is the position of the *lower lid margin*—higher than normal in blepharospasm, and normal in ptosis and involuntary levator inhibition (see Fig. 14-1). In patients with involuntary inhibition of levator contraction, lid elevation is often delayed after normal or forced eyelid closure. We acknowledge that sometimes differentiating blepharospasm from involuntary levator inhibition is not possible; furthermore, in some cases, the two conditions may coexist.

## A Decision Tree Approach to the Evaluation of Blepharospasm (Chart 14-2)

If narrowing of the lid fissure is due to blepharospasm, the first consideration is trigeminal irritation.

### ▨ Trigeminal irritation present

Trigeminal irritation is caused by **anterior ocular inflammation** (keratitis, uveitis), **meningitis,** or **subarachnoid hemorrhage.** These conditions may produce narrowing of the palpebral fissure, but not complete involuntary eyelid closure. Patients typically exhibit painful aversion to bright lights *(photophobia)* and secondary squinting. They can always open their eyes to command—at least briefly. Ocular or meningeal inflammatory signs and symptoms are nearly always evident, and accompanying involuntary, stereotyped facial movements or tics are not present. Patients with this type of blepharospasm are generally more troubled by the primary inflammatory symptoms than by the resulting eyelid closure.

### ▨ Trigeminal irritation not present

If ocular or meningeal irritative signs are absent, the examiner should look for the presence of unilateral facial weakness.

### ▨ Unilateral facial weakness present

Unilateral facial weakness and blepharospasm suggest two possibilities: facial nerve abnormalities following (1) Bell's palsy or (2) intrinsic pontine disease.

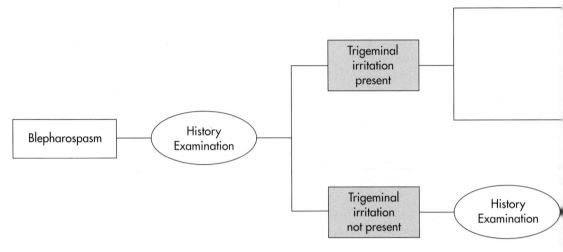

*Chart 14-2*

☐ Facial nerve abnormalities after Bell's palsy

In the recovery phase of a lower motor neuron facial (Bell's) palsy, the facial muscles on the involved side may be slightly contracted as compared with those on the normal side (Fig. 14-6). On attempted voluntary facial movements, a residual paresis of the contracted side will be evident, as well as some synkinesis of facial muscles. Superimposed on this static facial paresis and contracture may be episodic spasms of the facial muscles on the affected side, termed *hemifacial spasm*. Hemifacial spasm occurring in a setting of facial paresis is termed *postparalytic hemifacial spasm* (Fig. 14-7).

☐ Facial nerve abnormalities in pontine disease

In some cases without a history of previous facial palsy, the contracture and paresis develop slowly, often unbeknownst to the patient. An additional feature of many of these cases is a periodic rippling of the facial muscles, visible to the keen observer as a wormlike movement of the skin. Known as *facial myokymia,* this vermiform movement represents grouped fasciculations of motor units. The combination of facial myokymia with contracture and weakness of facial muscles is termed *spastic paretic facial contracture.* It is often caused by intrapontine disease—multiple sclerosis (MS),[2] glioma,[3] metastatic neoplasm,[4] tuberculoma,[5] or stroke.[6] Extraaxial lesions may also be responsible, including cerebellopontine angle mass,[7] Bell's palsy, and Guillain-Barré syndrome.[8]

Imaging[9] and pathologic studies[4,5] have shown that the intraaxial lesions are located slightly rostral and ipsilateral to the seventh nerve nucleus, leading to the hypothesis that the clinical manifestations are due to disconnection of the nucleus from modulating corticobulbar tracts with resultant hyperexcitability. Given that facial contracture and myokymia also occur in Guillain-Barré syndrome, a lesion of the nerve axon can also be responsible for these findings.

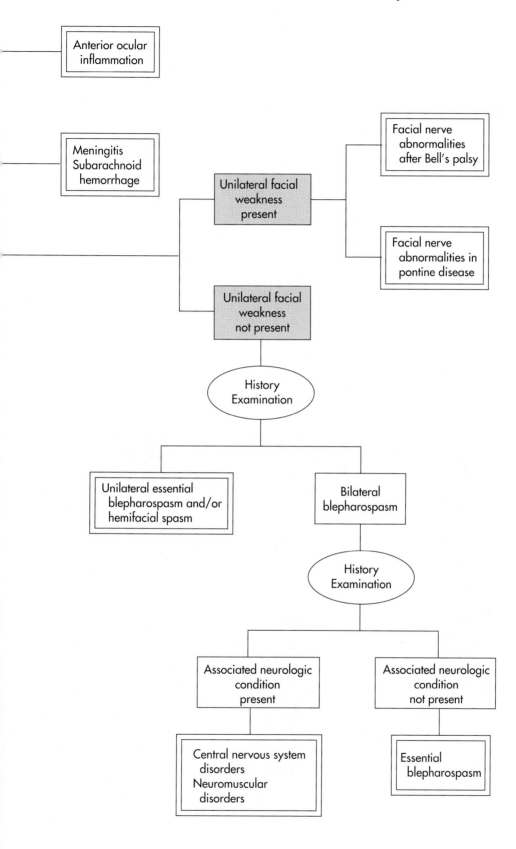

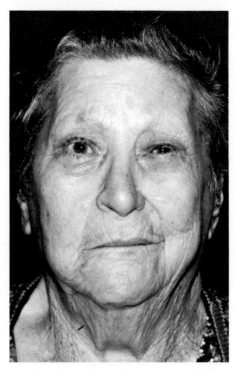

*Fig. 14-6.* Postparalytic facial contracture. Aberrant regeneration of facial nerve after left Bell's palsy has caused left facial contracture.

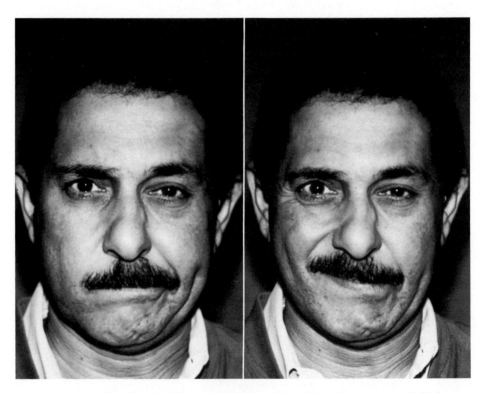

*Fig. 14-7.* Postparalytic hemifacial spasm. Patient with left hemifacial spasm *(left)* demonstrates left facial weakness when asked to smile *(right).*

Pathologic myokymia must be distinguished from the occasional but persistent and bothersome fasciculations that often occur in the eyelids of otherwise healthy individuals, known as *benign myokymia.* Benign myokymia is believed to reflect transient peripheral hyperexcitability of a small group of seventh nerve axons.

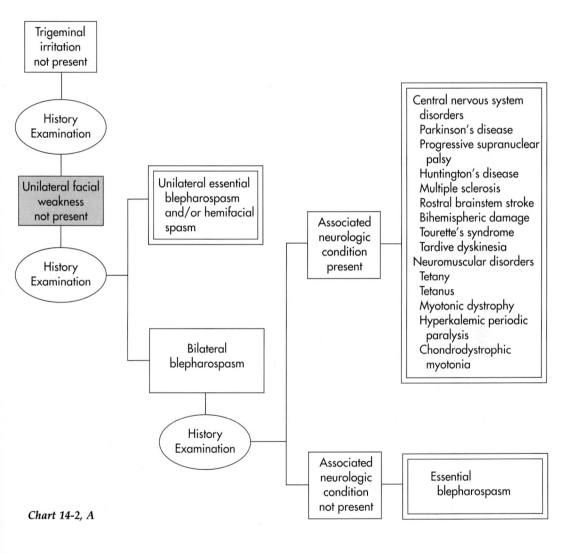

*Chart 14-2, A*

■ Unilateral facial weakness not present

If facial weakness is not present, the clinician should note whether the blepharospasm is unilateral or bilateral (Chart 14-2, *A*).

### ☐ Unilateral essential blepharospasm

Unilateral blepharospasm may represent the initial phase of what will later develop into **bilateral essential blepharospasm** (see Bilateral Blepharospasm). If it remains one sided and involves lower facial muscles, it probably represents hemifacial spasm.

### ☐ Hemifacial spasm

Hemifacial spasm is characterized by unilateral, involuntary bursts of tonic or clonic activity in the muscles of facial expression on one side that last seconds to minutes.[1,10] These episodes have no clear-cut precipitants and may occur during sleep. Although some patients have a history of an ipsilateral lower motor neuron facial paralysis (*postparalytic hemifacial spasm;* Fig. 14-7), many do not (*cryptogenic hemifacial spasm*). EMG has revealed synkinesis (simultaneous contraction) of orbicularis oculi and oris,[1] but hemifacial spasm is otherwise indistinguishable from voluntary facial muscle contraction. Patients with this disorder typically do not have facial myokymia.

The favored explanation for cryptogenic hemifacial spasm is that of Gardner and Sava,[11] who postulate that compression or other injury to the seventh nerve at its exit from the brainstem produces increased irritability and spontaneous firing. The synkinesis has been explained as spread of the impulse between neighboring axons within the nerve (neural "cross talk" or *ephaptic transmission*). Ferguson[12] suggests that proximal axonal damage results in deafferentation of the facial nucleus and unmasking of "automatic, associated and reflexive movements already present in the facial neuronal network."

In the past most cases of hemifacial spasm were considered idiopathic. However, improved imaging of the posterior fossa has revealed that many patients have large, aberrant arteries. In a review of 46 cases, Digre et al.[13] found that 36 patients (78%) had distended and malpositioned vertebral and/or basilar arteries (*dolichoectasia*) on computed tomography (CT) (Fig. 14-8). The authors postulated that hemifacial spasm resulted from compression of the dorsal root entry zone of the seventh cranial nerve, either by the trunk vessel or its branches. Other reports have also found a high prevalence of dolichoectasia in hemifacial spasm.[14,15] Although often associated with arteriosclerosis, dolichoectasia may be a surprising discovery in a patient without vasculopathic risk factors.

Hemifacial spasm is rarely associated with cerebellopontine angle masses (meningioma, epidermoid tumor) and temporal bone disease (cholesteatoma, metastatic tumor).[10] It has also been reported as a segmental myoclonic manifestation of rostral brainstem trauma, stroke, and demyelination.[16] Among the intraaxial causes is Whipple's disease, in which the facial contractions affect primarily the jaw and are synchronized to ocular convergence movements (*oculomasticatory myorhythmia*).[17]

Treatment of hemifacial spasm with medications has been disappointing. Although carbamazepine (Tegretol) may relieve the spasms in some cases,[18] in our experience the effect tends to be short lived and incomplete.

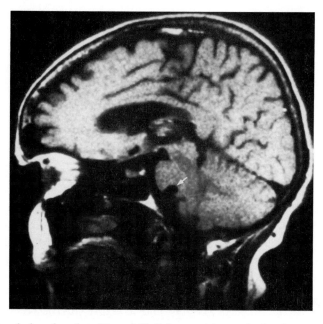

*Fig. 14-8.* Distended and malpositioned (dolichoectatic) vertebrobasilar artery compresses brainstem *(arrow)* to cause hemifacial spasm.

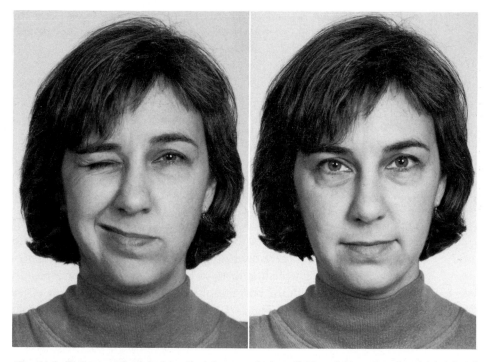

*Fig. 14-9.* Patient with right hemifacial spasm before *(left)* and 3 weeks after *(right)* facial injections of botulinum toxin.

## Management of Hemifacial Spasm

1. Perform brain (posterior fossa) imaging to rule out a treatable mass lesion.
2. If brain imaging is negative, inject botulinum toxin.
3. If botulinum fails and the patient is severely symptomatic and understands the risks, perform a suboccipital craniectomy.

Based on the hypothesis that an aberrant vessel compressing the nerve root entry zone is the cause of the spasms, surgeons have, via suboccipital craniectomy, placed nonabsorbable sponges between the offending vessel and the nerve. More than 500 such operations have now been reported, with an aggregate success rate of 85%.[19,20] Recurrences have been reported in up to 7% of cases, and complications in 15% to 25%, including facial palsy, deafness, and stroke.

Because of the potential risks of craniectomy, botulinum A toxin injection of the facial muscles has become a viable alternative for treating hemifacial spasm (Fig. 14-9). Preliminary reports reveal a success rate of over 90% without significant facial paresis or other complications.[21] Injections must be repeated approximately three times per year to maintain relief.

Spasmodic facial contractions exactly like those of hemifacial spasm may occur in the painful crises in up to 10% of patients with tic douloureux (tic convulsif).[22] We suggest that such patients be initially treated with carbamazepine, realizing that the spasms, unlike the pain, may be unresponsive to this medication.

### ☐ Bilateral blepharospasm

When involuntary eyelid closure affects both sides, the differential diagnosis is between isolated (essential) blepharospasm and blepharospasm associated with a variety of broader neurologic conditions.

### ☐ Associated neurologic condition present

### ☐ Central nervous system disorders

Blepharospasm was reported as a common feature of the dystonic facial grimacing found in patients with von Economo's encephalitis, which appeared in the decade following the 1919 influenza epidemic. Many of these patients went on to develop the postencephalitic form of parkinsonism. Blepharospasm is a documented feature of both the postencephalitic and idiopathic forms of parkinsonism **(Parkinson's disease)** (Fig. 14-10), as well as a characteristic in patients with **progressive supranuclear palsy.** These patients typically develop eyelid closure when their eyelids or brows are touched (reflex blepharospasm). Moreover, they often have delayed eyelid elevation after forced closure, a phenomenon that is mediated more by involuntary inhibition of levator contraction than by orbicularis spasm.[1]

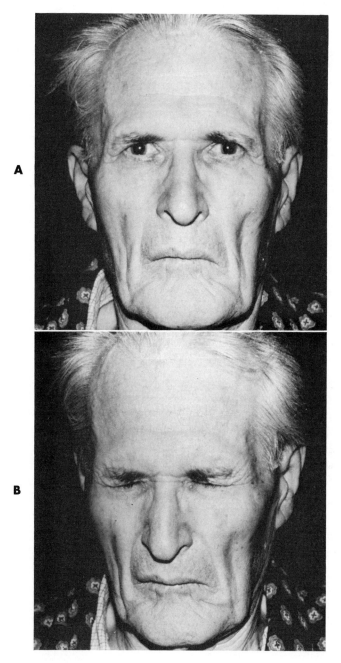

*Fig. 14-10.* Blepharospasm in Parkinson's disease. **A,** Expressionless facies. **B,** Blepharo-spasm after light tap on forehead.

Other central nervous system (CNS) conditions that manifest blepharospasm include **Huntington's disease,**[23] **multiple sclerosis,**[16,24] and **rostral brainstem stroke.**[16] Blepharospasm elicited by eyelid or brow contact is a common accompaniment of many disorders that cause extensive **bihemispheric damage** and should be regarded as a frontal release sign. Involuntary levator inhibition *(apraxia of lid opening),* which mimics blepharospasm, has been reported after a right parietal infarct[25] (see Part I).

Facial tics (including blepharospasm) occurring in childhood may be an initial manifestation of Gilles de la Tourette's syndrome.[26] Having its onset in the first decade, mainly in males, **Tourette's syndrome** consists of spasmodic contractions of facial, neck, or arm muscles, sometimes accompanied by vocal utterances (grunts, whistles), often including obscenities *(coprolalia).* These features are often accompanied by signs of attention deficit disorder (ADD).

Current management of disabling tics is with haloperidol (Haldol), pimozide (Orap), and clonidine (Catapres). The ADD must usually be approached separately with methylphenidate (Ritalin).[27]

Isolated stereotyped facial grimaces may simply represent "habit spasms," or compulsive gestures. They are usually brief and rarely disabling, although they may be a social embarrassment. The new tricyclic antidepressant clomipramine (Anafranil) may be helpful.

Blepharospasm has also been described as a rare manifestation of **tardive dyskinesia,** a movement disorder characterized by facial grimacing, intermittent jaw opening, lip smacking, and tongue protrusion.[28] Considered a manifestation of dopamine receptor supersensitivity, tardive dyskinesia is seen either spontaneously in the elderly, after levodopa treatment of Parkinson's disease, or, most commonly, after prolonged treatment of schizophrenia with neuroleptic medication (phenothiazines and butyrophenones). Discontinuation of the neuroleptic medication results in eventual remission in the majority, but in some patients dopamine-depleting agents may have to be used.

### Neuromuscular disorders

The neuromuscular conditions reported to cause blepharospasm are **tetany, tetanus, myotonic dystrophy,**[29] **hyperkalemic periodic paralysis,**[30] and **chondrodystrophic myotonia.**[31] In each of these conditions, the eyelid spasms are part of more widespread segmental or diffuse muscle contractions.

### Associated neurologic condition not present

Blepharospasm that appears to be unaccompanied by other neurologic abnormalities will usually be diagnosed as essential blepharospasm.

### Essential blepharospasm

The vast majority of adults who manifest blepharospasm have no evident underlying cause.[32] Patients are between 45 and 70 years at onset, and females outnumber males by about 2:1.[32,33] Dystonias affecting other facial and cervical muscles (and, rarely, more distant muscles) are found in more than 75% of patients.[32,33]

Patients who manifest prolonged bilateral (sometimes unilateral) contraction of mid and lower facial muscles along with their lid closure are said to have the syndrome of blepharospasm-orofacial dystonia, first described by Meige in 1910.[34] *Dystonia* implies a more sustained contraction than a spasm. Such sustained contractions lead to abnormal postures that change as different muscle groups become involved. Blepharospasm is often the initial sign, with progression to eyebrows, lips, tongue, jaw, larynx, pharynx, neck, and limbs.[35,36] Marsden[37] reported that of 30 cases of blepharospasm, 13 were isolated whereas 17 had dystonic features involving other facial and neck muscles. Significantly, none of the 13 patients with isolated cases developed dystonia elsewhere. No patients with this syndrome show neurologic deficits beyond the abnormal posturing. A single autopsy study of a patient with Meige's syndrome revealed no abnormalities.[38]

Excessive blinking is often the first symptom of essential blepharospasm. It may be written off as a habit spasm, nervousness, photosensitivity, or "dry eyes." Eventually blinking turns into uncontrolled eyelid spasms that interrupt activities of daily living—reading, watching television, cooking, and driving. The spasms are typically exacerbated by social interactions. Since the blepharospasm is sometimes unilateral at the outset, and since lower facial muscles may participate in the contractions, a misdiagnosis of hemifacial spasm is common. Whistling, humming, or other stereotyped acts may at first abort the blepharospastic attacks, but later nothing seems to help.

Controversy continues as to whether essential blepharospasm and Meige's syndrome (which we regard as components of the same illness) are based on a psychopathologic or neuropathologic disturbance. The psychopathologic theory holds that it is part of a conversion reaction.[39,40] In support of this theory is the frequent documentation of altered affect, especially depression.[41,42] Reports of relief of blepharospasm with placebos, tranquilizing medications, psychotherapy,[39,43] behavior modification,[44,45] and hypnosis[46] are also common. However, the frustratingly low success rate of psychotherapy has reinforced the neuropathologic theory of blepharospasm, which considers it a segmental dystonia.[37]

Further support for the "organic" basis of these dystonias is that they are also seen as part of well-defined CNS disorders, including brainstem stroke, MS, Parkinson's disease, and progressive supranuclear palsy. Another argument is that among patients with isolated blepharospasm, the prevalence of dystonias in family members is somewhat higher than expected (7% in the largest series).[47]

The medical treatment of blepharospasm and related dystonias has included nearly every available neurotransmitter or its analog. Despite anecdotal reports of improvement with every one of these agents, we remain unpersuaded of the lasting efficacy of any. On the other hand, we have had occasional, if sometimes short-term, success with sedative agents (principally benzodiazepines) and antidepressants (principally amitriptyline). We have been disappointed in the effects of psychotherapy, hypnosis, acupuncture, and biofeedback, in limited numbers.

Accordingly, we have relied in the past on surgical solutions: facial nerve avulsion and orbicularis myectomy.[48] Both procedures have a high initial suc-

## Management of Blepharospasm

1. Rule out any underlying neurologic condition such as Parkinson's disease or progressive supranuclear palsy.
2. Try an anxiolytic agent if stress is a factor and the patient is willing.
3. If the anxiolytic agent fails, inject botulinum toxin.
4. If botulinum toxin injections fail and the patient is sufficiently symptomatic, perform orbicularis myectomy.

cess rate, but also considerable morbidity (facial palsy, ectropion following neurectomy; facial anesthesia, periocular edema following myectomy). For this reason, we now prefer botulinum injection, which achieves substantial reduction in symptoms in greater than 90% of patients, albeit for a period of only 9 to 12 weeks.[49-51] Poor eyelid closure with resultant exposure keratitis is common but disappears within 2 weeks and can be managed with lubricants. Ptosis and diplopia, formerly common side effects, may be avoided by not injecting into the medial lower or central upper eyelid, and by using high-strength, low-volume injections. Curiously, patients with facial-cervical dystonias will often obtain relief merely from the orbicularis injections. Although initial experience suggested that the duration of toxin effect lessened with repeated injections, a recent report of 76 treated patients found a lengthening of effect.[50]

## REFERENCES

1. Lepore FE, Duvoisin RC. "Apraxia" of eyelid opening: an involuntary levator inhibition. Neurology 1985;35:423-7.
2. Gutmann L, Thompson JG Jr, Martin JD. Transient facial myokymia: an uncommon manifestation of multiple sclerosis. JAMA 1969;209:389-91.
3. Sogg RL, Hoyt WF, Boldrey E. Spastic paretic facial contracture: a rare sign of brain stem tumor. Neurology 1963;13:607-12.
4. Sethi PK, Smith BH, Kalyanaraman K. Facial myokymia: a clinicopathological study. J Neurol Neurosurg Psychiatry 1974;37:745-9.
5. Boghen D, Filiatraut R, Descarries L. Myokymia and facial contracture in brainstem tuberculoma. Neurology 1977;27:270.
6. Radu EW, Skorpil V, Kaeser HE. Facial myokymia. Eur Neurol 1975;13:499-512.
7. Espinosa RE, Lambert EH, Klass DW. Facial myokymia affecting the electroencephalogram. Mayo Clin Proc 1967;42:258-70.
8. Mateer JE, Gutmann L, McComas CF. Myokymia in Guillain-Barré syndrome. Neurology 1983;33:374-6.
9. Merchut MP, Biller J, Brumlik J, et al. Isolated facial myokymia and facial contracture: computed tomography and magnetic resonance imaging correlation. J Clin Neuro Ophthalmol 1985;5:120-3.
10. Digre K, Corbett JJ. Hemifacial spasm: differential diagnosis, mechanism, and treatment. Adv Neurol 1988;49:151-76.
11. Gardner WJ, Sava GA. Hemifacial spasm—a reversible pathophysiologic state. J Neurosurg 1962;19:240-7.
12. Ferguson JH. Hemifacial spasm and the facial nucleus. Ann Neurol 1978;4:97-103.
13. Digre KB, Corbett JJ, Smoker WRK, et al. CT and hemifacial spasm. Neurology 1988;38:1111-3.
14. Carlos R, Fukui M, Hasuo K, et al. Radiological analysis of hemifacial spasm with special reference to angiographic manifestations. Neuroradiology 1986;28:288-95.

15. Smoker WRK, Corbett JJ, Gentry LR, et al. High-resolution computed tomography of the basilar artery. II. Vertebrobasilar dolichoectasia: clinical-pathologic correlation and review. AJNR 1986;7:61-72.
16. Jankovic J, Patel SC. Blepharospasm associated with brainstem lesions. Neurology 1983;33:1237-40.
17. Schwartz MA, Selhorst JB, Ochs AL, et al. Oculomasticatory myorhythmia: a unique movement disorder occurring in Whipple's disease. Ann Neurol 1986;20:677-83.
18. Alexander GE, Moses H III. Carbamazepine for hemifacial spasm. Neurology 1982;32:286-7.
19. Loeser JD, Chen J. Hemifacial spasm: treatment by microsurgical facial nerve decompression. Neurosurgery 1983;13:141-6.
20. Wilson CB, Yorke C, Prioleau G. Microsurgical vascular decompression for trigeminal neuralgia and hemifacial spasm. West J Med 1980;132:481-7.
21. Mauriello JA Jr. Treatment of benign essential blepharospasm and hemifacial spasm with botulinum toxin: a preliminary study of 68 patients. In: Bosniak SL, Smith BC, eds. Advances in ophthalmic plastic and reconstructive surgery. Vol. 4. Blepharospasm. New York: Pergamon Press, 1985:283-89.
22. Maurice-Williams RS. Tic convulsif: the association of trigeminal neuralgia and hemifacial spasm. Postgrad Med J 1973;49:742-5.
23. Martin JB, Gusella JF. Huntington's disease: pathogenesis and management. N Engl J Med 1986;315:1267-76.
24. Keane JR. Gaze-evoked blepharoclonus. Ann Neurol 1978;3:243-5.
25. Johnston JC, Rosenbaum DM, Piccone CM, et al. Apraxia of eyelid opening secondary to right hemisphere infarction. Ann Neurol 1989;25:622-4.
26. Shapiro AK, Shapiro E, Wayne HLS. The symptomatology and diagnosis of Gilles de la Tourette's syndrome. J Am Acad Child Psychiatry 1973;12:702-23
27. Jankovic J, Rohaidy H. Motor, behavioral and pharmacologic findings in Tourette's syndrome. Can J Neurol Sci 1987;14:541-6.
28. Crane GE. Persistent dyskinesia. Br J Psychiatry 1973;122:395-405.
29. Van Allen MW, Blodi FC. Electromyographic study of reciprocal innervation in blinking. Neurology 1962;12:371-7.
30. Layzer RB, Lovelace RE, Rowland LP. Hyperkalemic periodic paralysis. Arch Neurol 1967;16:455-72.
31. Scaff M, Mendonca L, Levy JA, et al. Chondrodystrophic myotonia: electromyographic and cardiac features of a case. Acta Neurol Scand 1979;60:243-9.
32. Grandas F, Elston J, Quinn N, et al. Blepharospasm: a review of 264 patients. J Neurol Neurosurg Psychiatry 1988;51:767-72.
33. Jordan DR, Patrinely JR, Anderson RL, et al. Essential blepharospasm and related dystonias. Surv Ophthalmol 1989;34:123-32.
34. Meige H. Les convulsions de la face, une forme clinique de convulsion faciale, bilatérale et médiane. Rev Neurol 1910;20:437-43.
35. Paulson GW. Meige's syndrome: dyskinesia of the eyelids and facial muscles. Geriatrics 1972;27:69-73.
36. Tolosa ES. Clinical features of Meige's disease (idiopathic orofacial dystonia): a report of 17 cases. Arch Neurol 1981;38:147-51.
37. Marsden CD. Blepharospasm-oromandibular dystonia syndrome (Brueghel's syndrome): a variant of adult onset torsion dystonia? J Neurol Neurosurg Psychiatry 1976;39:1204-9.
38. Garcia-Albea E, Franch O, Munoz O, et al. Brueghel's syndrome: report of a case with postmortem studies. J Neurol Neurosurg Psychiatry 1981;44:437-40.
39. Langworthy OR. Emotional issues related to certain cases of blepharospasm and facial tics. Arch Neurol Psychiatry 1952;68:620-8.
40. Lazare A. Current concepts in psychiatry: conversion symptoms. N Engl J Med 1981;305:745-8.
41. Diamond EL, Trobe JD, Belar CD. Psychological aspects of essential blepharospasm. J Nerv Ment Dis 1984;172:749-56.
42. Cavenar JO Jr, Brantley IJ, Braasch E. Blepharospasm: organic or functional? Psychosomatics 1978;19:623-8.
43. Reckless JB. Hysterical blepharospasm

treated by psychotherapy and conditioning procedures in a group setting. Psychosomatics 1972;13:263-4.

44. Hidar A, Clancy J. Case report of successful treatment of a reflex trigeminal nerve blepharospasm by behavior modification. Am J Ophthalmol 1973; 75:148-9.

45. Sharpe R. Behavior therapy in a case of blepharospasm. Br J Psychiatry 1974; 124:603-4.

46. Wickramasekera I. Hyponosis and broad-spectrum behavior therapy for blepharospasm: a case study. Int J Clin Exp Hypn 1974;22:201-9.

47. Jankovic J, Ford J. Blepharospasm and orofacial-cervical dystonia: clinical and pharmacological findings in 100 patients. Ann Neurol 1983;13:402-11.

48. Anderson RL, Patrinely JR. Surgical management of blepharospasm. Adv Neurol 1988;49:501-20.

49. Cole H. Botulinum toxin may help blepharospasm sufferers. JAMA 1985;254: 1688-90.

50. Engstrom PF, Arnoult JB, Mazow ML, et al. Effectiveness of botulinum toxin therapy for essential blepharospasm. Ophthalmology 1987;94:971-5.

51. Scott AB, Kennedy RA, Stubbs HA. Botulinum A toxin injection as a treatment for blepharospasm. Arch Ophthalmol 1985;103:347-50.

# CHAPTER 15

# Proptosis and Adnexal Masses

· · · · · · · · · · · · · · · · · · · ·

Proptosis is the pathologic forward displacement of one or both eyes. The normal range of ocular protrusion, as measured by exophthalmometry, is 14 to 21 mm in adults.[1] Blacks may have normal values greater than 21 mm.[2] While a 2 mm difference in protrusion between fellow eyes is generally considered "normal," any disparity between eyes in a patient being evaluated for orbital disease must be regarded as suspicious.

Measuring the amount of proptosis in millimeters may not be the most important maneuver in evaluating patients with proptosis. Ballottement of the eyes to determine the degree of retropulsion is a more useful test. The patient who has true proptosis without increased resistance to retropulsion probably does not harbor an orbital mass lesion. Graves' ophthalmopathy and other orbital inflammations, in addition to orbital tumors, usually produce marked resistance to retropulsion. The presence of resistance to retropulsion, therefore, does not necessarily indicate a mass lesion; however, its absence must make one seriously question whether true proptosis exists. The patient with unilateral high myopia may appear proptotic, since the myopic eye has a much greater axial length. The pseudoproptosis due to axial myopia is confirmed by the obvious anisometropia found on retinoscopy.[3]

## A Decision Tree Approach to the Evaluation of Proptosis

The most frequent cause of acquired proptosis reported in the majority of ophthalmic series is Graves' ophthalmopathy. Therefore the initial distinction to be made in the patient with true proptosis is between Graves' ophthalmopathy and all other causes of proptosis (Chart 15-1).

▨ Lid retraction present

▣ Graves' ophthalmopathy

DIAGNOSIS. It is estimated that clinically detectable ocular signs are present in 40% of patients with Graves' disease.[4] Graves' ophthalmopathy may appear at any time during the course of dysthyroidism[5,6] (Table 15-1) but seems to become

**379**

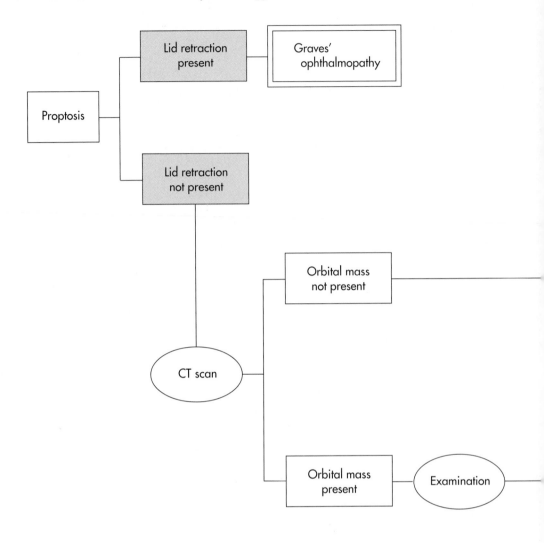

*Chart 15-1*

clinically evident within 18 months of the systemic manifestations of thyroid dysfunction.[5] The most frequent ophthalmic abnormality associated with Graves' disease is lid retraction (Fig. 15-1, *A* and *B*). In fact, for proptosis to occur without lid retraction would be unusual. This lid sign is so specific that it is used as a primary indicator of the proptosis of Graves' disease. Other clues to the diagnosis are previous treatment for hyperthyroidism or loss of weight without loss of appetite, palpitation, tremor, difficulty sleeping, and excessive perspiration. Even in patients who have euthyroid Graves' disease without a previous history or present evidence of thyroid dysfunction, proptosis is usually accom-

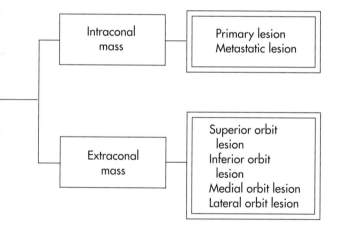

panied by other ocular signs such as lid edema, conjunctival chemosis, and injection over the horizontal rectus muscles.

A decreased blink rate and delay in inhibition of the upper lids on downgaze (lid lag) (Fig. 15-1, C) often accompany the lid retraction of Graves' ophthalmopathy. The retraction may be asymmetric, so that initially the patient may appear to have ptosis when in reality the problem is contralateral lid retraction. At times, however, the classic lid signs of Graves' ophthalmopathy may be masked by a concomitant true ptosis of myasthenia gravis. A significant association exists between thyroid disease and myasthenia.[7] Since both disorders may

TABLE 15-1	*Graves' Ophthalmopathy in Thyroid Dysfunction*

| | | Thyroid state | | | Time course of ophthalmopathy to systemic dysthyroidism | | |
|---|---|---|---|---|---|---|---|
| | No. of patients | Hyperthyroid | Hypothyroid | Euthyroid | Simultaneous | Precedes | Follows |
| Marcocci et al.[5] | 221 | 202 (91.4%) | 0 | 19 (8.6%) | 87 (43%) | 27 (13.4%) | 88 (43.6%) |
| Wiersinga et al.[6] | 125 | 96 (76.8%) | 3 (2.4%) | 26 (20.8%) | 39 (39%) | 37 (37%) | 23 (23%) |

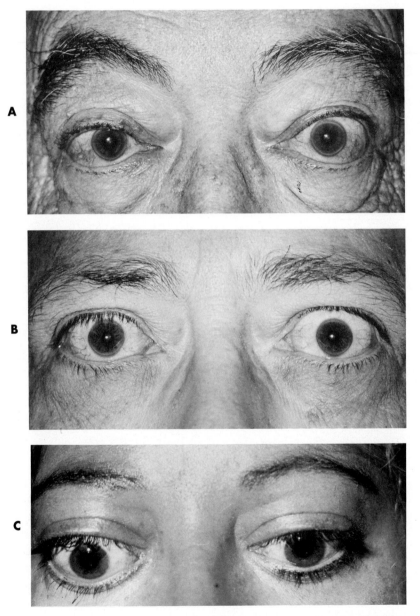

*Fig. 15-1.* **A,** Unilateral lid retraction *(left).* Right upper lid is in its normal position. **B,** Bilateral lid retraction; left greater than right. **C,** Bilateral lid retraction on downward gaze; right greater than left.

affect eyelid position and ocular motility, the clinical picture in patients with both disorders is often confusing (Fig. 15-2).

Mechanical restriction of the upper lid is proposed as the mechanism of lid lag by some authorities.[8-10] Relief of retraction following topical application of adrenergic blocking agents has led to the speculation by others that increased sympathetic tone is the underlying cause.[11] Retraction in the initial stages of the disorder is likely due to excessive sympathetic innervation to Müller's muscle. Adrenergic blocking agents will reverse the retraction at this stage. Cicatricial lid changes probably account for the chemically irreversible long-standing retraction.

If lid retraction is present, the diagnosis of Graves' ophthalmopathy is established. No further testing to uncover the cause of proptosis need be employed.

Conjunctival injection over the horizontal rectus muscles is another reliable sign of Graves' ophthalmopathy (Plate 9, *A* and *B*). However, other characteristic patterns of conjunctival injection should suggest alternative diagnostic possibilities. Carotid-cavernous fistulas cause arterialization of the conjunctival vessels (Plate 9, *C* and *D*), which is particularly distinctive on slit lamp examination. Orbital pseudotumor may be associated with an anterior scleritis/episcleritis, al-

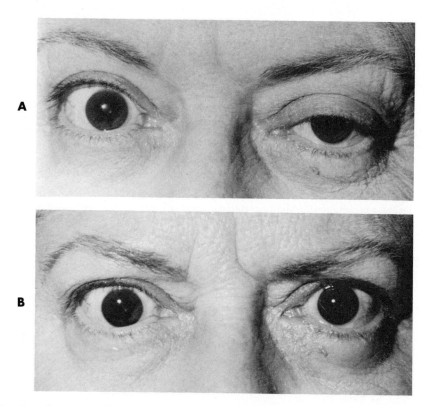

*Fig. 15-2.* Graves' ophthalmopathy and myasthenia gravis. **A,** Patient has retraction of right upper lid, but left upper lid is ptotic. **B,** After intravenous Tensilon, left ptosis disappears and both lids are retracted.

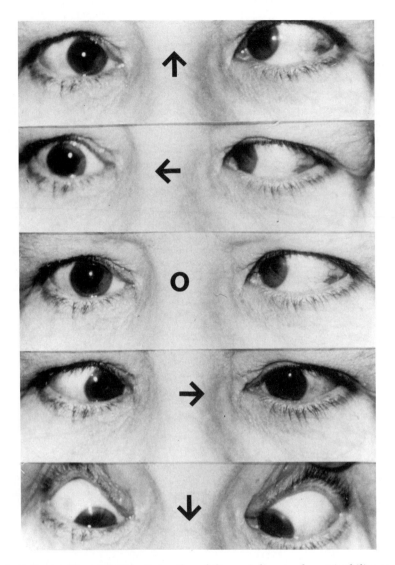

*Fig. 15-3.* Patient with restrictive myopathy of Graves' disease shows inability to elevate either eye, bilateral abduction defects, an esotropia in primary position, and decreased depression of left eye. Arrows indicate direction of gaze.

though more frequently a nonspecific conjunctival injection with chemosis is found (Plate 9, *E* and *F*).

Graves' ophthalmopathy also affects the extraocular muscles, resulting in troublesome and frequently permanent diplopia. This inflammatory myositis has a predilection for the inferior and medial rectus muscles; the lateral rectus is rarely affected. Reduced ocular elevation associated with an abduction deficit should suggest the restrictive myopathy of dysthyroidism (Fig. 15-3).

Graves' optic neuropathy is an infrequent yet treatable cause of visual loss. This optic neuropathy is due to compression of the optic nerve by markedly enlarged extraocular muscles at the orbital apex. Feldon et al.[12] used orbital computed tomography (CT) to determine that enlarged extraocular muscle volume was directly correlated with the development of Graves' optic neuropathy. The medial rectus muscle appeared disproportionately enlarged in patients with optic neuropathy. Barrett et al.[13] retrospectively reviewed orbital CT scans in 31 patients with Graves' ophthalmopathy and devised a muscular index, based on the percentage of orbital width occupied by the horizontal rectus muscles and the percentage of orbital height occupied by the vertical recti, to predict the risk of developing Graves' optic neuropathy. Orbits with optic neuropathy had a significantly higher muscular index than those without optic neuropathy. These two retrospective studies suggest that patients with enlarged extraocular muscles are at greater risk to develop Graves' optic neuropathy.

Visual loss may be associated with optic disc edema, optic atrophy, or a normal-appearing optic disc.[14] The pattern of visual field loss is a nerve fiber bundle defect that often involves fixation.

The clinical signs of Graves' ophthalmopathy are specific enough to establish the diagnosis. Further testing is aimed at determining the patient's metabolic status. Measurement of TSH levels by a sensitive immunoradiometric assay, combined with $T_3$ and $T_4$ determinations when required, will distinguish between the euthyroid and hyperthyroid patient.[15] We do not believe that the Werner suppression or thyrotropin-releasing hormone (TRH) stimulation tests are necessary in the evaluation of these patients. The diagnosis of Graves' ophthalmopathy must remain a clinical one and, aside from determining the patient's systemic metabolic state, requires no confirmatory diagnostic testing.

On imaging, Graves' ophthalmopathy shows bilateral extraocular muscle enlargement (Fig. 15-4). We have encountered patients with Graves' ophthalmopathy who do not show muscle enlargement. In our experience, however, when a restrictive myopathy or optic neuropathy is seen, muscle enlargment on imaging is invariably present. This bilaterality is so characteristic that if the fellow orbit is normal with high-resolution imaging, the diagnosis of Graves' ophthalmopathy is suspect. Less frequent signs of proptosis—optic nerve straightening and anterior septal bulging—are suggestive but not diagnostic of Graves' ophthalmopathy. If the diagnosis of Graves' ophthalmopathy can be established clinically, imaging is unnecessary and should not be employed as a routine confirmatory investigation.

Enlarged superior or inferior rectus muscles on CT scans have been mistaken for tumors at the orbital apex. The development of high-resolution imaging with multiple views has made this misdiagnosis less common.

**PATHOGENESIS.** The ocular manifestations of Graves' ophthalmopathy are in some unknown way associated with an underlying abnormality of the thyroid gland, generally developing when thyroid autoimmunity exists.[5,6] The precise immunologic mechanism, however, remains obscure. Antibodies against orbital connective tissue and extraocular muscle have been detected in the serum of patients with Graves' ophthalmopathy.[16] Serum antibodies against human eye muscle and porcine eye muscle have been identified in up to 70% of patients with Graves' disease without ophthalmopathy.[17] This antibody has also been

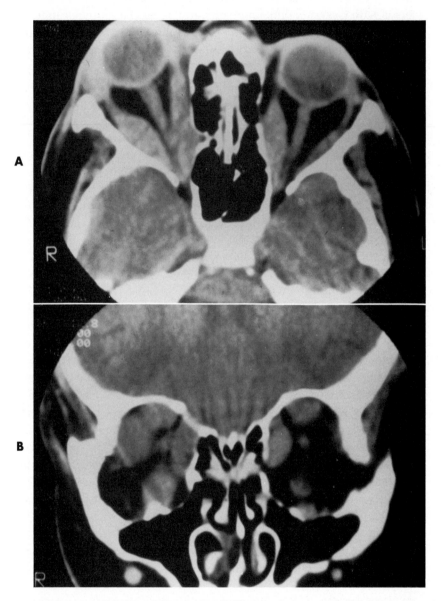

*Fig. 15-4.* Graves' ophthalmopathy. **A,** Axial CT scan shows marked enlargement of medial recti and right lateral rectus. Tendinous insertions are uninvolved. **B,** Optic nerve OD is crowded (patient developed a right optic neuropathy).

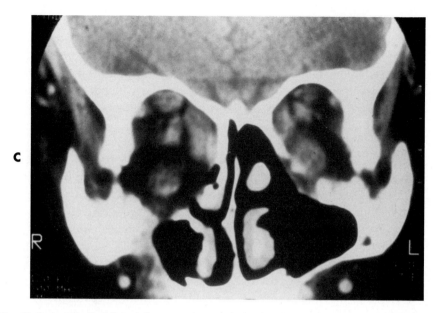

*Fig. 15-4, cont'd.* **C,** After right posterior medial orbital decompression, orbital volume is increased, with compression of optic nerve relieved.

found in high titers when CT scanning shows signs of extraocular muscle enlargement.[18]

However, Weetman et al.[19] claim that antibodies may be found in patients with thyroid autoimmunity irrespective of their eye signs. They suggest that T and B cell autoreactivity to striated (including skeletal) muscle antigens is frequent in these patients and unrelated to eye disease.

Campbell[20] postulates that whatever the mechanism, lymphocytic infiltration of the orbital tissue activates previously quiescent fibroblasts. These fibroblasts then secrete a mucopolysaccharide—glycosaminoglycan (GAG)—which results in muscle edema. This ultimately leads to fibrosis of muscle fibers and eventually to atrophy.

**TREATMENT.** The primary treatment of any patient with an abnormality of thyroid function must be directed at returning the patient to the euthyroid state. There appears to be no increased risk of developing ophthalmopathy with any treatment regimen for hyperthyroidism. In 288 hyperthyroid patients studied by Sridama and DeGroot,[4] ophthalmopathy developed anew in 6.7%, 7.1%, and 4.9% after treatment with antithyroid drugs, surgery, or radiation, respectively, and progressed in 19.2%, 19.8%, and 22.7%. The ophthalmopathy improved in 12% to 14% of patients in each treatment group. Conjunctival chemosis and lid edema may remit with systemic treatment of the hyperthyroid state. However, some patients may show progression of ocular signs when they become euthyroid.

The goal of therapy in patients with Graves' ophthalmopathy is visual rehabilitation. These patients are challenging to treat and are probably best approached in collaboration with other specialists. Rehabilitation often includes some form of systemic treatment (usually corticosteroids), orbital decompression, radiation therapy, strabismus surgery, and lid surgery. The rehabilitation routinely extends over many months, and the patients should be informed of this at the onset. Typically these are unhappy patients who are willing to persevere and who, in the end, are extremely grateful.

From a practical standpoint, determining if Graves' ophthalmopathy is in an acute or subacute active inflammatory phase or in a quiescent cicatricial phase is important. The patient with an active congestive orbitopathy must be treated differently from the patient with the same signs (lid retraction, proptosis, strabismus) but whose disease is stable and noncongestive.

Treatment of the abnormal thyroid state alone may improve some of the eye signs of Graves' disease.[4] Prummel et al.[21] also noted this trend in 87 patients not previously treated for systemic or ophthalmic Graves' disease. The improvement was noted only in soft tissue swelling and eye muscle involvement. If vision is threatened, more aggressive treatment is required. The intensity of treatment should be dictated by the severity of specific symptoms or signs. Visual loss due to Graves' optic neuropathy demands more urgent attention than does mild proptosis, which is a cosmetic blemish only.

### Active stage

*Lid retraction.* No local medical treatment for lid retraction is satisfactory. Should corneal exposure result from exaggerated widening of the interpalpebral fissure, a lateral tarsorrhaphy can provide temporary symptomatic relief, as well as an acceptable cosmetic appearance.

*Proptosis and ductional deficits.* In acute Graves' ophthalmopathy, proptosis is often associated with conjunctival injection and diplopia due to inflammation of the extraocular muscles. The use of systemic corticosteroids in this setting is controversial, being condemned by some and strongly advocated by others. Early use of systemic corticosteroids is aimed at the control of the inflammatory myositis to prevent or lessen the postinflammatory cicatricial restrictive myopathy. Some patients respond dramatically to corticosteroids, whereas others do not. Evidence suggests that this variable response to treatment reflects a difference in patients' immunologic status.[22] These immunologic disparities may eventually serve as a guide as to which patients should be treated with corticosteroids and which patients should be treated initially with various other modalities.

Proptosis is a stable sign of Graves' ophthalmopathy; Streeten et al.[23] reported that it worsened following treatment of hyperthyroidism in only 19 (15.6%) of 122 patients followed continually for 3 to 19 years. Patients with proptosis alone and no ductional deficits therefore should be observed without treatment.

Intraorbital corticosteroid injections have been suggested as an alternative to systemic medication. Thomas and Hart[24] reported that 12 of their 19 patients experienced full restoration of ocular motility following retrobulbar injection of repository steroids. In another study, intraorbital corticosteroids were used in

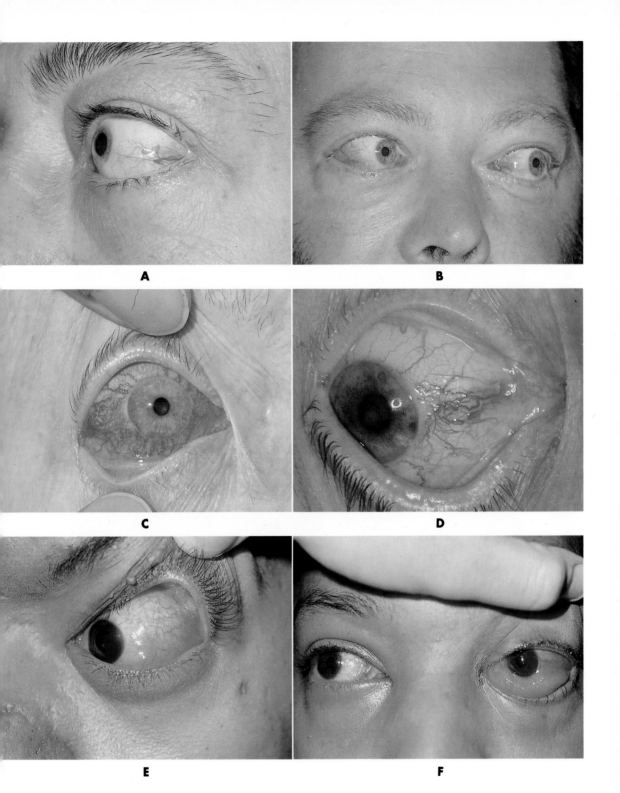

*Plate 9.* **A** and **B,** Graves' ophthalmopathy with injection localized over horizontal rectus muscles. **C,** Carotid-cavernous fistula with markedly arterialized conjunctival blood vessels. **D,** Dural fistula with conjunctival signs much less severe. **E,** Diffuse scleral injection with orbital pseudotumor. **F,** Marked conjunctival chemosis accompanying injection in orbital pseudotumor.

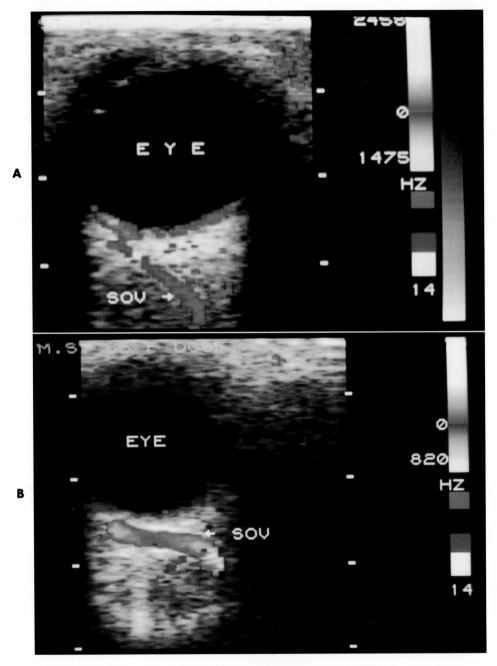

*Plate 10.* Color Doppler orbital image. **A,** Normal superior ophthalmic vein *(SOV)* with blue indicating normal venous direction of blood flow. **B,** In patient with carotid-cavernous fistula, SOV is red, indicating arterial direction of flow.

*Management of Graves' Disease Ductional Deficits*

1. Administer oral prednisone, 80 to 100 mg/day. Discontinue steroids if no clinical improvement occurs within 2 weeks.
2. If steroids relieve the patient's symptoms, taper the steroid dosage slowly (10 mg/day/week).
3. Steroid therapy should not last longer than 3 months.
4. Should the orbitopathy worsen during the period of steroid reduction, increase the dose.
5. No definitive tapering schedule exists; thus titrate the steroid dosage against clinical signs.
6. Chronic administration of high-dose systemic corticosteroids is to be discouraged.

conjunction with orbital radiotherapy for Graves' ophthalmopathy but proved to be less effective than systemic corticosteroid treatment with orbital radiation.[25] Intraorbital corticosteroid therapy has not gained popularity and is rarely used in the treatment of Graves' ophthalmopathy.

Orbital radiation is effective in treating Graves' ophthalmopathy.[26,27] Orbital decompression also has been advocated as a primary treatment in acute orbitopathy. The philosophy behind this suggestion is that less permanent ophthalmic problems will result if more room is available in the orbit during the acute inflammatory phase. No controlled study is available to prove this hypothesis, and we would not support primary orbital decompression in the absence of severe corneal or optic nerve involvement.

*Optic neuropathy.* The consensus is that treatment is both necessary and urgent when Graves' optic neuropathy occurs. This is a true ophthalmic emergency for which several modes of treatment are available.

*Antiinflammatory and immunosuppressive drugs.* The administration of systemic corticosteroids (up to 200 mg of prednisone daily) may result in dramatic reversal of visual loss.[28] Guy et al.[29] have suggested much larger doses—up to 1 g daily administered intravenously for 3 days. If no improvement occurs after 5 days of systemic corticosteroid administration, another treatment modality should be instituted at once. During tapering of the corticosteroids, the optic neuropathy may become reactivated. Chronic steroid therapy may control the inflammation, but the prolonged use of these drugs with all their well-known side effects should be avoided.

Cyclosporine is less effective than corticosteroids in treating Graves' ophthalmopathy. However, Prummel et al.[30] reported that combined therapy with the two agents produced improvement in 13 (59%) of 22 patients who did not respond to either drug alone. Conversely, in an earlier study, Kahaly et al.[31] found that cyclosporine alone was more effective than corticosteroids in treating acute Graves' ophthalmopathy and in preventing recurrence after drug withdrawal. However, combined corticosteroid and cyclosporine therapy again had the greatest beneficial effect on Graves' ophthalmopathy.[31]

*Orbital decompression surgery.* Many surgical procedures have been proposed over the years, but we believe that transantral orbital decompression into the ethmoid and maxillary sinuses is the treatment of choice. This approach has the advantage of having no external incisions, while providing reduction of proptosis of up to 12 mm. In experienced hands the surgery is relatively free of complications. Ogura and Thawley[32] described two instances of postoperative sinusitis, one oroantral fistula, and one cerebrospinal fluid (CSF) leak resulting in meningitis in 252 surgical patients. In a series of 200 patients Desanto[33] described the following complications: CSF rhinorrhea (4), nasolacrimal duct obstruction (9, 5 of whom required surgical repair), oroantral fistula requiring closure (7), blindness of one eye (2), and numb lip temporarily (200, with only 8 patients having a permanent deficit). Because this approach may result in a higher incidence of postoperative ocular misalignment, it should be abandoned. However, the exact effect of transantral decompression on ocular muscle balance is unknown, since no study has measured the ocular alignment preoperatively and postoperatively.

Inferior and medial orbital decompression through an orbital incision,[34] inferior and medial decompression combined with lateral decompression,[35] and even four-wall decompression[36] have been suggested as alternatives to transantral decompression. It appears certain that the inferior and medial orbital confines must be decompressed for maximal therapeutic effect (Fig. 15-4, *C*). The particular approach used to achieve this is less important.

*Orbital radiation.* Supravoltage orbital radiation at 1500 to 2000 cGy administered over 10 days is effective and is a viable treatment alternative in patients with optic neuropathy.[26,37,38] Kinyoun et al.[39] described disastrous visual loss due to radiation retinopathy following orbital radiation for Graves' ophthalmopathy. In three of four patients, the complication was attributed to dosage miscalculation or errors in radiotherapeutic technique. The eventual occurrence of malignant neoplasm in the radiated field remains a theoretical concern but, to our knowledge, has not been reported.

*Plasmapheresis.* Removal of circulating immunoglobulins by plasma exchange appeared to improve Graves' orbitopathy in individual case reports. However, one clinical trial of plasmapheresis in 18 patients showed no evidence of immediate or delayed improvement in any eye signs of the disorder.[40]

Improvement in the acute signs of Graves' ophthalmopathy was recorded in another group of 15 patients treated with plasmapheresis.[41] However, their improvement was not sustained unless they were treated for 3 to 6 months with prednisone and azathioprine. Although plasma exchange may be effective in treating acute Graves' ophthalmopathy, we do not recommend it as a first-line treatment of this disease.

### Inactive stage

*Extraocular muscle imbalance.* Attempts at surgical correction of the diplopia of Graves' ophthalmopathy should not be performed until the patient is euthy-

---

### Management of Graves' Optic Neuropathy

1. Give systemic corticosteroids (80 to 120 mg/day or high-dose pulse steroids) for 2 to 3 days, followed by transantral orbital decompressive surgery.
2. If surgery is to be delayed even for several days, continue systemic corticosteroids if the patient has no contraindication to these drugs.

---

roid and until the measured ocular misalignment has been unchanged for 4 to 6 months. Muscle surgery should precede lid surgery.

The diplopia of Graves' ophthalmopathy is due to a restrictive myopathy wherein the normally elastic extraocular muscle becomes a fibrotic band. Since the inferior and medial rectus muscles are involved most frequently, patterns of esotropia and hypertropias alone or in combination are the rule. Recession is the surgical procedure of choice. Resections in these situations may cause a restrictive pattern in the opposite direction and should be employed only in extraordinary circumstances.

The success rate of muscle surgery in these patients does not approach that of congenital strabismus surgery. A single operation was effective in correcting the diplopia of Graves' ophthalmopathy in only 50% to 65% of patients reported by Dyer.[42] Of 45 patients reported by Evans and Kennerdell,[43] 30 (67%) had binocular single vision restored in the primary position by one surgical procedure, and 27 (60%) experienced binocular single vision in the reading position.

Prior treatment for Graves' disease does not appear to influence the surgical outcome. Mourits et al.[44] achieved useful binocular single vision using a fixed suture technique in 27 (71%) of 38 patients with one operation independent of previous treatment modalities. The advent of the adjustable suture technique, where final placement of a recessed muscle is done with the patient awake and cooperating for prism cover testing, seems to decrease the incidence of reoperations. Using this technique, Scott and Thalacker[45] achieved primary position fusion in 18 (82%) of 22 patients without the aid of prisms after one operation.

Binocular single vision over a wide range of gaze is an unrealistic therapeutic expectation in the majority of patients with the strabismus of Graves' ophthalmopathy. The elimination of diplopia in primary position and the reading position is the basic goal of surgery. Because of the incomitance of deviations, prism glasses (possibly only in a bifocal segment following inferior rectus recession) may be necessary after surgery. The patient who can be rehabilitated visually with any combination of surgery and prism glasses has a successful result.

*Lid retraction.* The correction of long-standing lid retraction or other lid abnormalities is beyond the scope of this text. Lid surgery should be undertaken as the last step in the patient's rehabilitation following orbital and muscle surgery.

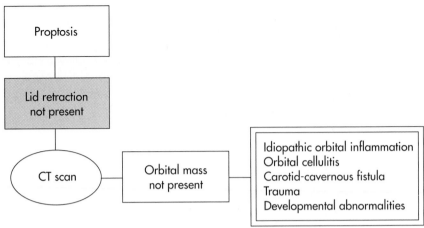

**Chart 15-1, A**

## ▓ Lid retraction not present

The absence of lid retraction and other clinical signs of thyroid dysfunction requires that orbital imaging be obtained as the next step in the evaluation of the patient with proptosis (Chart 15-1, *A*).

○ *CT scan.* Presently we prefer CT to magnetic resonance imaging (MRI) as the initial imaging procedure for proptosis for the following reasons:

1. CT provides better detail of orbital and periorbital bony structures.
2. CT may detect an unsuspected intraorbital metallic foreign body that may have been put in motion by high-field MRI.
3. Special techniques such as surface coil receptors or fat suppression are required to obtain adequate MR orbital images. These techniques are not universally available.
4. Radiologists at present have more expertise interpreting orbital CT.

If CT reveals a lesion, the examiner can determine if subsequent MRI should be done to further define the disease process.

This one imaging study will answer the next crucial question: Is a mass lesion present in the orbit or periorbital area? If no mass is found, clinical signs and symptoms must be used to differentiate between the nontumorous entities that produce proptosis.

## ☐ Orbital mass not present

Two of the nontumorous causes of proptosis are idiopathic orbital inflammation (pseudotumor) and orbital infection (orbital cellulitis). The two disorders often are confused with each other and with Graves' ophthalmopathy. Carotid-cavernous fistulas and trauma are less frequent causes of nontumorous proptosis.

### ☐ Idiopathic orbital inflammation

Proptosis, orbital congestion, periorbital edema, diplopia, and visual loss are the signs of orbital inflammation. Specific causes such as syphilis, tuberculosis, sarcoidosis, Wegener's granulomatosis, or collagen vascular disease must be sought but are not frequently found. What remains is orbital inflammation without a specific etiology—orbital pseudotumor.

In this condition any orbital structure may be selectively affected, resulting in the preeminence of one symptom or sign. At other times all orbital structures appear to be involved equally, making the diagnosis less confusing. The "lumpers" refer to this disorder as pseudotumor, whereas the "splitters" sometimes divide pseudotumor into different entities based on the structure involved:

| | |
|---|---|
| Sclera | Posterior scleritis (sclerotenonitis) |
| Lacrimal gland | Dacryoadenitis |
| Extraocular muscle | Myositis |
| Cavernous sinus/superior orbital fissure | Tolosa-Hunt syndrome |

Distinguishing between idiopathic orbital inflammation and orbital lymphoma is frequently difficult.[46-48] Retrospective correlation of clinical and pathologic data has shown that even experienced ophthalmic pathologists cannot consistently distinguish inflammatory lesions from lymphoma.[49-50] However, light microscopy remains important, since unequivocally inflammatory lesions do not behave like neoplasms even after extended clinical follow-up.[51]

Immunochemical techniques have demonstrated that lymphomas are more likely to be composed of monoclonal B lymphocytes, whereas inflammatory pseudotumors are composed of polyclonal B lymphocytes. However, in an updated review of the subject, Jakobiec et al.[52] stress that both monoclonality and polyclonality may be associated with extraocular lymphoma. Medeiros et al.[53] studied 61 patients with orbital and conjunctival lymphoid infiltrates and found that lymphocytic infiltrates that express monotypic immunoglobulins are predictive of their clinical behavior. These lesions behave as low-grade B cell lymphomas. The authors stress that the immunohistologic classification of these lymphoid lesions is useful especially in lesions in which standard histology is not definitely diagnostic.

The CT pattern of orbital pseudotumor varies depending on the orbital region that is preferentially affected (Fig. 15-5). The CT characteristics of 21 patients with the clinical diagnosis of orbital pseudotumor included contrast enhancement (95%), retrobulbar fatty infiltration (76%), proptosis (71%), extraocular muscle enlargement (57%), apical fat edema (48%), muscle tendon sheath involvement (43%), optic nerve thickening (38%), and uveoscleral thickening (33%).[54] While extraocular muscle enlargement may resemble that of Graves' ophthalmopathy, myositis will generally involve the area of the tendinous insertion to the globe, and Graves' myopathy usually spares this region.[55] Orbital pseudotumor is also more likely to be unilateral. The paranasal sinuses may rarely be opacified with orbital pseudotumor.[56]

MRI may be useful in further distinguishing orbital pseudotumor from more invasive lesions. Atlas et al.[57] used surface coil MRI studies in orbital pseudotumor. The lesions were hypointense to fat and isointense to muscle on T1-weighted images. On T2-weighted images the lesions were isointense or only minimally hyperintense to fat. By contrast, orbital metastasis appeared markedly hyperintense to fat on T2-weighted images.

The investigation of the patient with signs of noninfectious orbital inflam-

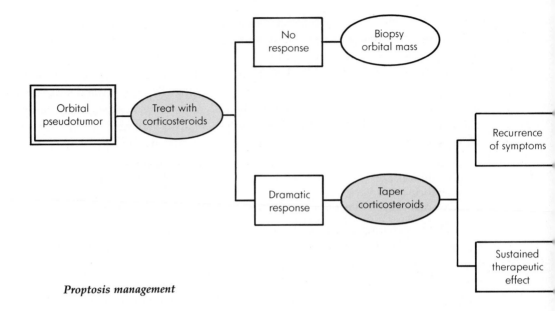

*Proptosis management*

mation must also seek to rule out underlying systemic disease. In the investigation of these patients, we perform a complete blood count (CBC) and erythrocyte sedimentation rate (ESR), VDRL-RPR, urinalysis, SMA-12, and chest x-ray study.

MANAGEMENT. In the patient with proptosis, periorbital edema, ophthalmoplegia, imaging consistent with the diagnosis of orbital pseudotumor, and a negative systemic evaluation, we defer orbital biopsy pending a trial of systemic corticosteroid treatment (see chart above). So dramatic is the inflammatory improvement with 80 to 100 mg of oral prednisone that a 24- to 48-hour course of the drug has been suggested as a specific "therapeutic trial." The lesion that does not abate dramatically is probably not pseudotumor and should be biopsied. If the expected initial response to treatment occurs, the steroid dose is tapered, being titrated to the clinical signs and symptoms. Should a recurrence develop, increasing the steroid dosage will often be all that is needed. Should the orbital signs persist or a second recurrence develop despite the increased steroid dosage, CT should be repeated and orbital biopsy performed.

Some patients with orbital pseudotumor have contraindications to systemic corticosteroids, or these drugs are ineffective. Orbital radiotherapy, in doses as low as 1000 to 2000 cGy, is an acceptable alternative treatment.[48] Some patients with chronic recurrent orbital pseudotumor (myositis) may be treated effectively with azathioprine[58] or cyclosporine[59] as an alternative to radiotherapy.

Some rare forms of orbital pseudotumor do not respond to conventional

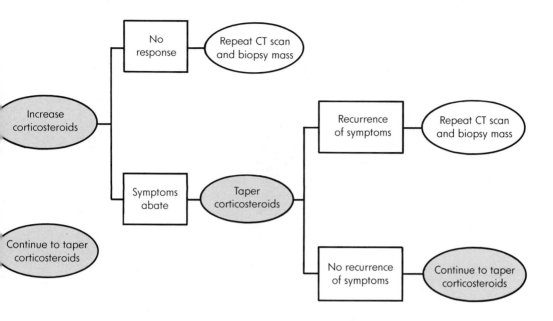

treatment. Garrity et al.[58] described three such patients with a particularly aggressive form of orbital inflammatory disease. These patients had a primary vasculitis, which was angiocentric as well as angiodestructive. Despite the inflammation being centered histopathologically within the walls of small blood vessels, no systemic vasculitis was ever identified. All of these patients had bilateral involvement, which was resistant to treatment with up to 100 mg of prednisone daily. Cyclophosphamide provided relief from inflammation and led to drug-free remission periods in all patients. Although this is a relatively uncommon form of orbital inflammatory disease, it does respond to aggressive treatment and therefore must be considered in the evaluation of these disorders.

## ▢ Orbital cellulitis

Proptosis, periorbital swelling, and ophthalmoplegia in a febrile patient suggest orbital cellulitis. The presence of ophthalmoplegia implies true orbital involvement by the infection, whereas periorbital edema alone suggests that the infection is limited to the preseptal area.

Patients with cellulitis are almost invariably febrile and have a leukocytosis. The absence of fever in any untreated immunocompetent patient militates strongly against orbital cellulitis. Most patients will have contiguous sinus disease, with the ethmoid sinus involved most often. The maxillary and frontal sinuses are less frequently affected, although pansinusitis is not unusual[60-61] (Fig. 15-6).

In case of trauma, a retained intraorbital foreign body may be serving as a nidus for continued infection. Because of the potential presence of a metallic in-

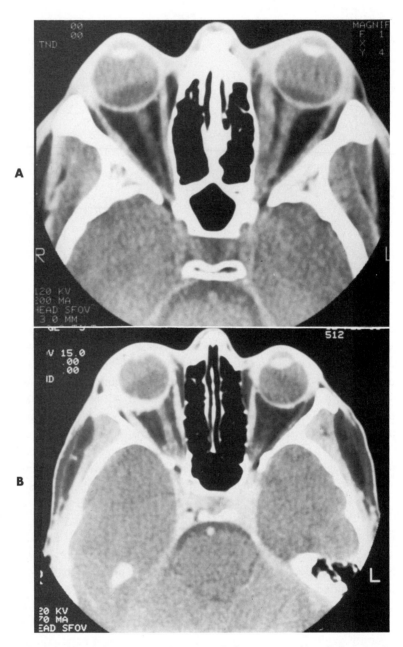

*Fig. 15-5.* Orbital pseudotumor. **A,** Myositis. Enlargement of medial rectus is unilateral and involves tendinous insertion as well. **B,** Scleritis. Entire right sclera enhances after contrast administration.

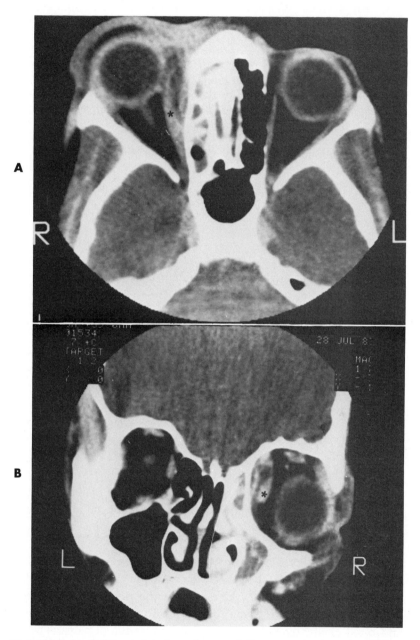

*Fig. 15-6.* Orbital cellulitis. Axial, **A,** and coronal, **B,** views of cellulitis of right orbit with right ethmoid and maxillary opacification. Right eye is displaced laterally and down. Right medial rectus (*) is elevated by a subperiosteal abscess.

## Management of Mucormycosis

1. Early definitive diagnosis is crucial! Biopsy is critical at an early stage, often before the black eschars appear in the nose or on the face.
2. Correct the underlying metabolic disorder.
3. Perform wide local excision and debridement of devitalized oral, nasal, sinus, and orbital tissues.
4. Provide adequate sinus and orbital drainage.
5. Use local irrigation, packing the sinus and orbit with amphotericin B. This approach seems to have a rationale,[68] since many times the area involved by mucormycosis is ischemic and intravenous amphotericin B may not reach this area.
6. Administer intravenous amphotericin B.
7. Reserve orbital exenteration for patients who, despite the above measures, show definite disease progression.

## Management of Orbital Cellulitis Unresponsive to Antibiotics

1. If an immunocompetent patient fails to respond to appropriate antibiotic therapy within 3 to 4 days, repeat the CT scan.
2. If CT reveals no mass in the orbit or paranasal sinuses and the patient shows no signs of systemic infection, the correct diagnosis is probably orbital pseudotumor. Discontinue antibiotics and begin systemic corticosteroids.
3. If CT reveals an intraorbital, subperiosteal, or sinus abscess, institute surgical drainage.
4. If a mass has developed or become more prominent, immediately perform a biopsy to rule out neoplasm (e.g., rhabdomyosarcoma, neuroblastoma).

traocular or infraorbital foreign body, CT is the first imaging study to perform in all patients who have sustained trauma. A nonmetallic foreign body such as wood may be difficult to visualize with high-resolution CT, but with MRI it may be detected.[62] The foreign body must be removed.[63]

The initial investigation of suspected nontraumatic orbital cellulitis must be aimed at identifying the causative organism. Cultures of the blood and of purulent wound drainage may be done, but the yield of positive cultures is low.[64]

The blood culture is the most critical of these tests, since the conjunctiva and nasal cavity are not sterile and noncausative organisms may grow in culture. The most likely organisms to be found on blood culture are *Haemophilus influenzae* (in children), *Staphylococcus aureus*, and *Streptococcus pneumoniae*. Once an organism is identified, specific intravenous antibiotic therapy is prescribed. After cultures have been obtained, intravenous broad-spectrum antibiotics are used initially to ensure that each of the most common causative organisms is covered.

While bacteria are the organisms that invade the orbit most frequently, the

| TABLE 15-2 | Ophthalmic Signs/Symptoms of Carotid Cavernous Fistula | | | | | |
|---|---|---|---|---|---|---|
| | Palestine et al.[70] (74 cases) | | Kupersmith et al.[71] (34 cases) | | Barrow et al.[72] (14 cases) | |
| Symptoms/signs | No.* | % | No. | %* | No. | %* |
| Conjunctival injection | 64 | 86 | 30 | 88 | 14 | 100 |
| Proptosis | 63 | 85 | 29 | 85 | 10 | 71 |
| Sixth nerve palsy | 37 | 51 | 28 | 82 | 10 | 71 |
| Third nerve palsy | 28 | 38 | 22 | 65 | 4 | 29 |
| Bruit | 61 | 82 | 29 | 85 | 8 | 57 |
| Intraocular pressure elevated | 28 | 38 | 24 | 71 | 10 | 71 |
| Decreased acuity | 10 | 14 | 8 | 23 | 12 | 86 |
| Dilated retinal veins | 30 | 41 | 11 | 32 | Not recorded | |

*Calculated from data.

presence of more exotic microbes should not be overlooked. Fungal infection may exist alone or in combination with bacterial cellulitis, especially following perforating orbital trauma with organic matter. In these instances specific cultures must be done to detect these organisms.

Any diabetic or immunologically compromised patient who develops signs of orbital inflammation should be considered to have orbital mucormycosis until proved otherwise. Diabetic patients need not be in ketoacidosis.[65] The nonseptate hyphae of mucormycosis cause an obliterative arteritis with necrotic lesions in the orbit and nasal cavity. If mucormycosis is suspected, a complete nasal examination should be performed to detect the typical black eschars of mucor. Recent reports link the appearance of mucormycosis with deferoxamine, a drug used to treat iron or aluminum excess.[66,67] Although most of these patients have developed systemic mucormycosis, any patient taking deferoxamine who develops orbital signs should be investigated for orbital mucormycosis.

The time-honored treatment of orbital mucormycosis infection begins with orbital exenteration. However, Kohn and Hepler[68] have described eight patients with mucormycosis who were successfully treated without orbital exenteration.

In patients with mucormycosis, CT scanning often shows abnormalities of paranasal sinuses or of the nasal fossa. However, the early changes may be impossible to distinguish from benign mucosal thickening.[69]

Immunocompetent patients with bacterial cellulitis usually begin to respond to appropriate antibiotic treatment within 3 to 4 days. If the condition fails to respond to appropriate antibiotic therapy, we recommend that CT be repeated.

### ☐ Carotid-cavernous fistula

Proptosis associated with chronic conjunctival injection and an audible bruit is highly suggestive of a fistula between the carotid artery and the cavernous sinus. Review of three studies shows the relative frequency of these and other signs and symptoms of carotid fistula[70-72] (Table 15-2). Arterialization of con-

| TABLE 15-3 | *Anatomic Classification of Carotid-Cavernous Fistula* |
|---|---|
| **Type** | **Description** |
| Type A | Direct tears |
| | High flow |
| | Communication between ICA and CS |
| Type B | Dural AVM |
| | Slow flow |
| | Communication between meningeal branches of ICA and CS |
| Type C | Dural AVM |
| | Slow flow |
| | Communication between meningeal branches of ECA and CS |
| Type D | Dural AVM |
| | Slow flow |
| | Communication between meningeal branches of ICA, ECA, and CS |

From Barrow DL, Spector RH, Braun IF, et al. Classification and treatment of spontaneous carotid-cavernous sinus fistulas. J Neurosurg 1985; 62:248-56.
*AVM*, Arteriovenous malformation; *ECA*, external carotid artery; *ICA*, internal carotid artery; *CS*, cavernous sinus.

junctival veins is the response to sustained arterial blood flow directly into venous channels (Plate 9, *C*). The intraocular pressure may be elevated as a result of the increased episcleral venous pressure. Machinelike bruits, synchronous with the pulse, may be detected with a stethoscope placed over the patient's eye or temporal area.

The marked differences in the percentages of visual loss in the three series in Table 15-2 indicate that the true prevalence of this problem remains in doubt.

Six potential causes of visual loss with carotid-cavernous fistulas have been reported[70,73]:

1. Glaucoma due either to increased episcleral venous pressure or, rarely, to iris neovascularization
2. Anterior segment ischemia
3. Corneal decompensation from exposure
4. Cystoid macular edema, hemorrhage in the macula, or macular ischemia
5. Retinal artery occlusion
6. Optic nerve ischemia

Improved angiography has resulted in the reclassification of fistulas according to the velocity of blood flow through the shunt into *low-* and *high*-flow fistulas. This information is combined with specific details of the anatomic origin of the arteries supplying the fistula (Table 15-3). Finally, the etiology may be *spontaneous* or *traumatic*, with type A usually being traumatic whereas types B, C, and D are spontaneous. While the ocular signs are usually ipsilateral to the fistula, bilateral signs may appear with a unilateral fistula, and rarely the ocular manifestions may be contralateral to the fistula (Plate 9, *D*).

Spontaneous resolution of these fistulas may occur, especially if they are of the low-flow variety. However, Sattler[74] collected 16 examples of spontaneous

## Management of Carotid Cavernous Fistula

1. Perform selective arteriography in all patients with signs suggestive of a carotid cavernous fistula if they are candidates for therapeutic intervention.
2. Attempt detachable balloon occlusion of direct carotid-cavernous (high-flow) fistulas, with preservation of carotid flow.
3. Treat (low-flow) fistulas from the external carotid circulation by embolization of the fistulous artery with particulate material or intravascular adhesives.

thrombosis in 322 cases of a probable high-flow fistula. Henderson and Schneider[75] reported one instance of regression of an untreated direct carotid-cavernous fistula in 17 cases. Phelps et al.[76] reported spontaneous closure of the fistula in 9 of their 19 patients with dural fistulas, and Barrow et al.[72] reported spontaneous closure in 5 of 14 patients with dural fistulas.

Imaging may assist in correctly identifying the process. The most consistent sign of carotid fistula is enlargement of the superior ophthalmic vein. However, this sign may be present in orbital pseudotumor, cavernous meningioma, and Graves' ophthalmopathy.[77] Color Doppler technology may assist in identifying a fistulous cause by showing the characteristics of arterial blood flow instead of venous flow in the enlarged superior ophthalmic vein[78] (Plate 10). Enlargement of the extraocular muscles usually seen in Graves' ophthalmopathy also may be found on imaging with carotid-cavernous fistulas.

The definitive diagnosis of carotid-cavernous fistula is made by selective cerebral angiography. While digital subtraction intravenous techniques are sufficient to document the presence of a fistula, intraarterial angiography with selective catheterization is needed to detect all fistulous communications before treatment may be attempted.

The most serious long-term consequence of carotid-cavernous fistulas is loss of vision. We recommend treatment of carotid-cavernous fistulas in the following instances:

1. When danger of loss of vision is imminent
2. When the continuous noise produced by the intracranial bruit is a severe disturbance to the patient
3. When intractable or incapacitating periocular pain or corneal exposure is present
4. When the cosmetic blemish is producing functional limitation

Several sophisticated methods of closing a carotid-cavernous fistula while preserving carotid patency are available. Detachable balloons introduced endoarterially through the internal carotid artery or endovenously through the internal jugular vein and inferior petrosal sinus, or both, are used in carotid cavernous fistulas. Debrun et al.[79] have reported successful occlusion of the fistula with this technique while retaining internal carotid artery patency in 68% of their first 54 cases and in 80% of their last 37 cases. Injection of isobutyl cyanoacrylate (glue) or particles of polyvinyl alcohol foam, or the insertion of steel coils[80] is used to treat slow-flow dural fistulas. Thrombogenic needles or wires also may be introduced into the cavernous sinus through a temporal craniotomy.[81] Direct surgical repair of a fistula is possible but technically difficult.[82,83]

Cerebral and ocular ischemia can result from these treatment attempts. We urge that these procedures be performed only by experienced interventional neuroradiologists.

### ☐ Trauma

Trauma to the orbital region may produce acute proptosis with varying amounts of ophthalmoplegia. The cause of this clinical picture is usually retrobulbar accumulations of blood, which are easily detectable by neuroimaging. An expanding retrobulbar hemorrhage may result in progressive proptosis. The increasing intraorbital pressure can raise intraocular pressure to the point where the central retinal artery pulsates. In this circumstance immediate opening of the orbital septum through an inferior cul-de-sac approach is recommended. This is more safely performed using a controlled incision. Needling of the retrobulbar space is to be discouraged.

Orbital hemorrhage may cause acute proptosis without preceding trauma. Spontaneous orbital hemorrhage is usually a dramatic event characterized by pain, proptosis, ophthalmoplegia, ecchymosis of the eyelids, and loss of vision in some patients. The most frequently discovered underlying abnormality in these patients is a congenital venous anomaly (varix).[84]

### ☐ Developmental anomalies

Exophthalmos may occur in developmental anomalies of the skull, especially craniostenosis.[85,86] Abnormal fusion of the bones of the skull results in shallow orbits and proptosis. In some instances raising intraorbital pressure (as in crying) may result in forward luxation of the eye, with the lids coming to rest behind the globe. This is not a difficult diagnosis to make if severe malformation of the skull is present. However, a spectrum does exist, so that minimal skull anomalies causing proptosis may go undetected. Oxycephaly ("tower skull") and dysostosis craniofacialis (Crouzon's disease) are the developmental anomalies that most often produce proptosis. The use of modern neurosurgical techniques of midfacial reconstruction has improved the cosmetic appearance of many of these individuals.

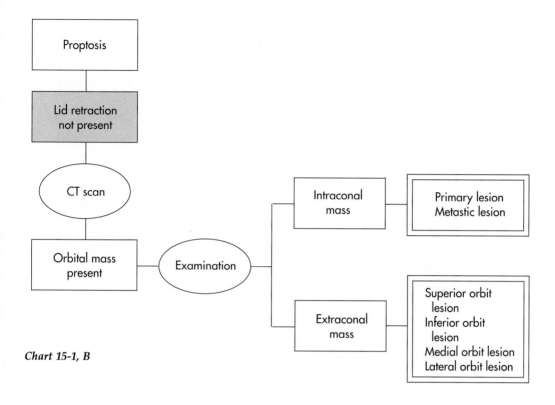

*Chart 15-1, B*

☐ Orbital mass present

A large number of different mass lesions may exist in the orbit or invade it from without. The types of tumors will vary with the age of the patient. The location of the mass in the orbit is frequently a clue to its nature (Chart 15-1, *B*). We will consider separately those masses that are intraconal (within the cone of the extraocular muscles), those that are extraconal, and those that are outside the orbit but impinge on it (periorbital).

☐ Intraconal mass

Intraconal mass lesions produce forward displacement of the globe. This is true whether the lesion is primary or metastatic, benign or malignant. Primary masses arise from structures normally found in the orbit. Imaging cannot establish the histology of orbital tumors, although the sharpness of margins, the presence of a capsule, and the degree of vascularity make certain lesions more likely than others.

▣ Primary lesion

Hemangiomas, among the most common orbital tumors, may occur anywhere in the orbit but have an affinity for the intraconal space. Cavernous hemangiomas are found mainly in adults and enlarge slowly over a period of many years. A well-encapsulated mass that enhances markedly after intravenous contrast injec-

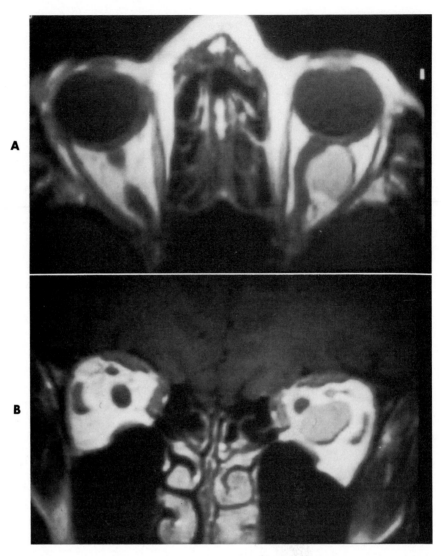

*Fig. 15-7.* Intraconal hemangioma. Axial, **A,** and coronal, **B,** MRI scans show intraconal mass lesion causing proptosis and medial deviation of optic nerve.

tion on CT is characteristic of these lesions (Fig. 15-7). Hemangiomas usually produce an MRI picture of a well-circumscribed mass that is isointense to muscle on short TR/TE. Regions of high intensity on long TR/TE images probably represent thrombosis.[87] While proptosis is usually the only sign, at times optic nerve compression with visual loss can result. Complete surgical excision of hemangiomas within their capsule is the treatment of choice.

Venous anomalies (varices) may also cause proptosis. Some patients experience increased proptosis on Valsalva maneuver or bending forward. Bleeding from orbital varices may produce painful proptosis, which may be associated with a subconjunctival hemorrhage. The imaging picture of a venous varix is usually distinctive enough to establish the diagnosis, although orbital venography may be necessary in rare instances. Surgical removal of a venous varix is seldom necessary and usually not possible. We advise nonintervention in these patients.

Primary tumors of the optic nerve also result in forward proptosis. In children gliomas are more frequent, whereas in adults meningiomas are found with greater regularity. Children with orbital meningiomas may manifest other evidence of neurofibromatosis (3 of 25 patients in one series[88]).

Meningiomas of the optic nerve sheath produce proptosis and progressive visual loss over a period of months to years. In a review of 22 patients with optic nerve meningiomas, Sibony et al.[89] found 17 patients (77%) had visual loss. Transient visual obscurations were noted by 5 patients (23%), but other ophthalmic symptoms, including proptosis, were infrequent. The optic disc appearance included disc elevation in 13 patients (59%) and atrophy in 9 (41%). Optociliary shunts were detected in 5 patients (23%) (Plate 8, *A*).

Enlargement of the optic nerve with increased density peripherally and decreased density centrally ("tram track" sign) is said to be the characteristic CT finding of an optic nerve sheath meningioma (Fig. 15-8, *A*). Diffuse enlargement of the optic nerve, at times with angulation, is also consistent with meningioma. The meningioma may involve the entire intraorbital optic nerve or any portion thereof. Meningiomas manifest variable signal intensity characteristics with MRI, the exact cause of which is unknown. The optic nerve may be seen as a linear structure coursing through the perioptic mass. The advantage of MRI is the ability to visualize the tumor's extent through the optic canal, since MRI does not visualize bone. Gadolinium-DTPA will cause mild enhancement of intraorbital and intracanalicular meningiomas. Its great benefit is the enhancing of otherwise invisible intracranial meningiomas, which are isointense to cortical gray matter.[90] A disadvantage of MRI is the inability to detect calcium, which these tumors often contain.[87]

Experience suggests that retaining useful vision following surgery for an optic nerve sheath meningioma is the exception and not the rule.[91,92] Clark et al.[93] recommend attempted surgical resection of all these tumors, although they admit that only small anterior orbital tumors may be removed with preservation of vision (as occurred in only one of their nine patients).

Radiation therapy appears to halt visual loss in optic nerve meningiomas. Eleven patients treated in two series have experienced improvement of vision or halting of progressive visual loss after orbital radiotherapy.[94,95]

Childhood orbital meningiomas are thought to be more aggressive than the adult variety, prompting the suggestion that extensive surgical extirpation be performed in younger patients.[96] We do not agree with this treatment and urge that optic nerve meningiomas in children be treated the same way as optic nerve meningiomas in adults.

Enlargement of an optic nerve on a CT scan in a child is more likely to be caused by a glioma than a meningioma. As in the case of meningiomas, other stigmata of neurofibromatosis should be sought. Great controversy continues about the treatment of optic nerve gliomas. Some have suggested observation of these tumors, which they consider to be benign hamartomas.[97] Others, who

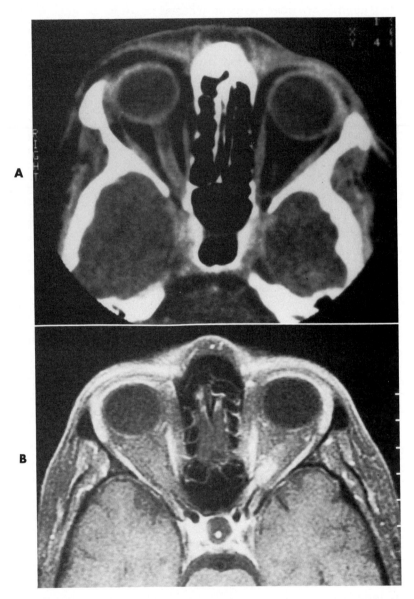

*Fig. 15-8.* Perioptic meningioma. **A,** CT scan shows enhancement at periphery of optic nerve resembling a tram track. **B,** MRI scan with gadolinium shows meningioma extending as highlight to intracranial optic nerve.

## Management of Optic Nerve Sheath Meningioma

1. Clinically reevaluate the patient every 6 months, including visual field examination.
2. Repeat MRI with gadolinium-DTPA studies every 6 months for 2 years, then yearly if no growth is indicated clinically or by imaging.
3. If visual function deteriorates, administer 5000 cGy of radiation.
4. Surgical intervention is considered only if intracranial extension through the optic canal occurs.
5. Biopsy of these lesions is unnecessary unless atypical clinical behavior or imaging findings occur.

view these lesions as potentially more aggressive, suggest complete surgical removal to prevent extension to the optic chiasm.

A small minority suggests primary radiation.[98] The weight of neuro-ophthalmic opinion presently seems to favor observation as long as the tumor is localized to the orbit and has not caused blindness. The answers, however, are by no means clear.

### ☐ Metastatic lesion

Metastatic tumors to the orbit from breast cancer are estimated to be the most frequent (42%), followed by lung (11%) and prostate (8.3%) cancer.[99] Metastatic neuroblastoma to the orbit may produce rapidly progressing proptosis. Neuroblastoma may be bilateral in up to 50% of patients, and frequently radiologic evidence of metastasis to the bones of the skull is found. Like rhabdomyosarcomas, neuroblastomas should be treated with a combination of radiation and chemotherapy once biopsy has provided the histologic diagnosis.

Enophthalmos, and not proptosis, may be produced by scirrhous breast carcinoma when it metastasizes to the orbit. Enophthalmos was present in 9 (24%) of 38 patients with metastatic orbital lesions.[100]

Any proptotic patient who has a history of treatment for cancer must be suspected of having orbital metastasis. However, Goldberg et al.[99] estimated that the orbital tumor is the first sign of an underlying malignancy in 42% of cases. Histologic verification is mandatory before treatment is begun, since other causes of proptosis are possible in these patients.

Fine-needle aspiration biopsy of orbital tumors is an alternative to biopsy through an orbitotomy in selected patients. The technique involves using imaging or B scan echography as a guide to needle placement in the mass and then aspirating cells from the mass.[98] This method of obtaining a tissue diagnosis is especially useful in patients with suspected metastatic orbital tumors. Once tissue verification is obtained by fine-needle aspiration biopsy, appropriate treatment alternatives may be selected.

☐ Extraconal mass

Orbital mass lesions in the extraconal space are likely either to be extending into the orbit from surrounding structures or to be metastatic from distant sources. It is estimated that 39% of metastases are to the lateral orbital space, whereas 32% are superior, 20% are medial, and 12% are inferior.[99] Of course, not all extraconal masses are metastatic, hemangiomas and rhabdomyosarcomas being examples of extraconal tumors primary to the orbit.

Rapidly progressive proptosis in a child must be considered to be caused by orbital rhabdomyosarcoma until proved otherwise. This is the most frequent primary malignant orbital tumor of childhood. It may be located at any point in the orbit, including the intraconal space. Usually a severe accompanying adnexal reaction is present, involving eyelid edema, lid injection, and conjunctival chemosis, which may be confused with orbital cellulitis or pseudotumor. At other times the only sign is progressive proptosis. CT scanning will reveal the mass lesion, which in many instances shows bony destruction.

A child suspected of harboring a rhabdomyosarcoma should have an immediate biopsy to confirm the diagnosis. The encouraging results of a combination of radiation and chemotherapy have spared many children the disfigurement of orbital exenteration.[101] Once the diagnosis has been established, these children should be treated in a center with experience with these malignant but potentially curable tumors.

☐ Superior orbit lesion

A mass lesion of the superior orbital space will cause downward displacement of the globe (Fig. 15-9, *A*). Lesions frequently encountered in the superior nasal quadrant are dermoid tumors and mucoceles.

**Dermoid tumors** are the most frequent developmental masses found in children. They cause slowly progressive proptosis with downward ocular displacement. Lesions located anteriorly often have extension into the deeper portions of the orbit. CT scanning will reveal the typical cystic lesion of the dermoid. Simple excision of the lesion is the treatment of choice.

Another benign mass of the superior medial orbit is the **mucocele.** This slowly expanding sinus (usually frontal) lesion gradually erodes the orbital roof to extend into the orbital space. Downward proptosis and inability to elevate the eye are the typical findings. Radiologic investigation will reveal marked sinus opacification with disruption of the bony orbitofrontal boundary. Surgical correction requires obliteration of the frontal sinus with fat to prevent recurrence.

When a superior orbital mass is suspected, adequate neuroradiologic visualization of the orbital roof must be obtained to ensure that an orbital encephalocele with protrusion of the brain through a defect in the orbital roof is not present. More than one unwary surgeon has performed a biopsy on a superior orbital mass only to have the pathologic report return a diagnosis of "brain tissue."

**Fibrous dysplasia,** an abnormality of bone formation, typically involves the frontal bones with resultant proptosis and downward ocular displacement.

This is a disorder of the young and tends to be slowly progressive. Progressive stenosis of the optic canal may result in visual loss. Heroic surgical procedures by a skilled plastic surgery team have been advocated as the only "cure" for this disorder.[102] The diagnosis is usually apparent on imaging.

The downward and medial displacement of an eye suggests a lesion in the area of the **lacrimal gland.** In this situation a benign mixed tumor of the lacrimal gland must be suspected. These encapsulated tumors are curable only if they are resected en bloc initially. Excisional biopsy with rupture of the capsule may cause seeding of tumor into the orbit, producing continued growth and eventually death from this locally aggressive tumor.

The duration of proptosis and the radiographic features of the lacrimal fossa may serve as guides to the diagnosis of lacrimal gland masses (Fig. 15-9, *B*). If the patient's signs and symptoms have been present for under 12 months or if destructive changes are visualized in the lacrimal fossa, a carcinoma of the lacrimal gland should be suspected, and incisional biopsy of the mass may be performed. However, if the history is longer than 12 months and imaging through the lacrimal fossa is either normal or shows only pressure changes, then a benign mixed tumor is likely and en-bloc excision of the mass is required.[103]

Jakobiec et al.[104] have supplemented the guidelines of Stewart et al.[103] by considering the CT findings of various lacrimal fossa lesions. On CT scans inflammatory lacrimal fossa lesions are often oblong and anteriorly located. Other signs of orbital inflammation (scleral enhancement, myositis) are also seen. In this setting, biopsy through the eyelid without violating the periosteum is recommended. Benign mixed lacrimal gland tumors have a more rounded CT appearance and extend toward the posterior orbit. When this pattern is encountered, total excision of the mass through a lateral orbital approach is suggested. Lesions other than lacrimal gland tumors may occur in the lacrimal fossa; however, all lesions in this area should be considered benign mixed tumors until proved otherwise. No evidence exists that orbital exenteration, followed by radiation therapy, is more effective than radiation therapy alone in the long-term survival of patients with lacrimal gland carcinoma.

### ⬜ Inferior orbit lesion

An eye displaced upward signifies pathology in the maxillary sinus or in the orbital floor (Fig. 15-9, *C*). Maxillary sinus mucoceles and tumors of the superior antrum are the two most frequent sinus causes of superior ocular displacement. CT scans of the orbital floor and maxillary sinus will define the exact location of the process.

Mass lesions in the inferior orbital space also may be primary or secondary, benign or malignant. The answer again is provided by a combination of imaging and surgical exploration. An inferior orbitotomy should not be performed until detailed evaluation of the maxillary sinus has been completed.

Fungal infectious processes in the paranasal sinuses may cause orbital signs suggestive of a mass lesion. A combination of imaging and biopsy will lead to the correct diagnosis even in these unusual cases.[105]

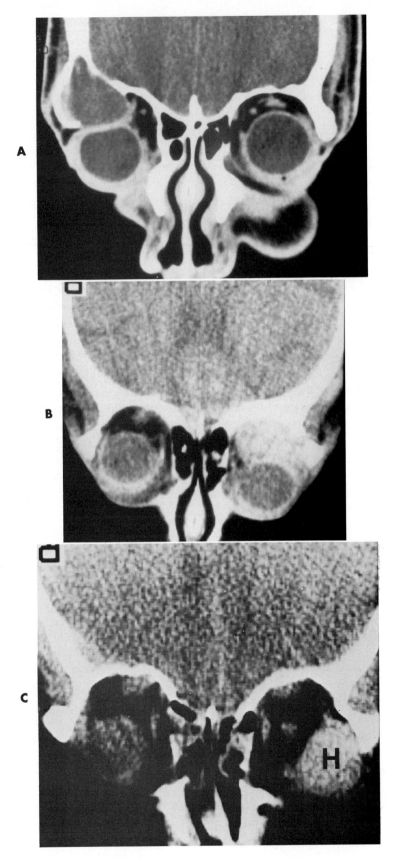

*Fig 15-9.* For legend see opposite page.

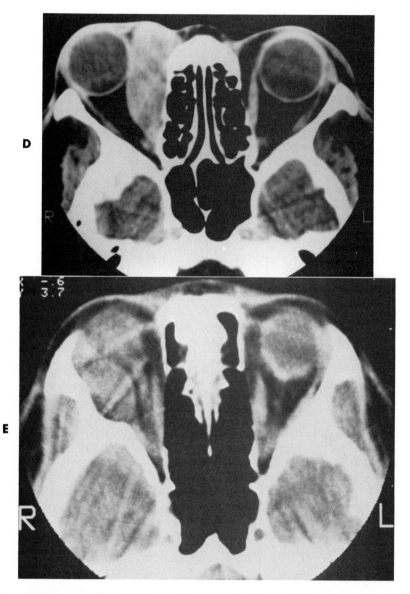

*Fig. 15-9.* Extraconal orbital mass lesions. **A,** Superior orbit: epidermoid tumor displaces right globe downward. **B,** Malignant lacrimal gland tumor displaces eye inferiorly and is eroding bony orbital rim. **C,** Inferior orbit: hemangioma *(H)* in inferior left orbit displaces globe upward and out of plane of scan. **D,** Medial orbital mass (lymphoma) involves medial rectus muscle and displaces globe laterally. **E,** Lateral orbital mass displaces globe medially and has scalloped out lateral orbital wall. Note medial bowing of right optic nerve.

### ☐ Medial orbit lesion

Lateral displacement of the eye results from mass lesions in the medial orbital space (Fig. 15-9, *D*). This is a particularly ominous sign, since it often signals extension of an aggressive process from the ethmoid-sphenoid complex into the medial orbital space. In children rhabdomyosarcoma must be considered. In adults carcinoma of the sinus is a frequent cause. These carcinomas are very aggressive and almost invariably lead to death following a protracted course despite all attempts at treatment.

Ethmoid sinus mucoceles also may displace the eye laterally. Modern imaging techniques usually can distinguish this benign cause of ocular displacement.

### ☐ Lateral orbit lesion

The lateral orbital space is the least frequent location for all orbital mass lesions, although metastatic lesions are found here with increased frequency.[99] When the eye is moved nasally, a mass lesion is most likely present in the pterygopalatine fossa or temporally within the orbit (Fig. 15-9, *E*). Knochel et al.'s review[106] of 227 orbital CT scans performed over a 5-year period revealed only 23 lateral orbital masses. The most frequent masses were metastatic (5), pseudotumor (4), hemangioma (2), meningioma (2), and rhabdomyosarcoma (2). Other causes were arteriovenous malformations, encephalocele, fibrous dysplasia, and trauma with hemorrhage. The nature of two masses was unknown.

**REFERENCES**

1. Henderson JW. Orbital tumors. Philadelphia: WB Saunders, 1973:28.
2. de Juan E Jr, Hurley DP, Sapira JD. Racial differences in normal values of proptosis. Arch Intern Med 1980: 140:1230-1.
3. Osher RH, Shields JA, Schatz NJ. Axial myopia: a neglected cause of proptosis. Arch Neurol 1978;35:237-41.
4. Sridama V, DeGroot LJ. Treatment of Graves' disease and the course of ophthalmopathy. Am J Med 1989; 87:70-3.
5. Marcocci C, Bartalena L, Bogazzi F, et al. Studies on the occurrence of ophthalmopathy in Graves' disease. Acta Endocrinol 1989;120:473-8.
6. Wiersinga WM, Smit T, van der Gaag R, et al. Temporal relationship between onset of Graves' ophthalmopathy and onset of thyroidal Graves' disease. J Endocrinol Invest 1988; 11:615-9.
7. Kiessling WR, Pflughaupt KW, Ricker K, et al. Thyroid function and circulating antithyroid antibodies in myasthenia gravis. Neurology 1981;31:771-4.
8. Feldon SE, Levin L. Graves' ophthalmopathy. V. Aetiology of upper eyelid retraction in Graves' ophthalmology. Br J Ophthalmol 1990;74:484-5.
9. McLean JM, Norton EWD. Unilateral lid retraction without exophthalmos: a manifestation of thyroid system dysfunction. Arch Ophthalmol 1959; 61:681-6.
10. Miller NR. Walsh and Hoyt's clinical neuro-ophthalmology, vol 2. 4th ed. Baltimore: Williams & Wilkins, 1985: 953.
11. Dixon RS, Anderson RL, Hatt MU. The use of thymoxamine in eyelid retraction. Arch Ophthalmol 1979; 97:2147-50.
12. Feldon SE, Lee CP, Muramatsu SK, et al. Quantitative computed tomography of Graves' ophthalmopathy: extraocular muscle and orbital fat in development of optic neuropathy. Arch Ophthalmol 1985;103:213-5.
13. Barrett L, Glatt HJ, Burde RM, et al. Optic nerve dysfunction in thyroid

eye disease: CT. Radiology 1988;167: 503-7.

14. Trobe JD, Glaser JS, Laflamme P. Dysthyroid optic neuropathy: clinical profile and rationale for management. Arch Ophthalmol 1979;96:1199-209.

15. Toft AD. Use of sensitive immunoradiometric assay for thyrotropin in clinical practice. Mayo Clin Proc 1988; 63:1035-42.

16. Kendall-Taylor P, Perros P.: Circulating retrobulbar antibodies in Graves' ophthalmopathy. Acta Endocrinol 1989; 121(suppl 2);31-7.

17. Nauman J, Adler G, Faryna M, et al. Eye muscle membrane antibodies. Acta Endocrinol 1989;121(suppl 2):90-8.

18. Chang TC, Huang KM, Chang TJ, et al. Correlation of orbital computed tomography and antibodies in patients with hyperthyroid Graves' disease. Clin Endocrinol 1990;32:551-8.

19. Weetman AP, Fells P, Shine B. T and B cell reactivity to extraocular and skeletal muscle in Graves' ophthalmopathy. Br J Ophthalmol 1989;73:323-7.

20. Campbell RJ. Immunology of Graves' ophthalmpathy: retrobulbar histology and histochemistry. Acta Endocrinol 1989;121(suppl 2):9-16.

21. Prummel MF, Wiersinga WM, Mourits MP, et al. Amelioration of eye changes of Graves' ophthalmopathy by achieving euthyroidism. Acta Endocrinol 1989;121(suppl 2):185-9.

22. Sergott RC, Felberg NT, Savino PJ, et al. Graves' ophthalmopathy—immunologic parameters related to corticosteroid therapy. Invest Ophthalmol Vis Sci 1981;20:173-82.

23. Streeten DHP, Anderson GH Jr, Reed GF, et al. Prevalence, natural history and surgical treatment of exophthalmos. Clin Endocrinol 1987;27:125-33.

24. Thomas ID, Hart JK. Retrobulbar repository corticosteroid therapy in thyroid ophthalmopathy. Med J Aust 1974;2:484-7.

25. Marcocci C, Bartalena L, Panicucci M, et al. Orbital cobalt irradiation combined with retrobulbar or systemic corticosteroids for Graves' ophthalmopathy: a comparative study. Clin Endocrinol 1987;27:33-42.

26. Sandler HM, Rubenstein JH, Fowble BL, et al. Results of radiotherapy for thyroid ophthalmopathy. Int J Radiat Oncol Biol Phys 1989;17:823-7.

27. Kriss JP, Petersen IA, Donaldson SS, et al. Supervoltage orbital radiotherapy for progressive Graves' ophthalmopathy: results of a twenty-year experience. Acta Endocrinol 1989;121(suppl 2):154-9.

28. Klingele TG, Hart WM, and Burde RM. Management of dysthyroid optic neuropathy. Ophthalmologica 1977; 174:327-35.

29. Guy JR, Fagien S, Donovan JP, et al. Methylprednisolone pulse therapy in severe dysthyroid optic neuropathy. Ophthalmology 1989;96:1048-53.

30. Prummel MF, Mourits MP, Berghout A, et al. Prednisone and cyclosporine in the treatment of severe Graves' ophthalmopathy. N Engl J Med 1989;321:1353-9.

31. Kahaly G, Schrezenmeir J, Krause U, et al. Cyclosporine and prednisone v. prednisone in treatment of Graves' ophthalmopathy: a controlled, randomized and prospective study. Eur J Clin Invest 1986;16:415-22.

32. Ogura JH, Thawley SE. Orbital decompression exophthalmos. Otolaryngol Clin North Am 1980;13:29-38.

33. DeSanto LW. The total rehabilitation of Graves' ophthalmopathy. Laryngoscope 1980;90:1652-78.

34. Linberg JV, Anderson RL. Transorbital decompression: indications and results. Arch Ophthalmol 1981;99:113-9.

35. Trokel SL, Cooper WC. Orbital decompression: effect on motility and globe position. Ophthalmology 1979; 86:2064-70.

36. Stranc M, West M. A four-wall orbital decompression for dysthyroid orbitopathy. J Neurosurg 1988;68:671-7.

37. Donaldson SS, Bagshaw MA, Kriss JP. Supervoltage orbital radiotherapy for Graves' ophthalmopathy. J Clin Endocrinol Metab 1973;37:276-85.

38. Palmer D, Greenberg P, Cornell P, et al. Radiation therapy for Graves' ophthalmopathy: a retrospective analysis. Int J Radiat Oncol Biol Phys 1987; 13:1815-20.

39. Kinyoun JL, Kalina RE, Brower SA, et

al. Radiation retinopathy after orbital irradiation for Graves' ophthalmopathy. Arch Ophthalmol 1984;102:1473-6.

40. Kelly W, Longson D, Smithard D, et al. An evaluation of plasma exchange for Graves' ophthalmopathy. Clin Endocrinol 1983;18:485-93.

41. Glinoer D, Schrooyen M. The treatment of severe Graves' ophthalmopathy with plasma exchange and immunosuppression. Acta Endocrinol 1989; 121(suppl 2):149-53.

42. Dyer JA. Ocular muscle surgery in Graves' disease. Trans Am Ophthalmol Soc 1978;76:125-39.

43. Evans D, Kennerdell JS. Extraocular muscle surgery for dysthyroid myopathy. Am J Ophthalmol 1983;95:767-71.

44. Mourits MP, Koornneef L, van Mourik-Noordenbos AM, et al. Extraocular muscle surgery for Graves' ophthalmopathy: does prior treatment influence surgical outcome? Br J Ophthalmol 1990;74:481-83.

45. Scott WE, Thalacker JA. Diagnosis and treatment of thyroid myopathy. Ophthalmology 1981;88:493-8.

46. Chavis RM, Garner A, Wright JE. Inflammatory orbital pseudotumor: a clinicopathologic study. Arch Ophthalmol 1978;96:1817-22.

47. Mottow-Lippa L, Jakobiec FA, Smith M. Idiopathic inflammatory orbital pseudotumor in childhood. II. Results of diagnostic tests and biopsies. Ophthalmology 1981;88:565-74.

48. Sergott RC, Glaser JS, Charyulu K. Radiotherapy for idiopathic inflammatory orbital pseudotumor. Arch Ophthalmol 1981;99:853-6.

49. Jakobiec FA, McLean I, Font RL. Clinicopathologic characteristics of orbital lymphoid hyperplasia. Ophthalmology 1979;86:948-66.

50. Knowles DM II, Jakobiec FA. Orbital lymphoid neoplasma: a clinicopathologic study of 60 patients. Cancer 1980;46:576-89.

51. White V, Rootman J, Quenville N, et al. Orbital lymphoproliferative and inflammatory lesions. Can J Ophthalmol 1987;22:362-73.

52. Jakobiec FA, Neri A, Knowles DM II.

Genotypic monoclonality in immunophenotypically polyclonal orbital lymphoid tumors: a model of tumor progression in the lymphoid system. Ophthalmology 1987;94:980-94.

53. Medeiros LJ, Harmon DC, Linggood RM, et al. Immunohistologic features predict clinical behavior of orbital and conjunctival lymphoid infiltrates. Blood 1989;74:2121-9.

54. Flanders AE, Mafee MF, Rao VM, et al. CT characteristics of orbital pseudotumors and other orbital inflammatory processes. J Comput Assist Tomogr 1989;13:40-7.

55. Trokel SL, Jakobiec FA. Correlation of CT scanning and pathologic features of ophthalmic Graves' disease. Ophthalmology 1981;88:553-64.

56. Eshaghian J, Anderson RL. Sinus involvement in inflammatory orbital pseudotumor. Arch Ophthalmol 1981; 99:627-30.

57. Atlas SW, Grossman RI, Savino PJ, et al. Surface-coil MR of orbital pseudotumor. AJR Am J Roentgenol 1987; 148:803-8.

58. Garrity JA, Kennerdell JS, Johnson BL, et al. Cyclophosphamide in the treatment of orbital vasculitis. Am J Ophthalmol 1986;102:97-103.

59. Diaz-Llopis M, Menezo JL. Idiopathic inflammatory orbital pseudotumor and low-dose cyclosporine. Am J Ophthalmol 1989;107:547-8.

60. Gellady AM, Shulman ST, Ayoub EM. Periorbital and orbital cellulitis in children. Pediatrics 1978;61:272-7.

61. Watters EC, Waller H, Hiles DA, et al. Acute orbital cellulitis. Arch Ophthalmol 1976;94:785-8.

62. Green BF, Kraft SP, Carter KD, et al. Intraorbital wood: detection by magnetic resonance imaging. Ophthalmology 1990;97:608-11.

63. Weisman RA, Savino PJ, Schut L, et al. Computed tomography in penetrating wounds of the orbit with retained foreign bodies. Arch Otolaryngol 1983;109:265-8.

64. Powell KR, Kaplan SB, Hall CB, et al. Periorbital cellulitis: clinical and laboratory findings in 146 episodes, including tear countercurrent immuno-

electrophoresis in 89 episodes. Am J Dis Child 1988;142:853-7.

65. Van Johnson E, Kline LB, Julian BA, et al. Bilateral cavernous sinus thrombosis due to mucormycosis. Arch Ophthalmol 1988;106:1089-92.

66. Boelaert JR, Fenves AZ, Coburn JW. Mucormycosis among patients on dialysis. N Engl J Med 1989;321:190-1.

67. Daly AL, Velazquez LA, Bradley SF, et al. Mucormycosis: association with deferoxamine therapy. Am J Med 1989;87:468-71.

68. Kohn R, Hepler R. Management of limited rhino-orbital mucormycosis without exenteration. Ophthalmology 1985;92:1440-4.

69. Gamba JL, Woodruff WW, Djang WT, et al. Craniofacial mucormycosis: assessment with CT. Radiology 1986; 160:207-12.

70. Palestine AG, Younge BR, Piepgras DG. Visual prognosis in carotid-cavernous fistula. Arch Ophthalmol 1981; 99:1600-3.

71. Kupersmith MJ, Berenstein A, Flamm E, et al. Neuroophthalmologic abnormalities and intravascular therapy of traumatic carotid cavernous fistulas. Ophthalmology 1986;93:906-12.

72. Barrow DL, Spector RH, Braun IF, et al. Classification and treatment of spontaneous carotid-cavernous sinus fistulas. J Neurosurg 1985;62:248-56.

73. Sanders MD, Hoyt WF. Hypoxic ocular sequelae of carotid-cavernous fistulae: study of the causes of visual failure before and after neurosurgical treatment in a series of 25 cases. Br J Ophthalmol 1969;53:82-97.

74. Sattler CH: Pulsierender exophthalmus. In Graefe A, Saemisch TH, eds. Handbuch der gesamten Augenheilkunde. Berlin: Julius Springer, 1930:chap 13.

75. Henderson JW, Schneider RC. The ocular findings in carotid-cavernous fistula in a series of 17 cases. Am J Ophthalmol 1959;48:585-97.

76. Phelps CD, Thompson HS, Ossoinig KC. The diagnosis and prognosis of atypical carotid-cavernous fistula (red-eyed shunt syndrome). Am J Ophthalmol 1982;93:423-36.

77. Peyster RG, Savino PJ, Hoover ED, et al. Differential diagnosis of the enlarged superior ophthalmic vein. J Comput Assist Tomogr 1984;8:103-7.

78. Flaharty PM, Lieb WE, Sergott RC, et al. Color Doppler imaging: a new noninvasive technique to diagnose and monitor carotid cavernous fistulas. Arch Ophthalmol 1991;109:522-6.

79. Debrun GM, Viñuel F, Fox AJ, et al. Indications for treatment and classification of 132 carotid-cavernous fistulas. Neurosurgery 1988;22:285-9.

80. Teng MMH, Guo WY, Huang CI, et al. Occlusion of arteriovenous malformations of the cavernous sinus via the superior ophthalmic vein. AJNR 1988; 9:539-46.

81. Mullan S. Treatment of carotid-cavernous fistulas by cavernous sinus occlusion. J Neurosurg 1979;50:131-44.

82. Dolenc V. Direct microsurgical repair of intracavernous vascular lesions. J Neurosurg 1983;58:824-31.

83. Parkinson D, Downs AR, Whytehead LL, et al. Carotid cavernous fistula: direct repair with preservation of carotid. Surgery 1974;76:882-9.

84. Krohel GB, Wright JE: Orbital hemorrhage. Am J Ophthalmol 1979;88:254-8.

85. Howell SC. The craniostenosis. Am J Ophthalmol 1954;37:359-79.

86. Koziak PH. Craniostenosis: report of 22 cases. Am J Ophthalmol 1954;37:380-90.

87. Atlas SW. Magnetic resonance imaging of the orbit: current status. Magn Reson Q 1989;5:39-96.

88. Karp LA, Zimmerman LE, Borit A, et al. Primary intraorbital meningiomas. Arch Ophthalmol 1974;91:24-8.

89. Sibony PA, Krauss HR, Kennerdell JS, et al. Optic nerve sheath meningiomas: clinical manifestations. Ophthalmology 1984;91:1313-26.

90. Zimmerman CF, Shatz NJ, Glaser JS. Magnetic resonance imaging of optic nerve meningiomas: enhancement with gadolinium-DTPA. Ophthalmology 1990;97:585-91.

91. Ebers GC, Girvin JP, Canny CB. A "possible" optic nerve meningioma. Arch Neurol 1980;37:781-3.

92. Mark LE, Kennerdell JS, Maroon JC, et al. Microsurgical removal of a primary intraorbital meningioma. Am J Ophthalmol 1978;86:704-9.

93. Clark WC, Theofilos CS, Fleming JC. Primary optic nerve sheath meningiomas: report of nine cases. J Neurosurg 1989;70:37-40.

94. Kennerdell JS, Maroon JC, Malton M, et al. The management of optic nerve sheath meningiomas. Am J Ophthalmol 1988;106:450-7.

95. Smith JL, Vuksanovic MM, Yates BM, et al. Radiation therapy for primary optic nerve meningiomas. J Clin Neuro Ophthalmol 1981;1:85-99.

96. Walsh FB. Meningiomas primary within the orbit and optic canal. In: Glaser JS, Smith JL, eds: Neuro-Ophthalmology: symposium of the University of Miami and the Bascom Palmer Eye Institute, vol 8. St Louis: Mosby–Year Book, 1975:166-90.

97. Wright JE. Primary optic nerve meningiomas: clinical presentation and management. Trans Am Acad Ophthalmol 1977;83:617-25.

98. Dubois PJ, Kennerdell JS, Rosenbaum AE, et al. Computed tomographic localization for fine needle aspiration biopsy of orbital tumors. Radiology 1979;131:149-52.

99. Goldberg RA, Rootman J, Cline RA. Tumors metastatic to the orbit: a changing picture. Surv Ophthalmol 1990;35:1-24.

100. Goldberg RA, Rootman J. Clinical characteristics of metastatic orbital tumors. Ophthalmology 1990;97:620-4.

101. Raney RB, Handler SD. Management of neoplasms of the head and neck in children. II. Malignant tumors. Head Neck Surg 1981;3:500-10.

102. Munro IR, Chen YR. Radical treatment for fronto-orbital fibrous dysplasia: the chain-link fence. Plast Reconstr Surg 1981;67:719-30.

103. Stewart WB, Krohel GB, Wright JE. Lacrimal gland and fossa lesions: an approach to diagnosis and management. Ophthalmology 1979;86:886-95.

104. Jakobiec FA, Yeo JH, Trokel SL, et al. Combined clinical and computed tomographic diagnosis of primary lacrimal fossa lesions. Am J Ophthalmol 1982;94:785-807.

105. Nielsen EW, Weisman RA, Savino PJ, et al. Aspergillosis of the sphenoid sinus presenting as orbital pseudotumor. Otolaryngol Head Neck Surg 1983;91:699-703.

106. Knochel JQ, Osborn AG, Wing SD. Differential diagnosis of lateral orbital masses. J Comput Assist Tomogr 1981;5:11-5.

# CHAPTER 16

# Headache

• • • • • • • • • • • • • • • • • •

Of all of the ailments that plague humankind, headache is among the most ubiquitous. Most headaches do not reflect serious pathology. Their importance lies in the fact that they prevent the suffering individual from functioning in everyday life. The evaluation of headache patients is time consuming. Because of the pressures of practice, and because their personalities make interacting with chronic headache sufferers difficult, these patients often do not receive the extended attention required and leave the physician's office less than satisfied, wandering from office to office seeking help.

Patients with headaches are commonly referred to the ophthalmologist in the belief that inappropriate optical corrections are the source of many headaches, or to the neurologist because of concern for the existence of intracranial pathology. To deal with these patients, physicians must be able to recognize and categorize certain characteristic symptom complexes. Nonetheless, a number of patients do not seem to fall easily into a specific diagnostic group. The approach to these patients requires asking a sequence of historical questions. In the vast majority of headache patients, the physical examination is normal.

Ray and Wolff[1] determined that the pain-sensitive structures within the cranium included (1) the great venous sinuses and their tributaries, (2) parts of the dura on the floor of the skull, and (3) the dural arteries and the cerebral arteries at the base of the brain. They formulated six basic sources of intracranial headache: (1) traction on tributary veins passing to the great venous sinuses or displacement of the great venous sinuses, (2) traction on the middle meningeal artery, (3) traction on the large cerebral arteries or their branches at the base of the brain, (4) distention and dilatation of the intracranial arteries, (5) inflammation in or around any of the pain-sensitive structures, and (6) direct pressure on the cranial or cervical nerves containing afferent pain fibers from these structures, which include the fifth cranial nerve above the tentorium cerebelli and the ninth, tenth, eleventh, twelfth, and upper cervical nerves below the tentorium. The opinion that the brain itself is insensitive to pain has held sway since the reports of Penfield[2] and Ray and Wolff.[3] However, Raskin et al.[4] have reported that 15 patients developed headache syndromes after electrode implantation in the region of the thalamus or periaqueductal gray matter.

Extracranial sources of head pain include skin, mucous membranes, tympanic membrane, fascia, muscles and galea, and the extracranial arteries and veins of the head and neck. Headaches may be classified using this neuroanatomic background,[5] but for practical purposes categorizing headaches based on their clinical presentations is easier (see box). We have adapted the classification of the Headache Classification Committee of the International Headache Society.[6]

Raskin[7] offers the theory that most headaches represent a migraine variant due to unstable serotoninergic neurotransmission. This dismodulation of serotonin receptors is present both centrally (leading to an increased firing rate of serotonin-containing nuclei [midline raphe] to produce head pain) and peripherally in the myenteric plexus of the intestine, accounting for the common occurrence of gastrointestinal upset. Compelling arguments against this hypothesis include the lack of major changes in plasma serotonin in most headache patients and the differential effect of serotonin on the intracerebral and extracerebral vessels. On the other hand, Doenicke et al.[8] demonstrated, at least in migraineurs, that the intravenous infusion of a novel serotonin receptor agonist (GR43175) relieved symptoms in 17 of 24 severe attacks in patients with migraine. In the other seven attacks, the severity of the pain was reduced to that of a mild headache.

## Distinctive Headache Syndromes

Certain headache syndromes are so characteristic that the diagnosis is obvious from listening to the history. These types of headaches fall into one of two major categories (see box): (1) those recognized by classic historical features, which can be subdivided into those with or without definable triggers, and (2) those recognized by physical features associated with systemic, central nervous system (CNS), or local disease. The classification of the remaining patients with headache complaints is based on determining the time-intensity curve (variation in intensity of pain with the duration) of the headache and finding the relation, if any, of the headache to other events. The aim of this chapter is not to be encyclopedic about each entity, but to offer a clinical classification system that allows for categorization.

### HEADACHES RECOGNIZED BY CLASSICAL HISTORICAL FEATURES

The following headache patterns are easily recognized by history alone. The first group is not associated with a defined trigger mechanism.

#### HEADACHES ASSOCIATED WITH NO OBVIOUS EXOGENOUS TRIGGER MECHANISM

Cluster headache. Patients with a *typical cluster headache* are awakened from sleep in the early morning (1 to 3 AM; 75% of attacks occur between 9 PM and 10 AM[9]) by the onset of excruciating head pain, usually unilateral. The pain is described as being in the distribution of the external carotid artery and its branches (frontal or frontotemporal pain). The headache is accompanied by lacrimation (84%), conjunctival edema and injection (58%), ipsilateral Horner's syndrome

## Classification of Headache

I. Distinctive headache syndromes
   A. Recognized by classical historical features
      1. No obvious exogenous trigger mechanism
         a. Cluster headache
            (1) Typical cluster headache
            (2) Chronic paroxysmal hemicrania
            (3) Hemicrania continua
         b. Migraine with aura
            (1) Typical aura
            (2) Prolonged aura
            (3) Familial hemiplegic migraine
            (4) Migraine with infarction
            (5) Basilar artery migraine
            (6) Ophthalmoplegic migraine
         c. Cranial neuralgias
            (1) Trigeminal neuralgia
            (2) Glossopharyngeal neuralgia
         d. Idiopathic stabbing headache (ice pick–like pain)
         e. Giant cell arteritis
         f. "Thunderclap" headache
         g. "Exploding" headache
      2. Obvious exogenous trigger mechanism
         a. "Ice cream" headache
         b. Dietary headache
         c. Altitude headache
         d. Posttraumatic headache
         e. Low intracranial pressure headache
         f. Asthenopia
         g. Headache associated with sexual activity
   B. Recognized by physical features and associated with other disease states
      1. Herpetic neuralgia
      2. Sinus disease
      3. Dental disease
      4. Temporomandibular joint pain
      5. Fever
      6. Arterial hypertension
         a. Sudden rise in blood pressure
         b. Essential hypertension
      7. Central nervous system disease
         a. Raised intracranial pressure
         b. Coughing
         c. Raeder's syndrome
             (1) Type 1
            (2) Type 2
      8. Ocular inflammation
      9. Ocular ischemia
II. Nondistinctive headache syndromes
   A. Migraine without aura
   B. Migraine equivalents
   C. Retinociliary migraine
   D. Childhood migraine
   E. Tension-type headaches
   F. Ocular neurosis
   G. Atypical facial pain
   H. Greater occipital neuralgia

(51%), and rhinorrhea (43%).[10] The pain is described as boring or burning and as being of such severity that the patient usually paces the floor until the pain subsides in 30 minutes to 1 to 2 hours. The patient is asymptomatic until the attack recurs at the same time the next day, but multiple attacks (one to three) in 1 day may occur. The headaches may recur daily for days or weeks, then disappear, and then return on a regular basis once or twice a year. In about 10% of patients they may become chronic.[9] The onset is usually in the third or fourth decade (later onset in women) and is more common in men. These headaches are often triggered by even minimal alcohol ingestion during the cluster phase. Patients tolerate alcohol well during the asymptomatic phase. Some[7] consider this variation in response to alcohol to be diagnostic of cluster headache.

If the patient has a typical history of cluster headache and the only neurologic finding is postganglionic Horner's syndrome (see Chapter 13), then no further investigation is needed. Cluster headache is believed to be a vascular headache, possibly migrainous in nature. Some have found the antimigraine ergotamine tartrate to be effective in aborting the paroxysm.[11] Kudrow[11] recommends the use of ergotamine aerosol and states that it is effective in 80% of cases. Raskin[7] states that the intravenous use of dihydroergotamine rarely fails to abort an episode within 5 minutes.

Once the diagnosis has been made, prophylactic treatment to "break the cluster" should sequentially include systemic corticosteroids (first-line drug; dosage 40 to 150 mg orally each day for 10 to 14 days), methysergide (4 to 16 mg p.o. daily), and lithium chloride. Lithium chloride should be used in a dose of 300 to 1500 mg daily, with the "cluster" breaking in about 1 to 2 weeks after initiation of therapy. Lithium is especially effective in the chronic form of the disease. None of these drugs is universally effective when used prophylactically. Chlorpromazine (Thorazine) has been reported to be effective in 93% (12 of 13) of patients with cluster headache.[12]

*Chronic cluster headache* is divided into two subcategories: chronic paroxysmal hemicrania and hemicrania continua. *Chronic paroxysmal hemicrania* was first described by Sjaastad and Dale[13] in 1974. This condition is characterized by excruciating unilateral oculotemporal pain associated with ipsilateral lacrimation, rhinorrhea, ptosis, miosis, and conjunctival edema. The attacks are brief (1 to 20 minutes), with a high frequency of daily attacks (up to 30/day). The attacks usually start in childhood and last for 2 to 3 weeks with a variable interlude of remission. Almost all patients respond to indomethacin.[14] Aspirin may be effective as well.[15]

Medina and Diamond[16] described *hemicrania continua* in 54 patients with three characteristic complaints: (1) lateralized continuous dull aching pain, (2) superimposed daily jabbing, ice pick–like head pain often associated with exercise, and (3) focal lateralized intense pain, lasting 5 to 50 minutes and recurring four to five times daily. The focal pain often awakened patients from sleep and was triggered by alcohol or exercise. The syndrome had been present for 1 to 12 years. No particular age predilection was found, and men and women were affected equally. Eighty percent of patients responded to indomethacin (>100 mg daily) with alleviation of pain. Those who did not respond to indomethacin responded to tricyclic antidepressants.

**Migraine with aura.** Migraine (from the Greek *hemikranios:* "half skull") as a nosologic entity has defied simple definition.[6,17] Migraine consists of the paroxysmal occurrence of a constellation of symptoms, including severe unilateral headache (30% will be generalized) accompanied by gastroenterologic dysfunction (90% of patients have anorexia, nausea, vomiting, and/or diarrhea). The headache may be preceded, accompanied, or followed by neurologic (usually visual) or somatic phenomena. Migraine can occur with or without an aura. Characteristic subtypes of migraine with aura can easily be recognized, whereas the diagnosis of migraine without aura is often one of exclusion. From our vantage, the migraine syndrome represents a "final common pathway" for a heterogenous group of disorders with different etiologies. This heterogeneity can be inferred by the large number of different triggers such as food, wine, stress, alleviation of stress, hormonal changes, and the variable response to medications. Although migraine has been classified in many different ways, we are using a modification of the classification of the International Headache Society.[6]

*Migrane with typical aura.* Migraine with typical aura is the most stereotypic of all the migraine syndromes but is found in only about 20% of patients with migraine. Attacks are characterized by a sharply defined aura that is usually visual but may be sensory or motor, lasting for 5 to 40 minutes before fading as the headache phase begins. The pain, which is usually unilateral and throbbing, lasts for hours. The neurologic manifestations of the aura occur contralateral to the pain. Anorexia, nausea, and extreme sensitivity to light (not eye pain) and noise are concomitant features of the headache phase.

Historically, in migraine with typical aura, investigators have held that the aura phase is associated with intracranial vasoconstriction, producing localized ischemia. This phase is followed by vasodilatation of the extracranial arteries, producing the typical headache. Unfortunately, this simplistic view does not explain a multitude of observations. In many patients intracranial vasoconstriction occurs in one area and vasodilatation in another. Olesen[18] has demonstrated that in migraine with aura, a spreading oligemia moves occipitofrontally at the rate of 2 mm/minute. This decrease in the regional blood supply posteriorly precedes the onset of the aura.[19] The migration of the oligemia does not follow the topography of the cerebral circulation, thus precluding a primary vascular pathogenesis. This finding is more compatible with the neurogenic hypothesis based on the spreading depression of Leão.[20] However, investigators have emphasized that the oligemic spread and clinical symptomatology develop much faster than the neurologic wave of migrating depression and that the latter is thus an unlikely explanation of events. In addition, a few patients with migraine with aura and those without aura fail to demonstrate spreading oligemia, reinforcing the probable heterogeneity of the process underlying the migraine syndrome.

The aura is usually visual, although it may take a hemiparetic, hemisensory, or dysphasic form. The most common symptom is the scintillating scotoma. This visual disturbance usually begins as a small, gray, ill-defined area just eccentric to fixation. Individual letters or words may seem to break up. The area then slowly expands while tending to drift peripherally. The scotoma may consist of an area of totally absent sight or an area of reduced sensitivity, which may be outlined by bright shimmering lights in a zigzag configuration (fortification specter). Scintillations may consist of brilliantly colored or iridescent shimmering highlights surrounding the scotoma along the leading edge of the zigzag pattern. The visual symptoms may assume other forms, including eccentric scotomas, awareness of brightness in the peripheral field, apparent pulsation of the intensity of ambient illumination, flashes, heat waves, distortions, and hallucinations of movement of stationary objects involving one or both hemifields simultaneously or consecutively. After the age of 40, patients may lose the headache phase but still experience the aura (*acephalgic migraine* or *migraine equivalent*). The aura may consist of motor or sensory deficits that clear with the onset of the headache, paralleling the course of the visual phenomena.

*Migraine with prolonged aura.* Patients with migraine may experience paroxysmal neurologic deficits that persist into and after the headache phase. Neurologic dysfunction may begin before, during, or following the headache. The deficits, which may persist for hours to weeks, include both motor and sensory systems (hemipareses, dysarthria, automatisms,[21] hemianesthesias, teichopsia).

*Familial hemiplegic migraine.* A well-recognized subset of migraine with prolonged aura occurs in families (familial hemiplegic migraine).[22] In this group the attacks of motor deficit always occur on the same side, and complete recovery is the rule.

*Migraine with infarction.* In one nonfamilial variety of hemiplegic migraine (migraine with infarction), incomplete recovery is not unusual. Permanent homonymous or quadrantic visual field defects have been well documented in patients who have previously experienced classic migraine attacks with scintillating scotomas.[23] Permanent hemisensory disturbances (e.g., paresthesias of hands, arm, face, tongue, or lips) have been reported. With the exception of familial hemiplegic migraine, all of these patients should be evaluated for the presence of a structural lesion by magnetic resonance imaging (MRI), including the use of gadolinium. Angiography, if considered necessary, is not contraindicated in patients with migraine.[24]

*Basilar artery migraine.* Basilar artery migraine is a disorder that mimics the transient ischemic attacks of vertebrobasilar insufficiency seen in elderly individuals—the sudden onset of transient visual disturbances, vertigo, gait ataxia, dysarthria, and acroparesthesias.[25] The neurologic aberrations persist for 10 to 30 minutes and are followed by severe headache and vomiting.[25] The visual symptoms include vivid flashes of light throughout the visual field, transient bilateral blindness, bilateral blurred vision, formed visual hallucinations, and diplopia.[26] Transient alterations in consciousness have also been reported. This was believed to be an affliction of adolescent girls and young women until Golden and French[27] noted its occurrence in preschool children. Their findings were extended by Lapkin and Golden,[26] who reported 30 children from 7 months to 14 years old with basilar artery migraine. The vast majority of children had frequent attacks (three per week), and the headache tended to be nonlateralized. Such attacks are less frequent in adults.

Differentiating vertebrobasilar insufficiency from migraine in children with brainstem symptoms and signs is difficult. The points supporting the diagnosis of migraine are (1) a strong family history of migraine (86%) and (2) exclusion of persistent or progressive neurologic disease.[26] The prognosis, despite recurrent attacks, is excellent, although cerebellar[28] and brainstem[29] infarction have been reported.

Basilar artery migraine may also occur in patients in their sixties, at which time it may be confused with vertebrobasilar insufficiency. However, most patients experience the onset of this syndrome complex before age 25 and will have a personal or strong family history of migraine.

*Ophthalmoplegic migraine.* Ophthalmoplegic migraine is a rare disorder, usually having its onset before age 10.[30] The third cranial nerve is affected more often than the sixth (10:1),[30] and the paralysis can involve the extraocular muscles, as well as the pupillary and ciliary muscles. Some degree of pupillary sparing is present in two thirds of patients. The paralysis begins either at the height of the pain or at the cessation of the pain and lasts for days to weeks.[31] Recovery is gradual and tends to become less complete with repeated attacks. The ophthalmoplegia tends to be on the same side as the headache.

Strict criteria should be met before the diagnosis of ophthalmoplegic migraine is made:

1. Onset in the first decade.
2. History of typical migraine headaches (i.e., severe throbbing headache or equivalent).
3. Normal cerebral angiogram, dynamic computed tomography (CT), or thin-section MRI. The likelihood of an aneurysm is so low in children under age 15 that we consider dynamic CT scanning[32] or thin-section MRI (2 mm) adequate substitutes for angiography, acknowledging that this is a controversial issue.

The treatment of migraine is discussed in the Appendix at the end of the chapter.

**Cranial neuralgias.** Cranial neuralgias include two distinct entities: trigeminal neuralgia and glossopharyngeal neuralgia. Each of these syndromes is characterized by paroxysms of pain occurring in the distribution of a particular cranial nerve.

*Trigeminal neuralgia.* Trigeminal neuralgia (tic douloureux) is marked by the sudden onset of severe pain in the distribution of one division of the fifth nerve—usually the third, occasionally the second, and rarely the first. The pain is so intense that the facial muscles typically contract and distort the face during an attack, and the patient anticipates with dread the ensuing bouts of pain. The pain is most often described as electric shock–like in nature. Occasionally the pain may spread to involve a second or third division during a paroxysm. The paroxysms are usually short (20 to 30 seconds) but may be repetitive and closely spaced, and under these circumstances last up to an hour. In time the spontaneous attacks, which initially may be intermittent (separated by days or weeks), tend to occur at closer intervals (one or two attacks per day).

A typical attack can occur spontaneously or be triggered by various stimuli such as light touch, a cool breeze on the face, biting, chewing, brushing teeth, shaving, and sudden changes in oral temperatures when eating hot or cold substances. Trigger mechanisms occur in approximately 50% of patients, and one or more stimuli may induce an attack in any individual. Patients are asymptomatic between paroxysms. The neurologic examination is normal. This syndrome tends to occur in individuals over the age of 50 years. If present in a younger individual, or if sensory abnormalities or other accompanying neurologic deficits are found, underlying pathology such as an intracranial mass lesion, multiple sclerosis, or dental disease must be excluded. In patients with the classic syndrome of trigeminal neuralgia, diagnostic procedures are unnecessary.[21]

Carbamazepine has been considered to be the mainstay of prophylactic treatment for patients with trigeminal neuralgia. This drug should be administered at mealtime in gradually increasing doses.[33] Patients rarely respond to less than 600 mg daily, and a maximum therapeutic dosage is 1600 mg per day. Because of the notable side effects of carbamazepine, including drowsiness, dizziness, bone marrow suppression, and hepatic toxicity, Fromm[34] has recommended that baclofen (40 to 80 mg daily) should be the first drug used in treating trigeminal neuralgia. Phenytoin, valproic acid, and clonazepam also have been used successfully.

Not infrequently, surgical intervention will be warranted if medical treatment is unsuccessful. The most common surgical procedure is percutaneous radiofrequency trigeminal gangliolysis. Suboccipital craniectomy to relieve vascular compression of the trigeminal nerve at its exit from the brainstem is becoming more popular. Evidence suggests that the cause of trigeminal neuralgia is focal demyelination of the trigeminal nerve due to aberrant blood vessels compressing the root entry zone in the pons.[35]

*Glossopharyngeal neuralgia.* Glossopharyngeal neuralgia is seen less frequently than is trigeminal neuralgia (1:200) and is characterized by the sudden onset of stabbing and jolting pain in the posterior half of the tongue, the tonsils, and the pharynx. Some patients appear to have a trigger zone in the pharynx, and the paroxysms are initiated by swallowing. The pain may occur at night and is of such severity that the patient bolts out of bed.[36] The pathophysiology underlying glossopharyngeal neuralgia is analogous to that for trigeminal neuralgia, and thus the treatment is basically the same; however, medical therapy is less successful.

**Idiopathic stabbing headache.** Ice pick–like pain is a benign syndrome that consists of lancinating, momentary, shooting pain.[37] It can occur anywhere in the head, as well as within the eye. These pains are infrequent, can occur in groups or as single shocks, and are not associated with any known disease. This syndrome has been reported to be more frequent in migraineurs. A typical history of momentary, lancinating pains supported by a negative examination precludes the need for further diagnostic evaluation. Recognition of this syndrome is important, since it frightens both patient and physician who are not aware of its benignity.[38]

**Giant cell arteritis.** The onset of headaches in a patient over the age of 55 should alert the clinician to the possibility that the patient has giant cell arteritis. In the more typical form these headaches are generally localized over areas of inflammatory involvement of the temporal arteries or its branches, which may be associated with nodular excrescences.

Often these patients do not complain of headache but are aware of scalp tenderness exacerbated by combing or brushing their hair, wearing a hat, or leaning their head on a pillow or chair. Accompanying symptoms may include jaw claudication with chewing or talking, and polymyalgia rheumatica. The concomitant or sequential development of sudden visual loss or diplopia in an elderly patient helps make the diagnosis obvious. An immediate Westergren erythrocyte sedimentation rate followed by the administration of systemic corticosteroids is indicated in these patients. (See Chapter 9.)

**"Thunderclap" headache.** Apoplectic excruciating headache, depressed consciousness, and signs of meningeal irritation are diagnostic of subarachnoid hemorrhage. Similar headaches without neurologic signs have been reported.[39,40] Some have suggested that they represent migraine precursors and that they are benign. Our feeling, and that of others,[41-43] is that in such cases aneurysm must be excluded.

**"Exploding" headache.** A small group of elderly patients will be awakened from sleep by loud bangs in their head often accompanied by a flash of light. On awakening they are in a cold sweat accompanied by labored breathing and tachycardia. This event was first reported 100 years ago and was referred to as "sensory shocks."[44,45] It is a benign occurrence, but subarachnoid hemorrhage must always be excluded.

## HEADACHES ASSOCIATED WITH AN OBVIOUS EXOGENOUS TRIGGER MECHANISM

**"Ice cream" headache.** When eating or drinking extremely cold substances, certain patients develop a sharp, deep pain in the periocular and frontal region. This pain abates gradually over a period of 20 to 60 seconds. It arises from applying the cold substances to the roof of the mouth (palate) and not to the esophagus or stomach, thus representing referred pain from one area subserved by the fifth cranial nerve to another. This syndrome is benign.

**Dietary headache.** Some headaches are clearly associated with the ingestion of certain foods or abuse of certain medications, such as butalbital, aspirin, and caffeine (BAC).[46] The exclusion of certain substances from the diet after prolonged daily use (such as caffeine) can also produce headaches. Nitrite or nitrate compounds, which are used as additives or preservatives in certain foods, are potent vasodilating agents, and they can induce vascular headaches in susceptible individuals.[47] These additives are found in smoked fish and in preserved meats such as bologna, sausage, salami, and frankfurters. Similarly, after ingesting nitroglycerin for angina pectoris, patients often develop a headache within minutes to an hour, often lasting about 20 minutes.

Monosodium glutamate is another food additive that can trigger vascular headaches in susceptible individuals, either immediately following ingestion (20 to 30 minutes) or 12 to 18 hours later. Some of these individuals also experience bloating and peripheral edema. Monosodium glutamate is used as a flavoring agent in freshly prepared oriental dishes and as an additive in instant and canned soups, potato chips, dry-roasted nuts, processed meats, and TV dinners. The headache is severe and is typically throbbing. It often responds to analgesic combinations containing a fast-acting barbiturate and caffeine (BAC).

The post-alcohol or "hangover" headache occurs the morning after the consumption of alcoholic beverages to excess. This headache has a generalized throbbing quality that increases in intensity with exertion. It is often accompanied by nausea and vomiting. Aspirin or acetaminophen compounds containing caffeine are effective in easing the head pain.

Alcohol in minimal amounts may act as a trigger in certain patients who have either cluster or migraine headaches. In those patients with cluster headache, alcohol acts as a trigger only during the cluster phase (see earlier under Cluster Headache).

Individuals who have ingested caffeine in coffee, tea, cola, or medications on a daily basis predictably develop a headache if they suddenly discontinue the use of this substance.[48] These people become irritable and initially experience a generalized dull aching headache that may, with time, develop into either a throbbing headache or a muscle contraction–type headache. These headaches are relieved by ingestion of caffeine or mild analgesics without caffeine. Continued abstinence for 3 to 5 days is also curative.

**Altitude headache.** Altitude headaches occur in individuals who travel directly from sea level to 8000 feet or above. The headache is usually delayed in onset and may be accompanied by other symptoms of mountain sickness, including nausea, vomiting, and shortness of breath. Altitude headache is throbbing and usually generalized but frequently is more severe frontally. These patients are often most comfortable when they are active. Evidence indicates that mountain sickness can be prevented by the prophylactic use of acetazolamide[49] (250 mg four times a day) for 3 days prior to and during the period of high-altitude exposure.

**Posttraumatic headache.** The complaint of headache or neck pain following direct or indirect (whiplash) head trauma is common. Headache is just one symptom of the posttraumatic syndrome, which includes dizziness, insomnia, concentration difficulties, and mood and personality changes. These patients complain of prolonged localized tenderness of muscle groups, splinting, and typical muscle contraction headaches. The diagnosis of posttraumatic headache is made on the basis of the history and by excluding organic structural damage. Despite improved diagnostic techniques, the mechanism of persistent posttraumatic headaches remains an enigma. Effective treatment of these patients includes the use of analgesics, sedatives, and tricyclic antidepressants, as well as physiotherapy and psychotherapy.

Persistent headache following mild to moderate head trauma suggests a chronic subdural hematoma. We believe all such patients deserve imaging studies.

**Low intracranial pressure headache.** Headaches due to decreased cerebrospinal fluid (CSF) pressure generally follow lumbar puncture but also occur in cases of spontaneous or traumatic CSF rhinorrhea. These headaches are positional, being induced by sitting or standing and relieved by lying down. The approach to a patient with persistent CSF rhinorrhea and headache necessitates pa-

**Sources of Asthenopia**

I. Uncorrected refractive errors
   A. Hyperopia
   B. Presbyopia
II. Acquisition of new glasses
   A. With appropriate prescription
      1. Initial correction of an astigmatic error
      2. Induced heterophorias
      3. Change in accommodative or vergence requirements as a result of the glasses
   B. With inappropriate prescription
      1. Incorrect refraction or filling of the prescription
      2. Induced heterophoria: horizontal or vertical misplacement of optical center
      3. Change in base curve
         a. Reflective changes, eikonic changes
         b. Change in speed of movement of objects across the retina
III. Heterophorias
IV. No identifiable cause

tience. If therapeutic intervention is believed to be warranted, nucleotide localization of the leaking area can be followed by surgery. Persistent headache following lumbar puncture may require a blood patch.[50,51]

**Asthenopia.** Asthenopia is the ocular and periocular discomfort associated with prolonged ocular use (usually for near visual tasks). The initial symptom is usually a feeling of lid heaviness, which gradually progresses to a feeling of somnolence. The eyes feel "tired," hot, or uncomfortable, and some relief may be obtained by rubbing the eyes or discontinuing the ocular task. If the work is continued, the vague discomfort may give rise to an aching feeling of the eyes and the development of various headache symptoms (e.g., brow ache, temporal pain, or neck tenderness).[52,53]

Initially the headache tends to be described as a brow ache that with continued ocular use becomes more generalized. Occasionally patients complain of frontal, temporal, or occipital discomfort. Ultimately these patients may develop a severe muscle contraction or combined muscle contraction–throbbing headache with neck and shoulder discomfort. Late in the evolution of the syndrome, associated visceral symptoms, such as nausea, are not unusual. The symptom complex of lid heaviness, sleepiness, ocular discomfort, and headache is generally referred to as eyestrain.

Among the many causes of eyestrain (see box) is the presence of uncorrected refractive errors, such as hyperopia (including presbyopia) and heterophoria. The clinical syndrome can be reproduced experimentally with the use of myopic lenses in emmetropic individuals.[54] Uncorrected myopia does not produce asthenopia.

One of the most frequent causes of asthenopia is the prescription of new glasses. Eyestrain can occur whether the correction is appropriate or inappropriate. In the former case, prescribing a cylindric correction for the first time or altering the power or axis of a previously prescribed refraction induces the asthenopic symptoms. In the correction of anisometropia, a substantial difference in the refractive error of each eye may also produce asthenopia. A small group of these patients will have *aniseikonia*, a difference in the retinal image size perceived by each eye. The discomfort can be alleviated by an eikonic correction. A significant increase in myopic correction or hyperopic correction, either distance or reading addition, can produce a change in the accommodative and vergence requirements, resulting in asthenopia.

The prescription of an inappropriate refractive correction (e.g., excessive minus sphere or a cylinder correction at the wrong axis) also can cause asthenopia. Similarly, a change in the base curve of the corrective lenses in a myopic individual almost always induces asthenopia. In patients with high refractive corrections, horizontal or vertical misplacement of the optical center of a corrective lens can induce a heterophoria and thus asthenopia. In all these cases symptoms begin after a new spectacle correction is worn.

Although experimentally[54] the induction of heterophorias has inconsistently produced asthenopia, little doubt exists clinically that in some individuals heterophoria is associated with asthenopia.[55] Patients with heterophorias obtain binocular vision by maintaining an appropriate distribution of tone to the extraocular muscles by using various fusional mechanisms. Burian and von Noorden[55] state that the appearance of symptoms depends on the individual's sensorimotor state and not on the absolute amount of heterophoric deviation; that is, "what matters is the presence or absence of a discrepancy between the deviation and the amplitudes of motor fusion." Asthenopia often occurs in patients in whom a latent vertical deviation begins to break down and become manifest. Examples are congenital superior oblique palsy and convergence insufficiency as an aftermath of a serious systemic illness in patients with normal vergence amplitudes.

A certain number of individuals have no identifiable cause of the asthenopia. Since the treatment of asthenopia requires identifying an inducing factor, for patients in whom such evidence is lacking, the examiner must investigate situational, emotional, or psychiatric factors contributing to the symptoms. The correction of asthenopia may require spectacles of various types, including bifocals and prisms, replacement of inappropriate refractive corrections, and, rarely, eye muscle surgery. Orthoptic training has been variably effective in treating convergence insufficiency.

**Headache associated with sexual activity.** The distinctive occurrence of coital headache and the psychologic stress it imposes necessitates calling attention to this underreported event.[56,57] Some believe it to be a form of migraine. It is more common in men. Most often (70% of cases) the headache is explosive, of a throbbing quality, and begins at or shortly before orgasm. It persists for minutes to a few hours and may be associated with a confused state. It may be associated with stroke.[7,58] The question of how to evaluate such a patient should be dictated by the presence of neurologic signs. Propranolol and indomethacin are effective prophylactically in approximately 80% of cases.[7]

# HEADACHES RECOGNIZED BY PHYSICAL FEATURES AND ASSOCIATED WITH OTHER DISEASE STATES

**HERPETIC NEURALGIA.** The pain of herpes zoster is described as being steady and severe with a burning and aching quality. The pain is in the distribution of a given dermatome, usually the first division of the fifth cranial nerve, although it may involve the seventh nerve (external ear) with ipsilateral facial palsy (Ramsay Hunt syndrome.)[59] The pain precedes the onset of the typical rash by 4 to 7 days, and during this period the diagnosis cannot be made. The patient may be febrile during the prodromal period. The typical herpetiform lesion is associated with hyperalgesia and paresthesias, and later examinations often show hypoesthesia and paresthesias in the involved areas. The patient may develop a concurrent ipsilateral keratouveitis. Although some have stated that keratouveitis is more common if the nasociliary branch of the frontal division is involved, in our experience this finding is not consistent. During the acute phase the judicious use of analgesics of varying strengths is necessary.

Although the pain usually regresses within a week or two, it may persist for months or years, especially in the elderly. The overall incidence of postherpetic neuralgia is 10%,[60,61] but the incidence increases with age (75% > 70 years).[62] In the postherpetic phase dysesthesias such as crawling and pricking sensations become prominent. These sensory experiences are often exacerbated by pressure on the involved skin, as from wearing eyeglasses. These patients are often so distracted by dysesthesia that they are unable to be productive. Amitriptyline is effective in alleviating the discomfort in about 50% of patients.[63,64] Some patients have a therapeutic window, which must be reached by titration.[64] Others of the tricyclics may also be effective.

The use of additional agents such as valproic acid or fluphenazine may provide symptomatic relief in patients with resistant pain.[63] The topical application of capsaicin ointment may also be effective.[61] This ointment should not be used until the rash has cleared.

Although preliminary observation suggested that systemic corticosteroids[65] prescribed during the eruptive phase may prevent the development of postherpetic neuralgia, more recent data[66] have demonstrated that they are ineffective. Acyclovir has been recommended as being useful in preventing postherpetic neuralgia, but the available data would belie this conclusion.[60,61]

**SINUS DISEASE.** The headache of nasal and paranasal sinus disease is usually described as being dull, aching, and constant, with tenderness almost universally found over the involved sinus. These headaches are generally aggravated by changes in atmospheric pressure. The headache of frontal sinus disease is generally located in the frontal region and is commonly present on awakening and becomes less severe as the day goes on. The pain of sphenoid and ethmoid sinus disease is localized behind the eyes and over the vertex of the head. Maxillary sinus pain has a bandlike distribution below the eye, extending laterally over the temporal region. This headache usually starts in the early afternoon and becomes progressively worse toward the evening. Chronic sinus headaches can induce a superimposed muscle contraction–type headache. A history of allergies, chronic upper respiratory tract infections, or sensitivity to changes in atmospheric pressure (flying, diving) should provide the clue to order appropriate imaging studies and to refer the patient to an otolaryngologist.

**DENTAL DISEASE.** The pain experienced with dental disease is exquisitely localized to the disease area and has a burning and aching quality. The pain may be induced or exacerbated by chewing or exposure to hot or cold foods. With a prolonged toothache, remote pain described as having an aching quality and often mimicking a muscle contraction headache can develop.

**TEMPOROMANDIBULAR JOINT PAIN.** Degenerative disease of the temporomandibular joint can irritate the auriculotemporal nerve and chorda tympani nerves, inducing a characteristic pain syndrome.[67,68] This syndrome is usually seen in middle-aged or elderly adults and is described as an aching, steady pain that increases in severity from morning to evening. The accompanying headache may involve the vertex, occiput, and supraorbital regions. Because the pain is distributed over the vertex and occiput, the diagnosis often is overlooked. Many of these patients develop a secondary muscle contraction headache.

**FEVER.** The headache associated with fever accompanying systemic disease is usually dull, deep, aching, and generalized. It is often worse in the back of the head. The headache is exacerbated by standing and exertion.

**ARTERIAL HYPERTENSION.** Headaches associated with elevation of systemic blood pressure may be divided into those associated with an acute rise in blood pressure and those associated with essential hypertension, in which the incidence of muscle contraction and migraine headaches is also increased.[48,69]

    **Sudden rise in blood pressure.** The systemic arterial pressure often rises at times of violent exercise, sexual excitement, or anger. Similar acute elevations can be produced by the secretion of vasoactive substances by a pheochromocytoma or the ingestion of tyramine by patients using monoamine oxidase inhibitors. These headaches have a sudden onset and are excruciating and throbbing in nature. They are generally bilateral. The duration of the headache parallels the duration of the acute elevation in blood pressure, usually lasting less than 15 minutes.

    **Essential hypertension.** Headaches associated with essential hypertension are dull, diffuse, and of a deep aching nature. They are usually intermittent and characteristically throb at the onset. Patients are commonly awakened in the early hours of the morning with a generalized headache that is somewhat relieved by sitting up. These headaches are exacerbated by any activity that produces a Valsalva maneuver. They often may be complicated by the development of superimposed muscle contraction or migraine headaches.

**CENTRAL NERVOUS SYSTEM DISEASE**

    **Raised intracranial pressure.** Headache may be a feature of increased intracranial pressure (ICP) whether the increase is due to a mass lesion or to an alteration of CSF dynamics. No direct correlation exists between the severity of the headache and the absolute level of CSF pressure. Dalessio[48] states that the headaches associated with raised ICP are due either to traction on or displacement of pain-sensitive intracranial structures. Northfield[70] suggests that the headache is produced by sudden alterations in pressure. Neither explanation is totally satisfactory.

Headaches associated with raised ICP are deep and boring and frequently tend to be worse in the early morning. They may be associated with vomiting, which is often projectile in nature because it is unaccompanied by nausea and is therefore unexpected. These headaches are aggravated by any activity that includes a Valsalva maneuver. Cataclysmic onset of headache with relatively spontaneous immediate relief suggests a ball-valve effect.

**Coughing.** Following coughing, bending, or exercise, headache that may be severe and last for seconds to minutes can be experienced. Although 10% of such patients will have an intracranial disorder or skeletal anomaly, the vast majority have a benign syndrome.[71] All such patients should have an imaging study. In those patients with no intracranial pathology, the paroxysms tend to disappear spontaneously within a few years and are indomethacin responsive.[14]

**Raeder's syndrome.** Grimson and Thompson[72] have defined Raeder's syndrome as a headache accompanied by postganglionic Horner's syndrome. Essentially two types of Raeder's syndrome exist[73]: type 1 Raeder's syndrome, in which cranial nerve involvement is present, and type 2 Raeder's syndrome, in which cranial nerves are not involved. We have extracted cluster headache from this latter group because of its stereotyped clinical course.

*Type 1 Raeder's syndrome* includes patients with lesions involving multiple parasellar cranial nerves (cranial nerves III, IV, V, and VI). In the face of such a symptom complex, an MRI scan should be obtained to rule out parasellar mass lesions such as pituitary adenomas, chordomas, meningiomas, internal carotid artery aneurysms, or intracranial spread of sinus or nasopharyngeal tumors.

*Type 2 Raeder's syndrome* includes patients in whom neurologic involvement is limited to pain in the ophthalmic division of the trigeminal nerve associated with postganglionic Horner's syndrome. The headache is variable in duration, lasting for hours or days, or it may be continuous over weeks to months with exacerbations in intensity. It is often periocular in location. These headaches usually occur in middle-aged men and resolve spontaneously.

If the headaches are persistent, or if the patient gives a history of neck trauma, including chiropractic manipulation, the possibility of a dissecting aneurysm of the carotid artery in the neck should be considered. In the face of ischemic symptoms (e.g., neuropathy of the ninth or twelfth cranial nerves; dysgusia may be an accompanying symptom), arteriography may be indicated. Some investigators believe that anticoagulation with heparin followed by coumadin is efficacious in treating dissecting aneurysm.[74]

**OCULAR INFLAMMATION.** The cornea and conjunctiva are richly endowed with pain-sensitive nerve endings. Minor inflammatory diseases or irritative phenomena (e.g., an exposed suture, foreign body in the cul-de-sac or on the cornea) may produce a constant foreign body sensation. With time this can cause the development of deep-seated frontal or fronto-occipital headaches that may mimic muscle contraction headaches. More severe corneal dysfunction such as occurs with "overwear syndrome" in contact lens patients, ultraviolet keratitis (welder's keratitis, sunlamp or solar exposure), or bullous keratopathy produces intense ocular discomfort that slowly spreads to become a generalized headache if the primary process continues unabated for some time. Corneal ulceration of almost any type produces ocular pain and headache with the exception of those cases in which corneal sensation is decreased.

Inflammatory disease of the iris and ciliary body is associated with an almost continuous, deep, aching sensation exacerbated by ocular use and accompanied by true photophobia or pain on exposure to light.[75] Acute angle-closure glaucoma and some secondary angle-closure glaucomas can also produce severe acute monocular pain associated with nausea and vomiting. If the attack remains untreated, a severe generalized headache develops with time. The diagnosis of ocular pain or headaches due to ocular pathology is usually obvious and easily made during the history and physical examination.

**OCULAR ISCHEMIA.** Orbital or ocular ischemia secondary to occlusive artery disease or to temporal or Takayasu's arteritis may cause periocular or retrobulbar pain and headache. This ocular ischemic syndrome can include such diverse signs as conjunctival injection, anterior segment ischemia with cell and flare, rubeosis iridis, and hypotony, as well as an ischemic retinopathy and optic neuropathy. Patients with this syndrome may complain of decreased vision in bright light.[76] (See Chapter 5.)

# Nondistinctive Headache Syndromes

A group of unrelated headache syndromes that are not clearly definable remains. Some of these headaches constitute atypical variants of characteristic headache syndromes (see box on p. 419).

## MIGRAINE WITHOUT AURA

**EPIDEMIOLOGY.** Although migraine with aura is a distinctive syndrome, migraine without aura, which makes up 80% of all migraine headaches, is not. The borders between all the varieties of migraine are not distinct. Migraine overall affects 15% to 19% of men and 25% to 29% of women.[77] Fifty percent of migraine attacks begin before age 20; 13% begin before age 10.[78] Although the onset of migraine in middle-aged individuals over age 45 is not rare, the diagnosis should be made without investigation only when the syndrome is stereotypically classical. While migraine is generally agreed to be genetically determined, the exact mode of inheritance has not been clearly defined. Familial incidence has been estimated at between 65% and 90%[21]; thus a family history of migraine may help secure the diagnosis of migraine headache in patients with nonclassic presentation.

Evidence supports that the underlying cause of migraine is an inherited disorder of platelet aggregation.[79-83] Platelets contain all of the serotonin (5-hydroxytryptamine) present in the blood. During aggregation, platelets release serotonin, adenosine diphosphate (ADP), and adenosine triphosphate (ATP), all of which are thought to play a role in control of the tone of cerebral vessels.[81] Abnormalities of platelet metabolism can be correlated with ultrastructural abnormalities.[84] In addition, in patients with oral contraceptive–induced migraine, a reversible change in platelet response to serotonin-induced platelet aggregation has been demonstrated.[85]

Platelet aggregation substantially increases during the preheadache phase of migraine, paralleling the increase in plasma serotonin. Platelets of migraine patients have been shown to (1) be hyperaggregable and demonstrate increased stickiness to ADP induction,[79] (2) have a decrease in platelet monoamine oxidase activity during attacks,[30,85] and (3) have higher spontaneous aggregation and adhesion during the headache-free period and a decreased serotonin release and mild deficit in serotonin uptake for 3 days following an attack.[81] These findings suggest a role for platelet antiaggregants in the prophylaxis of migraine.[86] Raskin[7] invokes a theory of serotoninergic dysfunction with perturbation of underlying serotoninergic tone.

Much has been made of the so-called migraine personality. The migraine patient has been described as compulsive, overconscientious, ambitious, and highly intelligent. No psychologic studies using appropriate control groups to substantiate this description have been published.[21] If a relationship to stress does exist, migraine tends to occur after the stressful situation is over (in a period of letdown, such as on weekends or during the first few days of vacation).

Migraine attacks, especially without aura, seem to be related to hormonal changes in women. Migraine headaches have been induced de novo or increased in severity in women who begin taking oral contraceptive pills.[2] These women appear to be at increased risk of developing cerebrovascular accidents.[87] Similar exacerbations of migraine are noted during periods of endogenous hormonal change, such as puberty, menstruation, ovulation, pregnancy, and menopause. The converse may also be true, with a decrease in headaches being associated with pregnancy and menopause.

Some patients with migraine can have headaches triggered by food substances containing tyramine or phenylalanine, such as aged cheeses, chocolate, yogurt, and buttermilk. In others the ingestion of red wines or a reduction in caffeine intake can act as a trigger. Dietary factors are probably not important in more than a few patients with migraine.[88] The literature contains two cases in which nonmigraineurs received bone marrow transplants from HLA-matched relatives who suffered from migraine.[89] The patients not only developed migraine, but developed a sensitivity to red wine as an inducing agent as well. In these cases a platelet hypothesis seems more plausible than a perturbation of a serotoninergic tone and speaks for an inherited susceptibility. When specifically questioned, patients with migraine may report stripe-induced visual discomfort (82%).[90] This aversive reaction makes it difficult for individuals to read certain magazines or newspapers.

**CLINICAL PRESENTATION.** The prodromal phase of migraine without aura is not well defined.[17] The aural phase may precede the onset of headache by hours or days and take many forms, including mood disorders, gastrointestinal distress, fatigue, and changes in fluid balance, especially in women. Occasional patients may experience an olfactory hallucination sometime preceding the headache, suggesting temporal lobe seizure activity. The headache may last for many hours to several days and is described as a pulsating pain, which may be either unilateral or generalized but in the latter case is usually more severe on one side. Other symptoms include anorexia, nausea and vomiting, and a desire to avoid light and noise, which seem to exacerbate the pain. Occasionally patients may experience a diuretic phase with polyuria if fluid retention is part of the prodrome. Patients with migraine without aura may occasionally experience attacks with aura.

Migraine without aura is often exacerbated by the onset of depression. Depressive patients also often have muscle contraction–type headaches. Thus in this group of patients, the onset of a migraine headache may induce a superimposed muscle contraction headache; the converse is also true, producing a combined-type headache symptom complex.

In migraineurs with active systemic lupus erythematosus, the headaches seem to occur with increased frequency.[91] Although an association of migraine in patients with so called low-tension glaucoma has been implied,[92] we believe that the evidence for this relationship is extremely poor.

## MIGRAINE EQUIVALENTS

The aura of migraine may occur without headache, in which case it is called a migraine equivalent or acephalgic migraine. Similarly, car sickness and periodic abdominal pain are considered by some to represent migraine equivalents in children.[93,94] The presence of a history of or symptoms of car sickness in an adult with the recent onset of headaches or sensory disturbances is diagnostically helpful. Periodic diarrhea, fever, and mood changes in children and adults in an inappropriate clinical setting are considered to represent migraine equivalents.

The occurrence of migraine scotomas without pain was first described by Gowers.[95] O'Connor and Tredici[96] reported 61 such patients, whose age range was 21 to 61 years, with the number of attacks in an individual varying between 1 and 100 and the attacks lasting from 15 minutes to 3 hours. Visual symptoms included scintillating scotomas, transient hemianopia, amaurosis fugax, altitudinal field loss, tunnel vision, temporal crescent loss, unilateral central scotoma with alteration in color perception, and diplopia. Other neurologic symptoms and signs included paresthesias, dysphasia, difficulty with mentation, dysarthria, and vertigo, which occurred in 29% of their patients. A positive family history of migraine was present in only 24%.

Fisher[97] has documented the onset of unexplained transient cerebral dysfunction in 120 patients over the age of 40, all of whom had normal cerebral angiograms and no evidence of epilepsy. He believes these transient episodes are best explained as neurologic accompaniments to migraine. The symptoms included scintillating scotomas, blurred vision, homonymous field defects, and blindness in isolation or accompanied by paresthesias, speech disturbances, or brainstem symptoms. Fifty percent of these patients had accompanying, nondescript headaches. The diagnosis of migraine can be made without angiography when the buildup and migration of visual scintillations, the march of the paresthesias, and the orderly change from one accompaniment to another are present. These attacks tend to be recurrent and without sequelae.

## RETINOCILIARY MIGRAINE

Tippin et al.[98] reviewed the records of 83 patients with atypical amaurosis with or without ocular infarction under age 45. The visual complaints were atypical in that the onset was gradual in 58% and not classically "window shade" in evolution. Cerebral transient ischemic attacks had occurred in 21% of these patients. Headache or orbital pain was a prominent associated symptom in 41% of patients, and another 25% had severe headaches at times not associated with visual loss. Of 42 patients followed for a mean of 5.8 years, none developed a stroke. These authors concluded that amaurosis fugax in younger patients has a more benign clinical course than that found in an older population and that migraine is the likely underlying cause.

We believe that most bouts of transient visual loss in young individuals are probably migrainous in origin but also that in this circumstance migraine must be a diagnosis of exclusion (see Chapter 5). Kline and Kelly,[99] as well as Kline and Glaser,[100] have witnessed attacks of so-called ocular migraine in which patients have lost vision in one eye either instantaneously or with progressive peripheral contraction (similar to visual loss from hypoperfusion) of their visual field. These patients had an associated amaurotic pupil and an absent visually evoked response. Ophthalmoscopic examination revealed an isolated narrowing of the retinal veins. In addition, arteriolar narrowing, segmentation of the blood column, and optic disc pallor can be seen (Fig. 16-1). Fluorescein angiography revealed delayed filling of the central retinal artery circulation. Similarly, ophthalmic artery hypoperfusion has been reported in the same setting with delayed filling of the entire ocular vascular bed, including the disc.[101,102]

## CHILDHOOD MIGRAINE

Migraine is the most common cause of periodic headaches in childhood. Although similar to those that occur in the adult, these headaches tend to be generalized and shorter in duration and often are associated with more severe visceral symptomatology.

The treatment of migraine is discussed in the Appendix at the end of this chapter.

## TENSION-TYPE HEADACHES

**ACUTE MUSCLE CONTRACTION HEADACHE.** Acute muscle contraction headache, the most frequent type of headache (90% of all headaches[103]), commonly occurs during periods of emotional or physical stress. It is produced by sustained contraction of the neck and scalp muscles. The pain is usually dull and

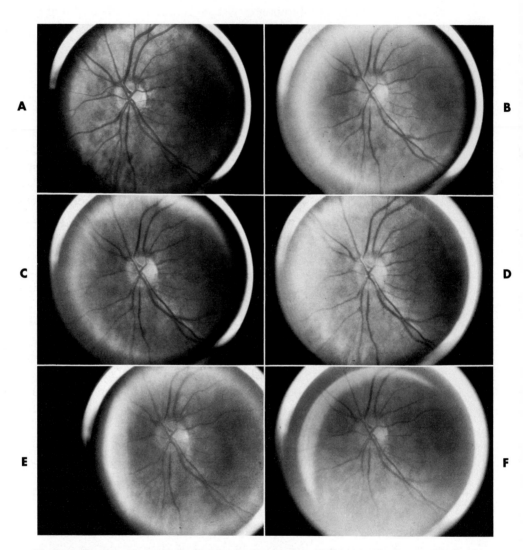

*Fig. 16-1.* Fundus photographs demonstrating sequence of events during an attack of retinal migraine. **A,** Normal vision control fundus. **B,** Total amaurosis (patient describes this as a "tan out" or "like grease covering a surface"—about 8 minutes into the attack): decreased venous caliber, slight decrease in arteriolar diameter. **C, D,** and **E,** Attack continues unabated for about 7 to 8 minutes. **F,** Vision begins to return with "breaking up of the grease"; no apparent change in fundus.

nonthrobbing, with tenderness and knotting noted in the strap muscles of the neck. This type of headache may be superimposed on almost any other type of headache and can act as a trigger for vascular headaches in susceptible patients. It is treated most effectively with analgesics in combination with a fast-acting barbiturate, although simple analgesics eventually relieve the pain.

**CHRONIC MUSCLE CONTRACTION HEADACHE.** Chronic muscle contraction headaches are characterized by feelings of tightness, bands, head-in-a-vise, caps of pressure, or crawling sensations associated with knotting and tenderness of the neck muscles. The pain may last for days, weeks, months, or years and is present on awakening. The patients often complain of temporal and masseter discomfort secondary to bruxism. Occasionally these people may develop symptoms of a superimposed vascular headache including intolerance to light and sound, nausea and vomiting, and an exacerbation of the pain with a throbbing quality.

Most patients with chronic muscle contraction headache tend to be anxious and depressed. In fact, depression can be considered to be a hallmark of this syndrome. A headache that has been present for years without a change in character may be considered to be benign; however, any change in the character of the headache requires excluding the presence of organic pathology. The diagnostic workup depends on the history and signs noted on physical examination.

Although these patients are difficult to treat because of their tendency to abuse medication, gratifying success has been found with the use of tricyclic antidepressants. Often as little as 10 to 25 mg of amitriptyline at bedtime may break the chronic cycle.

## OCULAR NEUROSIS

Some patients complain of ocular symptoms with or without pain. These patients may state that they are unable to glance at print, drive, or be out in the sun without developing severe ocular pain. Such patients may also complain of being unable to read for more than a short period without resting. Careful examination will fail to reveal any ocular or neurologic pathology. As a group these patients are resistant to therapy.

## ATYPICAL FACIAL PAIN

Atypical facial pain is a unilateral pain syndrome that does not localize to a particular division of the fifth or ninth cranial nerve. It is likely to involve the entire side of the head and face and extend into the neck. Unlike "tic," this pain is not paroxysmal in nature; it tends to be constant and of long duration. The pain is often described as aching or burning and of such intensity that the patient cannot function. These patients do not complain of paresthesias, and no neurologic findings are evident. This diagnosis can be made only by excluding a malignancy involving contiguous structures. Atypical facial pain syndromes are resistant to treatment, often requiring the constant use of narcotic agents. These patients are unlikely to have spontaneous remissions.

Evidence indicates that patients with atypical facial pain may develop psychologic dependence on their pain.[104] Despite a report on the efficacy of psychoactive agents,[105] most of these patients require a multidisciplinary approach offered by "pain clinics."

## GREATER OCCIPITAL NEURALGIA

In some patients who complain of chronic periocular or retro-ocular pain, examination reveals a point of exquisite tenderness between the mastoid process and the occipital protuberance. Relief of pain by local infiltration of lidocaine into the area of point tenderness is diagnostic. Permanent pain relief[106,107] has been claimed with subsequent local injections of depocorticosteroids. The pain is believed to be due to traumatic irritation and inflammation of the greater occipital nerve as it pierces the tendinous insertion of the splenius capitis at the base of the skull. The retro-orbital and periocular pain is considered to be referred pain in the distribution of the trigeminal nerve. An overflow of impulses from the fascicles of C2 as it enters the cord to ascend and descend in the dorsal spinothalamic tract is believed to trigger activity in the spinal root of the trigeminal nerve. These patients frequently develop superimposed muscle contraction–type headaches.

A similar headache syndrome consisting of chronic occipital or suboccipital pain with radiation of pain to the orbit or forehead can be experienced by patients with osteoarthritis of the C2-C3 zygapophyseal joint.[108] Entrapment of the superficial medial branch of the third cervical nerve is considered to be causative, and relief of pain by an anesthetic block in the C2-C3 joint is considered diagnostic. Unfortunately, no recommended therapeutic approach has been totally successful.

# Appendix

## TREATMENT OF MIGRAINE HEADACHE

Treatment of migraine can be divided into two major categories: abortive (once the attack has begun) and prophylactic.

**ABORTIVE TREATMENT.** The treatment of migraine attack, once it has begun, may include a variety of analgesic, sedative, or specific vasoactive substances (Table 16-1).

Simple analgesics such as aspirin or acetaminophen, either alone or in combination with phenacetin and caffeine, should be tried first, but most often these drugs are ineffective. A combination of a fast-acting barbiturate, caffeine, and aspirin (Fiorinal) or acetaminophen (Fioricet) is extremely effective, especially in cases in which a muscle-contraction component serves as a trigger mechanism. These drugs should be prescribed in a dose of two capsules every 4 to 6 hours, not to exceed six capsules in a 24-hour period. This combination of drugs is habit forming and, if abused, can cause a chronic headache syndrome.[46] These compounds may be prescribed with codeine as a single prescription.

**TABLE 16-1**    *Treatment of Migraine (Acute Attack) in Adults*

| Drug | Generic composition | Dosage |
|---|---|---|
| Analgesics | | |
|   Aspirin | — | 2 tablets every 4-6 hours as needed |
|   Acetaminophen | — | 2 tablets every 4-6 hours as needed |
|   Aspirin or acetaminophen combined with 30 or 60 mg codeine | — | 2 tablets every 4-6 hours as needed |
|   Fiorinal | Butalbital<br>Aspirin<br>Caffeine | 2 tablets every 4-6 hours as needed; not to exceed 6 tablets in 24 hours |
|   Fioricet | Butalbital<br>Caffeine<br>Acetaminophen | 2 tablets every 4-6 hours as needed; not to exceed 6 tablets in 24 hours |
| Nonsteroidal antiinflammatory agents | | |
|   Motrin | Ibuprofen | 400-600 mg every 4-6 hours as needed |
|   Dolobid | Diflunisal | 500 mg every 6-12 hours as needed |
|   Naprosyn | Naproxen | 250-500 mg every 4-6 hours as needed |
| Vasoactive compounds | | |
|   Gynergen | 1 mg ergotamine tartrate | 2 tablets initially; then 1 tablet every 30 minutes; not to exceed 6 tablets in 24 hours or 10 tablets in 1 week |
| | 0.50 mg/ml ergotamine tartrate | 0.5 subcutaneously or intramuscularly; repeat every 40-60 minutes; not to exceed 2 ml in 1 week |
|   Cafergot | 1 mg ergotamine tartrate<br>100 mg caffeine | 2 tablets initially; then 1 tablet every 30 minutes; not to exceed 6 tablets in 24 hours or 10 tablets in 1 week |
|   Cafergot-PB | 1 mg ergotamine tartrate<br>100 mg caffeine<br>0.125 mg belladonna alkaloid | 2 tablets initially; then 1 tablet every 30 minutes; not to exceed 6 tablets in 24 hours or 10 tablets in 1 week |
|   Cafergot-PB suppositories | 2 mg ergotamine tartrate<br>100 mg caffeine<br>30 mg phenobarbital<br>0.125 belladonna alkaloid | Rectally; 1 suppository initially and in 1 hour; not to exceed 10 in 1 week |
|   Ergomar | 2.0 mg ergotamine tartrate | 1 tablet sublingually at onset; then 1 tablet every 30 minutes to a total of 3; not to exceed 10 in 1 week |
|   Medihaler-Ergotamine aerosol | 9.0 mg/ml ergotamine tartrate | Single inhalation at onset to be repeated in 5 minutes as needed; not to exceed 6 inhalations in 24 hours |
|   Midrin | 65 mg isometheptene mucate<br>100 mg dichloralphenazone<br>325 mg acetaminophen | 2 tablets every 4 hours; not to exceed 8 tablets in 24 hours |
| Antiemetics | | |
|   Reglan | 65 mg metoclopramide hydrochloride | Tablets or injectable |
|   Compazine | 25 mg prochlorperazine | Rectally; 1 suppository every 12 hours |

The chronic use of compounds containing phenacetin should be avoided, since this drug may cause renal failure. Various nonsteroidal antiinflammatory agents such as ibuprofen, disulfanyl, and naproxen have been shown to be effective, especially in women who experience exacerbation in the migraine syndrome in the premenstrual period.

If these nonspecific analgesic drugs do not relieve the headache, the vasoactive ergotamine derivatives should be prescribed. These agents have an effect both directly on vascular muscle as well as on central serotoninergic tone. With respect to vascular tone, they have both alpha-adrenergic agonist and alpha-adrenergic antagonist activity, a beta-adrenergic blocking effect, and a direct effect on smooth muscle. Thus their vascular action would seem to depend on the vasomotor tone present at the time of treatment; that is, those arteries that are constricted tend to dilate, and vice versa.[109]

The ergotamine compounds are absorbed rapidly and completely after parenteral administration but are poorly absorbed orally and sublingually. The poor absorption of sublingual preparations is partly explained by variation in the oral pH of the individual being treated. The decreased absorption of the oral compounds is caused by the action of the drug, which reduces the gastric motility, and by the effects of nausea and induced vomiting that accompany the migraine attack itself. Most commonly used antiemetic agents are not effective in treating the nausea and vomiting associated with a migraine attack. Metoclopramide[110] has been shown to be an effective agent for this purpose. A potent antiemetic, this drug increases gastric motility and therefore increases absorption of antimigraine medication, as well as having intrinsic antimigraine activity. Caffeine has been known for years to increase the absorption of ergotamine compounds.

Ergotamine tartrate and caffeine, and ergotamine tartrate, caffeine, belladonna alkaloids, and phenobarbital in tablet or suppository form have been used to treat migraine. Drugs containing ergotamine compounds are most effective when administered during the prodromal stage before the onset of the headache. Once the headache is fully established, treatment with the ergotamine compounds is less effective unless they are administered parenterally. Raskin[7] has advocated intravenous dihydroergotamine to treat severe untractable migraine. The dosages and routes of administration for the more widely used drugs are listed in Table 16-1. The drugs can be taken orally, sublingually, rectally, parenterally, or by inhalation. Two other drugs that may be effective in patients who do not get relief with the ergotamine compounds are isometheptene (a postganglionic alpha- and beta-adrenergic antagonist) and cyproheptadine (a histamine and serotonin antagonist with anticholinergic and sedative effects).

The side effects of the ergotamine compounds are generally mild, but ergotamine abuse may produce drowsiness, depression, anorexia, peripheral pulseless disease, and migraine exacerbation. Because of their potent vasoconstrictive effects, they are contraindicated in pregnancy.

During an attack, patients with migraine are most comfortable in a dark room, protected from noise, with an ice pack or cold cloth on their head. They will usually seek these conditions themselves and remain there until the head-

| TABLE 16-2 | *Prophylactic Treatment of Migraine in Adults* | |
|---|---|---|

| Drug | Generic | Dosage |
|---|---|---|
| Tranquilizers | | |
| Valium | Diazepam | 2-4 mg q.i.d. |
| Xanax | Alprazolam | 0.25-0.50 mg t.i.d. |
| Platelet inhibitors | | |
| Aspirin | | 65-325 mg daily |
| Nonsteroidal antiinflammatory agents | | |
| Indocin | Indomethacin | 25-50 mg t.i.d. |
| Tricyclic antidepressants | | |
| Elavil | Amitriptyline | 25-200 mg h.s. or q.12h. |
| Beta blockers | | |
| Inderal | Propranolol | 10-80 mg t.i.d. |
| Inderal LA | | 120 mg q.12h. |
| Calcium channel blockers | | |
| Cardizem | Diltiazem | 30-60 mg t.i.d. |
| Procardia | Nifedipine | 10-30 mg t.i.d. |
| Isoptin | Verapamil | 80-160 mg t.i.d. |
| Serotonin antagonists | | |
| Sansert | Methysergide | 2 mg b.i.d. to q.i.d. |

ache abates. Abatement usually occurs with sleep, and the patient awakens with a feeling of extreme clear headedness.

**PROPHYLACTIC TREATMENT.** For patients whose headaches occur with intolerable frequency, are disabling or prolonged, or are associated with transient or permanent neurologic deficits, prophylactic therapy should be considered (Table 16-2).

**General considerations.** The patient should be made aware of any emotional or stress factors that may precipitate the migraine attack. Frequently muscle contraction headaches can act as a migraine trigger. Avoidance of identifiable specific inducer substances such as particular foods or alcohol should be encouraged. If the headaches are related to menstruation, the use of nonsteroidal antiinflammatory agents perimenstrually is often effective.

The use of oral contraceptives or any agents containing estrogen should be discontinued as soon as possible.[87,111] If the patient tends to be very anxious, a tranquilizing agent such as diazepam may be helpful. Various classes of drugs have been shown to be effective in certain individuals, but none universally so.[112,113] These drugs include platelet inhibitors, nonsteroidal antiinflammatory drugs (NSAIDs), tricyclic antidepressants, beta blockers, calcium channel blockers, and serotonin antagonists.

**Platelet inhibitors.** Both aspirin and dipyridamole have been demonstrated in double-blind crossover trials to be effective in reducing the frequency of migraine syndromes.[114] As would be expected, a greater effect was seen in patients with demonstrated platelet hyperaggregability. An overall decrease in frequency of headaches occurred in 65% of patients.[114] The use of 325 mg of aspirin every other day has been shown to reduce the incidence of migraine by 20%.[115]

**Indomethacin.** Indomethacin is a nonsteroidal antiinflammatory agent that has been demonstrated to be the specific treatment in patients with various subsets of cluster headache and in migraine patients not responding to other prophylaxis.[14,16]

**Tricyclic antidepressants.** The use of tricyclic antidepressants to treat migraine headache and its variants is widely accepted. The major tricyclic antidepressant used in migraine therapy is amitriptyline. The antimigraine response to amitriptyline is independent of its antidepressant activity.[116] It is generally used in dosages of 25 to 200 mg daily in a single bedtime dose, thus obviating one of the major side effects, sedation. Amitriptyline has been shown to be effective in 72% of migraineurs.[116] The drug may be discontinued after a 2-month headache-free interval, with treatment being reinitiated if migraine attacks recur. Some of the newer agents in this class of drugs have fewer side effects and are purported to have less of a sedative effect, but their efficacy in migraine has not been demonstrated.

**Beta blockers.** Propranolol, a nonspecific beta blocker, has been shown to be an effective agent in reducing the frequency and severity of the migraine syndrome. Beta blockers are contraindicated in patients with asthma, heart block, or congestive heart failure. Propranolol is prescribed in divided doses of 10 to 80 mg four times daily. The use of low doses of propranolol may, in the proper milieu, induce or aggravate vasospasm,[117,118] producing arterial occlusion. At a dosage level of 320 mg daily, 84% of patients are symptomatically improved: of these, 55% are headache free. Generally propranolol is well tolerated,[119,120] but in young adults it tends to reduce exercise tolerance. Although propranolol is widely used in the prophylactic treatment of all migraine syndromes, it is approved only for migraine without aura.[121]

**Calcium channel blockers.** The presynaptic release of CNS neurotransmitters such as serotonin is calcium dependent. Calcium increases the number of serotonin-binding sites. Thus one mode of action of the calcium blockers in treating migraine is to stabilize serotoninergic tone. The calcium channel blockers relax arterial muscle walls as well. They have been shown to be effective in a few controlled studies in reducing the frequency of migraine attacks.[122] Diltiazem, verapamil, and nifedipine have similar effectivity in ameliorating migrainous syndromes. These three drugs have similar side effects, which include hypotension, headache, and nausea. Of the three, diltiazem has the lowest incidence of side effects (13%).[122]

**Serotonin antagonists.** Methysergide is a semisynthetic ergotamine derivative. A beneficial response to methysergide has been demonstrated in 50% to 65% of a cohort of migraineurs.[119] Its usefulness is limited by its tendency to produce adverse reactions in 40% of patients. Prolonged use of this drug without interruption may promote retroperitoneal, pulmonary, and cardiac subendothelial valvular fibrosis (most likely an idiosyncratic reaction). Investigators currently believe that these complications are avoidable by slowly tapering the drug over a period of 2 to 3 weeks and discontinuing its use for 3 to 4 weeks every 6 months. The usual dosage is 2 mg, taken two to four times daily.

## REFERENCES

1. Ray BS, Wolff HG. Studies on pain: "spread of pain"; evidence on site of spread within the neuraxis of effects of painful stimulation. Arch Neurol Psychiatry 1945;53:257-61.
2. Penfield W. A contribution to the mechanisms of intracranial pain. A Research Nerv Ment Dis Proc 1935; 15:399-416.
3. Ray BS, Wolff HG. Experimental studies on headache: pain-sensitive structures of the head and their significance in headache. Arch Surg 1940; 41:813-56.
4. Raskin NH, Nosobuchi Y, Lamb S. Headache may arise from perturbation of brain. Headache 1987;27: 416-20.
5. Burde RM. Headache. In: Symposium on neuro-ophthalmology: transactions of the New Orleans Academy of Opthalmology. St Louis: Mosby–Year Book, 1976:242.
6. Headache Classification Committee of the International Headache Society. Classification and diagnostic criteria for headache disorders, cranial neuralgias and facial pain. Cephalalgia 1988;8(suppl 7).
7. Raskin NH. Headache. 2nd ed. New York: Churchill Livingstone, 1988.
8. Doenicke A, Brand J, Perrin VL. Possible benefit of GR43175, a novel 5-HT$_1$–like receptor agonist, for the acute treatment of migraine. Lancet 1988;1: 1309-11.
9. Russell D. Cluster headache: severity and temporal profiles of attacks and patient activity prior to and during attacks. Cephalalgia 1981;1:209-16.
10. Manzoni GC, Terazano MG, Bono G, et al. Cluster headaches—clinical findings in 180 patients. Cephalalgia 1983;3:21-30.
11. Kudrow L. Cluster headache: mechanisms and management. Oxford: Oxford University Press, 1980.
12. Caviness VS Jr, O'Brien P. Cluster headache: response to chlorpromazine. Headache 1980;20:128-31.
13. Sjaastad O, Dale I. Evidence for a new(?), treatable headache entity. Headache 1974;14:105-8.
14. Mathew NT. Indomethacin responsive headache syndromes. Headache 1981; 21:147-50.
15. Kudrow DB, Kudrow L. Successful aspirin prophylaxis in a child with chronic paroxysmal hemicrania. Headache 1989;29:280-1.
16. Medina JL, Diamond S. Cluster headache variant: spectrum of a new headache syndrome. Arch Neurol 1981; 38:705-9.
17. Rose CF. Clinical characterization of migraine. In: Olesen J, Edvinsson L, eds. Basic mechanisms of headache. Amsterdam: Elsevier, 1988:chap 1.
18. Olesen J. The pathophysiology of migraine. In: Vinken PJ, Bruyn GW, Klawans HL, eds. Handbook of clinical neurology. Vol 48. Headache. Amsterdam: Elsevier, 1986:59-83.
19. Olesen J, Friberg L, Olsen TS, et al. Timing and topography of cerebral blood flow, aura, and headache during migraine attacks. Ann Neurol 1990;28:791-8.
20. Leão AAP. Spreading depression of activity of the cerebral cortex. J Neurophysiol 1944;7:359-90.
21. Appenzeller O, Feldman RG, Friedman AP. Migraine, headache, and related conditions—panel 7. Arch Neurol 1979;36:784-805.
22. Heyck H. Varieties of hemiplegic migraine. Headache 1973;12:135-42.
23. Featherstone HJ. Clinical features of stroke in migraine: a review. Headache 1986;26:128-33.
24. Shuaib A, Hachinski VC. Migraine and risks from angiography. Arch Neurol 1988;45:911-2.
25. Bickerstaff ER. Basilar artery migraine. Lancet 1961;1:15-7.
26. Lapkin ML, Golden GS. Basilar artery migraine: a review of 30 cases. Am J Dis Child 1978;132:278-81.
27. Golden GS, French JH. Basilar artery migraine in young children. Pediatrics 1975;56:722-6.
28. McDonald JV. Basilar artery migraine: case report. J Neurosurg 1990;72:289-91.
29. Bickerstaff ER. Migraine variants and complications. In: Blau JN, ed. Migraine: clinical and research aspects. Baltimore: John Hopkins University Press, 1987:55-75.

30. Friedman AP, Harter DH, Merritt HH. Ophthalmoplegic migraine. Arch Neurol 1962;7:320-7.

31. Vijayan N. Ophthalmoplegic migraine: ischemic or compressive neuropathy? Headache 1980;20:300-4.

32. Teasdale E, Statham P, Straiton J, et al. Non-invasive radiological investigation for oculomotor palsy. J Neurol Neurosurg Psychiatry 1990;53:549-53.

33. Blom S. Trigeminal neuralgia: its treatment with a new anticonvulsant drug (G32883). Lancet 1962;1:839-40.

34. Fromm GH. Trigeminal neuralgia and related disorders. Neurol Clin 1989; 7:305-19.

35. Fromm GH, Terrence CF, Maroon JC. Trigeminal neuralgia: current concepts regarding etiology and pathogenesis. Arch Neurol 1984;41:1204-7.

36. Rushton JG, Stevens JC, Miller RH. Glossopharyngeal (vago-glossopharyngeal) neuralgia: a study of 217 cases. Arch Neurol 1981;38:201-5.

37. Raskin NH, Schwartz RK. Ice pick-like pain. Neurology 1980;30:203-5.

38. Olesen J. The classification and diagnosis of headache disorders. Neurol Clin 1990;8:793-9.

39. Abbott RJ, van Hille P. Thunderclap headache and unruptured cerebral aneurysm [Letter]. Lancet 1986;2:1459.

40. Wijdicks EFM, Kerkhoff H, van Gijn J. Long-term follow-up of 71 patients with thunderclap headache mimicking subarachnoid haemorrhage. Lancet 1988;2:68-70.

41. Day JW, Raskin NH. Thunderclap headache: symptom of unruptured cerebral aneurysm. Lancet 1986;2: 1247-8.

42. Clarke CE, Shepherd DI, Chishti K, et al. Thunderclap headache [Letter]. Lancet 1988;2:625.

43. Pearce JMS. Thunderclap headache [Letter]. Lancet 1988;2:625.

44. Oswald I. Exploding head [Letter]. Lancet 1988;2:625.

45. Pearce JMS. Exploding head syndrome. Lancet 1988;2:270-1.

46. Sands GH. A protocol for butalbital, aspirin and caffeine (BAC) detoxification in headache patients. Headache 1990;30:491-6.

47. Henderson WR, Raskin NH. "Hot dog" headache: individual susceptibility to nitrite. Lancet 1972;2:1162-3.

48. Dalessio DJ, ed. Wolff's headache and other head pain. 4th ed. New York: Oxford Press, 1980.

49. Greene MK, Kerr AM, McIntosh IB, et al. Acetazolamide in prevention of acute mountain sickness: a double-blind controlled cross-over study. Br Med J 1981;283:811-3.

50. Balagot RC, Lee T, Liu C, et al. The prophylactic epidural blood patch [Letter]. JAMA 1974;228:1369-70.

51. Cass W, Edelist G. Postspinal headache: successful use of epidural blood patch 11 weeks after onset. JAMA 1974;227:786-7.

52. Duke-Elder S. The practice of refraction. 8th ed. St Louis: Mosby–Year Book, 1969:1.

53. Walsh FB, Hoyt WF. Clinical neuro-ophthalmology, vol 1. 3rd ed. Baltimore: Williams & Wilkins, 1969:423.

54. Eckardt LB, McLean JM, Goodell H. Experimental studies on headache: the genesis of pain from the eye. A Research Nerv Ment Dis Proc 1943; 23:209-27.

55. Burian HM, von Noorden GK. Binocular vision and ocular motility: theory and management of strabismus. St Louis: Mosby–Year Book, 1974:167.

56. Renshaw DC, Joynt RJ. Coital cephalalgia. JAMA 1985;253:253-4.

57. Silbert PL, Edis RH, et al. Benign vascular sexual headache and exertional headache: interrelationships and long term prognosis. J Neurol Neurosurg Psychiatry 1991;54:417-21.

58. Levy RL. Stroke and orgasmic cephalgia. Headache 1981;21:12-3.

59. Hunt JR. Geniculate neuralgia (neuralgia of the nervus facialis). Arch Neurol Psychiatry 1937;37:253-85.

60. Watson CPN, Evans RJ. Postherpetic neuralgia: a review. Arch Neurol 1986;43:836-40.

61. Watson CPN. Post-herpetic neuralgia. Neurol Clin 1989;7:231.

62. de Moragas JM, Kierland RR. The outcome of patients with herpes zoster. Arch Dematol 1957;75:193-6.

63. Watson CPN, Evans RJ, Reed K, et al.

Amitriptyline versus placebo in post-herpetic neuralgia. Neurology 1982; 32:671-3.

64. Watson CPN. Therapeutic window for amitriptyline analgesia [Letter]. Can Med Assoc J 1984;130:105-6.

65. Keczkes K, Basheer AM. Do corticosteroids prevent post-herpetic neuralgia? Br J Dermatol 1980;102:551-5.

66. Esmann V, Kronn S, Peterslund NA, et al. Prednisolone does not prevent post-herpetic neuralgia. Lancet 1987; 2:126-9.

67. Coston JB. A syndrome of ear and sinus symptoms dependent upon disturbed function of the temporomandibular joint. Ann Otol Rhinol Laryngol 1934;43:1-15.

68. Howell FV. The teeth and jaws as sources of headache. In: Dalessio DJ, ed. Wolff's headache and other head pain. 4th ed. New York: Oxford University Press, 1980:385.

69. Traub YM, Korczyn AD. Headache in patients with hypertension. Headache 1978;17:245-7.

70. Northfield DWC. Some observations on headache. Brain 1938;61:133-62.

71. Symonds C. Cough headache. Brain 1956;79:557-68.

72. Grimson BS, Thompson HS. Raeder's syndrome: a clinical review. Surv Ophthalmol 1980;24:199-210.

73. Boniuk M, Schlezinger NS. Raeder's paratrigeminal syndrome. Am J Ophthalmol 1962;54:1074-84.

74. McNeill DH Jr, Dreisbach J, Marsden RJ. Spontaneous dissection of the internal carotid artery: its conservative management with heparin sodium. Arch Neurol 1980;37:54-5.

75. Au YK, Henkind P. Pain elicited by consensual pupillary reflex: a diagnostic test for acute iritis. Lancet 1981;2:1254-5.

76. Furlan AJ, Whisnant JP, Kearns TP. Unilateral visual loss in bright light: an unusual symptom of carotid artery occlusive disease. Arch Neurol 1979; 36:675-6.

77. Water WE, O'Connor PJ. Prevalence of migraine. J Neurol Neurosurg Psychiatry 1975;38:613-6.

78. Heyck H. Kopfschmerz und vegetatives Nervensystem (Migräne und verwandte Kopfschmerzformen). Bibl Psychiatr Neurol 1966;130:167-201.

79. Couch JR, Hassanein RS. Platelet aggregability in migraine. Neurology 1977;27:843-8.

80. Glover V, Sandler M, Grant E, et al. Transitory decrease in platelet monoamine-oxidase activity during migraine attacks. Lancet 1977;1:391-3.

81. Hannington E, Jones RJ, Amess JAL, et al. Migraine: a platelet disorder. Lancet 1981;2:720-3.

82. Hannington E, Jones RJ, Amess JAL. Platelet aggregation in response to 5-HT in migraine patients taking oral contraceptives [Letter]. Lancet 1982; 1:967-8.

83. Hanington E, Jones RJ, Amess JAL. Migraine and platelets [Letter]. Lancet 1982;1:1248.

84. D'Andrea G, Welch KMA, Riddle JM, et al. Platelet serotonin metabolism and ultrastructure in migraine. Arch Neurol 1989;46:1187-9.

85. Sandler M, Youdim MBH, Hanington E. A phenylethylamine oxidising defect in migraine. Nature 1974;250:335-7.

86. Dalessio DJ. Migraine, platelets, and headache prophylaxis [Editorial]. JAMA 1978;239:52-3.

87. Salmon ML, Winkelman JZ, Gay AJ. Neuro-ophthalmic sequelae in users of oral contraceptives. JAMA 1968; 206:85-91.

88. Ryan RE Jr. A clinical study of tyramine as an etiological factor in migraine. Headache 1974;14:43-8.

89. Lönnqvist B, Ringdén O. Migraine precipitated by red wine after bone marrow transplantation [Letter]. Lancet 1990;1:364.

90. Marcus DA, Soso MJ. Migraine and stripe-induced visual discomfort. Arch Neurol 1989;46:1129-32.

91. Brandt KD, Lessell S. Migrainous phenomena in systemic lupus erythematosus. Arthritis Rheum 1978;21:7-16.

92. Phelps CD, Corbett JJ. Migraine and low-tension glaucoma: a case-control study. Invest Ophthalmol Vis Sci 1985;26:1105-8.

93. Cullen KJ, Macdonald WB. The peri-

odic syndrome: its nature and prevalence. Med J Aust 1963;2:167-73.

94. Symon DNK, Russell G. Abdominal migraine: a childhood syndrome defined. Cephalalgia 1986;6:223-8.

95. Gowers WR. Subjective visual sensations: Being the Baoman Lecture. Trans Ophthalmol Soc UK 1895; 15:1-38.

96. O'Connor PS, Tredici TJ. Acephalgic migraine: fifteen years experience. Ophthalmology 1981;88:999-1003.

97. Fisher CM. Late-life migraine accompaniments as a cause of unexplained transient ischemic attacks. Can J Neurol Sci 1980;7:9-17.

98. Tippin J, Corbett JJ, Kerber RE, et al. Amaurosis fugax and ocular infarction in adolescents and young adults. Ann Neurol 1989;26:69-77.

99. Kline LB, Kelly CL. Ocular migraine in a patient with cluster headaches. Headache 1980;20:253-7.

100. Kline LB, Glaser JS. Visual evoked response in moncular visual loss. Br J Ophthalmol 1982;66:382-5.

101. Burde RM. Editorial comment. J Clin Neuro Ophthalmol 1983;3:75-6.

102. Fujino T, Akiya S, Takagi S, et al. Amaurosis fugax for a long duration. J Clin Neuro Opthalmol 1983;3:9-12.

103. Goldor H. Headache and eye pain. Int Ophthalmol Clin 1967;7:697-705.

104. Szasz TS. The painful person. Lancet 1968;88:18-22.

105. Lascelles RG. Atypical facial pain and depression. Br J Psychiatry 1966;112: 651-9.

106. Bode DD Jr. Ocular pain secondary to occipital neuritis. Ann Ophthalmol 1979;11:589-94.

107. Knox DL, Mustonen E. Greater occipital neuralgia: an ocular pain syndrome with multiple etiologies. Trans Am Acad Ophthalmol Otolaryngol 1975;79:OP513-9.

108. Bogduk N, Marsland A. On the concept of third occipital headaches. J Neurol Neurosurg Psychiatry 1986; 49:775-80.

109. Fanchamps A. Pharmacodynamic principles of anti-migraine therapy. Headache 1975;15:79-90.

110. Pinder RM, Brodgen RN, Sawyer PR, et al. Metoclopramide: a review of its pharmacological properties and clinical use. Drugs 1976;12:81-131.

111. Ramcharan S, Pellegrin FA, Ray RM, et al. The Walnut Creek Contraceptive Study: a prospective study of the side effects of oral contraceptives. J Reprod Med 1980;25(suppl):346-72.

112. Atkinson R, Appenzeller O. Pharmacologic rationale for the management of recurrent headaches. In: Palmer GC, ed. Neuropharmacology of the central nervous system and behavioral disorders. New York: Academic Press, 1981:317.

113. Raskin NH, Schwartz RK. Interval therapy of migraine: long-term results. Headache 1980;20:336-40.

114. Masel BE, Chesson AL, Peters BH, et al. Platelet antagonists in migraine prophylaxis: a clinical trial using aspirin and dipyridamole. Headache 1980;20:13-8.

115. Buring JE, Peto R, Hennekens CH. Low dose aspirin for migraine prophylaxis. JAMA 1990;264:1711-3.

116. Couch JR, Hassanein RS. Amitriptyline in migraine prophylaxis. Arch Neurol 1979;36:695-9.

117. Burde RM. Migraine [Editorial]. J. Clin Neuro Ophthalmol 1986;6:72-3.

118. Katz B. Migrainous central retinal artery occlusion. J Clin Neuro Ophthalmol 1986;6:69-71.

119. Saper JR. Migraine. II. Treatment. JAMA 1978;239:2480-4.

120. Scheife RT, Hills JR. Migraine headache: signs and symptoms, biochemistry, and current therapy. Am J Hosp Pharm 1980;37:365-74.

121. Physicians desk reference. 43rd ed. Oradell, NJ: Medical Economics, 1989: 2306.

122. Winniford MD, Hillis LD. Calcium antagonists in patients with cardiovascular disease: current perspectives. Medicine 1985;64:61-73.

# Index

**A**

Abducens nerve palsy, 260-263
  combined, 265-266
  Duane's syndrome and, 264-265
Abducens nucleus, 264
Abduction deficits, 264
Aberrant regeneration of oculomotor nerve, 253-254
Aberrations, refractive, diplopia and, 229
Abnormal retinal correspondence, 230-232
Abortive treatment for migraine, 438, 440-441
Abscess, pituitary, 95
Accommodative esotropia, 283-284
Acephalgic migraine, 434
Acetazolamide, 188
Acetylcholine-receptor antibody levels in myasthenia gravis, 358
ACTH-producing tumor, 82
Acuity; *see* Visual acuity
Adduction lag, 213
Adenoma, pituitary
  apoplexy and, 79-81
  malignant, 82
Adie's syndrome, 335-336
Adnexa, 126
Adnexal mass, 403-412
  extraconal, 408, 410-412
  intraconal, 403-407
Afferent visual system, abnormal, 304
Afterimage, prolonged, 156
Agnosia, topographic, 162
Agraphia, alexia without, 114
AION; *see* Anterior ischemic optic neuropathy
Alcohol abuse
  headache and, 420, 426
  optic neuropathy and, 61-63
Alexia without agraphia, 114
Altered color, 156, 161
Altered sensorium, 150

Alternating anisocoria, 340
Alternating gaze deviation, periodic, 314-315
Alternating nystagmus, periodic, 307
Altitude headache, 426
Amblyopia, unexplained visual loss and, 20-22
Aminoglycosides
  myasthenia gravis and, 359
  oscillopsia and, 311
Amplitudes, fusional, in decompensated phoria, 283
Amsler grid, maculopathy and, 22
Analgesics for migraine, 439
Anemia, optic neuropathy and, 63
Aneurysm
  chiasmal syndrome and, 95
  circle of Willis and, 95
  third nerve palsy and, 249
    child and, 256
Angiography for transient visual loss, 120, 136
Aniseikonia, 237-238
  asthenopia and, 428
Anisocoria, 325-338
  abnormal light reaction and, 333-336
  constriction and, 338
  intraocular pressure and, 336-337
  light reaction in, 338
  ptosis and, 328-333
Anisometropia, amblyopia and, 20-22
Antagonist, inhibitional palsy of, 269, 272
Anterior ischemic optic neuropathy, 50-51
Anterior segment, transient visual loss and, 126
Anterior visual pathway
  pituitary apoplexy and, 81
  radiation injury to, 86
Antiaggregation, platelet, 138-139
Antibody
  Graves' ophthalmopathy and, 385
  myasthenia gravis and, 358

**447**

Anticholinesterase agent, 246
Anticoagulation, 138
Anticonvulsant drug, 308-309
Antidepressant for migraine, 442
Antiinflammatory drug, 389
Aortic stenosis, calcific, 132
Aphakia, 156
Apoplexy, pituitary, 79-81
Applanation pressure, 336-337
Apraxia
    of lid opening, 347
    ocular motor, 208-209
Arachnoiditis, chiasmal, 96
Arcuate scotoma, 15, 18
Arterial hypertension
    central retinal vein occlusion and, 194
    headache and, 430
Arteriography
    homonymous hemianopia and, 106-107
    migraine caused by, 105
Arteriosclerosis, 125
Arteriovenous malformation, 105
Arteritic ischemic optic neuropathy, 51-56
Arteritis
    giant cell
        diplopia and, 250
        headache and, 424-425
    optic neuropathy and, 49
    Takayasu's, 432
Artery
    chiasm and, 76
    hemifacial spasm and, 370
    mesencephalic, 211
    retinal, occlusion of, 66-67
Artifact in unexplained visual loss, 34
Aspiration biopsy of orbital tumor, 407
Aspirin
    for migraine, 441-442
    platelet antiaggregation and, 138-139
Asthenopia, headache and, 427-428
Astigmatism, 232
Astrocytoma, 299
Asymmetric binocular oscillations, 297-301
Atheroma, vertebrobasilar, 118
Atheromatous carotid disease, 137
Atherosclerosis, 118
Atrial fibrillation, 128-129
Atrial myxoma, 133
Atrophy, optic, 176
    hereditary, 64
Aura of migraine, 421-423; *see also* Migraine
    as hallucination, 105
    illustration of, 168
Autoimmune optic neuritis, 48

Automated perimetry, 38
Avulsion of facial nerve for blepharospasm, 374-375

**B**

Basilar artery migraine, 422-423
Behçet's disease, 48
Bell's palsy, 366, 368
Benedikt's syndrome, 261
Benign episodic pupillary dilatation, 339
Benign paroxysmal positional nystagmus, 311
Best-corrected acuity, 4
Beta blocking agent for migraine, 442
Bielschowsky head tilt test, 272-273
Big blind spot syndrome, 194
Bilateral condition
    blepharospasm as, 372-376
    homonymous hemianopia as, 33-34
        postchiasmal visual loss and, 104
    horizontal gaze deficit as, 212
    internuclear ophthalmoplegia as, 213
    nerve fiber bundle defects as, 33
    optic neuritis as, 47-48
    papilledema as, 183
    pursuit paresis as, 210
    reduced pupillary light reactions and, 340-341
    saccadic paresis as, 208
    sixth nerve palsy as
        in adult, 261
        in child, 263
    uveitis as, 195
    visual cortex lesions as, 31
Binocular condition
    diplopia as, 234-236
    symmetric oscillations and, 301-311
    transient visual loss as, 124
Binocular hallucinations, 167-169
Binocular illusions, 157-163
Biopsy
    giant cell arteritis and, 54
    of orbital tumor, 407
Birth control pills
    migraine and, 433
    transient visual loss and, 126
Birth trauma, Horner's syndrome and, 332
Bitemporal hemianopia, 13
    chiasmal compression and, 78
    unexplained visual loss and, 33
Blepharospasm, 347, 365-378
    bilateral, 372-376
    facial weakness and, 365-369
    hemifacial spasm and, 370-372
    trigeminal irritation and, 365

Blepharospasm-orofacial dystonia, 374
Blind spot, big, 194
Blindness, cortical, 112
Blinking, blepharospasm and, 374
Blood pressure, hypertensive
  central retinal vein occlusion and, 194
  headache and, 430
  pseudotumor cerebri and, 187
  retinopathy and, 192
Blood-brain barrier, 106
Bobbing, ocular, 314
Body, hyaline, 180
Body temperature in multiple sclerosis, 226
Botulinum toxin
  for hemifacial spasm, 371, 372
  for sixth nerve palsy, 261
Botulism, 266
Brainstem
  glioma of, 262-263
  pontine gaze deficits and, 212
Brainstem ptosis, 359-360
Branch retinal artery occlusion, 66-67
Brightness, decreased, 156
Brightness comparison test, 9
Bromocriptine, pituitary tumor and, 84
Brown's superior oblique tendon sheath
      syndrome, 243
Bruns' nystagmus, 309

**C**

Calcific aortic stenosis, 132
Calcium channel blockers for migraine, 442
Caloric nystagmus, 310-311
Cancer; *see* Tumor
Carbamazepine
  nystagmus caused by, 308
  trigeminal neuralgia and, 424
Carbonic anhydrase inhibitors, pseudotumor
      cerebri and, 188
Carcinoma; *see* Tumor
Cardiac disease in transient visual loss, 125
Cardiac embolus, 127-135
Cardiomyopathy, 133
Carotid artery
  echography of, 135
  stenosis of, 135
  transient visual loss and, 118, 119-120
Carotid endarterectomy, 136-139
Cataract, 156
Cavernous sinus–carotid fistula, 399-402
Cellulitis, orbital, 395, 397-399
Central disruption of fusion, 286-287
Central nervous system disease
  blepharospasm and, 372-374

Central nervous system disease—cont'd
  headache and, 430-431
Central positional nystagmus, 311
Central retinal artery occlusion, 66-67
Central retinal vein occlusion, 140
  disc elevation and, 193-194
Central scotoma
  chiasmal compression and, 76, 77
  retrobulbar optic nerve lesion and, 15, 16
Central vestibular nystagmus, 306
Centrocecal scotoma, 15, 17
Centronuclear myopathy, 219
Cerebellar artery infarction, 306
Cerebral angiography, 136
Cerebral diplopia, 158
Cerebral dyschromatopsia, 112
Cerebral hemispheric ptosis, 359
Cerebral ischemia, 124-125
Cerebral metamorphopsia, 158
Cerebral polyopia, 234
Cerebrospinal fluid in multiple sclerosis, 44
Cervical carotid echography, 135
Chemical-induced optic neuropathy, 60-61
Chemotherapy, glioma and, 94
Chiasmal prolapse into empty sella, 86, 96
Chiasmal syndrome, 74-103
  craniopharyngioma and, 88-90
  glioma and, 92-95
  imaging for, 78-79
  meningioma and, 90-92
  nontumorous causes of, 95-97
  pituitary tumor and, 79-87
    apoplexy and, 79-81
    endocrinologic symptoms of, 81-82
    follow-up care in, 87
    recurrent visual loss and, 85-86
    special forms of, 82-83
    treatment of, 83-85
  signs of, 75-78
  symptoms of, 74-75
  unexplained visual loss and, 33
Child
  esotropia in, 284
  fourth nerve palsy in, 259-260
  Horner's syndrome and, 332
  meningioma and, 405
  migraine and, 435
  pseudotumor cerebri and, 186
  rhabdomyosarcoma and, 408
  sixth nerve palsy in, 262-263
  third nerve palsy in, 255-257
Cicatricial lid retraction, 362, 364
Ciliary muscle paresis, 335-336
Circle of Willis, aneurysm in, 95

Claude Bernard syndrome, 340, 364
Cluster headache, 418, 420
Cocaine test for anisocoria, 328-329
Cogwheeling in Parkinson's disease, 217
Collier's sign, 364
Coloboma, 178
Color alteration, 156, 161
Color of iris, 331-332
Color saturation test, 9
Color testing, 26
Coma
    nystagmus and, 311
    pituitary apoplexy and, 81
Comitant ocular misalignment, 282-288
    accommodative esotropia and, 283-284
    central disruption of fusion and, 286-287
    decompensated phoria and, 282-283
    esotropia of childhood and, 284
    foveal displacement and, 286
    skew deviation and, 286
    vergence paresis and, 284-286
Compression, transient visual loss and, 120-121
Compression optic neuropathy, disc elevation
        and, 192
Compressive ocular motor palsy, myasthenia
        gravis and, 244
Compressive optic neuropathy, 56
Computed tomography
    chiasmal syndrome and, 78-79
    Graves' ophthalmopathy and, 385
    orbital inflammation and, 393
    sphenoid ridge meningioma and, 57
Cone-rod dystrophy, 26-27
Confrontation testing, procedure for, 37-38
Congenital disorder
    elevated optic disc as, 179-182
    horizontal gaze deficits as, 211-212
    ocular motor apraxia as, 208-209
    ptosis as, 352
Conjugate eye movement, 200-203
Conjugate gaze, spasticity of, 109
Conjugate nystagmus, 303-311
    jerk, 305-311
    pendular, 303
Conjugate system, 203-205
Conjunctival injection, Graves'
        ophthalmopathy and, 383
Constricted visual fields, 28-33
Constriction
    anisocoria and, 338
    pilocarpine test and, 334-336
    pupillary, 322-323
Contact lens
    lid deformity from, 351

Contact lens—cont'd
    overwear syndrome and, 432
Contraction, muscle, headache and, 435, 437
Contracture, facial, 368
Contralateral antagonist, inhibitional palsy of,
        269, 272
Contralateral lid retraction, 348
Contrast sensitivity test, 9
Convergence nystagmus, 302-303
Convergence paresis, 284-285
Convergence-retraction nystagmus, 302
Corectopia, midbrain, 342
Cornea
    inflammation of, headache and, 431-432
    surface abnormality of, 6
Cortex, visual, bilateral lesions of, 31
Cortical blindness, 112
Corticosteroid; *see* Steroid
Coughing, headache and, 431
Cover-uncover test, diplopia and, 236
Cranial arteritis, optic neuropathy and, 51
Cranial nerve
    third nerve palsy and, 247-257; *see also*
        Third nerve palsy
    fourth nerve palsy and, 257-260
    sixth nerve palsy and, 260-263
        diplopia and, 224
    eccentric gaze and, 301
    facial nerve avulsion and, 374-375
    neuralgia and, 423-424
    tic douloureux and, 423-424
    trigeminal irritation and, 365
Craniopharyngioma, 88-90
Crescent, temporal, 109-110, 111
Crisis, oculogyric, 217
Crossed eyes, 283-284
Crouzon's disease, 402
Cryptogenic hemifacial spasm, 370
Cupping of optic disc, 173, 176
Cyanopsia, 156
Cyclic oculomotor paresis in child, 256
Cyclosporine for Graves' optic neuropathy,
        389-390
Cystic craniopharyngioma, 90

**D**

Dazzle, 166
Decision tree
    for abnormal optic disc, 174-175, 190-191
    for anisocoria, 326-327, 334
    for blepharospasm, 366-367, 369
    for diplopia, 230-231
    for illusions and hallucinations, 148-149,
        152-154, 157, 164-167

Decision tree—cont'd
　for nystagmus, 292-293, 302, 304-305
　for ocular misalignment, comitant, 282
　for ocular misalignment, incomitant,
　　240-241
　for prechiasmal visual loss, 42-43, 52-53
　for proptosis, 380-381
　for ptosis, 348-349, 351, 353, 355
　for transient visual loss, 122-123, 125, 127,
　　134
　for unexplained visual loss, 2-3, 21, 25
Decompensated phoria, 282-283
　diplopia and, 227
Decompression for pituitary apoplexy, 81
Deformity of lid, 351
Degeneration
　of mitral valve, 130-132
　retinal, 28
　spinocerebellar, 65
Dehydrating agents for pseudotumor cerebri,
　188
Dehydration, transient visual loss and, 126
Dementia, 150
Demyelinating polyradiculoneuropathy, 266
Demyelination of optic nerve, 41; *see also*
　　Optic neuritis
Dental disease, headache and, 430
Depression, migraine and, 434
Deprivation, visual
　hallucinations from, 151
　monocular, 298
　nystagmus and, 304
Dermatochalasis, 348
Dermoid tumor, 408
Developmental anomaly, proptosis and, 402
Diabetes
　hypoplasia of optic disc and, 177
　mucormycosis and, 399
　papillopathy and, 193
Dietary headache, 425-426
　migraine and, 433
Dilatation, benign episodic pupillary, 339
Dilator muscle of iris, 323
Diltiazem for migraine, 442
Diplopia, 224-238
　binocular, 234-236
　cerebral, 158
　chiasmal syndrome and, 74
　comitant misalignment and, 282-288
　diagnosis of, 224-229
　Graves' ophthalmopathy and, 391
　incomitant ocular misalignment and,
　　239-282
　　abducens nerve and, 260-263

Diplopia—cont'd
　incomitant ocular misalignment and—cont'd
　　combined palsies and, 265-266
　　decision tree for, 240-241
　　forced duction test for, 239, 242-243
　　isolation of paretic muscles and, 267-276
　　nonisolated palsies and, 263-265
　　oculomotor nerve and, 247-257; *see also*
　　　Oculomotor nerve palsy
　　Tensilon test for, 244-247
　　trochlear nerve and, 257-260
　　intermittent, 224, 226-229
　　monocular, 229-234
　　no misalignment with, 237-238
　　pituitary apoplexy and, 80
Dipping, ocular, 314
Dipyridamole for migraine, 441-442
Disc elevation
　retinopathy and, 192, 193-194
　and optic neuropathy, 192-193
Disconjugate nystagmus, 301-303
Disconnection syndrome, 114
Disjunctive eye movement, 205, 207
Dissociation, light-near, 333
Divergence nystagmus, 303
Divergence paresis, 285-286
DNA, Leber's optic neuropathy and, 64
Dolichoectasia, 370
Dominant optic atrophy, 64
Dorsolateral pontine nuclei, 205
Dot, white, 24
Double vision; *see* Diplopia
Downbeat nystagmus, 309
Downgaze deficits, 214
Drug
　for Graves' optic neuropathy, 389
　for migraine, 439, 440
　nystagmus of multiple sclerosis and, 299
Drug-induced condition
　illusions or hallucinations as, 147, 149
　nystagmus as, 308-309
　ophthalmoplegia as, 338
　oscillations and, 291
　ptosis as, 353
Drusen, 180
Duane's syndrome, 264-265
Duction test, forced, 239, 242-243
Ductional deficits, 388
Dyschromatopsia, cerebral, 112
Dyskinesia, tardive, 374
Dysmetria, 313
Dysostosis craniofacialis, 402
Dysplasia
　fibrous, orbital, 408-409

Dysplasia—cont'd
optic disc and, 176-179
Dystonia, blepharospasm-orofacial, 374
Dystrophy
cone-rod, 26-27
muscular, gaze disturbance and, 219

**E**

Eccentric gaze
jerk nystagmus and, 308
monocular oscillations and, 299-301
Echography, carotid, 135
Edema, optic disc, 50
Efferent nystagmus, 299
Electromyography in myasthenia gravis, 357
Electroretinography, 26
Elevated optic disc, 179-195
congenitally, 179-182
papilledema and, 182-189
Elevation paresis, monocular, 215
Embolus, 119-120, 127-135
Empty sella syndrome, 86, 96
Encephalomyopathy, 217-218
Encephalopathy, Wernicke's, 261
Endarterectomy, carotid, 136-138
Endocarditis, emboli and, 129-130
Endocrine disorder
pituitary tumor and, 81-82
pseudotumor cerebri and, 184, 186
Enhanced ptosis, 356
Enophthalmos, 407
Epilepsy, 167, 169
Episodic pupillary dilatation, 339
Epitheliitis, retinal pigment, 24
Epithelium, retinal pigment, 180
Ergotamine tartrate for migraine, 439, 440
Erythrocyte sedimentation rate, 51, 54
Erythropsia, 156
Esotropia
accommodative, 283-284
thalamic, 211
Esthenopia, 283
Ethambutol-induced optic neuropathy, 60
Evanescent white dot syndrome, 24
Exophthalmos, 402; *see also* Proptosis
"Exploding" headache, 425
External ophthalmoplegia, progressive, 218
Extraaxial palsy, 265
Extraconal mass, 408, 410-411
Extracranial vessels, emboli of, 119
Extraocular muscle
Graves' ophthalmopathy and, 384, 390-391
myasthenia gravis and, 244
surgery on, diplopia after, 230-232

Eye movement
conjugate, 200-203
fast, 203-205
disorders of, 207-209, 211-217
velocity and, 200
flashes induced by, 166
slow, 205
disorders of, 210, 211-217
types of movement and, 200
Eyelid
anisocoria and, 328
blepharospasm and, 365-378; *see also*
Blepharospasm
deformity of, ptosis and, 351
nystagmus of, 312
ptosis and, 347-361; *see also* Ptosis
retraction of, 362-365
Graves' ophthalmopathy and, 379-391,
391; *see also* Graves' ophthalmopathy
Eyestrain, headache from, 427-428

**F**

Facial contracture, 368
Facial nerve avulsion for blepharospasm,
374-375
Facial pain, atypical, 437-438
Facial weakness, blepharospasm and, 365-369
Familial hemiplegic migraine, 422
Fasciculus, medial longitudinal, 299-300
Fast eye movement system, 203-205
disorders of, 207-209
slow eye movement disorder with, 211-217
velocity and, 200
Fever, headache and, 430
Fiber
oculomotor nerve and, 248-249
pupillomotor, 322
retinal, 76
Fiber bundle defect, nerve, 33
Fibrillation, atrial, 128-129
Fibromyxomatous degeneration of mitral
valve, 130-132
Fibrous dysplasia, orbital, 408-409
Fifth cranial nerve, 423-424
Fine-needle aspiration biopsy of orbital tumor,
407
First order neuron, 323-324
Horner's syndrome and, 333
Flashes, 166
Flickering lights, 166
Floppy infant syndrome, 266
Fluid, cerebrospinal, 44
Fluorescein angiography
maculopathy and, 23-24

Fluorescein angiography—cont'd
   papilledema and, 183
Flutter, 313
Food, migraine and, 433
Food additives, headache from, 425-426
Forced duction test, 239, 242-243
Foster-Kennedy syndrome, 91
Fourth nerve palsy, 257-260
   combined, 265-266
   intraaxial, 261-262
Foveal displacement syndrome, 286
Foveation, superior colliculus and, 204
Foville's syndrome, 264
Frontal eye fields, 204
Fundus, Leber's optic neuropathy and, 64
Fungal infection, 398, 399
Fusion, central disruption of, 286-287
Fusional amplitudes in decompensated
         phoria, 283

**G**

Gadolinium-DTPA, chiasmal syndrome and,
      78-79
Gaze, 200-223
   conjugate, spasticity of, 109
   eccentric
      jerk nystagmus and, 308
      monocular oscillations and, 299-301
   myasthenia gravis and, 245
   myopathic, 217-219
   ocular motor system and, 200-207
      conjugate systems and, 203-205
      vergence systems and, 205, 207
   supranuclear control pathways and, 207-217
      fast eye movement systems and, 207-209,
         211-217
      slow eye movement systems and, 210,
         211-217
      vergence system and, 210-211
Gaze-paretic nystagmus, 308
Geniculate nucleus, lateral, 107
Gentamicin, oscillopsia and, 311
Ghosting
   diplopia and, 232
   as illusion, 155
   unexplained visual loss and, 6
Giant cell arteritis
   diplopia and, 250
   headache and, 424-425
   optic neuropathy and, 51
Gilles de la Tourette's syndrome, 374
Glaucoma
   headache and, 432
   optic disc and, 173

Glioma
   optic, 92-95
   sixth nerve palsy and, 262-263
Glossopharyngeal neuralgia, 424
Gradenigo's syndrome, 263, 265
Graves' ophthalmopathy, 379-391
   compressive optic neuropathy and, 192
   diagnosis of, 379-385
   diplopia and, 226
   forced duction test and, 242-243
   myasthenia gravis and, 357
   pathogenesis of, 385, 387
   treatment of, 387-391
Greater occipital neuralgia, 438
Growth hormone, 177
Guillain-Barré-Strohl syndrome, 266

**H**

Hallucinations, 163-169
   binocular, 167-169
   in homonymous field, 105-106
   illusions versus, 145-147
   monocular, 166
   occipital lobe disease and, 114
   Parinaud's syndrome and, 215
Hangover headache, 426
Head nodding, 297
Head posture in strabismus, 239
Head tilt test, 272-273
Headache, 417-446
   atypical facial pain and, 437-438
   chiasmal syndrome and, 75
   classification of, 419
   cluster, 418, 420
   cranial neuralgia and, 423-424
   disease state and, 429-432
   exogenous trigger for, 425-428
   giant cell arteritis and, 424-425
   greater occipital neuralgia and, 438
   migraine; *see* Migraine
   ocular ischemia and, 432
   ocular neurosis and, 437
   pituitary apoplexy and, 80
   tension, 435, 437
Heart disease, 125, 127-135
Heimann-Bielschowsky phenomenon, 298
Hemangioma, orbital, 403-404
Hemianopia
   bitemporal
      chiasmal compression and, 78
      unexplained visual loss and, 33
   homonymous; *see* Homonymous
         hemianopia
   unexplained visual loss and, 12-15

Hemianopic illusions, binocular, 159
Hemicrania, paroxysmal, 420
Hemicrania continua, 420
Hemifacial spasm, 368, 370-372
Hemifield slide phenomenon, 74
Hemifield slip, 227
Hemispheric ischemia, 137
Hemispheric ptosis, 359
Hemorrhage, subarachnoid, 80
Hereditary disease
    Huntington's disease as, 209
    motor sensory neuropathy as, 341
    myasthenia gravis as, 352
    optic neuropathy as, 63-66
        disc elevation and, 193
Herniation, uncal, 339
Herpes zoster ophthalmicus, 259
Herpetic neuralgia, 429
Heterochromia iridis, 331-332
Heterophoria
    asthenopia and, 428
    diplopia and, 227
Homonymous field, illusions on, 151
Homonymous hemianopia
    bilateral, 33-34
    chiasmal compression and, 78
    postchiasmal visual loss and, 104-116
        decreased visual acuity and, 104
        hallucinations and, 105
        lateral geniculate nucleus and, 107
        occipital lobe lesions and, 109-114
        optic tract lesions and, 107
        parietal lobe lesions and, 109
        reduced visual perception and, 105
        temporal lobe lesions and, 108-109
    relative afferent pupillary defect and, 12
Horizontal eye movement, 201-203
Horizontal gaze deficits, 211-212
Horizontal misalignment, 267, 268
Horizontal nystagmus
    jerk, 307
    rotary, 309
Hormone
    growth, 177
    migraine and, 433
Horner's syndrome, 330-333
Human immunodeficiency virus, 195
Huntington's disease, 209
Hyaline bodies, 180
Hydroxyamphetamine test, 330-333
Hypertension
    central retinal vein occlusion and, 194
    headache and, 430
    pseudotumor cerebri and, 187

Hypertensive retinopathy, 192
Hyperthyroidism; *see* Graves' ophthalmopathy
Hyperviscosity, transient visual loss and, 121
Hypoplasia, optic disc and, 176-177
Hypotony, disc elevation and, 195
Hysterical conversion reaction, 234

**I**

Ice cream headache, 425
Illusions, 145-163
    binocular, 157-163
    decision tree for, 148, 152-154
    hallucinations versus, 145-147
    mental state and, 150
    monocular, 154-156
Immunosuppressive drug, Graves' optic
        neuropathy and, 389
Impaired vision, hallucinations and, 150-151
In situ thrombosis, transient visual loss and,
        120
Inborn errors of metabolism, optic neuropathy
        and, 65
Incomitant ocular misalignment, 239-281
    abducens nerve and, 260-263
    combined palsies and, 265-266
    decision tree for, 240-241
    definition of, 234
    forced duction test for, 239, 242-243
    isolation of paretic muscles and, 267-276
    nonisolated palsies and, 263-265
    oculomotor nerve and, 247-257; *see also*
        Oculomotor nerve palsy
    Tensilon test for, 244-247
    trochlear nerve and, 257-260
Indomethacin for migraine, 442
Induced jerk nystagmus, 309-311
Infant
    botulism and, 266
    nystagmus in, 294-295
    pupils of, 342
Infarction
    of lateral medullary plate, 161-162
    midbrain, 169
    migraine with, 422
    myocardial, 133
    occipital lobe, 113
    peripheral nerve, 249-250
    of posterior inferior cerebellar artery, 306
    retinal artery, 66-67
    thalamic esotropia and, 211
Infection
    cellulitis and, 395, 397-399
    chiasmal syndrome and, 95
    fungal, 398, 399

Infection—cont'd
  herpes zoster ophthalmicus and, 259
  herpetic neuralgia and, 429
  uveitis and, 195
Infectious polyradiculoneuropathy, 266
Infective endocarditis, 129
Inferior arcuate scotoma, 18
Inferior cerebellar artery, posterior, 306
Inferior division paresis, 255
Inferior oblique muscle, 255
Inferior orbit lesion, 409, 412
Inferior rectus muscle, 255
Infiltrative optic neuropathy, 56-58
  disc elevation and, 192
Inflammation
  chiasmal syndrome and, 96
  combined nerve palsies and, 265
  compressive optic neuropathy and, 192
  headache and, 431-432
  ischemic ocular, 140
  orbital, 392-394
Inhibitional palsy of contralateral antagonist,
    269, 272
Interferometer, laser, 5-6
Intermittent diplopia, 224, 226-229
Intermittent pupillary syndromes, 339-342
Intermittent tropia, 227
Internuclear ophthalmoplegia, 213
  diplopia and, 224
  eccentric gaze and, 299-300
Intraaxial palsy, 261-262
Intracanalicular optic nerve, trauma to, 65
Intraconal mass, 403-407
Intracranial pressure
  headache and, 426-427, 430-431
  papilledema and, 182-189
  pseudotumor cerebri and, 187
Intraocular pressure
  anisocoria and, 336-337
  glaucoma and, 173
Inverse bobbing, 314
Iris, dilator muscle of, 323
Irradiation
  anterior visual pathway injury from, 86
  pituitary tumor and, 83-84
Ischemia
  chronic ocular, 139-140
  headache and, 432
  optic neuropathy and, 49-56
    disc elevation and, 193
  prolonged afterimage and, 156
  transient visual loss and, 124-125, 137
  vertebrobasilar atheroma and, 118
Isoniazide-induced optic neuropathy, 60-61

**J**

Jaw-winking phenomenon, 352
Jerk nystagmus, 305-311
  congenital, 296
  definition of, 289, 291
Joint, temporomandibular, 430
Junction scotoma, 76, 77
Junctional hemianopia, 14

**K**

Kestenbaum procedure for congenital
    nystagmus, 295
Koerber-Salus-Elschnig syndrome, 214-215

**L**

Labyrinthine dysfunction, nystagmus and, 291
Labyrinthine nystagmus, 306
Laser interferometer, 5-6
Latent nystagmus, 296
Lateral geniculate nucleus, 107
Lateral medullary plate infarction, 161-162
Lateral medullary syndrome, Wallenberg's,
    306
Lateral orbit lesion, 412
Leber's optic neuropathy, 64
Lens, contact
  lid deformity from, 351
  overwear syndrome and, 432
Lens capsule, opacified, 6
Lenticular abnormality, 6
Lenticular nuclear sclerosis, 232
Lid; *see* Eyelid
Lid nystagmus, 312
Lid-twitch sign, 356
Light
  flickering, 166
  swinging light pupil test and, 1, 7-9
Light reaction, pupillary, 322, 325
  abnormal, 333-336
  anisocoria and, 328
Light-near dissociation, 333
Lipohyalinosis, 118
Lithium chloride for cluster headache, 420
Longitudinal fasciculus, medial, 299-300
Lumbar puncture, 187-188
Lupus erythematosus, 48
Lyme disease, 49
Lymphoma, 393

**M**

Macropsia, 155
Macrosaccadic oscillations, 314
Macrosquare wave jerks, 313-314
Macular neuroretinopathy, 24

Macular sparing, 111
Maculopathy
    illusions and, 155
    normal visual acuity and, 35
    prolonged afterimage and, 156
    tests for, 22-24
Maddox rod, 274
Magnetic resonance imaging
    chiasmal syndrome and, 78-79
    multiple sclerosis and, 44
    orbital inflammation and, 393
    septo-optic dysplasia and, 177
Magnified ophthalmoscopy, 22-23
Malformation, arteriovenous, 105
Malignancy; *see* Pituitary tumor; Tumor
Malingering, diplopia and, 234
Mass; *see also* Tumor
    extraconal, 408, 410-412
    intraconal, 403-407
    superior oblique myokymia and, 299
    third nerve palsy and, 256
Medial longitudinal fasciculus, 204, 248,
        299-300
    internuclear ophthalmoplegia and, 213
Medial orbit lesion, 412
Medial rectus muscle, 261
Medication-induced illusions or
        hallucinations, 147, 149
Medullary plate infarction, 161-162
Medullary syndrome, Wallenberg's lateral, 306
Megalopapilla, 178
Meige's syndrome, 374
Meningioma, 90-92, 405
    sphenoid ridge, 57
Mental status, Huntington's disease and, 209
Mesencephalic artery, thalamic esotropia and,
        211
Metabolic disorder, optic neuropathy and,
        61-63
Metabolic lid retraction, 364
Metamorphopsia, 237
    cerebral, 158
    retinal, 156
Metastasis
    orbital, 407
    sixth nerve palsy and, 261
Methylsergide for migraine, 442
Micropsia, 155
Midbrain corectopia, 342
Midbrain infarct, hallucinations and, 169
Midbrain lid retraction, 364
Migraine
    aura and, 421-423
    childhood, 435

Migraine—cont'd
    hallucinations and, 167, 168
        in homonymous field, 105
    illusion and, 161
    ophthalmoplegic, 256-257, 423
    pupillary mydriasis and, 339-340
    retinociliary, 435, 436
    third nerve palsy and, 256-257
    transient visual loss and, 121, 124
    treatment of, 438-442
    without aura, 432-434
Migraine equivalents, 434-435
Millard-Gubler syndrome, 264
Miosis
    extreme, 342
    relative, 341
Misalignment, ocular
    comitant, 282-288
    incomitant, 239-281; *see also* Incomitant
        ocular misalignment
Mitochondrial DNA in Leber's optic
        neuropathy, 64
Mitochondrial myopathy, 217-218
Mitral valve, fibromyxomatous degeneration
        of, 130-132
Möbius syndrome, 211
Monocular condition
    diplopia as, 229-234
    elevation paresis as, 215
    hallucinations as, 166
    illusions as, 154-156
    nystagmus as, 297-301
    ocular deprivation as, 298
    oscillations as, 300
    transient visual loss as, 124
Monosodium glutamate, headache from,
        425-426
Moore's lightning flashes, 166
Morning glory disc, 178
Motor nystagmus, 304
Motor sensory neuropathy, hereditary, 341
Mucocele, chiasmal syndrome and, 95
Mucormycosis, 398, 399
Multiple evanescent white dot syndrome, 24
Multiple images, illusion and, 154-155, 159; *see
        also* Diplopia
Multiple sclerosis
    diplopia and, 226
    nystagmus of, 299
    optic neuritis and, 42-46
    visual evoked potentials and, 36
Muscle
    ciliary, 335-336
    dilator, of iris, 323

Muscle—cont'd
  diplopia after surgery on, 230-232
  Graves' ophthalmopathy and, 384, 390-391
  medial rectus, 261
  myopathic gaze disorders and, 217-219
  paretic
    isolation of, 267-276
    sphincter, 336
    third nerve palsy and, 255
  tension headache and, 435, 437
Muscular dystrophy, gaze disturbance and,
    219
Myasthenia gravis
  diplopia and, 226-227
  gaze disturbance and, 219
  Graves' ophthalmopathy and, 381, 383
  neonatal, 352
  ptosis and, 354-359
  Tensilon test and, 244-247
Myasthenic movements, 312-313
Mydriasis
  migraine and, 339-340
  relative, 341
Myectomy for blepharospasm, 374-375
Myocardial infarction, cerebral emboli and, 133
Myoclonus, ocular, 304
Myokymia, superior oblique, 291, 298-299
Myopathic gaze disorder, 217-219
Myopathy, ptosis and, 352
Myorhythmia, oculomasticatory, 302-303
Myotonic dystrophy, 219
Myotubular myopathy, 219
Myxoma, atrial, 133

N

Nasal sinus, headache and, 429-430
Near reaction, pupillary, 325
  anisocoria and, 333
Near reflex
  spasm of, 210-211
    diplopia and, 227
  synkinetic, 7
Nelson's syndrome, 82
Neovascular membranes, subretinal, 286
Nerve
  cranial; see Cranial nerve
  optic; see Optic nerve; Optic neuritis; Optic
    neuropathy
  peripheral, infarction of, 249-250
Nerve fiber bundle defect, 33
Neuralgia
  cranial, 423-424
  greater occipital, 438
  herpetic, 429

Neuritis, optic; see Optic neuritis
Neuroblastoma, metastatic, 407
Neuroborreliosis, Lyme, 49
Neurofibromatosis, glioma and, 93
Neuromuscular disorder, blepharospasm and,
    374
Neuromyotonia, diplopia and, 227, 229
Neurons of sympathetic pathway, 323-324
Neuropathy
  hereditary motor sensory, 341
  optic; see Optic neuropathy
Neuroretinal disturbance, 1
Neuroretinopathy, macular, 24
Neurosis, ocular, 437
Nifedipine for migraine, 442
Nodding of head, 297
Nonbacterial thrombotic endocarditis, 129-130
Nonhemianopic defect, 15-20
Nonsteroidal antiinflammatory drug for
    migraine, 439
Normotensive glaucoma, 173
Nothnagel's syndrome, 261
Nuclear sclerosis
  lenticular, diplopia and, 232
  unexplained visual loss and, 6
Nucleus
  abducens, 264
  dorsolateral pontine, 205
  lateral geniculate, 107
  pretectal, 321-322
  visceral, 247-248
Null point in nystagmus, 289, 295
Nystagmus, 289-311
  binocular, 301-311
    conjugate, 303-311
    disconjugate, 301-303
  chiasmal compression and, 78
  conditions mimicking, 312-315
  congenital, 294-296
  monocular, 297-301
  oscillopsia and, 163

O

Oblique tendon sheath syndrome, superior,
    243
Occipital lobe lesion, 109-116
  illusion and, 161
  infarction as, 113
Occipital neuralgia, 438
Occipital tumor, 105
Occlusion; see also Ischemia
  central retinal artery, 66-67
  retinal vein, 193-194
  transient visual loss and, 117-121

Ocular alignment; *see* Ocular misalignment
Ocular bobbing, 314
Ocular deprivation
  monocular, 298
  nystagmus and, 304
Ocular hypotony, 195
Ocular ischemia; *see also* Ischemia
  chronic, 139-140
  transient visual loss and, 137
Ocular migraine, 121, 124; *see also* Migraine
Ocular misalignment
  comitant, 282-288
  incomitant, 239-281
    abducens nerve and, 260-263
    combined palsies and, 265-266
    decision tree for, 240-241
    forced duction test for, 239, 242-243
    isolation of paretic muscles and, 267-276
    nonisolated palsies and, 263-265
    oculomotor nerve and, 247-257; *see also*
      Oculomotor nerve palsy
    Tensilon test for, 244-247
    trochlear nerve and, 257-260
  pseudoptosis and, 348
Ocular motility in myasthenia gravis, 356-357
Ocular motor apraxia, 208-209
Ocular motor palsy, compressive, 244
Ocular motor system, 200-217
  conjugate systems and, 203-205
  myopathic, 217-219
  supranuclear control centers and, 207-217;
    *see also* Supranuclear control pathway
  vergence systems and, 205, 207
Ocular myoclonus, 304
Ocular neuromyotonia, 227, 229
Ocular neurosis, 437
Ocular tilt reaction, 315
Oculogyric crisis, 217
Oculomasticatory myorhythmia, 302, 370
Oculomotor nerve palsy
  combined, 265-266
  incomitant misalignment and, 247-257
    in adults, 249-255
    in children, 255-257
Oculopathy, ischemic, 140
Oculopharyngeal muscular dystrophy, 219
Oculosympathetic pathway, 323-234
Opacified lens capsule, 6
Opening, lid, apraxia of, 347
Ophthalmopathy, Graves'; *see* Graves'
  ophthalmopathy
Ophthalmoplegia
  combined nerve palsies and, 265-266
  drug-induced, 338

Ophthalmoplegia—cont'd
  internuclear, 213
    diplopia and, 224
    eccentric gaze and, 299-301
  progressive external, 218
  pseudointernuclear, 300-301
Ophthalmoplegic migraine, 256-257, 423
Ophthalmoscopy
  congenitally elevated optic disc and, 180
  maculopathy and, 22-23
Opsoclonus, 313
Optic disc, 173-199
  decision tree for, 174-175
  edema of, 50
  elevated, 179-195
    congenitally, 179-182
    neuropathy and, 192-193
    papilledema and, 182-189
    retinopathy and, 192, 193-194
    uveitis and, 195
    vasculitis and, 194-195
  not elevated, 173-179
  transient visual loss and, 126
Optic glioma, 92-95
Optic nerve; *see also* Optic neuritis; Optic
    neuropathy
  altered motion and, 162-163
  retrobulbar lesion of, 15-20
  tumor of, 405
Optic neuritis, 41-73
  central retinal artery occlusion and, 66-67
  conditions mimicking, 49
  isolated, 46-48
  multiple sclerosis and, 42-46
  optic neuropathy and, 49-66; *see also* Optic
    neuropathy
  systemic disease and, 48-49
  visual evoked potentials and, 36
Optic neuropathy
  compressive, 56
  disc elevation and, 192-193
  Graves' ophthalmopathy and, 384-385,
    389-390
  hereditary, 63-66, 193
  infiltrative, 56-58, 192
  ischemic, 49-56, 193
  metabolic, 61-63
  normal visual acuity and, 34, 35
  radiation-induced, 58-60
  toxic, 60-61, 193
  unexplained visual loss and, 28
  visual evoked potentials and, 36
Optic tract syndrome, 107
  postchiasmal visual loss and, 104

Optical disturbance, definition of, 1
Optokinetic asymmetry, 109
Optokinetic nystagmus, 309-310
Oral contraceptives
  migraine and, 433
  transient visual loss and, 126
Orbicularis myectomy for blepharospasm,
    374-375
Orbit, 392-412
  carotid-cavernous fistula and, 399-402
  cellulitis and, 395, 397-399
  decompression surgery of, 390
  inflammation of, 392-394
    compressive optic neuropathy and, 192
  mass in, 403-412
    extraconal, 408, 410-412
    intraconal, 403-407
  trauma and, 402
Oscillations, 289-320; *see also* Nystagmus
  binocular symmetric, 301-311
    conjugate, 303-311
    disconjugate, 301-303
  macrosaccadic, 314
Oscillopsia, 163, 291; *see also* Nystagmus
Ovulation-stimulating agents, pituitary
    apoplexy and, 81
Oxycephaly, 402

**P**

Palinopsia, 114, 159, 160
  diplopia and, 234
Palsy
  fourth nerve, 257-260
    combined, 265-266
    intraaxial, 261-262
  progressive supranuclear, 216-217
    blepharospasm and, 372
  sixth nerve, 260-263
    combined, 265-266
    diplopia and, 224
    extraaxial, 265
    intraaxial, 264-265
  Tensilon test and, 244
  third nerve, 247-257
    in adults, 249-255
    in children, 255-257
  vertical gaze, 213-217
PAM; *see* Potential acuity meter
Panretinal photocoagulation, 140
Papilledema
  elevated optic disc and, 182-189
  Parinaud's syndrome and, 215
  transient visual loss and, 124
Papillopathy, diabetic, 193

Papillophlebitis, 194
Parachiasmal lesions; *see* Chiasmal syndrome
Paradoxical embolus, 133
Paradoxical pupillary light reaction, 343
Paralysis; *see* Palsy
Paramedian pontine reticular formation,
    204-205
  gaze deficits and, 212
Paranasal sinus, headache and, 429-430
Parasympathetic control of pupil, 321-323
Paresis; *see also* Palsy
  ciliary muscle, 335-336
  eccentric gaze and, 300
  horizontal gaze, congenital, 211-212
  monocular elevation, 215
  pursuit, 210
  saccadic, 207-208
  sphincter muscle, 336
  third nerve palsy and, 255
  vergence, 284-286
Parietal lobe, visual field defect and, 109
Parieto-occipital lobe lesion
  illusion and, 161
  spatial alterations and, 162
Parinaud's syndrome, 214-215
  nystagmus and, 302
Parkinson's disease, 217
  blepharospasm and, 372, 373
Paroxysmal hemicrania, 420
Paroxysmal positional nystagmus, 311
Passive duction test, 239, 242-243
Peduncular hallucinosis
  hallucinations and, 169
  Parinaud's syndrome and, 215
Pendular nystagmus, 303
  definition of, 289, 291
  multiple sclerosis and, 299
Penicillamine, myasthenia gravis and, 359
Perichiasmal lesions; *see* Chiasmal syndrome
Perimetry
  chiasmal syndrome and, 75-78
  papilledema and, 184
  unexplained visual loss and, 38
Periodic alternating gaze deviation, 314
Periodic alternating nystagmus, 307
Peripheral nerve infarction, 249-250
Peripheral positional nystagmus, 311
Peripheral vestibular nystagmus, 306
Pernicious anemia, optic neuropathy and, 63
Pharmacologic blockade of pupillary
    response, 338, 342
Phenothiazine-induced oculogyric crisis,
    217
Phenytoin, nystagmus caused by, 308

Phoria, decompensated, 282-283
  diplopia and, 227
Phosphenes, 166
Photocoagulation, 140
Photoreceptor
  color alteration and, 161
  eye movement–induced flashes and, 166
Photostress test, 23
Physiologic diplopia, 237
Pigment epitheliitis, retinal, 24
Pigment epithelium, retinal, 180
Pilocarpine test, 334-336, 337-338
Ping-Pong gaze, periodic alternating, 314-315
Pinhole tests, 4-5
Pituitary abscess, 95
Pituitary tumor, 75-76, 79-87
  apoplexy and, 79-81
  endocrine symptoms and, 81-82
  follow-up care in, 87
  special forms of, 82-83
  treatment of, 83-85
  tumor recurrence and, 85-86
Planum sphenoidale, 90
Plasmapheresis for Graves' ophthalmopathy, 390
Plate, medullary, infarction of, 161-162
Platelet aggregation in migraine, 433
Platelet inhibitors, 138-139, 441-442
Polycythemia, 121
Polymyalgia rheumatica, 51
Polyopia, cerebral, 234
Polyradiculoneuropathy, infectious, 266
Pontine disease, 366, 369
Pontine gaze disorder, 212-213
Pontine nuclei, dorsolateral, 205
Positional nystagmus, 311
Postchiasmal visual loss, 104-116
  decreased visual acuity and, 104
  hallucinations and, 105
  homonymous hemianopia and, 104-116
  lateral geniculate nucleus and, 107
  occipital lobe lesions and, 109-114
  optic tract lesions and, 107
  parietal lobe lesions and, 109
  reduced visual perception and, 105
  temporal lobe lesions and, 108-109
Posterior inferior cerebellar artery infarction, 306
Posterior lens capsule, opacified, 6
Posterior segment, 126, 140
Postganglionic lesion, 331
Postparalytic facial contracture, 368
Postpartum period, transient visual loss in, 126

Posttraumatic headache, 426
Posture, strabismus and, 239
Potential acuity meter, 5-6
Potential acuity tests
  subnormal acuity and, 1
  types of, 4-6
PPRF; *see* Paramedian pontine reticular formation
Prechiasmal visual loss, 41-73
  central retinal artery occlusion and, 66-67
  conditions mimicking optic neuritis, 49
  isolated optic neuritis and, 46-48
  multiple sclerosis and, 42-46
  optic neuropathy and
    compressive, 56
    hereditary, 63-66
    infiltrative, 56-58
    ischemic, 49-56
    metabolic, 61-63
    radiation-induced, 58-60
    toxic, 60-61
  systemic disease and, 48-49
Precocious puberty, Parinaud's syndrome and, 215
Prednisone for myasthenia gravis, 246
Preganglionic lesion, 331
Pregnancy
  pituitary apoplexy and, 81
  prolactin-secreting tumor and, 82
  transient visual loss and, 126
Premature infant, pupils of, 342
Pressure
  blood, hypertensive
    central retinal vein occlusion and, 194
    headache and, 430
    pseudotumor cerebri and, 187
    retinopathy and, 192
  intracranial, 430-431
    headache and, 426-427, 430-431
    papilledema and, 182-189
    pseudotumor cerebri and, 187
  intraocular
    anisocoria and, 336-337
    glaucoma and, 173
  venous, 187
Pretectal nucleus, 321-322
Prism, decompensated phoria and, 283
Progressive external ophthalmoplegia, 218
Progressive supranuclear palsy, 216-217
  blepharospasm and, 372
Prolactinoma, 85
Prolactin-secreting tumor, 82
Prolapse
  chiasmal, 86, 96

Prolapse—cont'd
  mitral valve, 130, 132
Prophylactic treatment for migraine, 441-442
Propranolol for migraine, 442
Proptosis, 379-416
  carotid-cavernous fistula and, 399-402
  cellulitis and, 395, 397-399
  developmental anomaly and, 402
  Graves' ophthalmopathy and, 379-391; *see also* Graves' ophthalmopathy
  orbital inflammation and, 392-395
  orbital mass and, 403-412
    extraconal, 408, 410-412
    intraconal, 403-407
  trauma and, 402
Prosopagnosia, 112
Prosthetic heart valve, 129
Pseudo-Horner's syndrome, 330
Pseudointernuclear ophthalmoplegia, 300
Pseudophakia, 156
Pseudoptosis, 347-350
Pseudotumor, orbital, 393, 394, 396
Pseudotumor cerebri, 184-189
Psychoactive drug, 147, 149
Psychogenic disorder
  blepharospasm and, 374
  diplopia as, 234, 237
  hallucinations and, 169
  illusion as, 155
  lenticular nuclear sclerosis and, 232
  near reflex spasm as, 210-211
  visual loss as, 31-33
    visual evoked potentials and, 36
Psychosis, hallucinations and, 150
PTC; *see* Pseudotumor cerebri
Ptosis, 347-361
  anisocoria and, 328, 331
  lid deformity and, 351
  myasthenia gravis and, 245, 354-359
  neurologic signs and, 359-360
  onset at birth of, 352
  pseudoptosis and, 347-350
  pupillary abnormality and, 353-354
  Tensilon test and, 243
Puberty, precocious, Parinaud's syndrome and, 215
Pulfrich stereo-illusion, 162
Puncture, lumbar, pseudotumor cerebri and, 187-188
Pupil, 321-346
  anisocoria and, 325-338
    abnormal light reaction and, 333-336
    constriction and, 338
    intraocular pressure and, 336-337

Pupil—cont'd
  anisocoria and—cont'd
    light reaction in, 338
    ptosis and, 328-333
  intermittent pupillary syndromes and, 339-342
  parasympathetic control and, 321-323
  ptosis and, 353-354
  size of, 324-325
  swinging light pupil test and, 1, 7-9
  sympathetic control of, 323-324
Pupillary light reaction, 322
  paradoxical, 343
  reduced bilateral, 340-341
Pupillary sparing in third nerve palsy, 252
Pursuit, smooth, 205
Pursuit paresis, 210
Pursuit pathway, 202
Pyridostigmine for myasthenia gravis, 246, 359

**Q**

Quick phases, 200
Quiverlike movements, 312-313

**R**

Radiation therapy
  anterior visual pathway injury from, 86
  craniopharyngioma and, 89
  glioma and, 93-94
  Graves' ophthalmopathy and, 389, 390
  meningioma and, 92
  optic neuropathy caused by, 58-60
  pituitary tumor and, 83-84
Raeder's syndrome, 431
Rebound nystagmus, 309
Recessive optic atrophy, 64
Recurrent pituitary tumor, 85-86
Red glass test, 235-236
Reflex
  near
    diplopia and, 227
    spasm of, 210-211
    synkinetic, 7
  pupillary light, 322
  vestibulo-ocular, 163
Reflex blepharospasm, 372
Refractive aberration, diplopia and, 229, 232
Refractive error, asthenopia and, 428
Regeneration, aberrant, of oculomotor nerve, 253-254
Relative afferent pupillary defect, 1
  swinging light pupil test and, 8-9
Repetitive divergence, 303

Restrictive disease
    forced duction test and, 242-243
    monocular oscillations and, 301
Retina
    color alteration and, 161
    degeneration of, 28
    disease of, 34
    ischemia of, 156
    pigment epitheliitis and, 24
Retinal correspondence, 230-232
Retinal embolus, 128
Retinal fibers, 76
Retinal metamorphopsia, 156
Retinal pigment epithelium, 180
Retinal vessels
    disc elevation and, 193-194
    hypoplasia of, 176
    occlusion of, 66-67
    sarcoidosis and, 48
    venous occlusion and, 140
Retinitis pigmentosa, 28
Retinociliary migraine, 121, 124, 435, 436
Retinopathy
    disc elevation and, 192, 193-194
    hypertensive, disc elevation and, 192
    venous stasis, 140
        disc elevation and, 193-194
Retraction of eyelid
    contralateral, 348
    Graves' ophthalmopathy and, 379-391; *see
        also* Graves' ophthalmopathy
Retrobulbar infiltrative optic neuropathy 56-58
Retrobulbar optic nerve lesion, 15-20
Retrogeniculate lesion, homonymous
        hemianopia and, 33-34
Reverse bobbing, 314
Rhabdomyosarcoma, 408
Rheumatic heart disease, 129
Rheumatologic disease, 125
Riddoch phenomenon, 112
Ridge, sphenoid, meningioma of, 57
Rod, Maddox, 274
Rotary nystagmus, horizontal, 309
Rotational nystagmus, 310

S

Saccades, 203
    vertical, 206
Saccadic paresis, 207-208
Saccadomania, 313
Sarcoidosis, retinal venulitis and, 48
Scarring of lid, 362, 364
Scintillations
    flickering, 166

Scintillations—cont'd
    migraine and, 421-422
    transient visual loss and, 121, 124
Sclerosis
    multiple
        diplopia and, 226
        nystagmus of, 299
        optic neuritis and, 42-46
        visual evoked potentials and, 36
    nuclear
        diplopia and, 232
        unexplained visual loss and, 6
Scotoma
    chiasmal compression and, 76-78
    hallucinations, migraine and, 105
    migraine and, 434
    retrobulbar optic nerve lesion and, 15-20
    tilted optic disc and, 179
Second order neuron, 324
    Horner's syndrome and, 333
    lesion of, 330
Seesaw nystagmus, 302
Segmental optic hypoplasia, superior, 177
Seizure disorder, pupillary dilatation and, 339
Sella, empty, 86, 96
Senile ptosis, 360
Sensorium, altered, 150
Sensory neuropathy, hereditary, 341
Septo-optic dysplasia, 177
Serotonin antagonist for migraine, 442
Sexual activity, headache from, 428
Single muscle paresis, 255
Sinus
    carotid-cavernous fistula and, 399-402
    headache and, 429-430
    optic neuritis and, 49
Sinus thrombosis, pseudotumor cerebri and,
        185
Sixth nerve nucleus, 264
Sixth nerve palsy, 260-263
    combined, 265-266
    diplopia and, 224
    extraaxial, 265
    intraaxial, 264-265
Size of pupil, 324-325
Sjögren's syndrome, optic neuropathy and, 48
Skew deviation, 286
Slide phenomenon, hemifield, 74
Slip, hemifield, 227
Slit lamp examination in anisocoria, 335-336
Slow eye movement system, 205
    disorders of, 210
        fast eye movement disorder with, 211-217
    types of movement and, 200

Smoking, optic neuropathy and, 61-62
Smooth eye movement, types of, 200
Smooth pursuit, 205
Sound-induced flashes, 166
Sparing
    macular, 111
    of pupil, 252
Spasm
    hemifacial, 368, 370-372
    of near reflex, 210-211
        diplopia and, 227
    vertical upgaze, 217
Spasmus nutans, 297-298, 304
Spastic contracture of medial rectus muscle,
        261
Spasticity of conjugate gaze, 109
Spatial relationships, altered, 161-162
Sphenoid ridge meningioma, 57
Sphincter muscle paresis, 336
Spinal fluid in multiple sclerosis, 44
Spinocerebellar degeneration, 65
Spontaneous jerk nystagmus, 305-309
Spot, big blind, 194
Spread, illusory, 159
Square wave jerks, 313-314
Stabbing headache, 424
Staring in Graves' ophthalmopathy, 362
Stasis retinopathy, venous, disc elevation and,
        193-194
Steele-Richardson-Olszewski syndrome,
        216-217
Stenosis
    aortic, 132
    carotid, 135
Steroid
    cluster headache and, 420
    giant cell arteritis and, 56
    Graves' disease and, 388, 389
    myasthenia gravis and, 359
    optic neuritis and, 58
    pituitary apoplexy and, 81
    pseudotumor cerebri and, 188
    ptosis induced by, 353
Strabismus, 282-288
    accommodative esotropia and, 283-284
    amblyopia and, 20-22
    central disruption of fusion and, 286-
        287
    compensatory head posture and, 239
    decompensated phoria and, 282-283
    diplopia after surgery for, 233
    esotropia of childhood and, 284
    foveal displacement and, 286
    skew deviation and, 286

Strabismus—cont'd
    vergence paresis and, 284-286
Streptomycin
    optic neuropathy caused by, 60-61
    oscillopsia and, 311
Stroke
    mitral valve prolapse and, 130, 132
    rare causes of, 133
    retinal, 66-67
    transient visual loss and, 128-132
Subarachnoid hemorrhage, 80
Subnormal acuity, 4-6
    amblyopia and, 20-22
    constricted visual fields and, 28-33
    electroretinography and, 26-28
    hemianopia and, 33-34
    maculopathy and, 22-24
    nerve fiber bundle defects and, 33
    potential acuity tests and, 6-11
    relative afferent pupillary defect and, 11-20
    visual field examination and, 26
Subnormal best-corrected acuity, 1
Subnucleus, superior rectus, innervation by,
        247
Subretinal neovascular membranes, 286
Superior colliculus, 204
Superior divisional paresis, 255
Superior oblique myokymia, 291, 298-299, 301
Superior oblique palsy in child, 259-260
Superior oblique tendon sheath syndrome,
        243
Superior orbital lesion, 408-409
Superior rectus subnucleus, 247
Superior segmental optic hypoplasia, 177
Supranuclear control pathway, 207-217
    fast eye movement systems and, 207-209,
        211-217
    slow eye movement systems and, 205, 210,
        211-217
    vergence system and, 210-211
Supranuclear palsy, progressive, 216-217
    blepharospasm and, 372
Swelling of optic disc, transient visual loss
        and, 126
Swinging light pupil test, 1, 7-9
Symmetric oscillations, binocular, 301-311
    conjugate, 303-311
    disconjugate, 301-303
Sympathetic pathway
    hydroxyamphetamine test and, 330-331
    lid retraction and, 364
    pupil and, 323-234
Synkinetic near reflex, 7
Syphilis, uveitis and, 195

**T**

Tadpole pupils, 339
Takayasu's arteritis, 432
Tardive dyskinesia, 374
Temperature in multiple sclerosis, 226
Temporal arteritis, 51
Temporal crescent, 109-110, 111
Temporal hemianopia, 12
Temporal lobe, 108-109
Temporal wedge defect, 19
Temporomandibular joint, 430
Tendon sheath syndrome, 243
Tensilon test
    incomitant misalignment and, 243-247
    ptosis and, 354-359
Tension-type headache, 435, 437
Thalamic esotropia, 211
Third nerve palsy
    combined, 265-266
    incomitant misalignment and, 247-257
        in adults, 249-255
        in children, 255-257
Third order neuron, 324
    hydroxyamphetamine test and, 331
    lesion of, 330
Thrombosis
    sinus, 185
    transient visual loss and, 117-120
Thrombotic endocarditis, 129-130
Thunderclap headache, 425
Thymus gland, myasthenia gravis and, 359
Thyroid disease; *see* Graves' ophthalmopathy
Tic douloureux, 423-424
Tilt reaction, ocular, 315
Tilt test, Bielschowsky, 272-273
Tilted optic disc, 179
Tobacco smoking, optic neuropathy and, 61-62
Tonic reaction, pupillary, 335
Topographic agnosia, 162
Torsional diplopia, 273, 276
Torticollis, spasmus nutans and, 297
Tourette's syndrome, 374
Toxic neuropathy, 193
Toxicity, optic neuropathy caused by, 60-61
Toxin, botulinum
    botulism from, 266
    for hemifacial spasm, 371, 372
    for sixth nerve palsy, 261
Traction, chiasmal syndrome and, 96-97
Tram track sign, 405
Trancelike state, 150
Transient ischemic attack
    mitral valve prolapse and, 130, 132
    transient visual loss and, 119-120

Transient visual loss, 117-144
    cardiac evaluation and, 127-135
    cerebral angiography and carotid
        endarterectomy and, 136-139
    heart disease and, 125
    mechanisms of, 117-121
    ocular ischemia and, 139-140
    rheumatologic disease and, 125
    risk factors for, 124-126
    scintillations and, 121, 124
Trauma
    chiasmal syndrome and, 96
    headache and, 426
    Horner's syndrome and, 332
    optic neuropathy and, 65-66
    proptosis and, 402
    ptosis and, 354
Tremor, superior oblique myokymia and,
    298-299
Tricyclic antidepressant for migraine, 442
Trigeminal nerve, blepharospasm and, 365
Trigeminal neuralgia, 423-424
Trochlear nerve palsy, 257-260
    combined, 265-266
    intraaxial, 261-262
Tropia, intermittent, 227
Tuberculum sellae, 90
Tumor
    compressive optic neuropathy and, 192
    craniopharyngioma and, 88-90
    extraconal, 408, 410-412
    glioma and, 92-95
    Horner's syndrome and, 333
    intraconal, 403-407
    meningioma and, 90-92
    occipital, 105
    optic nerve and, 405
    optic neuropathy and, 57
    pituitary, 79-87; *see also* Pituitary tumor
    sixth nerve palsy and, 262-263

**U**

Uhthoff's phenomenon in multiple sclerosis,
    226
Uncal herniation, 339
Uncorrected refractive error, 6
Unexplained visual loss, 1-40
    normal acuity and, 34-35
    subnormal acuity and, 4-6
        amblyopia and, 20-22
        constricted visual fields and, 28-33
        electroretinography and, 26-28
        hemianopia and, 33-34
        maculopathy and, 22-24

Unexplained visual loss—cont'd
  subnormal acuity and—cont'd
    nerve fiber bundle defects and, 33
    potential acuity tests and, 6-11
    relative afferent pupillary defect and,
      11-20
    visual field examination and, 26
  visual evoked potentials and, 36
Upgaze, vertical, spasms of, 217
Upgaze deficits, 214
Uveitis, disc elevation and, 195

**V**

Valvular disease, emboli and, 129
Varices, 404
Vascular system; *see* Vessels
Vasculitis, optic disc, 194
Vasoactive compounds for migraine, 439
Vasospasm, transient visual loss and, 120
Venous anomaly, 404
Venous pressure, pseudotumor cerebri and,
      187
Venous stasis retinopathy, 140
  disc elevation and, 193-194
Venulitis, retinal, sarcoidosis and, 48
Verapamil for migraine, 442
Vergence paresis, 284-286
Vergence systems, 205, 207
  abnormalities of, 203
Vertebrobasilar atheroma, 118
Vertebrobasilar insufficiency, 422-423
  hallucinations and, 169
  transient visual loss and, 124
Vertical gaze palsy, 213-217
Vertical jerk nystagmus, 307-308
Vertical misalignment, 267, 269-273
Vertical saccades, 206
Vertical upgaze spasms, 217
Vertigo, jerk nystagmus and, 306
Vessels
  carotid, 118-120, 135-139
  chiasm and, 76
  congenitally elevated optic disc and, 180
  fourth nerve palsy and, 258-259
  hemifacial spasm and, 370
  mesencephalic, 211
  retinal
    disc elevation and, 193-194
    hypoplasia and, 176
    occlusion of, 66-67
    sarcoidosis and, 48
    venous occlusion and, 140
Vestibular nystagmus, 306, 310-311
Vestibulo-ocular pathway, 203

Vestibulo-ocular reflex, oscillopsia and, 163
Vestibulopathy, 161-162
Virus, human immunodeficiency, 195
Visceral nucleus, 247-248
Visual acuity
  optic nerve hypoplasia and, 177
  papilledema and, 183-184
  postchiasmal visual loss and, 104
  subnormal, with unexplained visual loss,
      4-6
    amblyopia and, 20-22
    constricted visual fields and, 28-33
    electroretinography and, 26-28
    hemianopia and, 33-34
    maculopathy and, 22-24
    nerve fiber bundle defects and, 33
    potential acuity tests and, 6-11
    relative afferent pupillary defect and,
      11-20
    visual field examination and, 26
  unexplained visual field loss and, 34-35
Visual cortex, bilateral lesions of, 31
Visual deprivation
  monocular, 298
  nystagmus and, 304
Visual deprivation hallucinations, 151
Visual evoked potentials
  psychogenic visual loss and, 32-33
  unexplained visual loss and, 36
Visual field
  craniopharyngioma and, 88
  meningioma and, 90
  pseudotumor cerebri and, 187
  transient visual loss and, 126
  unexplained visual loss and
    constricted, 28-33
    maculopathy not present and, 26
    relative afferent pupillary defect and,
      11-12
Visual loss
  chiasmal, 73-103; *see also* Chiasmal
      syndrome
  postchiasmal, 104-116; *see also* Postchiasmal
      visual loss
  prechiasmal, 41-73; *see also* Prechiasmal
      visual loss
  transient, 117-144; *see also* Transient visual
      loss
  unexplained, 1-40; *see also* Unexplained
      visual loss
Visual perception, postchiasmal visual loss
      and, 105
Vitamin A, 184
Vitamin $B_{12}$, 62-63

Voluntary lid retraction, 364
Voluntary nystagmus, 312

**W**

Wallenberg's syndrome, 161-162, 306
Wall-eyed bilateral internuclear
        ophthalmoplegia, 213
Weakness, facial, 365-369

Weber's syndrome, 261
Wedge-shaped scotoma, 15, 19
Weight reduction in pseudotumor cerebri, 188
Wernicke's encephalopathy, 261
Whipple's disease, 370
White dot syndrome, multiple evanescent, 24
Willis' circle, aneurysm in, 95